BMA

D1576531

Core Topics in Neuroanaesthesia and Neurointensive Care

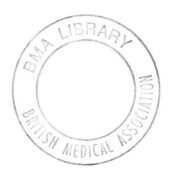

Core Topics in Neuroanaesthesia and Neurointensive Care

Edited by

Basil F. Matta
Divisional Director, Emergency and Perioperative Care, and Associate Medical Director,
Cambridge University Foundation Trust Hospitals, Cambridge, UK

David K. Menon
Head of the Division of Anaesthesia, University of Cambridge, and Consultant,
Neurosciences Critical Care Unit, Addenbrooke's Hospital, Cambridge, UK

Martin Smith
Consultant and Honorary Professor, Department of Neuroanaesthesia and Neurocritical Care,
The National Hospital for Neurology and Neurosurgery,
University College London Hospitals, London, UK

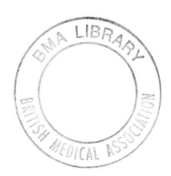

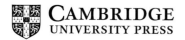

CAMBRIDGE UNIVERSITY PRESS
Cambridge, New York, Melbourne, Madrid, Cape Town,
Singapore, São Paulo, Delhi, Tokyo, Mexico City

Cambridge University Press
The Edinburgh Building, Cambridge CB2 8RU, UK

Published in the United States of America by Cambridge University Press, New York

www.cambridge.org
Information on this title: www.cambridge.org/9780521190572

First published 2011

Printed in the United Kingdom at the University Press, Cambridge

A catalogue record for this publication is available from the British Library

Library of Congress Cataloguing in Publication data
Core topics in neuroanaesthesia and neurointensive care / [edited by] Basil F. Matta,
David K. Menon, Martin Smith.
   p. ; cm.
   Includes bibliographical references and index.
   ISBN 978-0-521-19057-2 (hardback)
   1. Anesthesia in neurology.   2. Nervous system–Surgery.   3. Neurological intensive care.   I. Matta, Basil
F.   II. Menon, David K.   III. Smith, Martin, 1956–
   [DNLM: 1. Anesthesia–methods.   2. Brain–surgery.   3. Central Nervous System–physiopathology.
   4. Intensive Care–methods.   5. Monitoring, Physiologic–methods. WO 200]
   RD87.3.N47C67 2011   617.9'6748–dc23
   2011026296

ISBN 978-0-521-19057-2 Hardback

Contents

Contents

Contributors

Antony R. Absalom
University Department of Anaesthesia, Cambridge University Hospitals NHS Trust, Cambridge, UK

Lorenz Breuer
Department of Neurology, University Hospital Erlangen, Erlangen, Germany

Christoph S. Burkhart
Clinical Research Fellow, Department of Anesthesia, University Hospital Basel, Basel, Switzerland

Rowan M. Burnstein
Neurosciences Critical Care Unit, University of Cambridge, Addenbrooke's Hospital, Cambridge, UK

Ian Calder
Consultant Anaesthetist (retired),
The National Hospital for Neurology and Neurosurgery and The Royal Free Hospital, London, UK

Jonathan P. Coles
University Lecturer and Honorary Consultant, Department of Anaesthesia, Addenbrooke's Hospital, Cambridge, UK

Amanda Cox
Consultant Neurologist, University of Cambridge, Cambridge, UK

Marek Czosnyka
Reader in Brain Physics, Division of Academic Neurosurgery, Department of Clinical Neurosciences, Addenbrooke's Hospital, Cambridge, UK

Armagan Dagal
Assistant Professor, Department of Anesthesiology and Pain Medicine Harborview Medical Center, University of Washington, Seattle, USA

Judith Dinsmore
Consultant Neuroanaesthetist, Department of Anaesthesia, St George's Hospital, London, UK

Derek Duane
Consultant in Neuroanaesthesia and Neurointensive Care, Department of Neurosciences, Addenbrooke's Hospital, Cambridge, UK

Kristin Engelhard
Vice-Chair, Department of Anaesthesiology, Medical Center of the Johannes Gutenberg-University Mainz, Germany

Ari Ercole
Neurosciences Critical Care Unit, University of Cambridge, Addenbrooke's Hospital, Cambridge, UK

Rik Fox
Consultant Anaesthetist, Department of Anaesthesia, Royal National Orthopaedic Hospital, Stanmore, UK

Sabrina G. Galloway
Senior Vice President and Chief Operations Officer, Sentient Medical, Baltimore, USA

Arnab Ghosh
Clinical Research Fellow, Neurocritical Care Unit, The National Hospital for Neurology and Neurosurgery, University College London Hospitals, London, UK

Arun K. Gupta
Consultant in Neuroanaesthesia and Intensive Care, Neurosciences Critical Care Unit, University of Cambridge, Addenbrooke's Hospital, Cambridge, UK

Nicholas Hirsch
Consultant Neuroanaesthetist and Honorary Senior Lecturer, The National Hospital for Neurology and Neurosurgery, London, UK

Robin Howard
Consultant Neurologist, The National Hospital for Neurology and Neurosurgery, London, UK

Peter Hutchinson
Senior Academy Fellow, Reader and Honorary Consultant Neurosurgeon, Division of Academic Neurosurgery, Department of Clinical Neurosciences, Addenbrooke's Hospital, Cambridge, UK

Nicole C. Keong
Specialist Registrar in Neurosurgery, Department of Neurosurgery, Addenbrooke's Hospital, Cambridge, UK

Martin Köhrmann
Assistant Professor, Department of Neurology, University Hospital Erlangen, Erlangen, Germany

Arthur M. Lam
Medical Director of Neuroanesthesia and Neurocritical Care, Swedish Neuroscience Institute, Swedish Medical Centre, and Clinical Professor of Anesthesiology and Pain Medicine, University of Washington, Seattle, USA

Andrea Lavinio
Consultant in Anaesthesia and Critical Care, Neurosciences Critical Care Unit, Department of Anaesthesia, Cambridge University Hospitals NHS Foundation Trust, Cambridge, UK

Brian P. Lemkuil
Assistant Clinical Professor, Department of Anaesthesia, UCSD Medical Center, San Diego, USA

Luca Longhi
University of Milano, Neurosurgical Intensive Care Unit, Department of Anesthesia and Critical Care Medicine, Fondazione IRCCS Ospedale Maggiore Policlinico, Mangiagalli e Regina Elena, Milano, Italy

Craig D. McClain
Assistant Professor of Anaesthesia, Harvard Medical School, and Associate in Anesthesiology, Perioperative and Pain Medicine, Children's Hospital Boston, Boston, USA

Robert Macfarlane
Consultant Neurosurgeon, Department of Neurosurgery, Addenbrooke's Hospital, Cambridge, UK

Basil F. Matta
Divisional Director, Emergency and Perioperative Care, and Associate Medical Director, Cambridge University Foundation Trust Hospitals, Cambridge, UK

Stephan A. Mayer
Professor and Director of Neurocritical Care, Department of Neurology, Columbia University Medical Center, Neurological Institute, New York, USA

David K. Menon
Head of the Division of Anaesthesia, University of Cambridge, and Consultant, Neurosciences Critical Care Unit, Addenbrooke's Hospital, Cambridge, UK

Andrew W. Michell
Consultant in Clinical Neurophysiology, Department of Clinical Neurosciences, Addenbrooke's Hospital, Cambridge, UK

Dick Moberg
President, Moberg Research Inc., Ambler, PA, USA

Paul G. Murphy
Consultant and Honorary Senior Lectures, Department of Anaesthesia, The General Infirmary at Leeds, Leeds, UK

Clara Poon
University of Cambridge, Addenbrooke's Hospital, Cambridge, UK

Amit Prakash
Consultant, Department of Anaesthesia, Addenbrooke's Hospital, Cambridge, UK

Frank Rasulo
Institute of Anaesthesia and Intensive Care, Neurocritical Care Unit, Spedali Civili University Hospital, Brescia, Italy

Fred Rincon
Jefferson College of Medicine, Department of Neurological Surgery, Philadelphia, USA

Stefan Schwab
Chair and Professor, Department of Neurology, University Hospital Erlangen, Erlangen, Germany

Martin Smith
Consultant and Honorary Professor, Department of Neuroanaesthesia and Neurocritical Care, The National Hospital for Neurology and Neurosurgery, University College London Hospitals, London, UK

Sulpicio G. Soriano
Professor of Anesthesia, Harvard Medical School, Children's Hospital, Boston, and CHB Endowed Chair in Pediatric Neuroanesthesia, Boston, USA

Luzius A. Steiner
Médecin associé, Department of Anaesthesia, University Hospital Centre and University of Lausanne, Lausanne, Switzerland

Nino Stocchetti
Professor of Anaesthesia and Intensive Care, University of Milano, Neurosurgical Intensive Care Unit, Department of Anesthesia and Critical Care Medicine, Fondazione IRCCS Ospedale Maggiore Policlinico, Mangiagalli e Regina Elena, Milano, Italy

Stephan P. Strebel
Head of Neuroanesthesia, Department of Anesthesia, University Hospital Basel, Basel, Switzerland

Jane Sturgess
Consultant in Neuroanaesthesia, Addenbrooke's Hospital, Cambridge, UK

Magnus Teig
Specialist Trainee in Anaesthesia and Intensive Care Medicine, Neurocritical Care Unit, The National Hospital for Neurology and Neurosurgery, University College London Hospitals, London, UK

Tonny Veenith
Honorary Specialist Registrar and NIAA Clinical Research Fellow, Division of Anaesthesia, Cambridge University Hospitals NHS Foundation Trust, Cambridge, UK

Christian Werner
Chair, Department of Anesthesiology, Medical Center of the Johannes Gutenberg-University, Mainz, Germany

Christian Zweifel
Division of Academic Neurosurgery, Department of Clinical Neurosciences, Addenbrooke's Hospital, Cambridge, UK

Preface

Practice in related subspecialty areas of anaesthesia and critical care often relies on a common knowledge base and skill sets. Neuroanaesthesia and neurocritical care represent areas of subspecialty practice where such interdependence is arguably most relevant, the conceptual basis, research evidence and clinical ethos are perhaps most divergent from the parent specialties, and most closely related to each other. *Core Topics in Neuroanaesthesia and Neurointensive Care* is based on a recognition of this commonality of knowledge and skills. We see such shared knowledge as essential for the clinical care of patients in whom the nervous system has been injured (or who are at risk of such injury), regardless of whether the insult is the consequence of disease, or arises from operative or non-operative therapies.

An optimal utilization of such knowledge for patient benefit would underpin clear advances in clinical monitoring and treatment. Indeed, the last decade has seen an explosion of tools to monitor the at-risk brain, bringing fundamental understanding of disease biology to the bedside of individual patients. However, it is important to sound a cautionary note – these advances represent both an opportunity and a challenge. Modern imaging and monitoring modalities can provide exciting insights into the biology of disease, but it is important that we do not confuse the aim of improved clinical management with the technological means of achieving it. Despite increased knowledge, the margins of benefit that clinicians can produce in brain injury remain marginal. However, the good news is that, with better knowledge, these margins are increasing steadily. While the silver bullet of a neuroprotective intervention still eludes us, it is clear that we can make a difference, guided by rigorous outcome-based evidence (where this is available), supplemented by rational clinical care based on sound physiological principles (where it is not). Good clinical care in neuroanaesthesia and neurointensive care continues to be based on 'doing lots of little things very well'. Our hope is that this textbook provides a framework that allows meticulous attention to these details of clinical practice to be integrated into the wider perspective of improvements in patient care.

Basil F. Matta
David K. Menon
Martin Smith

Acknowledgements

This textbook represents the distillation of knowledge, experience and prejudices of individual authors. We dedicate this book to our families and friends who influenced our attitudes and opinions and made us the people we are; and to the patients and colleagues who crafted our practice and made us the clinicians that we have become.

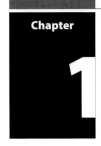

Anatomical considerations in neuroanaesthesia

Nicole C. Keong and Robert Macfarlane

Introduction

This chapter provides an overview of some of the key neuroanatomical considerations that may impact on neuroanaesthesia and neurointensive care. The topics and discussions are by no means exhaustive but serve as a platform for further exploration via standard neuroanatomical and neurosurgical texts.

Applied anatomy of the cranium

Anatomical considerations in planning surgical access

There are multiple factors that require consideration when planning an operative approach. All available imaging of the pathology should be reviewed to assess the surgical options. Further imaging, such as angiography or image-guidance sequences, may be appropriate. Where multiple surgical strategies are possible, the decision regarding the operative approach may be influenced by cosmesis, previous surgery and technical preference of the operating surgeon, as well as potential risks. The most direct route to pathology via the smallest possible exposure may not necessarily produce the best outcome. Other considerations are discussed below.

Pre-operative considerations

The ideal surgical approach to pathology should avoid eloquent areas of the brain in order to minimize the risk of producing further neurological deficit. In cases of extra-axial midline structures, surgical approaches are generally via the non-dominant side. Some areas of the brain, such as the temporal lobe, are more epileptogenic than others and this also needs to be taken into account. For example, approaching the lateral ventricle via an interhemispheric route through the corpus callosum is less likely to induce seizures than an approach via the frontal lobe.

Stereotactic or image-guided methods are useful in planning targets and trajectory, but some will require a form of rigid head fixation. Where pathology is within or adjacent to eloquent brain, pre-operative assessment using functional MRI (fMRI) may be indicated. Awake craniotomy may be the preferred surgical option for such pathology. The surgical approach will also determine patient positioning. It is important to be aware of particular risk factors of certain positions, for example, air embolism in the sitting position, or venous hypertension if there is excessive rotation of the neck. It is essential that the laterality of the pathology is confirmed before commencing the procedure.

Intraoperative considerations

If stereotactic or image-guidance methods are used, pre-operative planning and patient registration are necessary. These methods allow intraoperative navigation to target the lesion and may also assist with identification of resection margins (both soft tissue and bony). However, it must be appreciated that such methods range from among navigation based upon images acquired pre-operatively or intraoperatively to real time images, depending on the technical specification of the system. On-table localization of pathology does offer the option of fashioning a small bone flap directly over the lesion, which may be beneficial for cosmesis. However, a large bone flap is indicated in trauma or in other situations where the brain is swollen or likely to swell post-operatively. This provides the opportunity of not replacing the bone flap at the end of the procedure in order to provide a decompression, which reduces intracranial pressure. In this situation, the dura is also

Core Topics in Neuroanaesthesia and Neurointensive Care, eds. Basil F. Matta, David K. Menon and Martin Smith. Published by Cambridge University Press. © Cambridge University Press 2011.

left widely opened or only loosely tacked together. A large craniectomy is preferable to a small bony defect because there is less risk that brain herniation through the opening will obstruct the pial vessels at the dural margin and result in ischaemia or infarction of the prolapsing tissue.

In order to access the pathology, brain retraction may be required. A good anaesthetic is fundamental for providing satisfactory operating conditions that minimize the need for retraction. Patient positioning is also crucial to reduce venous pressure (for example, avoiding excessive neck rotation) and, where possible, to take advantage of the effect of gravity. The brain is intolerant of retraction, particularly if it is prolonged or over a narrow area. In addition to the risk of brain injury, inappropriate retraction may produce brain swelling or intraparenchymal haemorrhage. Early cerebrospinal fluid (CSF) drainage is another manoeuvre that may assist surgical exposure. This may be achieved by microsurgical dissection into various CSF cisterns at the operative site, access to lateral ventricles by means of a direct ventricular tap or via lumbar CSF drainage. Where appropriate, cortical incisions are made through the sulci rather than the gyri. Preservation of the draining veins is another factor that should be considered in order to minimize post-operative swelling and reduce the risk of venous infarction.

An appropriate size of craniotomy is fundamental in order to achieve good visualization of pathology while minimizing the need for retraction. In addition to this, various extended cranio-facial and skull base exposures have been developed to improve access to specific areas. Examples include the translabyrinthine approach to a large acoustic neuroma to minimize displacement of the cerebellum, or osteotomy of the zygomatic arch in the subtemporal approach to achieve good visualization of a basilar apex aneurysm.

Key aspects of functional neuroanatomy

Surface markings of the brain

The precise position of intracranial structures varies, but a rough guide to major landmarks is as follows. Draw an imaginary line across the top of the calvaria in the midline between the nasion and inion (external occipital protuberance). The Sylvian fissure runs in a line from the lateral canthus to three-quarters of the way from nasion to inion. The central sulcus (separating the motor from the sensory cortex) lies 2 cm behind the midpoint from nasion to inion and joins the Sylvian fissure at a point vertically above the condyle of the mandible.

Brain structure and function

The functional relevance of various cortical areas in the brain, such as language, has been well described, but it is important to note that these areas can vary considerably. However, disorders of different lobes of the brain generally produce characteristic clinical syndromes, dependent not only on site but also side. In terms of laterality, 93–99% of all right-handed patients are left-hemisphere dominant, as are the majority of left-handers and those who are ambidextrous (ranging from 50 to 92% in various studies). Large intracranial mass lesions may present with symptoms or signs of raised intracranial pressure. However, small mass lesions in anatomically eloquent areas may present early with specific focal deficits, particularly in cases of haemorrhage. Epilepsy may also occur as the presenting symptom.

Surgical resections may be undertaken in eloquent parts of the brain either by remaining within the confines of the disease process (intracapsular resection) or by employing some form of cortical mapping. This involves either cortical stimulation during awake craniotomy or pre-operative fMRI, which is then linked to an intraoperative image-guidance system. However, a good grasp of neuroanatomy is essential both in the operating room as well as the pre-operative stage in terms of assessing the relative likelihood of pathology causing the clinical symptoms and signs. A general discussion of the functional significance of the cerebral and cerebellar hemispheres is set out below. Figure 1.1 illustrates the lobes of the brain.

Frontal lobes

The frontal lobes are the cerebral hemispheres anterior to the Rolandic fissure (central sulcus; Fig. 1.1). Important areas within the frontal lobes are the motor strip, Broca's speech area (in the dominant hemisphere) and the frontal eye fields. Patients with bilateral frontal lobe dysfunction present typically with personality disorders, dementia, apathy and disinhibition. The anterior 7 cm of one frontal lobe can be resected without significant neurological sequelae, providing the contralateral hemisphere is normal. This may account for the relative late presentation and large size of some

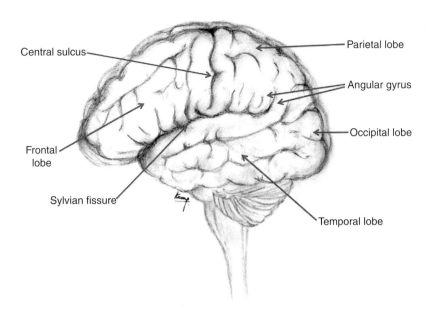

Central sulcus
Parietal lobe
Angular gyrus
Occipital lobe
Frontal lobe
Sylvian fissure
Temporal lobe

Fig. 1.1. Lobes of the brain (N. C. Keong, 2009).

frontal lesions. Resections more posterior than this in the dominant hemisphere are likely to damage the anterior speech area.

Temporal lobe

The temporal lobe lies anteriorly below the Sylvian fissure and becomes the parietal lobe posteriorly at the angular gyrus (Fig. 1.1). Its medial border is the uncus and is of particular clinical importance because it overhangs the tentorial hiatus adjacent to the midbrain. When intracranial pressure rises in the supratentorial compartment, it is the uncus of the temporal lobe that transgresses the tentorial hiatus, compressing the third nerve, midbrain and posterior cerebral artery. This is described as 'uncal herniation' to distinguish it from herniation of the tonsils through the foramen magnum (coning). In around 90% of cases, uncal herniation will produce dilation of the pupil on the same side as the pathology. In the remainder, it is a false localizing sign, where shift of the midbrain compresses the contralateral third nerve against the tentorial hiatus. It is also important to note another herniation syndrome, Kernohan's notch, where a space-occupying lesion produces midline shift of the midbrain and compresses the contralateral cerebral peduncle against the tentorium. This compression causes an ischaemic infarct in the corticospinal tract, resulting in a motor deficit ipsilateral to the pathology.

The temporal lobe has many roles including memory, the cortical representation of olfactory, auditory and vestibular information, some aspects of emotion and behaviour, Wernicke's speech area (in the dominant hemisphere) and parts of the visual field pathway. Like the frontal lobe, lesions in the temporal lobe may present with memory impairment or personality change. Seizures are common because structures in this lobe are particularly epileptogenic. Amygdalohippocampectomy with or without temporal lobectomy may be required for intractable forms of epilepsy with proven mesial temporal sclerosis on imaging. Temporal lobe seizures may be associated with vivid aura phenomena linked to the function of the temporal lobe (e.g. olfactory, auditory or visual hallucinations, unpleasant visceral sensations, bizarre behaviour or déjà vu).

The anterior portion of one temporal lobe (approximately at the junction of the Rolandic and Sylvian fissures) may be resected with low risk of neurodisability. Generally, this amounts to 4 cm of the dominant lobe or 6 cm of the non-dominant lobe. The upper part of the superior temporal gyrus is generally preserved to protect the branches of the middle cerebral artery (MCA) lying in the Sylvian fissure. More posterior resection may also damage the speech area in the dominant hemisphere. Care is needed if resecting the medial aspect of the uncus because of its proximity to the optic tract. In some patients undergoing temporal lobectomy, it may be appropriate to perform an fMRI investigation to confirm laterality of language and to establish whether the patient is likely to suffer significant memory impairment as a result of the procedure. Previously, patients would have undergone the Wada test prior to surgery. This investigation involves selective catheterization of each internal carotid artery in turn. While the hemisphere in question is anaesthetized with sodium amytal (effectiveness is confirmed by the onset of contralateral hemiplegia), the patient's ability to speak is evaluated. They are then presented with a series of words and images that they are asked to recall once the hemiparesis has recovered, thereby assessing the strength of verbal and non-verbal memory in the contralateral hemisphere.

Parietal lobes

These extend from the Rolandic fissure to the parieto-occipital sulcus posteriorly and to the temporal lobe inferiorly. The dominant hemisphere shares speech function with the adjacent temporal lobe, while both sides contain the sensory cortex and visual association areas. Parietal lobe dysfunction may produce cortical sensory loss or sensory inattention. In the dominant hemisphere, the result is dysphasia. Dysfunction in the non-dominant hemisphere produces dyspraxia (e.g. difficulty dressing, using a knife and fork) or difficulty with spatial orientation. Impairment of the visual association areas may give rise to visual agnosia (inability to recognize objects) or to alexia (inability to read).

Occipital lobes

Lesions within the occipital lobe typically present with a homonymous field defect without macular sparing. Visual hallucinations (flashes of light, rather than the formed images that are typical of temporal lobe epilepsy) may also be a feature. Resection of the occipital lobe will result in a contralateral homonymous hemianopia. The extent of resection is restricted to 3.5 cm from the occipital pole in the dominant hemisphere because of the angular gyrus, where lesions can produce dyslexia, dysgraphia and acalculia. In the non-dominant hemisphere, up to 7 cm may be resected.

Cerebellum

The cerebellum consists of a group of midline structures, the lingula, vermis and flocculonodular lobe, and two laterally placed hemispheres. Lesions affecting midline structures typically produce truncal ataxia, which may make it difficult for the patient to stand or even to sit. Obstructive hydrocephalus is common. Invasion of the floor of the fourth ventricle by tumour may give rise to vomiting or cranial nerve

dysfunction. Lesions within the hemispheres usually cause ipsilateral limb ataxia. Vertigo may result from damage to the vestibular reflex pathways. Nystagmus is typically the result of involvement of the flocculonodular lobe. Other features associated with disorders of the cerebellum include hypotonia, dysarthria and pendular reflexes.

Surgical anatomy of the cerebral circulation

Arterial

The cerebral circulation is made up of two components. The anterior circulation is fed by the internal carotid arteries, while the posterior circulation derives from the vertebral arteries (the vertebrobasilar circulation). The arterial anastomosis in the suprasellar cistern is named the 'circle of Willis' after Thomas Willis (Fig. 1.2), who published his dissections in 1664, with illustrations by the architect Sir Christopher Wren. This section is based on detailed accounts of the normal and abnormal anatomy of the cerebral vasculature, as described by Yasargil (1984) and Rhoton (2003).

The internal carotid artery (ICA) has no branches in the neck but gives off two or three small vessels within the cavernous sinus before entering the cranium just medial to the anterior clinoid process. It gives off the ophthalmic and posterior communicating

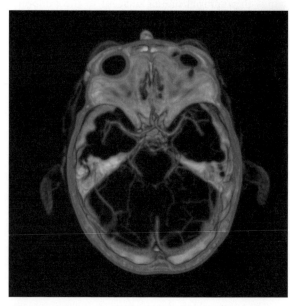

Fig. 1.2. CT angiogram of the circle of Willis. See colour plate section.

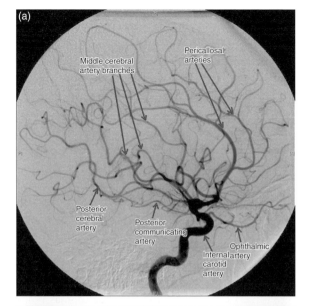

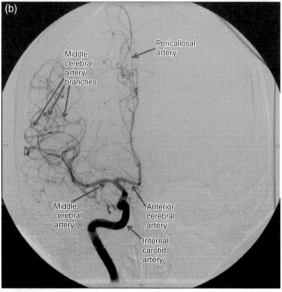

Fig. 1.3. Subtraction angiogram of the internal carotid circulation. (a) Lateral projection; (b) anteroposterior projection.

arteries (PComA) before reaching its terminal bifurcation, where it divides to become the anterior and middle cerebral arteries (Fig. 1.3). The anterior choroidal artery, the blood supply to the internal capsule, generally arises from the ICA nearer the origin of the PComA than the carotid bifurcation. It may arise as two separate arteries or as a single artery that divides into two trunks. The anterior cerebral artery (ACA) passes over the optic nerve and is connected with the vessel of the opposite side in the interhemispheric fissure by

the anterior communicating artery (AComA). The segment of the anterior cerebral artery proximal to the AComA is known as the A1 segment.

The distal ACA has four segments named according to their location in relation to the corpus callosum, the A2 (infracallosal), A3 (pre-callosal), A4 (supracallosal) and A5 (post-callosal) segments. The term pericallosal artery refers to the portion of the ACA beyond the A1 and therefore includes all the segments beyond that. In addition, the A2 also branches into the callosal marginal artery, which is variable in its presence and origin. The ACA supplies the orbital surface of the frontal lobe and the medial surface of the frontal lobe and the medial surface of the hemisphere above the corpus callosum back to the parieto-occipital sulcus. It extends onto the lateral surface of the hemisphere superiorly, where it meets the territory supplied by the MCA. The motor and sensory cortex to the lower limb are within the territory of supply of the ACA.

The MCA is the larger of the two terminal branches of the ICA. The MCA is divided into four segments, the M1 (sphenoidal), M2 (insular), M3 (opercular) and M4 (cortical) segments. The M1 segment begins at the origin of the MCA and passes laterally behind the sphenoid ridge and turns 90° at the genu. The M2 segment begins at the genu and gives off fronto-temporal branches before reaching the insula. The M3 segment begins at the insula and ends at the surface of the Sylvian fissure, giving off further branches whilst following a tortuous course in the process. The M4 segment refers to the branches to the lateral cerebral convexity. The MCA is responsible for the blood supply to most of the lateral aspect of the hemisphere, with the exception of the superior frontal (supplied by the ACA) as well as the inferior temporal gyrus and the occipital cortex (supplied by the posterior cerebral artery, PCA) (Fig. 1.4). Within its territory of supply are the internal capsule, speech and auditory areas, and the motor and sensory areas for the opposite side, with the exception of the lower limbs, which are supplied by the ACA.

The PComA arises from the posteromedial boundary of the ICA midway between the origin of the ophthalmic artery and the terminal bifurcation. The PComA and the proximal PCA form the posterior part of the circle of Willis. Embryologically, the PComA becomes the PCA, but, in the adult, the PCA is a branch of the basilar system. However, the PComA may remain the major origin of the PCA and this is termed a 'fetal' PComA. The posterior circulation comprises the vertebral arteries, which join at the clivus to form the

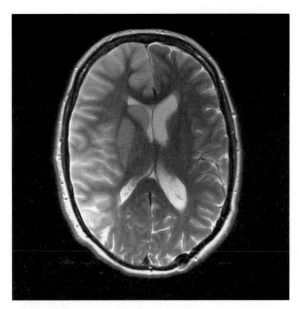

Fig. 1.4. Right middle cerebral artery (MCA) territory pathology. MRI brain scan demonstrating oedema following an infarct in the MCA territory.

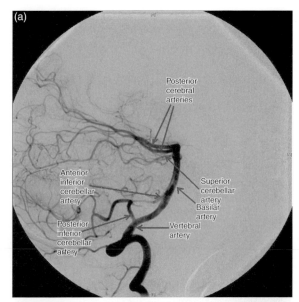

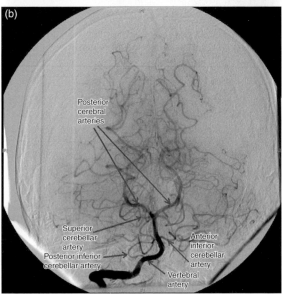

Fig. 1.5. Subtraction angiogram of the vertebral circulation. (a) Lateral projection; (b) anteroposterior projection.

basilar artery. This gives off multiple branches to the brainstem and cerebellum before the bifurcation of the basilar artery near the level of the posterior clinoids to become the PCAs. The PComA and PCA join at the lateral margin of the interpeduncular cistern, thus completing the circle of Willis and connecting the anterior and posterior circulations (Fig. 1.5).

The PCA is divided into four segments, P1 (pre-communicating), P2 (post-communicating), P3 (quadrigeminal) and P4 (cortical). The PCA gives off three kinds of branches: (i) central perforating branches to the diencephalon and midbrain; (ii) ventricular branches to the choroid plexus and walls of the lateral and third ventricles and adjacent structures; and (iii) cerebral branches to the cerebral cortex and splenium of the corpus callosum. The P1 segment extends from the basilar bifurcation to the junction with the PComA. The P2 lies in the crural and ambient cisterns and then terminates lateral to the posterior edge of the midbrain. The P2 is divided into anterior (P2A) and posterior (P2P) parts. The artery may be occluded as it crosses the tentorial hiatus when intracranial pressure is high (Fig. 1.6). The P3 segment courses from the lateral edge of the midbrain and ambient cistern to the lateral part of the quadrigeminal cistern and ends at the calcarine sulcus. The P4 segment begins at the calcarine sulcus and continues as branches to the cortical surface. Its territory of supply is the inferior and

inferolateral surface of the temporal lobe and the inferior and most of the lateral surface of the occipital lobe. The contralateral visual field lies entirely within its territory.

Arterial anomalies

In post-mortem series, a fully developed arterial circle of Willis exists in about 96% of cadavers, although the communicating arteries will be small in some.

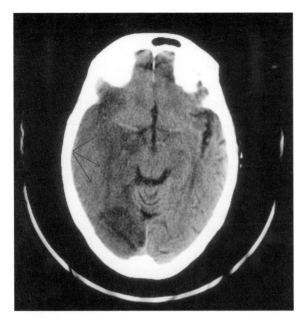

Fig. 1.6. CT head scan showing extensive infarction (low density) in the territory of the posterior cerebral artery (arrows). This was the result of compression of the vessel at the tentorial hiatus due to uncal herniation.

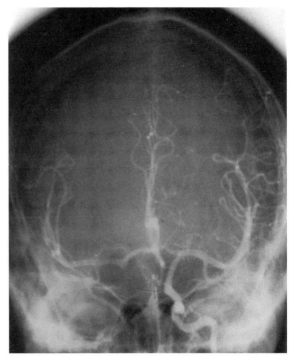

Fig. 1.7. The cross-compression test. Contrast has been injected into the left internal carotid artery while the right is occluded by external compression in the neck. This examination demonstrates good cross-filling of the distal vessels on the right from the left. The AComA and A1 segments are patent. However, this test alone is not a reliable way of determining that neurodisability will not ensue if the contralateral internal carotid artery is permanently occluded.

Because haemodynamic anomalies are associated with an increased risk of berry aneurysm formation, an incomplete circle of Willis is likely to be more common in neurosurgical patients than in the general population.

Hypoplasia or absence of one or more of the communicating arteries can be particularly important at times when one of the major feeding arteries is temporarily occluded. This is an important consideration for neurovascular procedures such as during carotid endarterectomy or when gaining proximal control of a ruptured intracranial aneurysm. Under such conditions, the circle of Willis cannot be relied upon to maintain adequate perfusion to parts of the ipsilateral or contralateral hemisphere. This situation will be compounded by atherosclerotic narrowing of the vessels or by systemic hypotension. The areas particularly vulnerable to ischaemia are the watersheds between vascular territories. Some estimate of flow across the AComA can be obtained angiographically by the cross-compression test. During contrast injection, the contralateral carotid is compressed in the neck, thereby reducing distal perfusion and encouraging flow of contrast from the ipsilateral side (Fig. 1.7). Transcranial Doppler provides a more quantitative assessment. Trial balloon occlusion in the conscious patient may be indicated for further evaluation of the presence of cross-flow and tolerance of permanent occlusion.

The A1 segments frequently vary in size (in 60–80% of patients). In approximately 5% of the population, one A1 segment will be severely hypoplastic or aplastic. The AComA is very variable in nature, having developed embryologically from a vascular network. It exists as a single channel in 75% of subjects but may be duplicated or occasionally absent (2%). The PComA is <1 mm in diameter in approximately 20% of patients. In almost 25% of people, the PComA is larger than the P1 segment and the PCAs are therefore supplied primarily (or entirely) by the internal carotid rather than the vertebral arteries. Because the posterior cerebral artery derives embryologically from the internal carotid artery, this anatomical variant is known as a persistent fetal-type posterior circulation (as described above).

If both the AComA and PComA are hypoplastic, then the middle cerebral territory is supplied only by the ipsilateral internal carotid artery (the so-called

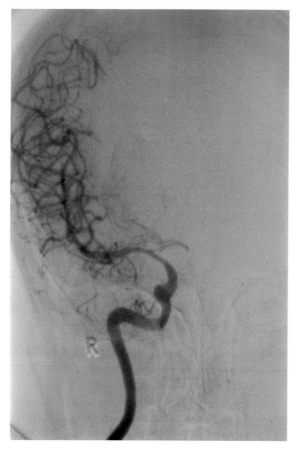

Fig. 1.8. Vasospasm in the A1 segment due to an AComA aneurysm. Only the right anteroposterior (MCA) territory fills following right internal carotid artery (ICA) angiography. In this instance, the circle of Willis would be unable to maintain right MCA blood flow if perfusion were to be reduced in the ipsilateral ICA. R, right side.

'isolated MCA'; Fig. 1.8). Such a patient will be very vulnerable to ischaemia if the internal carotid is temporarily occluded during surgery. Should it be necessary to occlude the internal carotid artery permanently, for example in a patient with an intracavernous aneurysm, some form of bypass graft will be required. Usually this is between the superficial temporal artery and a branch of the MCA (an extracranial–intracranial artery (EC–IC) bypass).

The small perforating vessels that arise from the circle of Willis to enter the base of the brain are known as the central rami. Those from the anterior and middle cerebral arteries supply the lentiform and caudate nuclei and internal capsule, while those from the communicating arteries and posterior cerebrals supply the thalamus, hypothalamus and mesencephalon. Damage to any of these small perforators at surgery may result in significant neurological deficit.

Microscopic anatomy

Cerebral vessels are different from their systemic muscular counterparts in that they possess only a rudimentary tunica adventitia. This is particularly relevant to subarachnoid haemorrhage. Whereas a clot surrounding a systemic artery will not result in the development of delayed vasospasm, it is likely that the lack of an adventitia allows blood breakdown products access to smooth muscle of the tunica media of the cerebral vessels, thereby giving rise to late constriction.

A second microscopic difference from systemic vessels is that the tunica media of both large and small cerebral arteries has its muscle fibres orientated circumferentially. This results in a point of potential weakness at the apex of vessel branches and may lead to aneurysm formation. Approximately 85% of berry aneurysms develop in the anterior circulation.

Venous

Cephalic venous drainage also differs from many other vascular beds in that it does not follow the arterial pattern. There are superficial and deep venous systems that, like the internal jugular veins, are valveless (Fig. 1.9). This is the basis for nursing patients with raised intracranial pressure such as traumatic brain injury and subarachnoid haemorrhage at a slight head elevation (30°). Anastomotic venous channels allow communication between intracranial and extracranial tissues via diploic veins in the skull. These may allow infection from the face or paranasal air sinuses to spread to the cranium, resulting in subdural empyema, cerebral abscess or a spreading cortical venous or sinus thrombosis.

The general pattern for venous drainage of the hemispheres is into the nearest venous sinus. The superior sagittal sinus occupies the convex margin of the falx and is triangular in cross-section. Because of its semi-rigid walls, the sinus does not collapse when venous pressure is low, resulting in a high risk of air embolism during surgery if the sinus is opened with the head elevated. Venous lakes are occasionally present within the diploë of the skull adjacent to the sinus, and can result in excessive bleeding or air embolus when a craniotomy flap is being turned.

The lateral margin of the superior sagittal sinus contains arachnoid villi responsible for the reabsorption of

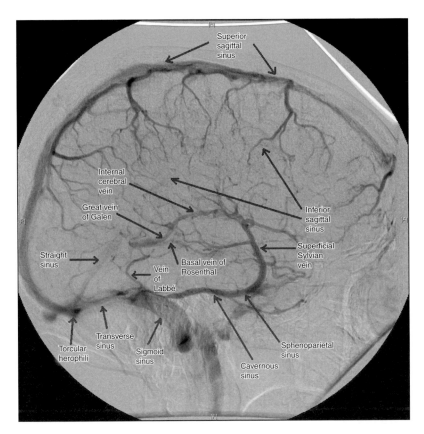

Fig. 1.9. The major superficial and deep venous drainage of the brain on venous phase angiography.

CSF into the venous circulation. It begins at the floor of the anterior cranial fossa at the crista galli and extends back in the midline, increasing progressively in size, until it reaches the level of the internal occipital protuberance. Here it turns to one side, usually the right, as the transverse sinus. The straight sinus turns to form the opposite transverse sinus at this point. An anastomosis of variable size connects the two and is known as the confluence of the sinuses or torcular Herophili.

The basal ganglia and adjacent structures drain via the internal cerebral veins, which lie in the roof of the third ventricle, and the basal veins, which pass around the cerebral peduncles. The internal cerebral and basal veins join to form the great cerebral vein of Galen beneath the splenium of the corpus callosum. This short vein joins the inferior sagittal sinus (which runs in the free edge of the falx) to form the straight sinus.

The superior cerebral veins (usually 8–12 in number) lie beneath the arachnoid on the surface of the cerebral cortex and drain the superior and medial surface of the hemisphere into the superior sagittal sinus. To do this, they must bridge the subdural space

(hence the alternative name of 'bridging veins'). If the hemisphere is atrophic and therefore relatively mobile within the cranium, these veins are likely to be torn by even minor head injury, giving rise to chronic subdural haematoma. A large acute subdural haematoma may also displace the hemisphere sufficiently to avulse the bridging veins, provoking brisk venous bleeding from multiple points in the sinus when the clot is evacuated. Tearing of bridging veins may also occur during or early after neurosurgical procedures in which there has been excessive shrinkage of the brain or loss of CSF. This phenomenon is thought to account for some cases in which post-operative haemorrhage develops in regions remote from the operative site.

Although venous anastomoses exist on the lateral surface of the hemisphere, largely between the superior anastomotic vein (draining upwards in the central sulcus to the superior sagittal sinus – the vein of Trolard), the Sylvian vein (draining downwards in the Sylvian fissure to the sphenoparietal sinus) and the angular or inferior anastomotic vein (draining via the vein of Labbé into the transverse sinus), sudden occlusion of large veins or a patent venous sinus may result in brain swelling or even venous infarction. As a general rule, the anterior one-third of the superior sagittal sinus may be ligated, but only one bridging vein should be divided distal to this if complications are to be avoided. If the sinus has been occluded gradually, for example by a parasagittal meningioma, then there is time for venous collaterals to develop. However, it then becomes all the more important that these anastomotic veins are not divided during removal of the tumour. Venous-phase angiography is particularly useful in planning the operative approach to tumours adjacent to the major venous sinuses or to the vein of Galen and thereby determining whether the sinus is completely occluded and can be resected *en bloc* with the tumour or whether the sinus is patent and requires reconstruction.

Innervation of the cerebral vasculature and neurogenic influences of cerebral blood flow

Sympathetic

The superior cervical ganglion largely supplies sympathetic innervation to the cerebral vasculature. In addition to the catecholamines, sympathetic nerve terminals contain another potent vasoconstrictor, neuropeptide Y. This 36 amino acid neuropeptide is found in abundance in both the central and peripheral nervous systems. Only minor (5–10%) reductions in cerebral blood flow (CBF) accompany electrical stimulation of sympathetic nerves, far less than that seen in other vascular beds. Although feline pial arterioles vasoconstrict in response to topical norepinephrine and the response is blocked by the α-blocker phenoxybenzamine, application of the latter alone at the same concentration has no effect on vessel calibre. This and other observations from denervation studies indicate that the sympathetic nervous system does not exert a significant tonic influence on cerebral vessels under physiological conditions. The sympathetic innervation also does not contribute to CBF regulation under conditions of hypotension or hypoxia.

However, Harper and colleagues (1972) observed that sympathetic stimulation does produce a profound fall in CBF if cerebral vessels have been dilated by hypercapnia. From this study came the 'dual-control' hypothesis, which proposed that the cerebral circulation comprises two resistances in series. Extraparenchymal vessels are thought to be regulated largely by the

autonomic nervous system, while intraparenchymal vessels are responsible for the main resistance under physiological conditions and are governed primarily by intrinsic metabolic and myogenic factors.

Sympathetic innervation has been shown to exert a significant influence on cerebral blood volume and protect the brain from the effects of acute severe hypertension. When blood pressure rises above the limits of autoregulation, activation of the sympathetic nervous system moderates the anticipated rise in CBF and reduces the plasma protein extravasation that follows breakdown of the blood–brain barrier. The autoregulatory curve is 'reset' such that both the upper and lower limits are raised. This is an important physiological mechanism by which the cerebral vasculature is protected from injury during surges in arterial blood pressure (Fig. 1.10). While cerebral vessels escape from the vasoconstrictor response to sympathetic stimulation under conditions of normotension, this does not occur during acute hypertension. It also follows from this that CBF is better preserved by drug-induced than haemorrhagic hypotension for the same perfusion pressure, because circulating catecholamine levels are high in the case of the latter.

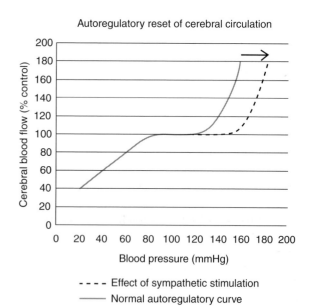

Fig. 1.10. Autoregulatory reset of the cerebral circulation. The normal curve illustrates the maintenance of cerebral blood flow as arterial blood pressure changes. Stimulation of the sympathetic nervous system results in a shift of the curve to the right, thereby protecting the cerebral vasculature from injury due to surges in blood pressure.

Sympathetic nerves are also thought to exert trophic influences on the vessels that they innervate. Sympathetectomy reduces the hypertrophy of the arterial wall that develops in response to chronic hypertension. Denervation has been shown to increase the susceptibility of stroke-prone spontaneously hypertensive rates to bleed into the cerebral hemisphere, which had been sympathectomized.

Parasympathetic

The cerebrovascular parasympathetic innervation is supplied from a variety of sources, which include the sphenopalatine and otic ganglia and small clusters of ganglion cells within the cavernous plexus, Vidian and lingual nerves. Vasoactive intestinal polypeptide (VIP), a potent 28 amino acid polypeptide vasodilator that is not dependent on endothelium-derived relaxant factor, has been localized immunohistochemically within parasympathetic nerve endings, as has nitric oxide synthase, the enzyme that forms nitric oxide from L-arginine.

Although stimulation of parasympathetic nerves does elicit a rise in CBF, there is, like the sympathetic nervous system, little to suggest that cholinergic mechanisms contribute significantly to CBF regulation under physiological conditions; nor are parasympathetic nerves involved in the vasodilatory response to hypercapnia. However, chronic parasympathetic denervation increases infarct volume by 37% in rats subjected to permanent MCA occlusion, primarily because of a reduction in CBF under situations when perfusion pressure is reduced. This suggests that parasympathetic nerves may help to maintain perfusion at times of reduced CBF and may explain in part why patients with autonomic neuropathy, such as diabetes, are at increased risk of stroke.

Sensory nerves and head pain

The anatomy of the sensory innervation to the cranium is important for an understanding of the basis of certain types of headache. The only pain-sensitive structures within the cranium are the dura mater, the dural venous sinuses and the larger cerebral arteries (>50 μm diameter). The structures that lie within the supratentorial compartment and rostral third of the posterior fossa are innervated predominantly by small myelinated and unmyelinated nerve fibres that emanate from the ophthalmic division of the trigeminal nerve (with a small contribution from the maxillary division). The caudal two-thirds of the posterior fossa is innervated by the C1 and C2 dorsal roots. With the exception of midline structures, innervation is strictly unilateral. Although each individual neuron has divergent axon collaterals that innervate both the cerebral vessels and dura mater, the extracranial and intracranial trigeminal innervations are separate peripherally. Centrally, however, they synapse onto single interneurons in the trigeminal nucleus caudalis.

This arrangement accounts for the strictly unilateral nature of some types of headache. The pain is poorly localized because of large receptive fields, and is referred to somatic areas. Referred cranial pain is similar to pain experienced in association with inflammation of other viscera, for example, referred pain to the umbilicus and abdominal muscle rigidity due to appendicitis. Headache is generally referred to the frontal (ophthalmic) or cervico-occipital (C2) regions and is associated with tenderness in the temporalis and cervical musculature. It is because of this arrangement that tumours in the upper posterior fossa may present with frontal headache and why patients with raised pressure within the posterior fossa and impending herniation of the cerebellar tonsils through the foramen magnum may complain of neck pain and exhibit nuchal rigidity or episthotonic posturing. This arching of the back and extension of the limbs may be mistaken for epilepsy, with potentially serious adverse consequences if diazepam is given due to its risk of causing respiratory depression. Central projections of the trigeminal nerve to the nucleus of the tractus solitarius account for the autonomic responses (sweating, hypertension, tachycardia and vomiting) that may accompany headache.

Sensory nerves form a fine network on the adventitial surface of cerebral arteries. Several neuropeptides, including substance P (SP), neurokinin A (NKA) and calcitonin gene-related peptide (CGRP), are contained within vesicles in the naked nerve endings. All three are vasodilators, while SP and NKA promote plasma protein extravasation and an increase in vascular permeability. Neurotransmitter release can follow both orthodromic stimulation and axon reflex-like mechanisms. Trigeminal perivascular sensory nerve fibres have been found to contribute significantly to the hyperaemic responses that follow reperfusion after a period of cerebral ischaemia and that accompany acute severe hypertension, seizures and bacterial meningitis. There is now considerable evidence to support the notion that neurogenic inflammation in the dura mater resulting from the release of sensory neuropeptides is the fundamental basis for migraine.

Cerebrospinal fluid pathways

Cerebrospinal physiology and anatomy

Approximately 80% of the CSF is produced by the choroid plexus in the lateral, third and fourth ventricles. The remainder is formed around the cerebral vessels and from the ependymal lining of the ventricular system. The rate of CSF production (500–600 ml day^{-1} in the adult) is independent of intraventricular pressure, until intracranial pressure is elevated to the point at which CBF is compromised. The lateral ventricles are C-shaped cavities within the cerebral hemispheres (Fig. 1.11). Each drains separately into the third ventricle via the foramen of Monro, which is situated just in front of the anterior pole of the thalamus on each side. The third ventricle is a midline slit, bounded laterally by the thalami and inferiorly by the hypothalamus. It drains via the narrow aqueduct of Sylvius through the dorsal aspect of the midbrain to open out into the diamond-shaped fourth ventricle. This has the cerebellum as its roof and the dorsal aspect of the pons and medulla as its floor. The fourth ventricle opens into the basal cisterns via a midline foramen of Magendie, which sits posteriorly between the cerebellar tonsils and laterally into the cerebellopontine angle via the foraminae of Lushka. The CSF circulates into the spinal canal and also over the subarachnoid spaces. Figure 1.12 illustrates CSF production and circulation.

Most of the CSF is reabsorbed via the arachnoid villi into the superior sagittal sinus, while some is reabsorbed in the lumbar theca. The exact mechanism for reabsorption is unknown, although it is thought to be via one-way bulk flow. Reabsorption may be dependent on the pressure differential between the CSF and venous systems, as well as the overlapping arrangement of endothelial cells of the arachnoid villi acting as a valve mechanism. Flow of CSF across the ventricular wall into the brain extracellular space is not an important mechanism under physiological conditions. However, this is seen in acute hydrocephalus as areas of periventricular lucency (PVL), normally at the frontal and occipital horns of the lateral ventricles.

Hydrocephalus

Obstruction to CSF flow results in hydrocephalus. This is divided clinically into communicating and non-communicating types depending on whether or not the ventricular system communicates with the subarachnoid space in the basal cisterns. The distinction between the two is important when considering treatment (see below). Examples of communicating hydrocephalus include subarachnoid haemorrhage (either traumatic or spontaneous, both of which silt up the arachnoid villi), meningitis and sagittal sinus thrombosis. In contrast, aqueduct stenosis, intraventricular

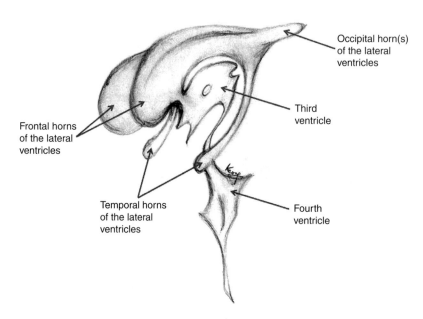

Fig. 1.11. An illustration of the three-dimensional shape of the ventricular system (N. C. Keong, 2010).

Occipital horn(s) of the lateral ventricles

Third ventricle

Frontal horns of the lateral ventricles

Temporal horns of the lateral ventricles

Fourth ventricle

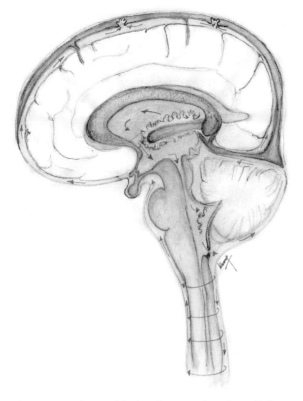

Fig. 1.12. Cerebrospinal fluid production and circulation (N. C. Keong, 2009).

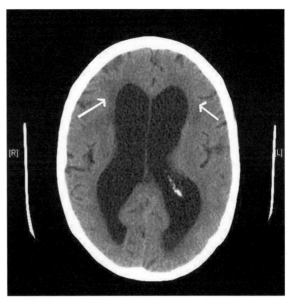

Fig. 1.13. CT head scan demonstrating dilation of the lateral ventricles and periventricular lucency (arrows).

haemorrhage and intrinsic tumours are common causes of non-communicating hydrocephalus. Other types of hydrocephalus are recognized such as normal pressure hydrocephalus, arrested hydrocephalus, long-standing overt ventriculomegaly in adults (LOVA), slit ventricles or unresponsive ventricles and slit ventricle syndrome. The descriptions, differentiation and investigation of these types are beyond the scope of this chapter (but are discussed by Keong *et al.*, 2011).

The diagnosis of hydrocephalus is usually made by the appearance on CT or MRI scan (Fig. 1.13). The features that suggest active hydrocephalus rather than *ex vacuo* dilation of the ventricular system secondary to brain atrophy are as follows:

- Dilation of the temporal horns of the lateral ventricles (>2 mm width).
- Rounding of the third ventricle or ballooning of the frontal horns of the lateral ventricles.
- Low density surrounding the frontal horns of the ventricles. This is caused by transependymal flow of CSF and is known as periventricular

lucency. However, in the elderly, this sign may be misleading, as it is also seen after multiple cerebral infarcts.

Management of hydrocephalus

In communicating hydrocephalus, CSF can be drained from either the lateral ventricles or the lumbar theca. Generally, this will involve the insertion of a permanent indwelling shunt unless the cause of the hydrocephalus is likely to be transient, infection is present or blood within the CSF is likely to block the shunt. Under such circumstances, either an external ventricular or lumbar drain, or serial lumbar punctures may be appropriate. Non-communicating or obstructive hydrocephalus requires CSF drainage from the ventricular system. Lumbar puncture is potentially dangerous because of the risk of coning if a pressure differential is created between the cranial and spinal compartments. A single drainage catheter is adequate if the lateral ventricles communicate with each other (the majority of cases), but bilateral catheters are needed if the blockage lies at the foramen of Monro.

Many forms of non-communicating hydrocephalus can now be treated by endoscopic third ventriculostomy, obviating the need for a prosthetic shunt with its attendant risk of blockage and infection (Fig. 1.14). An artificial outlet for CSF is created in the floor of the

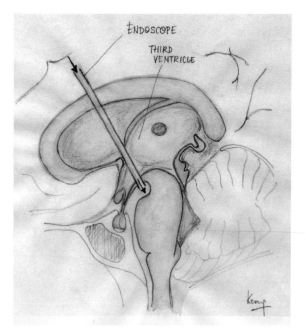

Fig. 1.14. Endoscopic third ventriculostomy (N. C. Keong, 2009).

third ventricle between the mamillary bodies and the infundibulum via an endoscope introduced through the frontal horn of the lateral ventricle and foramen of Monro. This allows CSF to drain directly from the third ventricle into the basal cisterns, where it emerges between the posterior clinoid processes and basilar artery.

Spinal anatomy

Assessing stability of the vertebral column

A stable spine is one in which normal movements will not result in displacement of the vertebrae. In an unstable spine, alterations in alignment may occur within movement. Instability can be a result of trauma, infection, tumour, degenerative changes or inflammatory disease. However, the degree of bone destruction or spinal instability does not always correlate with the extent of spinal cord injury.

The concept of the 'three-column' spine, as proposed by Holdsworth in 1970 and refined by Denis in 1983, is widely accepted as a means of assessing stability. The anterior column of the spine is formed by the anterior longitudinal ligament, the anterior annulus fibrosus of the intervertebral disc and the anterior part of the vertebral body. The middle column is formed by the posterior longitudinal ligament, the posterior

annulus fibrosus of the intervertebral disc and the posterior wall of the vertebral body. The posterior column is formed by the posterior arch and supraspinous and interspinous ligaments, as well as the ligamentum flavum. A single column disruption is stable, but a two- or three-column disruption should be managed as a potentially unstable injury until proven otherwise.

Plain radiographs showing normal vertebral alignment in a neutral position do not necessarily indicate stability, and views in flexion and extension may be necessary to assess the degree of ligamentous or bony damage (Fig. 1.15). While an unstable spine should generally be maintained in a fixed position, not all movements will necessarily risk compromising neurological function. For example, if a vertebral body has collapsed because of infection or tumour but the posterior elements are preserved, then the spine will be stable in extension, but flexion will increase the deformity and may force diseased tissue or the buckled posterior longitudinal ligament into the spinal canal. The mechanism of the injury has an important bearing on spinal stability after trauma. As a general rule, wedge compression fractures to the spine are stable, but flexion-rotation injuries cause extensive ligamentous damage posteriorly and are therefore unstable.

The spinal cord

The adult spinal cord terminates at about the lower border of L1 as the conus medullaris. Below this, the spinal canal contains peripheral nerves known as the cauda equina. Lesions above this level produce upper motor neuron signs and those below it a lower motor neuron pattern. Lesions of the conus itself may produce a mixed picture. A detailed account of the ascending and descending pathways is beyond the scope of this chapter but can be found in all standard anatomical texts. However, the following patterns of involvement may be a useful guide.

Extrinsic spinal cord compression

Classically, this produces symmetrical corticospinal ('pyramidal') involvement, with upper motor neuron weakness below the level of the compression (increased tone, clonus, little or no muscle wasting, no fasciculation, exaggerated tendon reflexes and extensor plantar responses), together with a sensory loss. If, however, the mass is laterally placed, then the pattern may initially be of hemisection of the cord – the Brown–Séquard syndrome. This produces ipsilateral

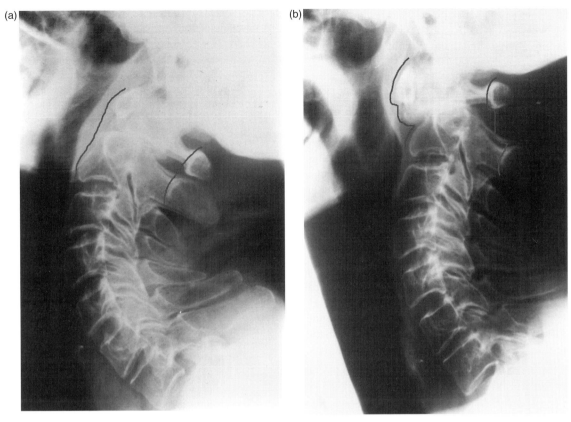

Fig. 1.15. Non-union of a fracture of the dens. (a) Satisfactory vertebral alignment in extension; (b) subluxation of C1 on C2 during neck flexion, resulting in severe spinal canal compromise.

pyramidal weakness, loss of fine touch and impaired proprioception but contralateral impairment of pain and temperature sensation. Examples of intrinsic spinal cord compression include a spinal meningioma or an epidural haematoma.

Central cord syndromes

Syringomyelia or intramedullary tumours affecting the cervicothoracic region will first involve the pain and temperature fibres, which decussate near the midline before ascending the lateral spinothalamic tracts. The result of central cord involvement is therefore a 'suspended' sensory loss, with a cape-type distribution of loss of sensitivity to pain in the upper limbs and trunk but with sparing of the lower limbs.

Cauda equina compression

This may result, for example, from a lumbar disc prolapse. Usually, but not invariably, it is accompanied by sciatica, which may be bilateral or unilateral and there may be weakness or sensory loss in a radicular distribution. In addition, there is perineal sensory loss in a saddle distribution, painless retention of urine with dribbling overflow incontinence and loss of anal tone.

Blood supply

The blood supply to the spinal cord is tenuous. The anterior and posterior spinal arteries form a longitudinal anastomotic channel that is fed by spinal branches of the vertebral, deep cervical, intercostals and lumbar arteries. In the neck, there is usually a feeder which comes from the thyrocervical trunk and accompanies either the C3 or C4 root. The largest radicular artery arises from the lower thoracic or upper lumbar region and supplies the spinal cord below the level of about T4. As in the cervical region, it accompanies one of the nerve roots and is known as the artery of Adamkiewicz. Its position is variable but is generally on the left side (two-thirds of cases) and arises between T10 and T12 in 75% of patients. In 15%, it lies between T5 and T8 and in 10% at L1 or L2.

It has a characteristic hairpin appearance on angiography because it ascends up the nerve root and then splits into a large caudal and a small cranial branch when it reaches the cord.

The artery of Adamkiewicz is vulnerable to damage during operations on the thoracic spine, particularly during excision of neurofibromas or meningiomas, or if an intercostal vessel is divided during excision of a thoracic disc. The artery is also vulnerable to injury during surgery to the descending thoracic aorta, during nephrectomy or even intercostals nerve blocks. Atherosclerotic disease of the radicular artery or prolonged hypotension may induce infarction of the anterior half of the cord up to mid-dorsal level, producing paraplegia, incontinence and spinothalamic sensory loss. However, joint position sense and light touch are preserved. Posterior spinal artery occlusion does not often produce a classic distribution of deficit because the vessel is part of a plexus and the territory of supply is variable. Because the arterial supply to the cord is not readily apparent at operation, surgery to the lower thoracic spine is often preceded by spinal angiography to determine the precise location of the artery of Adamkiewicz. However, this procedure itself carries a very small risk of spinal cord infarction.

Further reading

Denis, F. (1983). The three column spine and its significance in the classification of acute thoracolumbar spinal injuries. *Spine* **8**, 817–31.

Fawcett, E. and Blachford, J. V. (1905). The circle of Willis: an examination of 700 specimens. *J Anat Physiol* **40**, 63–70.

Hamani, C. (1997). Language dominance in the cerebral hemispheres. *Surg Neurol* **47**, 81–3.

Harper, A. M., Deshmukh, V. D., Rowan, J. O. and Jennett, W. B. (1972). The influence of sympathetic nervous activity on cerebral blood flow. *Arch Neurol* **27**, 1–6.

Heistad, D., Marcus, M., Busija, D. and Sadoshima, S. (1982). Protective effects of sympathetic nerves in the cerebral circulation. In Heistad, D. and Marcus, M. L., eds., *Cerebral Blood Flow: Effect of Nerves and Neurotransmitters*. New York: Elsevier, pp. 267–73.

Holdsworth, F. (1970). Fractures, dislocations, and fracture-dislocations of the spine. *J Bone Joint Surg Am* **52**, 1534–51.

Kano, M., Moskowitz, M. A. and Yokota, M. (1991). Parasympathetic denervation of rat pial vessels significantly increases infarction volume following middle cerebral artery occlusion. *J Cereb Blood Flow Metab* **11**, 628–37.

Keong, N., Czosnyka, M., Czosnyka, Z. and Pickard, J. D. (2011). Clinical evaluation of adult hydrocephalus. In Winn, R., ed., *Youmans Neurological Surgery*, 6th edn. Philadelphia, PA: Saunders/Elsevier.

Kobayashi, S., Waltz, A. G. and Rhoton, A. L. Jr (1971). Effects of stimulation of cervical sympathetic nerves on cortical blood flow and vascular reactivity. *Neurology* **21**, 297–302.

Macfarlane, R. and Moskowitz, M. A. (1995). The innervation of pial blood vessels and their role in cerebrovascular regulation. In Caplan, L., ed., *Brain Ischemia: Basic Concepts and Clinical Relevance*. London: Springer Verlag, pp. 247–59.

Macfarlane, R., Moskowitz, M. A., Sakas, D. E. *et al.* (1991). The role of neuroeffector mechanisms in cerebral hyperperfusion syndromes. *J Neurosurg* **75**, 845–55.

Moskowitz, M. A. and Macfarlane, R. (1993). Neurovascular and molecular mechanisms in migraine headaches. *Cerebrovasc Brain Metab Rev* **5**, 159–77.

Mueller, S. M. and Heistad, D. D. (1980). Effect of chronic hypertension on the blood–brain barrier. *Hypertension* **2**, 809–12.

Papanastassiou, V., Kerr, R. and Adams, C. (1996). Contralateral cerebellar hemorrhagic infarction after pterional craniotomy: report of five cases and review of the literature. *Neurosurgery*, **39**, 841–51; discussion 851–2.

Rhoton, A. (2003). The supratentorial arteries. In *Rhoton Cranial Anatomy and Surgical Approaches*. Neurosurgery Official Journal of the Congress of Neurological Surgeons. Baltimore, MD: Lippincott Wilkins and Williams, pp. 81–148.

Toczek, M. T., Morrell, M. J., Silverberg, G. A. and Lowe, G. M. (1996). Cerebellar hemorrhage complicating temporal lobectomy. Report of four cases. *J Neurosurg* **85**, 718–22.

Yasargil, M. (1984). *Microneurosurgery*, **vol. 1**. Stuttgard: Springer Verlag.

Chapter

2

The cerebral circulation

Tonny Veenith and David K. Menon

Introduction

Management strategies for the prevention of secondary brain injury are based on maintaining the cerebral perfusion pressure. Anaesthetic and surgical interventions alter cerebrovascular physiology profoundly; hence, a good understanding of these changes is crucial to limit the damage following a brain injury. The brain is unique with a high metabolic rate, and its oxygen demand exceeds that of all organs except the heart. It is approximately 2% of body mass and receives 20% of the basal oxygen consumption and 15% of the resting cardiac output (700 ml min^{-1} in the adult).

Mean resting cerebral blood flow (CBF) in young adults is about 50 ml (100 g brain tissue)$^{-1}$ min^{-1}. This mean value represents two very different categories of flow: 70 and 20 ml (100 g)$^{-1}$ min^{-1} for grey and white matter, respectively. Regional CBF (rCBF) and glucose consumption decline with age, along with marked reductions in brain neurotransmitter content, and less consistent decreases in neurotransmitter binding.

Applied anatomy of the cerebral circulation

Arterial supply

The blood supply to the brain originates from dorsal aorta, provided by the common carotid arteries, which branch into internal carotid arteries; and the basilar artery, formed by the union of the two vertebral arteries, which are branches of the subclavian artery. The anastomoses between these two sets of vessels give rise to the circle of Willis.

Anatomical variations and significance

From MRI and cadaveric studies, the 'normal' polygonal anastomotic ring is present in 40–50% of brains and is often incomplete in younger individuals and women. The presence of anatomical variants may substantially modify patterns of infarction following large-vessel occlusion. For example, in some individuals, the proximal part of one anterior cerebral artery is hypoplastic, and flow to the ipsilateral frontal lobe is provided largely by the contralateral anterior cerebral, via the anterior communicating artery. Occlusion of the single dominant anterior cerebral in such a patient may result in massive infarction of both frontal lobes: the unpaired anterior cerebral artery syndrome. In other patients, the posterior cerebral artery is the direct continuation of the posterior communicating artery, instead arising primarily from the basilar artery – a pattern that mimics the fetal pattern of circulation. In this setting, an internal carotid occlusion will result in a pan-hemispheric infarct.

Global cerebral ischaemia, such as that associated with systemic hypotension, classically produces maximal lesions in areas where the zones of blood supply from two vessels meet, resulting in 'watershed' infarctions, for example, following low flow states during cardiopulmonary bypass.

Venous drainage

The brain is drained by small veins, which join to form the pial veins; these coalesce to form the intra- and extracerebral venous sinuses, which are endothelialized folds of dura. These sinuses drain into the internal jugular veins, which, at their origin, receive minimal contributions from extracerebral tissues.

Measurement of oxygen saturation in the jugular bulb (SjO$_2$) provides a means of indirectly assessing the brain's ability to extract and metabolize oxygen. It has been suggested that the supratentorial compartment is preferentially drained by the right internal jugular vein, while the infratentorial compartment is preferentially

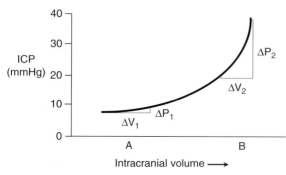

Fig. 2.1. An intracranial pressure (ICP)–volume curve. The curve shows the relationship between intracranial volume and ICP. Note that increases in intracranial volume produce a small change in intracranial pressure (ΔV_1 and ΔP_1, respectively) when initial intracranial volume is low and compensatory mechanisms are not exhausted. However, when compensatory mechanisms are exhausted, similar increases in intracranial volume (ΔV_2) result in large increases in ICP (ΔP_2).

drained by the left internal jugular vein. However, more recent data suggest considerable interindividual variation in cerebral venous drainage.

Cerebral blood volume: applied physiology and potential for therapeutic interventions

Most of the intracranial blood volume of about 200 ml is contained in the venous sinuses and pial veins, which constitute the capacitance vessels of the cerebral circulation; passive reduction in this volume can buffer rises in the volume of other intracranial contents (the brain and cerebrospinal fluid (CSF)). Conversely, when compensatory mechanisms to control intracranial pressure (ICP) have been exhausted, even small increases in cerebral blood volume (CBV) can result in steep rises in ICP (Fig. 2.1). The position of the system on this curve can be expressed in terms of the pressure–volume index (PVI), which is defined as the change in intracranial volume that produces a tenfold increase in ICP. This is normally about 26 ml, but may be markedly lower in patients with intracranial hypertension, who are on the steep part of the intracranial pressure–volume curve.

With the exception of oedema reduction by mannitol, the only intracranial constituent whose volume can readily be modified by physiological or pharmacological interventions is the parenchymal CBV, whose volume is set by vasomotor tone. Although the CBV forms only a small part of the intracranial volume, and such interventions produce only small absolute changes (typically ~10 ml or less), they may result in

marked reductions in ICP in the presence of intracranial hypertension.

Conversely, inappropriate clinical management may cause the CBV to increase. Again, although the absolute magnitude of such an increase may be small, it may result in steep rises in ICP in the presence of intracranial hypertension. The appreciation that pharmacological and physiological modulators may have independent effects on CBV and CBF is important for two reasons. Interventions aimed at reducing CBV in patients with intracranial hypertension may have prominent effects on CBF and result in cerebral ischaemia. Conversely, drugs that produce divergent effects on CBF may have similar effects on CBV, and using CBF measurement to infer effects on CBV and hence ICP may result in erroneous conclusions.

The cerebral microcirculation

The cerebral microcirculation is defined arbitrarily as the blood vessels of diameter <100 µm. The cerebrovascular microarchitecture is highly organized and follows the columnar arrangement seen with neuronal groups and physiological functional units. Pial surface vessels give rise to arterioles that penetrate the brain at right angles to the surface and give rise to capillaries at all laminar levels. Each of these arterioles supplies a hexagonal column of cortical tissue, with intervening boundary zones, an arrangement that is responsible for the columnar patterns of local blood flow, redox state and glucose metabolism seen in the cortex during hypoxia or ischaemia. Capillary density in the cortex is one-third of adult levels at birth, doubles in the first year and reaches adult levels at 4 years. At maturity, capillary density is related to the number of synapses, rather than the number of neurons or mass of cell bodies in a given region, and can be closely correlated with the regional level of oxidative metabolism. The cerebral circulation is protected from systemic blood pressure surges by a complex branching system and two resistance elements: the first of these lies in the large cerebral arteries, and the second in vessels of diameter <100 µm.

The blood–brain barrier

Endothelial cells in cerebral capillaries contain few pinocytic vesicles and are sealed with tight junctions, without any anatomical gap. Consequently, unlike other capillary beds, the endothelial barrier of cerebral capillaries presents a high electrical resistance and is

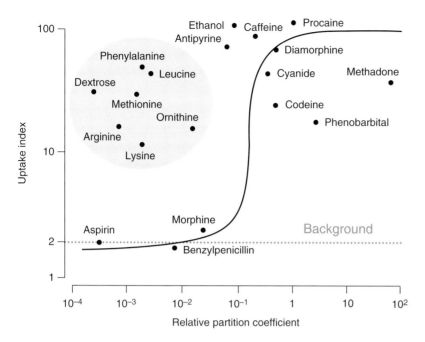

Fig. 2.2. Correlation between brain uptake index and oil/water partition coefficients for different substrates. While blood–brain barrier permeability, in general, increases with lipid solubility, note that several substances including glucose and amino acids show high penetration due to active transport or facilitated diffusion. (After Oldendorf, 1971.)

remarkably non-leaky, even to small molecules such as mannitol. This property of cerebral vasculature is termed the blood–brain barrier (BBB), and resides in its cellular components (the endothelial cell, astrocyte and pericyte) and its non-cellular structures (the endothelial basement membrane). A fundamental difference between brain endothelial cells and the systemic circulation is the presence of interendothelial tight junctions termed the zona occludens.

The BBB is a function of the cerebral microenvironment rather than an intrinsic property of the vessels themselves, as leaky capillaries from other vascular beds develop a BBB if they are transplanted into the brain or are exposed to astrocytes in culture. Passage through the BBB is not simply a function of molecular weight; lipophilic substances traverse the barrier relatively easily, and several hydrophilic molecules (including glucose) cross the BBB via active transport systems to enter the brain interstitial space (Fig. 2.2). In addition, the BBB maintains a tight control of relative ionic distribution in the brain extracellular fluid. These activities require energy and account for the high mitochondrial density in these endothelial cells, accounting for up to 10% of cytoplasmic volume. Several endogenous substances including catecholamines and vascular growth enhancing factor can dynamically modulate BBB permeability. Although the BBB is disrupted by ischaemia, this process takes hours to days rather than

minutes, and much of the cerebral oedema seen in the initial period after ischaemic insults is cytotoxic rather than vasogenic. Consequently, mannitol retains its ability to reduce cerebral oedema in the early phases of acute brain injury.

Physiological determinants of regional cerebral blood flow and cerebral blood volume

The concept of cerebral perfusion pressure

The driving pressure in most organs is the difference between arterial and venous pressure. However, in the brain, the downstream pressure is not the jugular venous pressure but the ICP. This is because the brain lies in a closed cavity, and when ICP is elevated, it results in collapse of the bridging pial veins and venous sinuses, which then act as Starling resistors. Consequently, the cerebral perfusion pressure (CPP) is defined as the difference between mean arterial pressure (MAP) and mean ICP:

$$CPP = MAP - ICP$$

Autoregulation

Autoregulation refers to the ability of the cerebral circulation to maintain CBF at a relatively constant level

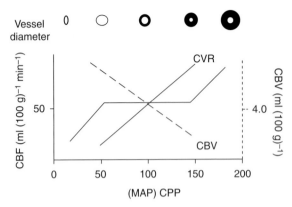

Fig. 2.3. Cerebrovascular resistance (CVR) changes in response to changes in the cerebral perfusion pressure (CPP) to maintain the cerebral blood flow (CBF). Cerebral vasodilation, and thus a decrease in CVR, maintains CBF with reductions in the CPP. This increases cerebral blood volume (CBV), which results in critical increases in intracranial pressure in patients with poor compliance (steep part of pressure–volume curve). MAP, mean arterial pressure.

during despite changes in CPP, by altering cerebrovascular resistance (CVR) (Fig. 2.3).

Static and dynamic autoregulation and their assessment

Classical cerebral autoregulation assessment does not consider the latency of autoregulatory mechanisms, focusing instead on the maintenance of CBF at different steady state levels of CPP (produced by vasopressors or postural alterations). Such measurement provides an indication of the efficiency of static autoregulation but does not address the time taken to re-establish baseline blood flow in response to a CPP alteration. This latency is assessed by techniques that specifically target dynamic autoregulation. One technique that is commonly used to assess dynamic autoregulation is transcranial Doppler ultrasonography (TCD), which quantifies real-time changes in beat-by-beat blood flow velocity in large cerebral arteries (typically the middle cerebral artery), following a range of interventions. One intervention is the production of a rapid drop in blood pressure by rapid deflation of a thigh cuff. An alternative is to measure the response middle cerebral artery flow velocity following a short period (3–5 s) of carotid compression – the transient hyperaemic response test (THRT). An increase in flow velocity during the recovery phase to suprabaseline levels is a marker of post-ischaemic hyperperfusion and suggests effective dynamic autoregulation. Some studies suggest that, especially in patients with impaired

autoregulation, the cardiac output and pulsatility of large-vessel flow may be more important determinants of rCBF than CPP itself.

Mechanisms of autoregulation

While autoregulation is maintained irrespective of whether changes in CPP arise from alterations in MAP or ICP, it tends to be preserved at lower levels when falls in CPP are due to increases in ICP rather than decreases in MAP due to hypovolaemia. One possible reason for this may be the vasoconstrictive effects of catecholamines secreted in haemorrhagic hypotension, as lower MAP levels are tolerated in hypotension if the fall in blood pressure is induced by sympatholytic agents or occurs in the setting of autonomic failure. Autoregulatory changes in CVR probably arise from myogenic reflexes in resistance vessels, but these may be modulated by activity of the sympathetic system or the presence of chronic systemic hypertension. Thus, sympathetic blockade or cervical sympathectomy shifts the autoregulatory curve to the left, while chronic hypertension or sympathetic activation shifts it to the right. These modulatory effects may also arise from angiotensin-mediated mechanisms. Animal studies, although inconclusive, suggest the importance of nitric oxide in this context. In reality, the clear-cut autoregulatory thresholds seen with varying CPP in Fig. 2.3 above are not observed; the autoregulatory 'knees' tend to be more gradual, and there may be wide variations in rCBF at a given value of CPP in experimental animals and even in neurologically normal individuals.

What are the safe limits for autoregulation?

It has been demonstrated that symptoms of cerebral ischaemia appear when the MAP falls below 60% of an individual's lower autoregulatory threshold. However, generalized extrapolation from such individualized research data to the production of 'safe' lower limits of MAP for general clinical practice is hazardous for several reasons. Firstly, there may be wide individual scatter in rCBF autoregulatory efficiency, even in normal subjects. For example, the efficiency of cerebral autoregulation declines with age, causing postural syncopal attacks. Secondly, the coexistence of fixed vascular obstruction (e.g. carotid atheroma or vascular spasm) may vary the MAP level at which rCBF reaches critical levels in relevant territories. Thirdly, the autoregulatory curve may be substantially modulated by mechanisms used to produce hypotension. Earlier discussion made the distinction between reductions in CPP produced by haemorrhagic hypotension, intracranial hypertension and pharmacological hypotension. The effects on autoregulation may also vary with the pharmacological agent used to produce hypotension. Thus, neuronal function is better preserved at similar levels of hypotension produced by halothane, nitroprusside or isoflurane in comparison with trimethaphan. Fourthly, the efficiency of autoregulation is compromised by disease, and dysautoregulation is associated with poor outcomes in traumatic brain injury (TBI), subarachnoid haemorrhage and after return of spontaneous circulation following cardiac arrest. Finally, autoregulatory responses are not immediate: estimates of the latency for compensatory changes in rCVR range from 10 to 60 s.

Flow–metabolism coupling

Increases in local neuronal activity are accompanied by increases in regional cerebral metabolic rate (rCMR). Until recently, increases in rCBF and oxygen consumption produced during such functional activation were thought to be closely coupled to the CMR of utilization of oxygen ($CMRO_2$) and glucose (CMRglu).

Clinical implications for flow metabolism: functional assessment of the brain

Functional activation in the brain results in capillary recruitment, as in other tissues. In the resting state, capillary flow is heterogeneous, and, as activation results in increased CBF, flow becomes more homogeneous across the capillary network. This mechanism is important for substrate transport across the BBB. However, some authorities still argue that all capillaries may be persistently open, and that 'recruitment' involves changes in capillary flow rates with homogenization of the perfusion rate in a network. There is a consistent ratio of about 5.6 between glucose and oxygen uptake in the resting brain. Increases in rCBF during functional activation tend to track glucose utilization but may be far in excess of the increase in oxygen consumption. Despite this revision of the proportionality between increased rCBF and $CMRO_2$ during functional activation, the relationship between rCBF and CMRglu is still linear, and glucose consumption is tightly coupled to neurotransmitter recycling and restoration of neuronal membrane potentials. However, the disproportionate increase in glucose utilization leads to regional anaerobic glucose utilization, with a consequent local decrease in oxygen extraction ratio and increase in local haemoglobin saturation. The

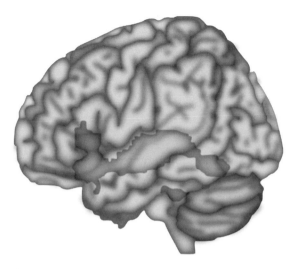

Fig. 2.4. Functional MRI of the brain for activation during spoken words. The blood oxygenation level-dependent (BOLD) contrast that is used to produce this image depends on the mismatch between increases in cerebral blood flow (CBF) and oxygen utilization during functional brain activation. The increase in CBF in excess of instantaneous oxygen utilization drops local deoxyhaemoglobin levels and increases the MR signal.

resulting local decrease in deoxyhaemoglobin levels provides the basis for functional neuroimaging using blood oxygenation level-dependent functional MFR (BOLD-fMRI; Fig. 2.4).

Other factors that alter flow–metabolism coupling

Use of anaesthetic agents and insults such as TBI alter flow–metabolism coupling. In TBI, flow may be uncoupled from metabolism; where blood flow is inadequate, ischaemia results, and where it is excessive, hyperaemia occurs. The efficiency of flow–metabolism coupling can also be modulated by hypo- and hyperthermia, seizures, sedation and by drugs that act directly on cerebrovascular tone (such as volatile anaesthetic agents or vasodilators).

Role of glial cells and the blood–brain barrier in flow–metabolism coupling

The brain is well organized into neurovascular units including neurons, glial cells and the cerebral microvasculature. Glial cells may be microglia, astrocytes and oligodendrocytes. The integration of neurovascular units is important for the maintenance of cerebral autoregulation and flow–metabolism coupling. Because of the large surface area contributed by the glial cells and the BBB ($\sim$20 m^2 per 1.3 kg brain), the glial/endothelial interface has an important role in regulating the brain microenvironment and blood

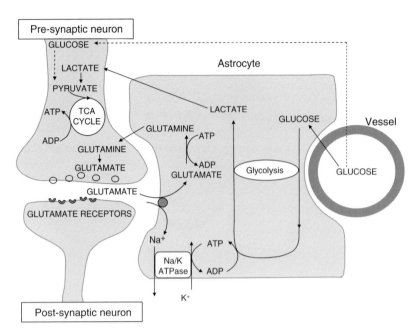

Fig. 2.5. Relationship of astrocytes to oxygen and energy metabolism in the brain. Glucose taken up by astrocytes undergoes glycolysis for generation of ATP to meet astrocytic energy requirements (for glutamate reuptake, predominantly). The lactate that this process generates is shuttled to neurons, which utilize it aerobically in the citric acid cycle.

flow. Astrocytes are multifunctional cells that perform various functions in various sites. Suggested cellular mechanisms by which astrocytes regulate cerebral metabolism (and hence CBF) are the glycolytic utilization of glucose with lactate production and maintenance of potassium homeostasis. Astrocytic glucose utilization and lactate production appear to be, in large part, coupled by the astrocytic reuptake of glutamate released at excitatory synapses, and the lactate produced by astrocytic glycolysis serves as a substrate for neuronal oxidative metabolism (Fig. 2.5).

The regulatory changes involved in flow–metabolism coupling that have a short latency (~1 s) are mediated either by metabolic or neurogenic pathways. The metabolic control is exerted by increases in perivascular potassium (regulated and maintained by astrocytes) or adenosine concentrations that follow neuronal depolarization. Neuronal control is enforced by a rich supply of nerve fibres. The mediators thought to play an important part in neurogenic flow–metabolism coupling are acetylcholine and nitric oxide, although roles have also been proposed for 5-hydroxytryptamine, substance P and neuropeptide Y.

Neurovascular modulation of cerebral circulation

Cerebral blood vessels receive an abundant nerve supply from the central and peripheral nerves. Autonomic and sensory supply arises from the sphenopalatine, trigeminal and superior cervical ganglia, innervating the extracranial and intracranial cerebral arteries. The dopaminergic neurons surrounding the large pial and penetrating vessels regulate the blood flow and are stimulated by the release of dopamine during nerve stimulation. This dopaminergic modulation may be important in the regulation of the blood flow during functional activation of the brain. The autonomic nervous system mainly affects tone in the larger cerebral vessels, up to and including the proximal parts of the anterior, middle and posterior cerebral arteries. β_2-Adrenergic stimulation results in vasodilation while α_2-adrenergic stimulation vasoconstricts these vessels. The effect of systemically administered α- or β-agonists is less significant. However, significant vasoconstriction can be produced by extremely high concentrations of catecholamines (e.g. in haemorrhage) or centrally acting α_2-agonists (e.g. dexmedetomidine).

Arterial carbon dioxide tension

Cerebral blood flow is proportional to arterial carbon dioxide tension ($PaCO_2$), subject to a lower limit below which vasoconstriction results in tissue hypoxia and reflex vasodilation, and an upper limit of maximal vasodilation (Fig. 2.6). On average, in the middle of the physiological range, each kPa change in $PaCO_2$ produces a change of about 15 ml $(100\,g)^{-1}$ min^{-1} in

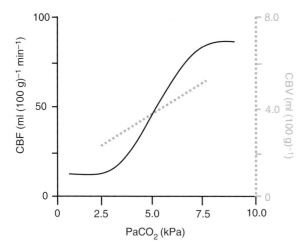

Fig. 2.6. Relative effects of PaCO₂ on cerebral blood flow (CBF) and cerebral blood volume (CBV). Hyperventilation is aimed at reducing CBV in patients with intracranial hypertension but may be detrimental because of its effects on CBF. Note that the slope of CBF reactivity to PaCO₂ is steeper than that for CBV (~25 vs. ~20% per kPa PaCO₂, respectively).

CBF. However, the slope of the $PaCO_2$/CBF relationship depends on the baseline normocapnic rCBF value, being maximal in areas where it is high (e.g. grey matter: cerebrum) and least in areas where it is low (e.g. white matter: cerebellum and spinal cord). $PaCO_2$ affects CBF by alteration of the extracellular pH, which, in turn, modulates intracellular calcium. One molecule implicated in part is nitric oxide (NO), which increases cyclic GMP (cGMP) and activates potassium channels directly, causing hyperpolarization and inhibiting voltage-gated calcium channels causing vasodilation. Prostaglandins may also mediate the vasodilation produced by carbon dioxide.

Moderate hypocapnia ($PaCO_2$ = 3.5–4.5 kPa) has long been used to reduce CBV in intracranial hypertension, but this practice is under review for two reasons. The carbon dioxide response is directly related to the change in perivascular pH; consequently, the effect of a change in $PaCO_2$ tends to be attenuated over time (hours) as brain extracellular fluid bicarbonate levels fall to normalize interstitial pH. Secondly, it has now been shown that 'acceptable' levels of hypocapnia in head-injured patients can result in dangerously low rCBF levels.

Effects of arterial carbon dioxide tension on cerebral blood volume and intracranial pressure

Grubb and colleagues studied the $CBF/PaCO_2$ response curve in primates and demonstrated that CBF changed by approximately 1.8 ml $(100 g)^{-1}$ min^{-1}

for each mmHg change in $PaCO_2$. However, in the same experiment, the $CBV/PaCO_2$ curve was much flatter (about 0.04 ml $(100 g)^{-1}$ per mmHg change (0.3 ml 100 g^{-1} kPa^{-1}) in $PaCO_2$). It follows from these figures that, while a reduction in $PaCO_2$ from 40 to 30 mmHg (5.3 to 4 kPa) would result in about a 40% reduction in CBF (from a baseline of about 50 ml $100g^{-1}$ min^{-1}), it would result in a 0.4% reduction in intracranial volume. This may seem trivial, but, in the presence of intracranial hypertension, the resultant 5 ml decrease in intracranial volume could result in a halving of ICP, as the system operates on the steep part of the intracranial compliance curve.

PaO₂ and CaO₂

The classical teaching is that CBF is unchanged until PaO_2 levels fall below approximately 7 kPa but rises sharply with further reductions. However, TCD data from humans suggests cerebral thresholds for cerebral hypoxic vasodilation as high as 8.5 kPa (~89–90% arterial oxygen saturation (SaO_2)). This non-linear behaviour is because tissue oxygen delivery governs CBF, and the sigmoidal shape of the haemoglobin–O_2 dissociation curve means that the relationship between CaO_2 (arterial oxygen content) and CBF is inversely linear. These vasodilator responses to hypoxaemia appear to show little adaptation with time but may be substantially modulated by $PaCO_2$ levels. Nitric oxide does not appear to play a role in the vasodilatory response to hypoxia. Some studies suggest that hyperoxia may produce cerebral vasoconstriction, with a 10–14% reduction in CBF with inhalation of 85–100% O_2, and a 20% reduction in CBF with 100% O_2 at 3.5 atmospheres. Human data suggest that this effect may not be clinically significant. Chronic hypoxia is a pathophysiological driver in conditions such as chronic obstructive airway disease and obstructive sleep apnoea, and may affect up to 2–4% of the general population. Such intermittent hypoxia accentuates systemic pressor responses, elevates baseline cerebral vascular resistance and may modulate cerebrovascular responses to hypercapnia.

Haematocrit

As in other organs, optimal oxygen delivery in the brain depends on a compromise between oxygen-carrying capacity and the rheological characteristics of blood; previous experimental work suggests that this may be best achieved at a haematocrit of about 40%. In the setting of vasospasm following subarachnoid haemorrhage, studies have suggested that modest haemodilution to a haematocrit of 30–35% may improve neurological outcome by improving rheological characteristics and increasing rCBF. However, this may result in a reduction in oxygen delivery if maximal vasodilation is already present and, as clinical results in the setting of acute ischaemia have not been uniformly successful, this approach must be viewed with caution.

Oxygen extraction ratios and jugular bulb oximetry

The cerebral oxygen extraction ratio (OER) is dependent on the balance between oxygen delivery (a product of arterial oxygen content and CBF) and oxygen utilization ($CMRO_2$). The OER changes with functional brain activation, which are the consequences of transient physiological uncoupling of flow and oxygen metabolism, are the basis of BOLD-fMRI contrast (as discussed above). Uncoupling of this balance can also reflect pathophysiology: reductions in CBF result in compensatory increases in OER, so as to maintain $CMRO_2$. This is manifest in jugular oximetry, with a fall in oxygen saturation providing a useful monitoring tool to detect inadequacy of CBF:

$$OER = (CaO_2 - CjO_2)/CaO_2 \text{ (expressed as a \% extraction)}$$

where CjO_2 is the jugular venous oxygen content. In the setting of TBI, such jugular desaturation to <50% has been associated with poor outcome.

Measurement of regional cerebral blood flow

All clinical and many laboratory methods of measuring CBF or rCBF are indirect and may not produce directly comparable measurements. It is also important to treat results from any one method with caution and to attribute any observed phenomena to physiological effects only when demonstrated by two or more independent techniques. Methods of measuring CBF may be regional or global, and may be applicable either to humans or primarily to experimental animals. All of these methods have advantages and disadvantages. All methods that provide absolute estimates of rCBF use one of two principles: they either measure the distribution of a tracer or estimate rCBF from the wash-in or wash-out curve of an indicator. Other techniques do not estimate rCBF directly but can be used either to measure a related flow variable (such as arterial flow

velocity) or to infer changes in flow from changes in metabolic parameters. These issues are addressed in detail elsewhere in this book.

Pharmacological modulation of cerebral blood flow

The importance of understanding drug effects on cerebrovascular physiology cannot be stressed enough. Drugs can exert changes in CBF, CMR and CPP, and therefore on CBV and ICP (Fig. 2.7). These effects may either be desirable (e.g. reducing intracranial volume (ICV) and ICP) or undesirable (e.g. increasing ICV and ICP thereby predisposing to brain herniation in patients with intracranial hypertension). In addition to causing changes in CPP, CBF, $CMRO_2$, CBV and ICP and altering production or reabsorption of CSF, pharmacological agents may modulate autoregulation, the flow–metabolism coupling and vascular responses to changes in $PaCO_2$ and PaO_2.

Halogenated volatile anaesthetic agents

Effects on cerebral blood flow, cerebral perfusion pressure, intracranial pressure and cerebral metabolic rate of oxygen

All potent fluorinated volatile anaesthetic agents affect CBF and CMR non-linearly and have been shown to increase CBF and ICP and reduce $CMRO_2$ (Fig. 2.8). The initial enthusiasm of halothane as a neuroanaesthetic agent was halted by the discovery of its potent vasodilatory effects, reducing CVR by 20–40% in normocapnic individuals at 1.2–1.5 minimum alveolar concentration (MAC). In another study, 1% halothane was shown to result in clinically significant elevations in ICP in patients with intracranial space-occupying lesions.

Studies with enflurane and isoflurane suggest that these agents might produce smaller increases in CVR at equivalent doses. As enflurane may produce epileptogenic activity, its use in the context of neuroanaesthesia has decreased. Several studies compared the effects of isoflurane and halothane on CBF, with conflicting results. While some studies showed that halothane produced larger decreases in CVR, others found no difference. Examination of the patterns of rCBF produced by these two agents provides some clues to the origin of this discrepancy. Halothane selectively increases cortical rCBF while markedly decreasing subcortical rCBF, while isoflurane produces a more

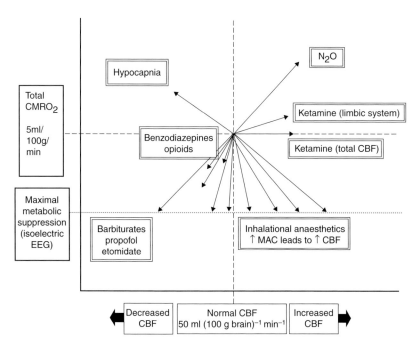

Fig. 2.7. Effect of drugs used in anaesthetic practice and hypocapnia on cerebral metabolic rate (CMR) and cerebral blood flow (CBF). Note that hyperventilation and the resulting hypocapnia can lead to vasoconstriction (decreased CBF) and an increase in CMR, a particularly unfavourable situation. Note also that increasing the inhalational anaesthetic agent concentration (minimum alveolar concentration, MAC) does not decrease CMR below a lower limit. However, it does increase CBF, thereby increasing CBV and intracranial pressure. This is hazardous for patients with poor intracranial compliance.

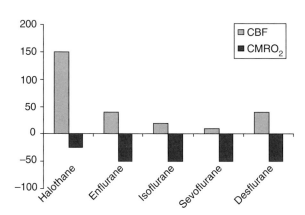

Fig. 2.8. Effects of fluorinated volatile anaesthetic agents on cerebral blood flow (CBF) and the cerebral metabolic rate of oxygen (CMRO$_2$).

generalized reduction in rCBF. Comparisons of the CBF effects of the two agents suggests that estimated CBF using techniques that preferentially looked at the cortex (e.g. ^{133}Xe wash-out) tended to show that halothane was a more potent vasodilator, while most studies that have used more global measures of hemispheric CBF (e.g. the Kety–Schmidt technique) have found little difference between the two agents at levels of around 1 MAC (Fig. 2.9).

Both agents tend to reduce global CMR, but the regional pattern of such an effect may vary, with

isoflurane producing greater cortical metabolic suppression (reflected by its ability to produce EEG burst suppression at higher doses). Both the rCBF and rCMR effects of the two anaesthetics are markedly modified by baseline physiology and other pharmacological agents. Thus, CBF increases produced by both agents are attenuated by hypocapnia (more so with isoflurane), and thiopentone attenuates the relative preservation of cortical rCBF seen with halothane. It is difficult to predict accurately what the effect of either agent would be on CBF in a given clinical situation, but this would be a balance of its suppressant effects on rCMR (with autoregulatory vasoconstriction) and its direct vasodilator effect (which is partially mediated via both endothelial and neuronal nitric oxide.

Although initial reports suggested that halothane could 'uncouple' flow and metabolism, more recent studies have clearly shown that, at concentrations commonly used for neuroanaesthesia, neither halothane, isoflurane nor desflurane completely disrupts flow–metabolism coupling, although their vasodilator effects may alter the slope of this relationship, due to changes in the flow/metabolism ratio with increases in anaesthetic concentration. Thus, although increases in metabolism are matched by increases in flow at all levels of anaesthesia, flow is higher at higher volatile anaesthetic concentrations at the same level of metabolism. In practice, the metabolic suppressant effects of

25

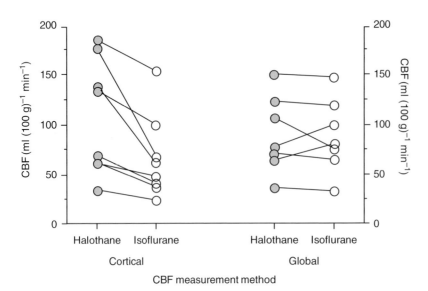

Fig. 2.9. Comparison of mean cerebral blood flow (CBF) in animals anaesthetized with 0.5–1.5 minimum alveolar concentration (MAC) of isoflurane or halothane, either in the same study or in comparable studies from a single research group with identical methodology within a single publication. In studies shown on the left, CBF was estimated using techniques likely to be biased towards cortical flow (e.g. [133]Xe wash-out), showing that halothane produces greater increases in CBF. In the studies on the right, CBF was estimated using techniques that measured global cerebral blood flow (e.g. the Kety–Schmidt method); the difference in effects on CBF between the two agents is much less prominent.

the anaesthetics are more prominent at lower concentrations and when no other metabolic suppressants are used. Conversely, these vasodilator effects may become more prominent at higher concentrations or when the volatile agents are introduced on a baseline of low or suppressed cerebral metabolism (such as that produced by intravenous anaesthesia).

While initial studies suggested that desflurane and sevoflurane had effects on the cerebral vasculature that appeared very similar to those of isoflurane, more recent studies have shown distinct differences between these agents. While high-dose desflurane, like isoflurane, can produce EEG burst suppression, this effect may be attenuated over time. It is not known whether this adaptation represents a pharmacokinetic or pharmacodynamic effect. Initial clinical reports suggest that desflurane may cause a clinically significant rise in ICP in patients with supratentorial lesions, despite its proven ability to reduce $CMRO_2$ as documented by EEG burst suppression. These increases in ICP, which are presumably related to cerebral vasodilation, appear to be independent of changes in systemic haemodynamics. In humans, sevoflurane produces some increase in TCD flow velocities at high doses (>1.5 MAC), but these appear to be less marked than desflurane, and were reported to be unassociated with increases in ICP in patients with supratentorial space-occupying lesions. In other studies, 1.5 MAC sevoflurane caused no increase in middle cerebral artery flow velocities and did not affect carbon dioxide reactivity or pressure autoregulation. This may be partially explained by

sevoflurane's weak direct vasodilator effect, especially in humans.

Effect on cerebrospinal fluid production

Most anaesthetic agents either increase the secretion or reduce the reabsorption of CSF. Halothane, up to a 0.5 MAC, reduces CSF production in haemodynamically stable animals, mediated by vasopressin-related mechanisms. Enflurane increases the production of CSF and provides increased resistance to the reuptake of CSF, partially explaining increases in ICP following its use. Isoflurane, on the other hand, reduces CSF production and enhances reabsorption.

Non-halogenated inhaled anaesthetic agents

Nitrous oxide

In equi-MAC doses, nitrous oxide (N_2O) is probably a more powerful vasodilator than either halothane or isoflurane. N_2O has been shown to produce cerebral stimulation with increases in $CMRO_2$, glucose utilization and a coupled increase in CBF. Furthermore, the vasodilation produced by N_2O is not decreased by hypocapnia, although the resulting increases in ICP can be attenuated by the administration of other CMR depressants such as the barbiturates. The increase in ICP reduces CPP and hence can compromise cerebral oxygen delivery, while the neural excitation increases oxygen demand, a combination that is particularly unfavourable in patients with raised ICP.

Xenon

Xenon has been used as an anaesthetic agent since 1950. However, its use was abandoned due to cost. Neverthless, since 1990, there has been renewed interest in its use. Xenon may offer a number of advantages for neuroanaesthesia, including rapid induction and emergence due to its low blood gas coefficient, possible neuroprotective effects (demonstrated in animal studies with focal ischaemia), probably via N-methyl-D-aspartate (NMDA) and α-amino-3-hydroxy-5-methyl-4-isoxazolole propionate (AMPA) antagonism. In healthy volunteers, xenon anaesthesia induces a uniform reduction in rCMRglu and a reduction in rCBF, but with an increase in rCBF/rCMRglu ratio, particularly in the insula, anterior and posterior cingulate, and in the somatosensory cortex.

Intravenous anaesthetics

Thiopentone, etomidate and propofol all reduce global CMR to a minimum of approximately 50% of baseline, with a coupled reduction in CBF. Reductions in CBV have been demonstrated with barbiturates, and probably occur with propofol and etomidate as well. Maximal reductions in CMR are reflected in an isoelectric EEG, although burst suppression is associated with only slightly less CMR depression. Initial doubts that CBF reductions produced by propofol were secondary to falls in MAP have proved to be unfounded. Even high doses of thiopentone or propofol do not appear to affect autoregulation, carbon dioxide responsiveness or flow–metabolism coupling.

Opiates

Although high doses (3 mg kg^{-1}) of morphine and moderate doses of fentanyl (15 μg kg^{-1}) have little effect on CBF and CMR, high doses of fentanyl (50–100 μg kg^{-1}) and sufentanil depress CMR and CBF. Results with alfentanil, in doses of 0.32 mg kg^{-1}, show no reduction in rCBF. These effects are variable and may be prominent only in the presence of N_2O, where CMR may be reduced by 40% from baseline. Bolus administration of large doses of fentanyl or alfentanil may be associated with increases in ICP in patients with intracranial hypertension, probably due to reflex increases in CBF that follow an initial decrease in CBF (due to reductions in MAP and cardiac output produced by large bolus doses of these agents). These effects are unlikely to be clinically significant if detrimental haemodynamic and blood gas changes can be avoided. Opioids do not appear to affect autoregulation.

Other drugs

Ketamine can increase global CBF and ICP, with specific increases in rCMR and rCBF in limbic structures, which may be partially attenuated by hypocapnia, benzodiazepenes or halothane. The ICP and CBF increases produced by ketamine are also attenuated by other general anaesthetic agents. Sedative doses of benzodiazepines tend to produce small decreases in CMR and CBF; however, there is a ceiling effect, and increasing doses do not produce greater reductions in these variables. α$_2$-Agonists such as dexmedetomidine reduce CBF in humans. There are good data, in animal models at least, that CBF reductions produced by intraventricular dexmedetomidine are probably due to direct vascular effects and are not exclusively the consequence of either systemic hypotension or coupled falls in rCBF arising from reductions in neuronal metabolism.

Most non-depolarizing neuromuscular blockers have little effect on CBF or CMR, although large doses of D-tubocurarine may increase CBV and ICP secondary to histamine release and vasodilation. In contrast, succinylcholine can produce increases in ICP, probably secondary to increases in CBF mediated via muscle spindle activation. However, these effects are transient and mild, and can be blocked by prior precurarization if necessary; they provide no basis for avoiding succinylcholine in patients with raised ICP when its rapid onset of action is desirable for clinical reasons.

Cerebral blood flow in disease

Ischaemia

Graded reductions in CBF are associated with specific electrophysiological and metabolic consequences, all of which are triggered at specific levels of CBF (Table 2.1). Some of these thresholds for metabolic events are well recognized, but others, such as the development of acidosis, cessation of protein synthesis and the failure of osmotic regulation, have only recently received attention. Ischaemia is thus a continuum between normal cellular function and cell death; cell death, however, is not merely a function of the severity of ischaemia but is also dependent on its duration and several other circumstances that modify its effects. Thus, the effects of ischaemia may be ameliorated by the CMR depression

Table 2.1 Electrophysiological and metabolic consequences of graded reductions in cerebral blood flow (CBF).

CBF (ml $(100\,g)^{-1}\,min^{-1}$)	Electrophysiological/metabolic consequence
>50	Normal neuronal function
?	Immediate-early gene activation
?	Cessation of protein synthesis
?	Cellular acidosis
20–23	Reduction in electrical activity
12–18	Cessation of electrical activity
8–10	ATP rundown, loss of ionic homeostasis
<8	Cell death (also depends on other modifiers: duration, cerebral metabolic rate, etc.)

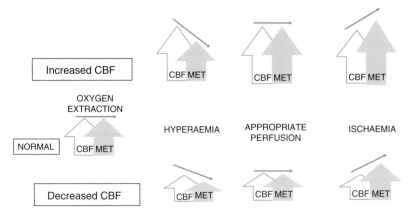

Fig. 2.10. Relationship of cerebral blood flow (CBF) to the presence of ischaemia under conditions of varying metabolism. Changes in CBF levels compared with physiological levels may be misleading, as a diagnosis of ischaemia or hyperaemia demands that CBF levels be assessed in the context of metabolic requirements. MET, cerebral oxygen metabolism.

produced by hypothermia or drugs, and exacerbated by increased metabolic demand associated with excitatory neurotransmitter release or compounded by other mechanisms of secondary injury (such as cellular calcium overload or reperfusion injury).

It is important to recognize that reductions in CBF do not always equate to ischaemia – a diagnosis of ischaemia depends on showing that CBF is inadequate to meet oxygen demands, and any given level of CBF needs to be interpreted in the light of metabolic requirements. For example, reductions in CBF associated with coupled reductions in $CMRO_2$ (e.g. following intravenous barbiturates) represent appropriate hypoperfusion. Indeed, in this setting, if CBF is increased (e.g. by hypercapnia), even if absolute levels of CBF are lower than normal, this represents hyperaemia. Conversely, increases in CBF that do not meet increased metabolic demand (e.g. with seizures in the context of intracranial hypertension) can be interpreted as hyperperfusion but in reality represent ischaemia. (Fig. 2.10)

Head injury

Severe head injury is accompanied by both direct and indirect effects on CBF and metabolism, which show both temporal and spatial variations. Cerebral blood flow may be high, normal or low soon after ictus but is typically reduced. Thirty per cent of patients undergoing CBF studies within 6–8 h of a head injury have significant cerebral ischaemia. Global hypoperfusion in these studies was associated with 100% mortality at 48 h, and regional ischaemia with significant deficits. Cerebral blood flow patterns also vary in relation to the time after injury. Initial reductions are replaced, especially in patients who achieve good outcomes, by a period of relative increase in CBF, which towards the end of the first week post-ictus may be replaced (in some patients) by reductions in CBF that are the consequence of vasospasm associated with traumatic subarachnoid haemorrhage (Fig. 2.11). Changes in CBF are non-uniform in the injured brain (see Chapter 10). Blood flow tends to be reduced in the immediate

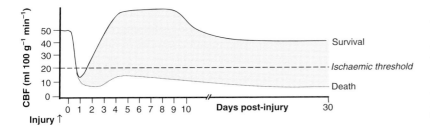

Fig. 2.11. Spectrum of cerebral blood flow (CBF) patterns following severe head injury. Following an initial period of ischaemia lasting <24 h, CBF begins to rise and may exceed normal values on days 2–4; CBF may fall to subnormal levels at later time points, chiefly due to the presence of vasospasm secondary to traumatic subarachnoid haemorrhage. The CBF levels may never rise in some patients, especially those who have a poor outcome.

vicinity of intracranial contusions, and cerebral ischaemia associated with hyperventilation may be extremely regional and not reflected in global monitors of cerebrovascular adequacy.

Elevations in ICP result in reductions in CPP and cerebral ischaemia, which lead to secondary neuronal injury. There is strong evidence than maintenance of a CPP above 60 mmHg improves outcome in patients with head injury and raised ICP. Traditionally, patients with intracranial hypertension have been nursed head up in an effort to reduce ICP. It is important to realize, however, that such manoeuvres will also reduce the effective MAP at the level of the head and run the risk of reducing CPP. It has been suggested that a 30° head-up elevation may provide the optimal balance by reducing ICP without decreasing CPP.

Hypertensive encephalopathy

Current concepts of the causation of hypertensive encephalopathy are based on the forced vasodilation hypothesis. Severe acute or sustained elevations in MAP overcome autoregulatory vasoconstriction in the resistance vessels and result in forced vasodilation. These vasodilated vessels, exposed to high intraluminal pressures, leak fluid and protein and result in cerebral oedema, which is multifocal and later diffuse.

Subarachnoid haemorrhage

Cerebral autoregulation and carbon dioxide responsiveness are grossly distorted after subarachnoid haemorrhage (SAH), more so in patients in worse clinical grades (Fig. 2.12). Such patients may be unable to compensate for reductions in MAP produced by anaesthetic agents and develop clinically significant deficits.

Clinically significant vasospasm after SAH occurs in up to 30–40% of patients, typically several days after the initial bleed, and may be due to one or more of several mechanisms. Nitric oxide may be taken up by haemoglobin in the extravasated blood or be

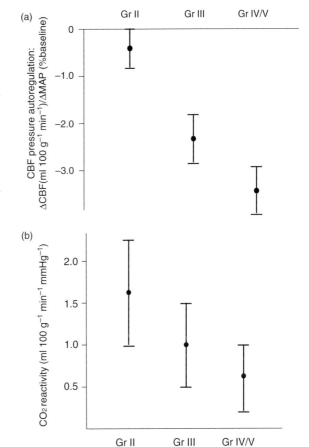

Fig. 2.12. Effect of Hunt and Hess grades of aneurysmal subarachnoid haemorrhage on (a) CBF reactivity to changes in $PaCO_2$ and (b) pressure autoregulation.

inactivated to peroxynitrite ($ONOO^-$) by superoxide radicals ($O^-\cdot$) produced during ischaemia and reperfusion. Alternatively, spasm may be secondary to lipid peroxidation of the vessel wall by various oxidant species including superoxide and peroxynitrite. Other authors have proposed a role for endothelin. Vasospasm tends to be worst in patients with the largest amounts of subarachnoid blood, suggesting that the blood in itself contributes to the phenomenon. Vasospasm is associated with parallel reductions in rCBF and $CMRO_2$ in the regions affected.

The clinical impact of late vasospasm has been substantially modified by the routine use of calcium-channel blockers such as nimodipine, and by the routine use of hypertensive–hypervolaemic–haemodilution (triple H) therapy. Triple H therapy involves the use of colloid administration (with venesection if needed) to increase filling pressures and reduce the haematocrit to 30–35%. If moderate hypertension is not achieved with volume loading, vasopressors and inotropes are used to maintain systolic blood pressures as high as 120–140 mmHg. The hypertensive element of this therapy protects non-autoregulating portions of the cerebral vasculature from hypoperfusion, while the haemodilution improves rheological characteristics of blood and facilitates flow through vessels whose calibre is reduced by spasm. Such interventions have been shown to produce clinically useful improvements in rCBF in regions of ischaemia in the setting of SAH but not in stroke.

Mechanisms of regional cerebral blood flow control

Some of the mechanisms involved in cerebrovascular control are shown in Fig. 2.13. Several of these have been referred to earlier. In addition, the level of free Ca^{2+} is important in determining vascular tone, and arachidonate metabolism can produce prostanoids that are either vasodilators (e.g. PGI_2) or vasoconstrictive (e.g. TXA_2). Endothelin (ET), produced by endothelin-converting enzyme in endothelial cells, balances the vasodilator effects of nitric oxide in a tonic matter by exerting its influences at ET_A receptors in the vascular smooth muscle.

Nitric oxide in the regulation of cerebral haemodynamics

Recent interest has focused on the role of NO in the control of cerebral haemodynamics. Nitric oxide is synthesized in the brain from the amino acid L-arginine by the enzyme NO synthase. This form of the enzyme is calmodulin dependent and requires Ca^{2+} and tetrahydrobiopterin for its activity, and differs from the inducible form of the enzyme that is present in mononuclear blood cells and is activated by cytokines. Under basal conditions, endothelial cells synthesize NO, which diffuses into the muscular layer and, via a cGMP-mediated mechanism, produces relaxation of vessels. There is strong evidence to suggest that NO exerts a tonic dilatory influence on cerebral vessels. It is important to emphasize that data on NO obtained from peripheral vessels cannot always be translated

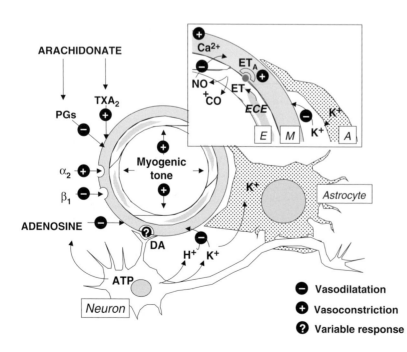

Fig. 2.13. Mechanisms involved in the regulation of rCBF in health and disease. The diagram shows a resistance vessel in the brain in the vicinity of a neuron and an astrocyte (A). E, endothelium; M, muscular layer; PGs, prostaglandins; TXA_2, thromboxane A_2; ET, endothelin; ECE, endothelin-converting enzyme; ET_A, ET_A receptor; NO, nitric oxide; CO, carbon monoxide; DA, dopamine. The inset box shows the detail of the vessel wall and adjacent glial cell process. See text for details.

to the cerebral vasculature; for example, some of the endothelium-derived relaxant factor activity in cerebral vessels may be due to compounds other than NO. There is growing evidence that carbon monoxide (CO) produced by haeme oxygenase may be responsible for significant cerebral vasodilation, especially when NO production is reduced. Nitric oxide plays an important role in cerebrovascular responses to functional activation, excitatory amino acids, hypercapnia, ischaemia and subarachnoid haemorrhage. Furthermore, it may also mediate the vasodilation produced by volatile anaesthetic agents, although other mechanisms, including a direct effect on the vessel wall, cannot be excluded.

Opioidergic mechanisms

A noxious stimulus (e.g. pain) increases CBF by sympathetic stimulation, which increases MAP and heart rate. However, the increase in CBF is more than that expected by a mere increase in MAP; the proposed mechanisms in animal models are opening of K^+_{ATP} channels, the L-arginine–NO pathway and cyclo-oxygenase products or endogenous opiates. Further research is needed to elucidate the exact mechanisms in humans. Endogenous opioid peptides present in cerebral perivascular nerves and in the CSF change in response to stimuli and activate regulatory mechanisms of the cerebral circulation. The μ and δ opiate receptors are implicated in the hypoxia- and hypercapnia-induced cerebral vasodilation.

Neurogenic flow–metabolism coupling

While the last 10 years have focused on flow–metabolism coupling being effected by a diffusible extracellular mediator, there is now accumulating evidence to suggest that dopaminergic neurons may play a major part in such events and, additionally, may control BBB permeability.

Further reading

Aaslid, R., Lindegaard, K. F., Sorteberg, W. and Nornes, H. (1989). Cerebral autoregulation dynamics in humans. *Stroke* **20**, 45–52.

Attwell, D., Buchan, A. M., Charpak, S. *et al.* (2010). Glial and neuronal control of brain blood flow. *Nature* **468**, 232–43.

Bentsen, N., Larsen, B. and Lassen, N. A. (1975). Chronically impaired autoregulation of cerebral blood flow in long-term diabetics. *Stroke* **6**, 497–502.

Benyó, Z. and Wahl, M. (1996). Opiate receptor-mediated mechanisms in the regulation of cerebral blood flow. *Cerebrovasc Brain Metab Rev* **8**, 326–57.

Bouma, G. J., Muizelaar, J. P., Stringer, W. A. *et al.* (1992). Ultra-early evaluation of regional cerebral blood flow in severely head-injured patients using xenon-enhanced computerized tomography. *J Neurosurg* **77**, 360–8.

Bundgaard, H., von Oettingen, G., Larsen, K. M. *et al.* (1998). Effects of sevoflurane on intracranial pressure, cerebral blood flow and cerebral metabolism. A dose-response study in patients subjected to craniotomy for cerebral tumours. *Acta Anaesthesiol Scand* **42**, 621–7.

Chakkarapani, E., Dingley, J., Liu, X. *et al.* (2010). Xenon enhances hypothermic neuroprotection in asphyxiated newborn pigs. *Ann Neurol* **68**, 330–41.

Chesnut, R. M. (1997). Hyperventilation in traumatic brain injury: friend or foe? *Crit Care Med* **25**, 1275–8.

Coles, J., Minhas, P., Fryer, T. *et al.* (2002). Effect of hyperventilation on cerebral blood flow in traumatic head injury: clinical relevance and monitoring correlates. *Crit Care Med* **30**, 1950–9.

Davis, D. H. and Sundt, T. M. (1980). Relationship of cerebral blood flow to cardiac output, mean arterial pressure, blood volume, and alpha and beta blockade in cats. *J Neurosurg* **52**, 745–54.

Diringer, M. N. (2009). Management of aneurysmal subarachnoid hemorrhage. *Crit Care Med* **37**, 432–40.

Dóczi, T. P. (1995). Comparison of static and dynamic cerebral autoregulation measurements. *Stroke* **26**, 2372–3.

Foster, G. E., Poulin, M. J. and Hanly, P. J. (2007). Intermittent hypoxia and vascular function: implications for obstructive sleep apnoea. *Exp Physiol* **92**, 51–65.

Fox, P. T., Raichle, M. E., Mintun, M. A. and Dence, C. (1988). Nonoxidative glucose consumption during focal physiologic neural activity. *Science* **241**, 462–4.

Göbel, U., Theilen, H. and Kuschinsky, W. (1990). Congruence of total and perfused capillary network in rat brains. *Circ Res* **66**, 271–81.

Grubb, R. L., Raichle, M. E., Eichling, J. O. and Ter-Pogossian, M. M. (1974). The effects of changes in $PaCO_2$ on cerebral blood volume, blood flow, and vascular mean transit time. *Stroke* **5**, 630–9.

Gupta, A. K., Menon, D. K., Czosnyka, M., Smielewski, P. and Jones, J. G. (1997). Thresholds for hypoxic cerebral vasodilation in volunteers. *Anesth Analg* **85**, 817–20.

Hamner, M. A., Möller, T. and Ransom, B. R. (2010). Anaerobic function of CNS white matter declines with age. *J Cereb Blood Flow Metab* (Epub ahead of print; doi:10.1038/jcbfm.2010.216).

Iadecola, C. (1998). Neurogenic control of the cerebral microcirculation: is dopamine minding the store? *Nat Neurosci* **1**, 263–5.

Koehler, R. C., Roman, R. J. and Harder, D. R. (2009). Astrocytes and the regulation of cerebral blood flow. *Trends Neurosci* **32**, 160–9.

Kolbitsch, C., Lorenz, I. H., Hörmann, C. *et al.* (2000). A subanesthetic concentration of sevoflurane increases regional cerebral blood flow and regional cerebral blood volume and decreases regional mean transit time and regional cerebrovascular resistance in volunteers. *Anesth Analg* **91**, 156–62.

Krabbe-Hartkamp, M. J., van der Grond, J., de Leeuw, F. E. *et al.* (1998). Circle of Willis: morphologic variation on three-dimensional time-of-flight MR angiograms. *Radiology* **207**, 103–11.

Magni, G., Rosa, I. L., Melillo, G., Savio, A. and Rosa, G. (2009). A comparison between sevoflurane and desflurane anesthesia in patients undergoing craniotomy for supratentorial intracranial surgery. *Anesth Analg* **109**, 567–71.

Maktabi, M. A., Elbokl, F. F., Faraci, F. M. and Todd, M. M. (1993). Halothane decreases the rate of production of cerebrospinal fluid. Possible role of vasopressin V1 receptors. *Anesthesiology* **78**, 72–82.

March, K. (1994). Retrograde jugular catheter: monitoring SjO2. *J Neurosci Nurs* **26**, 48–51.

Matta, B. F. and Lam, A. M. (1995). Nitrous oxide increases cerebral blood flow velocity during pharmacologically induced EEG silence in humans. *J Neurosurg Anesthesiol* **7**, 89–93.

Matta, B. F., Mayberg, T. S. and Lam, A. M. (1995). Direct cerebrovasodilatory effects of halothane, isoflurane, and desflurane during propofol-induced isoelectric electroencephalogram in humans. *Anesthesiology* **83**, 980–5; discussion 27A.

Matta, B. F., Heath, K. J., Tipping, K. and Summors, A. C. (1999). Direct cerebral vasodilatory effects of sevoflurane and isoflurane. *Anesthesiology* **91**, 677–80.

Oldendorf, W. H. (1971). Brain uptake of radiolabeled amino acids, amines, and hexoses after arterial injection. *Am J Physiol* **221**, 1629–39.

Oldendorf, W. H. (1974). Lipid solubility and drug penetration of the blood brain barrier. *Proc Soc Exp Biol Med* **147**, 813–15.

Origitano, T. C., Wascher, T. M., Reichman, O. H. and Anderson, D. E. (1990). Sustained increased cerebral blood flow with prophylactic hypertensive hypervolemic hemodilution ("triple-H" therapy) after subarachnoid hemorrhage. *Neurosurgery* **27**, 729–39; discussion 739.

Paulson, O. B., Hasselbalch, S. G., Rostrup, E., Knudsen, G. M. and Pelligrino, D. (2010) Cerebral blood flow response to functional activation. *J Cereb Blood Flow Metab* **30**, 2–14.

Pawlik, G., Rackl, A. and Bing, R. J. (1981) Quantitative capillary topography and blood flow in the cerebral cortex of cats: an in vivo microscopic study. *Brain Res* **208**, 35–58.

Pellerin, L. and Magistretti, P. J. (1994). Glutamate uptake into astrocytes stimulates aerobic glycolysis: a mechanism coupling neuronal activity to glucose utilization. *Proc Natl Acad Sci U S A* **91**, 10,625–29.

Pellerin, L. and Magistretti, P. J. (2004). Neuroenergetics: calling upon astrocytes to satisfy hungry neurons. *Neuroscientist* **10**, 53–62.

Raslan, A. and Bhardwaj, A. (2007). Medical management of cerebral edema. *Neurosurg Focus* **22**, E12.

Rozet, I., Vavilala, M. S., Lindley, A. M. *et al.* (2006). Cerebral autoregulation and carbon dioxide reactivity in anterior and posterior cerebral circulation during sevoflurane anesthesia. *Anesth Analg* **102**, 560–4.

Sokoloff, L. (1960). The metabolism of the central nervous system in vivo. In Field, J., Magoun, H. and Hall, V., eds. *Handbook of Physiology*, Section I, *Neurophysiology*. Washington, DC: American Physiological Society, pp. 1843–64.

The Brain Trauma Foundation (2000). The American Association of Neurological Surgeons. The Joint Section on Neurotrauma and Critical Care. Guidelines for cerebral perfusion pressure. *J Neurotrauma* **17**, 507–11.

Thompson, B. G., Pluta, R. M., Girton, M. E. and Oldfield, E. H. (1996). Nitric oxide mediation of chemoregulation but not autoregulation of cerebral blood flow in primates. *J Neurosurg* **84**, 71–8.

Ueda, Y., Walker, S. A. and Povlishock, J. T. (2006). Perivascular nerve damage in the cerebral circulation following traumatic brain injury. *Acta Neuropathol* **112**, 85–94.

Vazquez, A. L., Masamoto, K., Fukuda, M. and Kim, S. G. (2010). Cerebral oxygen delivery and consumption during evoked neural activity. *Front Neuroenergetics* **2**, 11.

Zakhary, R., Gaine, S. P., Dinerman, J. L. *et al.* (1996). Heme oxygenase 2: endothelial and neuronal localization and role in endothelium-dependent relaxation. *Proc Natl Acad Sci U S A* **93**, 795–8.

Zornow, M. H., Fleischer, J. E., Scheller, M. S., Nakakimura, K. and Drummond, J. C. (1990). Dexmedetomidine, an α2-adrenergic agonist, decreases cerebral blood flow in the isoflurane-anesthetized dog. *Anesth Analg* **70**, 624–30.

Mechanisms of neuronal injury and cerebral protection

Kristin Engelhard and Christian Werner

Introduction

Ischaemic and traumatic brain injuries are among the most common and important causes of disability and death worldwide. The end point of all cerebral injuries, such as stroke, global cerebral ischaemia during cardiac arrest, cardiac, vascular or brain surgery or head trauma, is the inadequate supply of the brain with oxygen and/or glucose, which triggers a characteristic pathophysiological cascade leading to neuronal death. Multiple neuroprotective strategies have been developed blocking one or more steps along this cascade. This chapter provides an overview of the mechanisms leading to neuronal cell death and the most important neuroprotective strategies.

Mechanisms of neuronal injury

Aetiology of neuronal injury

Cerebral ischaemia and/or hypoxia may occur as a consequence of shock, respiratory failure, vascular stenosis or occlusion, vasospasm, neurotrauma or cardiac arrest. These ischaemic/hypoxic insults evoke a cascade of pathophysiological processes that will result in neuronal damage, because the function and integrity of the brain depends on a constant supply of oxygen and glucose.

Primary and secondary lesions

Neurological outcome after cerebral injury is determined by two factors, the primary and the secondary injury. Primary injury is caused directly by the impact of energy or the initial cerebral hypoxic/hypoglycaemic event (core of infarction), leading to immediate cell loss. The incidence and dimension of primary damage will be minimized only by preventative measures (e.g. treatment of hypertension, diabetes mellitus or hyperlipidaemia and the use of helmet or air bags). Secondary brain damage represents the consecutive pathological processes initiated at the moment of injury with delayed clinical presentation. Within the first days after injury, these pathophysiological processes lead to an expansion of the primary lesion into challenged but still viable tissue. The area at risk of secondary brain damage is called the 'penumbra' and can account for up to 50% of the volume that later progresses to damage. The penumbra is a region of hypoperfused tissue surrounding the core, where the blood flow ranges between the thresholds of cell viability and functional activity. Metabolic derangement and neurochemical events within the penumbra lead to cell death unless reperfusion restores the metabolism/flow mismatch in the threatened area. The factors contributing to secondary brain damage in the penumbra represent the targets of potential neuroprotective therapies (Table 3.1). Therefore, strategies to protect the brain after trauma are based on an understanding of the pathophysiological processes of secondary brain damage.

Pathophysiological cascade

Energy failure

After the constant oxygen and glucose supply to the brain is interrupted, the electron transport chain within the mitochondria, and thereby oxidative phosphorylation, is inhibited. Within 1–2 min this is followed by decreased levels of high-energy phosphates (phosphocreatine), within 4 min by depletion of glucose and glycogen stores, and after 5–7 min the cellular ATP concentration rapidly drops to near zero. This initiates several detrimental effects, such as the accumulation of lactic acid due to anaerobic glycolysis or failure of the energy-dependent transmembrane ion pumps.

Core Topics in Neuroanaesthesia and Neurointensive Care, eds. Basil F. Matta, David K. Menon and Martin Smith. Published by Cambridge University Press. © Cambridge University Press 2011.

Table 3.1 Consequences of cerebral oxygen and energy failure.

Consequence	Leading to
Tissue acidosis	Neuronal damage
Membrane depolarization and excitotoxicity	Na⁺ influx (cerebral oedema)
	Ca^{2+} influx
Mitochondrial dysfunction	Free oxygen-radical formation
	Release of cytochrome c and apoptosis-inducing factor
Peri-infarct depolarization	Increased ATP consumption
Free oxygen-radical formation	Damage of cellular components
Cerebral inflammation	Pro-inflammatory cytokines
	Prostaglandin
	Reduced microcirculation
	Blood–brain barrier lesion
Systemic immunodepression	Systemic infection
Final consequence: apoptotic and necrotic cell death	

Permanent structural damage occurs within 5–15 min of oxygen deprivation, while hypoglycaemia can be tolerated for up to 60 min.

Tissue acidosis

During the initial minutes of cerebral ischaemia, brain metabolism switches from aerobic to anaerobic respiration, which rapidly produces lactic acid and acidifies the brain pH to 6.5–6.7. Hyperglycaemia aggravates this effect, leading to a tissue pH of 6.0. Acidosis itself might possess neuroprotective effects due to N-methyl-D-aspartate (NMDA) receptor blockade. However, in the presence of lactate presynaptic glutamate, reuptake is inhibited and excitotoxic neuronal damage is increased.

Membrane depolarization and cerebral oedema

A major consequence of the ATP shortage is a dysfunction of energy-dependent membrane ion pumps, allowing influx of Na⁺ and Ca^{2+} into the cell, and efflux of K⁺. High intracellular Na⁺ and Ca^{2+} concentrations are followed by Cl⁻ and H_2O influx into the neuron, leading to cytotoxic oedema and consecutively to an elevated intracranial pressure (ICP). Additionally, vasogenic brain oedema, which is caused by mechanical or autodigestive disruption or functional breakdown of the endothelial cell layer (an essential structure of the blood–brain barrier) of brain vessels, increases the volume of the extracellular space. Disintegration of the cerebral vascular endothelial wall allows uncontrolled ion and protein transfer from the intravascular to the extracellular (interstitial) brain compartments, with consecutive water accumulation and a further increase in ICP.

Excitotoxicity and intracellular Ca^{2+} overload

The general energy depletion leads to a massive influx of Ca^{2+} into the cell and a failure of the energy-dependent presynaptic reuptake of excitatory amino acids. Both mechanisms increase the accumulation of excitotoxic neurotransmitter glutamate in the extracellular space and thereby maintain the excitotoxic cell damage. Hyperactivation of NMDA, α-amino-3-hydroxy-5-methyl-4-isoxazolpropionate (AMPA) and metabotropic glutamate receptors further increases intracellular Ca^{2+} and Na⁺ concentrations. The intracellular Ca^{2+} overload appears to be one of the common pathways leading to irreversible cell damage and death. High intracellular Ca^{2+} concentrations trigger proteases that degrade cytoskeletal proteins (e.g. actin and spectrin) and extracellular matrix proteins (e.g. laminin). Furthermore, phospholipases A_1, A_2 and A_C are activated, thus hydrolysing phospholipids within mitochondrial and cell membranes and generating free fatty acids (e.g. arachidonic acid). These can be metabolized to free radicals, prostaglandins and leukotrienes, which will change membrane permeability and ion distribution. These enzymes do not require oxygen or energy and therefore function during cerebral ischaemia.

Mitochondrial damage

The major purpose of oxidative phosphorylation in mitochondria is the continuous production of ATP by the oxidation of glucose. Ischaemic or traumatic challenges affect both inadequate delivery of oxygen and glucose, and impairment of mitochondrial function, leading to inadequate production of ATP. One of the key events that causes mitochondrial injury is an abnormal increase in intracellular Ca^{2+}, which triggers the activation of degradative enzymes (e.g. calpain proteases and phospholipases) or the generation of enzymes that form reactive free oxygen radicals. Furthermore, high cellular Ca^{2+} levels activate the mitochondrial permeability transition where a non-selective, large conductance pore within the inner membrane opens, resulting in uncoupling of oxidative phosphorylation, osmotic swelling, release of matrix metabolites and even physical rupture of the mitochondrial outer membrane. Mitochondrial dysfunction leads to a loss of the mitochondrial membrane potential, a release of cytochrome *c* and apoptosis-inducing factor into the cytosol, and enhanced generation of free oxygen radicals, together promoting cell death.

Peri-infarct depolarization

Energy failure causes electrochemical and excitatory membrane depolarization of neurons and glial cells. This generates a wave of depolarization that moves away from the core lesion with a frequency up to eight events per hour. As repolarization is an energy-dependent process, which further stresses the metabolically compromised cells in the penumbra, peri-infarct depolarization and repolarization may contribute to the growth of the lesion.

Free oxygen radicals

Free oxygen radicals are physiologically produced in small amounts in cellular processes such as oxidative phosphorylation in the mitochondrial electron transport system. Under normal conditions, the generated superoxide radicals dismutate spontaneously or are enzymatically promoted (superoxide dismutase (SOD)) to hydrogen peroxide, which forms hydroxyl radicals. Hydroxyl radicals react with almost any intracellular molecule. Superoxide radicals can also react with nitric oxide (NO) creating the highly reactive peroxynitrite radical. The normal defence system against free radical damage includes enzymatic systems that quench or scavenge free radicals (e.g. SOD, catalase, glutathione peroxidase, and vitamins E and C). During cerebral ischaemia and reperfusion, the concentration of superoxide and hydroxyl radicals increases tremendously and the normal defence systems are overwhelmed. As radicals can react with and damage virtually any cellular component, this excessive free oxygen radical overload further promotes the disintegration of the cell.

Inflammation

Brain injury induces a complex array of immunological/inflammatory tissue responses and it is still unknown how the different cellular and molecular components interact to contribute to inflammatory responses in the neuronal tissue. Both primary and secondary insults activate the release of cellular mediators including pro-inflammatory cytokines, prostaglandins, free radicals and complement within hours. These processes induce chemokines and adhesion molecules and in turn mobilize immune and glial cells in a parallel and synergistic fashion. For example, activated polymorphonuclear leucocytes adhere to defective but also intact endothelial cell layers, as mediated through adhesion molecules (Fig. 3.1). These cells infiltrate injured tissue along with macrophages and T lymphocytes. Tissue infiltration of leucocytes is facilitated via upregulation of cellular adhesion molecules such as P-selectin, intercellular (ICAM-1) or vascular (VCAM-1) adhesion molecules, and integrins (CD11b/CD18). In response to these inflammatory processes, injured tissue will be eliminated, and within hours, days or weeks, astrocytes produce microfilaments and neutropines to ultimately synthesize scar tissue. Pro-inflammatory cytokines such as tumour necrosis factor (TNF), interleukin (IL)-1β and IL-6 are upregulated within hours of injury. The progression of tissue damage relates to direct release of neurotoxic mediators or indirectly to the release of NO in toxic concentrations and cytokines. The additional release of vasoconstrictors (prostaglandins and leukotrienes), the obliteration of microvasculature through adhesion of leucocytes and platelets, the blood–brain barrier lesion and the oedema formation further reduce tissue perfusion and – *summa summarum* – aggravate secondary brain damage.

Apoptotic and necrotic cell death

Two different types of cell death may occur following brain injury: necrosis and apoptosis (programmed cell death; Fig. 3.2). *Necrosis* takes place in response to severe mechanical or ischaemic/hypoxic tissue damage with excessive release of excitatory amino acid neurotransmitters and metabolic failure. Consecutively,

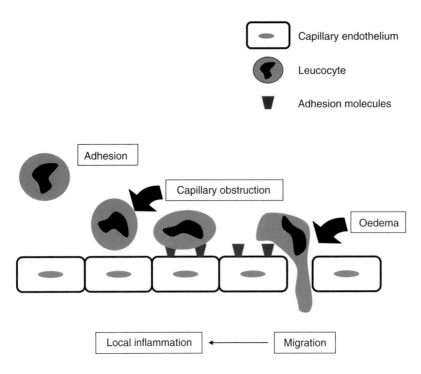

Fig. 3.1. After neuronal damage, cellular and endothelial adhesion molecules are expressed facilitating the adhesion and penetration of immunocompetent cells such as leucocytes. This leads to cellular oedema and local inflammation (upregulation of pro-inflammatory cytokines). (Adapted from a figure by Matthias David, University Medical Center of the Johannes Gutenberg University, Mainz, Germany, with the author's permission).

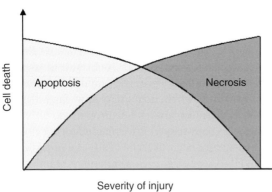

Fig. 3.2. Apoptotic cell death occurs after minor injury of the cell and is the active energy-consuming form of cell death involving a 'suicide programme'. The more severe an injury becomes, the less ATP is available and the more cells start to undergo necrotic cell death.

phospholipases, proteases and lipid peroxidases autolyse biological membranes. The resulting cell detritus is recognized as an 'antigen' and will be removed by inflammatory processes, leaving scar tissue behind.

In contrast, neurons undergoing *apoptosis*, an active form of cell death involving a 'suicide programme', are morphologically intact during the immediate post-traumatic period with adequate ATP production providing a physiological membrane potential. Apoptosis is triggered by release of cytochrome *c* from the

mitochondria into the cytoplasm (intrinsic pathway) or by activation of cell death receptors by their ligands (e.g. FasL or TNF-α; extrinsic pathway). Both pathways further mediate apoptotic cell death by the cleavage of different procaspases, which represent specific proteases of the IL-converting enzyme family. The most recently detected apoptosis-inducing factor is also released from the mitochondria and activates apoptosis by a caspase-independent pathway. Apoptosis becomes evident hours or days after the primary insult: translocation of phosphatidylserine initiates discrete but progressive membrane disintegration along with lysis of nuclear membranes, chromatin condensation and DNA fragmentation; likewise, very small particles derived from condensed intracellular material ('apoptotic bodies') are removed from the shrinking cell by exocytotic mechanisms. The nature of apoptosis generally requires energy supply and imbalance between naturally occurring pro- and anti-apoptotic proteins.

Experimental and clinical neuroprotection

Neuroprotection is defined as any strategy that antagonizes, interrupts or slows the sequence of injurious biochemical and molecular events that have the potency to cause irreversible cell death. In the past, more than

Table 3.2 Investigated neuroprotective strategies

General strategies

- Anti-excitotoxic interventions
- Anti-inflammatory interventions (cerebral)
- Protection against systemic infection
- Antioxidants
- Pre-/post-conditioning; remote conditioning
- Anti-apoptotic interventions
- Enhancing cerebral blood flow

Specific drug therapy

- Calcium-channel blocker
- Anaesthetic agents
- Glucocorticoids
- Nitric oxide
- Erythropoietin
- Magnesium
- Statins

160 clinical trials have been performed investigating more than 50 different neuroprotective approaches (e.g. calcium-channel blockers, free radical scavengers and glutamate antagonists) that were able to improve neurological outcome in experimental models (Table 3.2). However, due to multiple reasons, none of these clinical trials was able to translate the experimental neuroprotective strategy to clinical settings.

General strategies

Anti-excitotoxic interventions

Glutamate and aspartate are known as excitatory neurotransmitters that stimulate NMDA and AMPA receptors (Ca^{2+} and Na^+ influx, respectively). As the activation of these receptors initiates catabolic intracellular processes, blockade of NMDA and AMPA receptors may protect cerebral tissue. N-Methyl-D-aspartate receptors are generally comprised of NR1/NR2 subunits, which are hyperactivated during neuronal injury. The neonatal NR3 subunit reduces the excitability and the Ca^{2+} permeability of NMDA-associated ion channels, which makes exogenously added NR3 an interesting neuroprotective therapeutic.

Ketamine, MK-801 (dizocilpine), aptiganel, dextrorphan and Mg^{2+} represent *non-competitive* NMDA-receptor antagonists. In animal models of focal (but not global) cerebral ischaemia and head injury, ketamine as

well as MK-801 reduced neuronal injury and improved outcome. Likewise, infusion of the *competitive* NMDA-receptor antagonist CGS 19755 (selfotel) reduced infarct size following focal ischaemia. Clinical trials using MK-801 were terminated due to toxic side effects and the induction of mitochondrial vacuolization. The clinical development of the antitussive agent dextrorphan was also terminated because of side effects such as hallucination, agitation and sedation. In clinical phase III trials in patients with acute stroke using the *non-competitive* NMDA-receptor antagonist aptiganel (Cerestat, CNS-1102) or the *competitive* selfotel, side effects were minimized by choosing low drug concentrations (far below the protective dose range of preclinical studies). All trials showed no improvement in primary outcome and mortality was higher in the treatment groups. In contrast to the direct NMDA-receptor antagonists, the NMDA-receptor glycine site antagonist gavestinel had an acceptable safety profile; however, two phase III multicentre trials (GAIN Americas Trial and GAIN International Trial) in stroke patients were not able to show any neuroprotective effect. Another approach to minimize excitotoxic damage is blockade of the AMPA receptor. However, in a phase III trial, the AMPA antagonist YM872 (ARTIST+ trial) was abandoned after failing an interim futility analysis. Decreased excitotoxicity might also be achieved by activation of the inhibiting γ-aminobutyric acid (GABA) receptor. The GABA agonist clomethiazole, which has been promising in preclinical studies, unfortunately failed to improve neurological outcome when administered within 12 h after the onset of stroke. In summary, to date, no anti-excitotoxic drug has been effective in clinical multicentre trials.

Anti-inflammatory interventions

Poststroke inflammation is associated with progression of neuronal damage. Therefore, anti-inflammation represents a neuroprotective strategy, which includes inhibition of inflammatory mediators such as cytokines (e.g. IL-1, IL-6, nuclear factor-κB) and adhesion molecules (e.g. ICAM, VCAM, integrins). Despite many successful experimental studies, only a few clinical studies have been performed. The endogenous, highly selective IL-1 receptor antagonist (IL-1ra) suppressed markers of inflammation in 17 patients after stroke and improved clinical outcome at 3 months compared with 17 placebo-treated patients. The ICAM-1 antibody enlimomab reduced leucocyte adhesion and infarct size in many experimental stroke studies, but there was deteriorated neurological outcome in stroke patients after 90 days, causing significantly more infections and fever (Enlimomab Acute Stroke Trial). Hypoxia increases the in vitro expression of the neutrophil integrin CD11. In rats, administration of anti-CD11 monoclonal antibodies reduced infarct volume and apoptosis, which was associated with a decreased accumulation of neutrophils. Unfortunately, in a clinical trial in stroke patients, inhibition of neutrophils using an anti-integrin therapy with CD11/CD18 antibodies showed no protection and the study was prematurely terminated. To date, no multicentre trial has been able to prove the validity of anti-inflammatory therapeutic strategies in patients with neuronal injury. Possibly, cerebral inflammation after brain damage also has some beneficial effects. Inflammation seems to be important for clearing of damaged tissue, stimulating the process of angiogenesis, tissue remodelling and regeneration. Thus, it is possible that certain kinds of inflammatory reactions are neuroprotective and neuroregenerative. Therefore, an accurate balance between inflammation and anti-inflammation is necessary to assure the removal of cell debris and to avoid secondary cell damage. New therapeutic targets could be designed to obtain a correct modulation of the immune system and to reduce cerebral damage after brain injury.

In contrast to the inflammatory reaction of the brain, the systemic immune system is depressed after neuronal damage and thereby increases the susceptibility to infection. This central nervous system injury-induced immunodepression was first detected in mice, which showed that experimental stroke propagates bacterial aspiration from harmless intranasal colonization to harmful pneumonia due to systemic immunosuppression. Although the exact mechanism is unclear, it became evident that activation of the hypothalamic–pituitary axis and of the sympathetic nervous system triggers downregulation of the systemic immune response after brain damage. To prevent pneumonia as a consequence of stroke-induced immunodepression, three clinical trials tested the protective effect of antibiotic therapy with the fluocinolone levofloxacin (ESPIAS trial), the fluocinolone moxifloxacin (PANTHERIS trial) and the tetracycline minocycline. While the ESPIAS trial revealed that prophylactic administration of levofloxacin does not prevent infection in patients with acute stroke, the PANTHERIS trial suggested that preventative administration of moxifloxacin is superior in reducing infections after severe non-lacunar ischaemic stroke compared with

placebo. The conflicting results of both studies may be explained by patient selection and differences in antibiotics and dosages. Larger trials are needed to answer the question of whether survival of patients after neuronal trauma can be positively affected by preventative anti-infective therapy. The minocycline treatment in acute stroke improved outcome (Ranking Scale and Barthel Index), which was attributed to the prevention of infection but also blockade of other steps of secondary brain damage, such as reduction of microglial activation, an anti-NMDA effect and inhibition of apoptotic cell death. After a successful dose-finding study, the neuroprotective effect of minocycline after stroke is currently under investigation in two phase II studies, which should be completed in 2011.

Antioxidants

High concentrations of free radicals cause cellular degeneration and disruption of the brain–blood barrier. Antioxidants have been neuroprotective in several in vitro models of oxidative cell damage and in vivo models of cerebral ischaemia. However, none has been successfully translated into clinical practice. One of the most recent failures was disodium 4-[(tert-butylimino)methyl]benzene-1,3-disulfonate N-oxide (NXY-059), a nitrone-based free radical trapping agent, which initially appeared to be a promising compound, yet was later dismissed for not reaching predefined clinical goals. Consistently, in patients with intracerebral haemorrhage, NXY-059 also showed no neuroprotective potential. Similar failures of initially claimed promising compounds occurred with ebselen and edaravone, in spite of the fact that the latter compound has been approved for clinical use in Japan.

Superoxide dismutase is a physiological free radical scavenger that occurs in almost all organisms. Studies in cell cultures and transgenic mice overexpressing SOD have shown that SOD produces a maximum reduction in cellular oxidative stress. Unfortunately, SOD has an extremely low penetration through the blood–brain barrier and cellular membranes. Consequently, SOD has been conjugated with polyethylene glycol (PEG) to enhance the bioavailability. In patients with severe head injury (phase II trials), PEG–SOD reduced mortality when given in high concentrations. However, a consecutive phase III trial in 463 head-injured patients failed to confirm the neuroprotective effects of PEG–SOD.

Tirilazad mesylat (U-74006F), a non-glucocorticoid 21-aminosteroid, is a potent inhibitor of oxygen free radical-induced lipid peroxidation. Most laboratory investigations have shown that tirilazad reduces infarct size and improves neurological outcome in models of transient or permanent focal or global cerebral ischaemia, cardiopulmonary arrest, spinal cord injury and traumatic brain injury (TBI), even when infused after the insult. In contrast, phase III clinical trials in patients with acute stroke, subarachnoid haemorrhage (SAH) and head injury failed to confirm the experimental neuroprotective evidence.

Pre-/post-conditioning

An unconventional way to protect the brain seems to enhance its tolerance to ischaemic or anoxic insults by pre-conditioning. By a brief sublethal episode of ischaemia, cells become resistant to subsequent lethal events, which was first proven for the myocardium and later for the brain. Shortly after pre-conditioning (early pre-conditioning after minutes) or after a delay (delayed pre-conditioning after hours or days), the brain develops tolerance towards the same or even different subsequent injury. The pre-conditioning cascade includes stimuli that, via sensors and transducers, activate downstream transcription factors, ultimately modulating gene expression. Novel proteins may then act as effectors, enhancing the resistance of neurons to ischaemia, and/or pre-existing proteins may be modulated by post-translational modification acting as effectors. Tolerance induced by pre-conditioning changes the expression of genes involved in the suppression of metabolic pathways, immune responses, ion-channel activity and blood coagulation. These protection concepts include the antagonization of mechanisms of damage, increase in substrate delivery, decrease in energy use and improvement of recovery. Besides the classical pre-conditioning using short sublethal ischaemia drugs such as anaesthetic agents, molecules such as glutamate, inflammatory cytokines and caspases, or ATP-sensitive potassium (K_{ATP})-channel openers, can also pre-condition brain tissue and increase its tolerance towards injury.

If the concept of pre-conditioning is clinically valid, patients with transient ischaemic attacks should have an attenuated severity of subsequent stroke and an improved outcome compared with patients without a preceding event. Most prospective and retrospective clinical studies have been able to show this improvement. However, two more recent studies by Johnston in 2004 and Della Morte and colleagues in 2008 were not able to find a correlation between previous transient ischaemic attack and low stroke severity, thereby challenging the neuroprotective effects of pre-conditioning. The clinical benefit of pharmacological pre-conditioning might include patients undergoing cardiovascular or brain surgery or experiencing SAH (delayed ischaemic deficits due to vasospasm) who are at risk of developing brain injury in the near future. Of particular clinical and pharmacological interest are the mitochondrial K_{ATP}-channel openers, erythropoietin and volatile anaesthetics. The effect of pre-conditioning using erythropoietin after SAH has been under investigation. Although this study was terminated in February 2009 because of concerns about increased mortality in stroke patients, the results have not yet been published (http://clinicaltrials.gov/ct2/show/NCT00626574). Furthermore, in China a clinical trial on the pre-conditioning effects of sevoflurane in patients with intracranial aneurysm surgery was initiated (http://clinicaltrials.gov/ct2/show/NCT01204268). Slow intermittent reperfusion performed immediately after opening of the occluded vessel can reduce cerebral infarction after experimental stroke, which is described as post-conditioning. This concept of post-conditioning can be induced by a broad range of stimuli or triggers, and may even be performed as late as 6 h after focal ischaemia and 2 days after transient global ischaemia. Several clinical studies are currently being performed to investigate the protective effect of remote conditioning, which describes the fact that a 5 min ischaemia of a remote limb might protect the brain.

Specific drugs with multiple approaches

Calcium-channel blockers

The proposed mechanisms of neuronal protection by calcium-channel blockers include cerebral vasodilation, prevention of vasospasm, reduced Ca^{2+} influx and modulation of free fatty acid metabolism. Unfortunately, the results in animal models are rather contradictory. When calcium-channel blockers were infused within 15 min after the onset of cerebral ischaemia, neuronal injury and neurological outcome were positively influenced, while after that time window calcium-channel blockers have been ineffective.

Clinical trials have tested the neuroprotective effects of the L-type calcium-channel blocker nimodipine, especially the prevention of vasospasm, in patients with acute ischaemic stroke and aneurysmatic or traumatic SAH. According to a meta-analysis of nine placebo-controlled trials with a total of 3700 patients with acute stroke, oral administration of nimodipine appears to be associated with a favourable outcome as long as the treatment commences within the first 12 h following the onset of the symptoms. However, calcium-channel blockers may induce arterial hypotension below the individual ischaemic threshold of the patients, and any relevant decrease in arterial blood pressure will reverse the neuroprotective effects of the intended treatment. Consistently, recent analyses by the Cochrane Foundation identified no beneficial effect of nimodipine in patients with ischaemic stroke or traumatic haemorrhage. However, in patients with aneurysmal SAH, oral nimodipine reduces the risk of poor outcome and secondary ischaemia, while there is no evidence for intravenous nimodipine or other calcium-channel blockers.

Anaesthetic agents

The proposed mechanisms of anaesthetic protection include reduction of cerebral metabolism and ICP, and suppression of seizures and sympathetic discharge. Additionally, anaesthetics may be neuroprotective by inhibiting synaptic glutamate release, activating inhibitory GABA and glycine receptors, and minimizing intracellular Ca^{2+} concentration and free radical accumulation. While the protective effect of anaesthetic agents after neuronal injury in animals is quite evident, a multicentre trial in patients undergoing carotid endarterectomy with general or local anaesthesia revealed no difference in the occurrence of stroke at 30 days after surgery. Despite some limitations of this impressive trial such as statistical underpower, lack of standardization of the local anaesthetic used and varying levels of sedation in the local anaesthetic group, the data confirm the view that one single pharmacological approach may have little effect on the multiple pathological events in patients with parallel variability of coexisting disease.

Inhalational anaesthetics

Isoflurane, sevoflurane and desflurane produce cerebral metabolic suppression at end-tidal concentrations >0.5 minimum alveolar concentration (MAC), suggesting that volatile anaesthetics may correct for the imbalance between reduced oxygen supply and demand during focal cerebral ischaemia. Animal studies with focal or incomplete hemispheric ischaemia have shown that isoflurane, sevoflurane and desflurane may decrease infarct size and improve neurological outcome when given prior to the ischaemic challenge. These experimental data are consistent with studies in

sevoflurane-anaesthetized patients undergoing carotid endarterectomy showing increased tolerance to lower levels of cerebral blood flow with preserved neuronal function during carotid cross-clamping when compared with halothane or enflurane. In contrast, volatile anaesthetics have no neuroprotective properties in the setting of global cerebral ischaemia and when given after the insult. It is questionable whether the antinecrotic effects of volatile anaesthetics seen in different ischaemia models are permanent. As indicated above, neurons may die from apoptosis if the tissue is exposed to a lesser degree of hypoxia or ischaemia. Studies in rats subjected to focal cerebral or forebrain ischaemia have shown that necrotic cell death was substantially reduced at 2 or 5 days from ischaemia in isoflurane-anaesthetized rats compared with awake controls or fentanyl–NO-anaesthetized animals. However, cortical and subcortical damage was not different between isoflurane and awake state or fentanyl–NO anaesthesia at 14 days, 3 weeks or 3 months after ischaemia. This suggests that volatile anaesthetics economize ischaemic energy consumption with consecutive reduction in immediate necrotic cell death. However, the metabolic shift to less energy deprivation is insufficient to entirely restore neuronal integrity, and initiation of apoptosis (an energy-requiring process) will reverse the initial neuroprotection.

The noble gas xenon, which is currently undergoing trials as an anaesthetic agent in patients, reduces the extent of cerebral infarction in rodents subjected to focal ischaemia possibly by NMDA-receptor blockade. However, clinical trials investigating the neuroprotective potency of xenon are still lacking.

Barbiturates and propofol

Barbiturates as well as propofol reduce infarct size and improve neurological outcome following focal or incomplete global cerebral ischaemia as long as physiological variables are controlled during the experiments. Similar to volatile anaesthetics, this neuroprotective effect seems to be sustained in models of mild neuronal damage, while the neuroprotective effect after severe neuronal injury is not preserved after 1 week. While experimental data support the preventative neuroprotective effects of hypnotic agents, the clinical evidence is less convincing. In patients undergoing cardiac surgery with normothermic cardiopulmonary bypass, the infusion of thiopental (total dose during extracorporeal circulation: 39.5 ± 8.4 mg kg^{-1} IV) was able to minimize post-operative neuropsychological deficits. In contrast, barbiturates infused to comatose patients within the first hour following cardiopulmonary resuscitation were ineffective in reducing mortality as well as neurological deficits in survivors compared with standard ICU treatment. These data are consistent with the view that the infusion of hypnotics *prior* to focal but not global ischaemic insults may increase the ischaemic tolerance of neurons. Barbiturates may be also beneficial in patients with severe head injury and refractory intracranial hypertension. This conclusion is related to a series of clinical studies where infusion of barbiturates was effective in reducing ICP and probably the mortality rate following brain trauma as long as systemic haemodynamic stability was maintained. More recently, propofol was suggested as an alternative to barbiturates for sedation of patients with head injury due to a favourable context-sensitive half-time. Similar to barbiturates, propofol turned out to be effective in treating elevated ICP following head injury, and compared with an opioid-based sedative regimen, propofol was more effective in controlling ICP, although with a similar neurological outcome.

Glucocorticoids

Glucocorticoids ameliorate oedema associated with brain tumours and improve outcome in patients with bacterial meningitis. Besides these proven clinical indications, further neuroprotective effects of glucocorticoids have been investigated. After neuronal injury, the proposed neuroprotective mechanisms of glucocorticoids include an increased order of lipid bilayers, a decrease in intracellular Ca^{2+} concentration, free radical scavenging and prevention of free fatty acid accumulation by inhibition of lipid peroxidation. However, in patients with acute stroke, after traumatic head injury or following cardiac arrest, glucocorticoids (e.g. dexamethasone or methylprednisolone) did not reduce neuronal damage and even resulted in a deteriorated outcome. In contrast, following spinal cord injury, infusion of methylprednisolone ($30\,mg\,kg^{-1}$ bolus, $5.4\,mg\,kg^{-1}$ over $24\,h$ within $3\,h$ of injury; or $30\,mg\,kg^{-1}$ bolus, $5.4\,mg\,kg^{-1}$ over $48\,h$ within 3–$8\,h$ from injury) may slightly reduce motor deficit and improve function of sensory tracts.

Nitric oxide

Nitric oxide is a messenger molecule with impact on a variety of motor deficit intra-, extra- and intercellular processes. Nitric oxide occurs during the conversion of L-arginine to citrulline by the enzyme NO synthase (NOS). Three isoforms of NOS have been identified.

Constitutive NOS isoforms I (neuronal NOS, nNOS) and III (endothelial NOS, eNOS) are present in neurons, astrocytes, perivascular nerve fibres and endothelial cells. The inducible isoform NOS II (inducible NOS (iNOS)) is present in leucocytes and macrophages. Nitric oxide is a diffusible, highly reactive molecule with a half-life in the order of a few seconds. During hypoxic ischaemic conditions, NO exerts positive as well as negative effects on neuronal functions and structure. Endothelial NOS dilates cerebral vessels and is crucial for improving cerebral blood flow. The inducible NOS in leucocytes and macrophages may contribute to the formation of peroxynitrite and hydroxyl anions after neuronal damage, releasing NO at concentrations that are cytotoxic by inhibition of mitochondrial enzymes and DNA trauma. Experiments in nNOS knockout mice revealed a relevant reduction in infarct size following focal cerebral ischaemia compared with wild-type mice. In contrast, infarct size was increased in eNOS knockout animals. Lubeluzole, the S-isomer of a novel 3,4-difluorobenzothiazole, downregulates the glutamate-activated NOS pathway, thereby mediating neuroprotection in models of focal and global cerebral ischaemia models. However, a Cochrane Database meta-analysis reviewing five trials with 3510 stroke patients revealed no effect on functional outcome or mortality in the lubeluzole-treated patients.

Erythropoietin

In the brain, the glycoprotein erythropoietin is produced in the hippocampus, internal capsule, cortex, endothelial cells and astrocytes, and its receptors are expressed by neurons, microglia, astrocytes and cerebral endothelial cells. Hypoxia and ischaemia have been recognized as important driving forces of erythropoietin expression in the brain, suggesting that erythropoietin is part of a self-regulating physiological protection mechanism to prevent neuronal injury. Systemic application of the growth factor erythropoietin stimulates neurogenesis and neuronal differentiation, and activates brain neurotrophic, anti-apoptotic, anti-oxidant and anti-inflammatory signalling. Furthermore, erythropoietin seems to possess pre- and post-conditioning effects. These multiple protective approaches were confirmed in animal models of focal and global cerebral infarction and of TBI. In a small study in 13 patients with cerebral ischaemia, erythropoietin proved to be well tolerated and was associated with an improvement in clinical outcome after 1 month. Based on these promising results, the German Multicenter EPO Stroke Trial was started in 2003, aiming at the inclusion of over 500 patients. After the trial concluded in 2008, the authors realized that, during the study, the standard treatment of stroke changed and that over 60% of the patients additionally received recombinant tissue plasminogen activator (rtPA). Subgrouping the patients into rtPA and non-rtPA populations complicated the evaluation of the data. However, a preliminary analysis of the data showed that the results of the initial erythropoietin stroke trial can be reproduced. Another promising result derives from a single-centre study investigating 80 patients with aneurysmal SAH. In these patients, 90,000 IU of erythropoietin seemed to reduce delayed cerebral ischaemia following subarachnoidal haemorrhage by decreasing the severity of vasospasm and shortening of impaired autoregulation.

Magnesium

The potential neuroprotective mechanisms of magnesium include reduction of presynaptic glutamate release, blockade of NMDA receptors, improvement of mitochondrial calcium buffering, blockade of calcium entry via voltage-gated channels and relaxation of smooth muscles, which might be beneficial in patients with vasospasm after SAH.

After successful experimental studies in focal ischaemia models, a clinical study was performed in stroke patients (IMAGES), but magnesium infusion within 12 h after stroke failed to reduce the chances of death or disability. As a consequence, a shorter time window, 2 h after the onset of stroke symptoms, for magnesium infusion is currently being investigated (FAST-MAG trial, started in 2005). After a pilot study showing that intravenous magnesium might reduce the incidence of delayed cerebral ischaemia after SAH, a phase III trial failed to show any beneficial effect of magnesium infusion in aneurysmal SAH (IMASH trial). Continuous infusion of magnesium to patients within 8 h of TBI was not shown to be neuroprotective and might even have a negative effect in the treatment of significant head trauma. A promising innovative concept in the treatment of spinal cord injury might be the intrathecal application of magnesium sulfate, which improved neurological function in a model of spinal cord ischaemia.

Comment

In this chapter, the following potentially neuroprotective interventions were not discussed, because they are addressed in other chapters: (i) application of thrombolytic or antithrombotic agents to reverse vascular occlusion after stroke; (ii) management of physiological variables (e.g. cerebral perfusion pressure, cerebral oxygenation, plasma glucose concentration and therapeutic hypothermia) to improve neurological outcome; and (iii) treatment of intracranial hypertension (e.g. osmotherapy and hyperventilation).

Conclusion

Over the last few decades, the pathological mechanisms of neuronal damage have been characterized and many drugs have been tested successfully in reproducible and physiologically controlled animal models of cerebral ischaemia or brain trauma. However, translation from the bench to the bedside has failed and none of these drugs has proved its neuroprotective potency in clinical multicentre trials. Possibly, many agents were brought to clinical trial without a sufficient solid or relevant evidence-based preclinical foundation. In contrast to experimental studies, where the drug was administered shortly after or even before the ischaemic challenge, in most of the clinical trials, the drug was only applied as early as 6 h after the neuronal injury. Furthermore, in some cases, it is not possible to achieve the preclinical efficacious drug doses or plasma levels in humans due to unfavourable side effects or different pharmacokinetics. Another problem is the insufficiency of clinically available outcome measures. These and other pitfalls may be responsible for the lack of evidence for the effectiveness of potential neuroprotective drugs in clinical trials. To overcome these problems by improving the quality of the preclinical studies, guidelines for experimental studies have been established by the Stroke Therapy Academic and Industry Roundtable (STAIR). These criteria might help in future to choose the right drug for clinical investigations.

Further reading

Bosnjak, Z. J. and Sarantopoulos, C. D. (2009). Channels of preconditioning: potassium drain that protects the brain. *Anesthesiology* **110**, 961–3.

Bracken, M. B., Shepard, M. J., Holford, T. R. *et al.* (1997). Administration of methylprednisolone for 24 and 48 hours or tirilazat mesylate for 48 hours in the treatment of acute spinal-cord injury. Results from the third national acute spinal cord injury randomized controlled trial. *JAMA* **277**, 1597–1604.

Bullock, M. and Povlishock, J. (2007). Guidelines for the management of severe traumatic brain injury. *J Neurotrauma* **24** (Suppl. 1), S1–95.

Chamorro, A. and Hallenbeck, J. (2006). The harms and benefits of inflammatory and immune responses in vascular disease. *Stroke* **37**, 291–3.

Della Morte, D., Abete, P., Gallucci, F. *et al.* (2008). Transient ischemic attack before nonlacunar ischemic stroke in the elderly. *J Stroke Cerebrovasc Dis* **17**, 257–62.

Dirnagl, U., Klehmet, J., Braun, J. S. *et al.* (2007). Stroke-induced immunodepression: experimental evidence and clinical relevance. *Stroke* **38**, 770–3.

Dirnagl, U., Becker, K. and Meisel, A. (2009). Preconditioning and tolerance against cerebral ischaemia: from experimental strategies to clinical use. *Lancet Neurol* **8**, 398–412.

Emsley, H. C., Smith, C. J., Georgiou, R. F. *et al.* (2005). A randomised phase II study of interleukin-1 receptor antagonist in acute stroke patients. *J Neurol Neurosurg Psychiatry* **76**, 1366–72.

Enlimomab Acute Stroke Trial Investigators (2001). Use of anti-ICAM-1 therapy in ischemic stroke: results of the Enlimomab Acute Stroke Trial. *Neurology* **57**, 1428–34.

Fabricius, M., Fuhr, S., Bahtia, R. *et al.* (2006). Cortical spreading depression and peri-infarct depolarization in acutely injured human cerebral cortex. *Brain* **129**, 778–90.

Gidday, J. M. (2006). Cerebral preconditioning and ischaemic tolerance. *Nat Rev Neurosci* **7**, 437–48.

Ginsberg, M. (2008). Neuroprotection for ischemic stroke: past, present and future. *Neuropharmacology* **55**, 363–89.

Green, A. R. and Ashwood, T. (2005). Free radical trapping as a therapeutic approach to neuroprotection in stroke: experimental and clinical studies with NXY-059 and free radical scavengers. *Curr Drug Targets CNS Neurol Disord* **4**, 109–18.

Haley, E. C. Jr, Thompson, J. L., Levin, B. *et al.* (2005). Gavestinel does not improve outcome after acute intracerebral hemorrhage: an analysis from the GAIN International and GAIN Americas studies. *Stroke* **36**, 1006–10.

Harms, H., Prass, K., Meisel, C. *et al.* (2008). Preventive antibacterial therapy in acute ischemic stroke: a randomized controlled trial. *PLoS ONE* **3**, e2158.

Johnston, S. C. (2004). Ischemic preconditioning from transient ischemic attacks? Data from the Northern California TIA Study. *Stroke* **35**, 2680–2.

Kawaguchi, M., Furuya, H. and Patel, P. M. (2005). Neuroprotective effects of anesthetic agents. *J Anesth* **19**, 150–6.

Krams, M., Lees, K. R., Hacke, W. *et al.* (2003). Acute Stroke Therapy by Inhibition of Neutrophils (ASTIN): an adaptive dose–response study of UK-279276 in acute ischemic stroke. *Stroke* **34**, 2543–8.

Lampl, Y., Boaz, M., Gilad, R. *et al.* (2007). Minocycline treatment in acute stroke: an open-label, evaluator-blinded study. *Neurology* **69**, 1404–10.

Lewis, S. C., Warlow, C. P., Bodenham, A. R. *et al.* (2008). General anaesthesia versus local anaesthesia for carotid surgery (GALA): a multicentre, randomised controlled trial. *Lancet* **372**, 2132–42.

Low, C., Zheng, F., Lyuboslavsky, P. and Traynelis, S. (2000). Molecular determinants of coordinated proton and zinc inhibition of *N*-methyl-d-apartate NR1/NR2 receptors. *Proc Natl Acad Sci U S A* **97**, 11,062–7.

Lucas, S. M., Rothwell, N. J. and Gibson, R. M. (2006). The role of inflammation in CNS injury and disease. *Br J Pharmacol* **147**, S232–40.

Macleod, M. R., Fisher, M., O'Collins, V. *et al.* (2009). Reprint: Good laboratory practice: preventing introduction of bias at the bench. *J Cereb Blood Flow Metab* **29**, 221–3.

Mergenthaler, P., Dirnagl, U. and Meisel, A. (2004). Pathophysiology of stroke: lessons from animal models. *Metab Brain Disease* **19**, 151–67.

Mohr, J., Orgogozo, J., Harrison, M. *et al.* (1994). Meta-analysis of oral nimodipine trials in acute ischemic stroke. *Cerebrovascular Diseases* **4**, 197–203.

Muir, K. W., Lees, K. R., Ford, I. and Davis, S. (2004). Magnesium for acute stroke (Intravenous Magnesium Efficacy in Stroke trial): randomised controlled trial. *Lancet* **363**, 439–45.

Nakanishi, N., Tu, S., Shin, Y. *et al.* (2009). Neuroprotection by the NR3A subunit of the NMDA receptor. *J Neurosci* **29**, 5260–5.

Potts, M. B., Koh, S. E., Whetstone, W. D. *et al.* (2006). Traumatic injury to the immature brain: inflammation, oxidative injury, and iron-mediated damage as potential therapeutic targets. *NeuroRx* **3**, 143–53.

Prass, K., Braun, J. S., Dirnagl, U., Meisel, C. and Meisel, A. (2006). Stroke propagates bacterial aspiration to pneumonia in a model of cerebral ischemia. *Stroke* **37**, 2607–12.

Siesjo, B., Bengtsson, F., Grampp, W. and Theander, S. (1989). Calcium, excitotoxins, and neuronal death in the brain. *Ann N Y Acad Sci* **568**, 234–51.

Siren, A. L., Fasshauer, T., Bartels, C. and Ehrenreich, H. (2009). Therapeutic potential of erythropoietin and its structural or functional variants in the nervous system. *Neurotherapeutics* **6**, 108–27.

Slemmer, J. E., Zhu, C., Landshamer, S. *et al.* (2008). Causal role of apoptosis-inducing factor for neuronal cell death following traumatic brain injury. *Am J Pathol* **173**, 1795–805.

Starkov, A., Chinopoulos, C. and Fiskum, G. (2004). Mitochondrial calcium and oxidative stress as mediators of ischemic brain injury. *Cell Calcium* **36**, 257–64.

Verweij, B. H., Muizelaar, J. P., Vinas, F. *et al.* (2000). Impaired cerebral mitochondrial function after traumatic brain injury in humans. *J Neurosurg* **93**, 815–20.

Wegener, S., Gottschalk, B., Jovanovic, V. *et al.* (2004). Transient ischemic attacks before ischemic stroke: preconditioning the human brain? A multicenter magnetic resonance imaging study. *Stroke* **35**, 616–21.

Wong, G. K., Poon, W. S., Chan, M. T. *et al.* 2010). Intravenous magnesium sulphate for aneurysmal subarachnoid hemorrhage (IMASH): a randomized, double-blinded, placebo-controlled, multicenter phase III trial. *Stroke* **41**, 921–6.

Xiang, Z., Yuan, M., Hassen, G., Gampel, M. and Bergold, P. (2004). Lactate induced excitotoxicity in hippocampal slice cultures. *Exp Neurol* **186**, 70–7.

Zhang, Z., Artelt, M., Burnet, M., Trautmann, K. and Schluesener, H. J. (2006). Early infiltration of CD8+ macrophages/microglia to lesions of rat traumatic brain injury. *Neuroscience* **141**, 637–44.

Zhang, Z. G., Chopp, M., Tang, W. X., Jiang, N. and Zhang, R. L. (1995). Postischemic treatment (2–4 h) with anti-CD11b and anti-CD18 monoclonal antibodies are neuroprotective after transient (2 h) focal cerebral ischemia in the rat. *Brain Res* **698**, 79–85.

Zhao, H. (2009). Ischemic postconditioning as a novel avenue to protect against brain injury after stroke. *J Cereb Blood Flow Metab* **29**, 873–85.

Intracranial pressure

Christian Zweifel, Peter Hutchinson and Marek Czosnyka

Introduction

To cover the brain's metabolic demand, an adequate cerebral blood flow (CBF) is required. The brain is enclosed by the non-expandable skull and an increase in intracranial pressure (ICP) may reduce cerebral perfusion pressure (CPP), and impair CBF leading to cerebral ischaemia. Both CPP and ICP are established treatment targets in neurocritical care. Measurement of ICP has a high diagnostic and prognostic impact.

The Monro–Kelly doctrine

The brain weighs about 1400 g and occupies the majority of the intracranial compartment (83%). Cerebrospinal fluid (CSF) and cerebral blood volume (CBV) occupy approximately 11 and 6% of intracranial volume, respectively. We used to believe that the brain floats in the fluid, losing its relative weight according to Archimedes' law. In fact, there is not enough volume of CSF to make such a mechanism effective. However, because of the continuous fluid environment, all gradients of the ICP within the CNS are equilibrated according to Pascal's law. Therefore, under normal conditions, there is no risk of volume shifts or herniations. This role of CSF is important for understanding why, following head injury, there is a critical threshold for increased ICP in the range of above 20–25 mmHg. Following head injury, due to brain swelling, the normal pathways of CSF circulation are usually obstructed and pressure gradients may develop. Meanwhile, in communicating hydrocephalus, during pressure–volume studies, patients tolerate rises in ICP of up to 40–50 mmHg, usually without any symptoms or adverse effects.

In 1824, Kelly outlined the fundamental principle later applied to our understanding of the dynamics of ICP, known as the 'Monro–Kelly doctrine' (Dr Monro was Dr Kelly's teacher and at time of publication he was already deceased; the doctrine is a rare example in science of a pupil's gratitude extending beyond the grave). It states that the brain is enclosed in a non-expandable case of bone and the brain parenchyma is nearly incompressible. Furthermore, the CBV in the cranial cavity is therefore nearly constant, and a continuous outflow of venous blood from the cranial cavity is required to make room for continuous incoming arterial blood. In other words, the volume of the intracranial compartment must remain constant if ICP is to remain constant. It is worthwhile remembering that in the original Monro–Kelly doctrine, the volume of CSF was not taken into account.

The cerebrospinal pressure–volume curve is nonlinear (Fig. 4.1). Three parts of the ICP–volume curve are described. The curve is flat at lower intracranial volumes, where good compensatory reserve is found. The ICP remains low and stable despite changes in intracranial volume. This is due to the compensatory mechanisms of the reduction of volume of CBV and CSF. The venous blood and CSF pools are considered to have the highest compliance of all compartments and are the first to be affected by raising ICP. However, when these compensatory reserves are reduced or exhausted, the curve rapidly turns exponentially upwards. This part of the curve represents a phase of low compensatory reserve, where ICP increases considerably, even with relatively small increases in intracranial volume. At the end, at high levels of ICP, the curve flattens again, CPP is very low and ICP approximates to the mean arterial blood pressure (ABP). A further increase in ICP leads to a collapse of the cerebral arterial bed if Cushing's response is not able to keep CPP above the critical closing pressure of the cerebrovascular bed (20–30 mmHg).

Core Topics in Neuroanaesthesia and Neurointensive Care, eds. Basil F. Matta, David K. Menon and Martin Smith. Published by Cambridge University Press. © Cambridge University Press 2011.

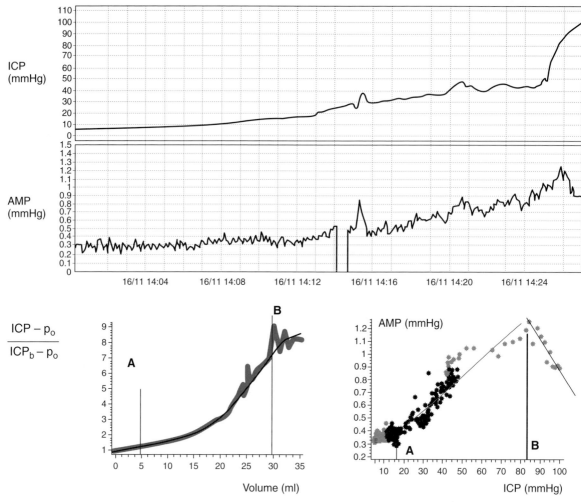

Fig. 4.1. Top panels: Experimental intracranial hypertension provoked by saline infusion into the lumbar subarachnoid space. In response to an increase in mean intracranial pressure (ICP), the pulse amplitude of ICP (AMP) starts to rise, until a level just above 80 mmHg is reached, above which a decrease in AMP is observed. Bottom left panel: The net volume of increasing CSF (i.e. infusion plus presumed production of CSF minus reabsorption integrated in time) is plotted against the relative increase in ICP (ICP$_b$, baseline pressure; p$_o$, reference pressure level), showing the full shape of the pressure–volume curve. Distinct regions are observed, delimited by the vertical lines A and B. Below A, pressure reacts weakly to changes of volume, indicating a good compensatory reserve. Between A and B, pressure increases exponentially with an increase in volume. Above B, the slope of the pressure–volume relationship decreases and finally saturates. This is a region of 'extra compensatory reserve', where the cerebral arterial bed collapses. Bottom right panel: The relationship between ICP and waveform amplitude provide a means of monitoring the physiology described above. Points A and B correspond to the lower and upper breakpoints of the relationship between AMP and mean ICP. Below A, the amplitude is constant; between A and B, it increases linearly with mean ICP, and above B, it decreases with a further increase in mean ICP.

Determinants of intracranial pressure

In most organs of the human body, the reference pressure for blood perfusion is either low or is coupled to atmospheric pressure. This does not apply to the intracranial space. The reference pressure (the outflow pressure) for brain perfusion is ICP, and in many pathological conditions it may be elevated. The ICP is derived from the circulation of cerebral blood and CSF. In the horizontal position, it may reach any value between right atrial pressure and ABP. In the vertical position, it usually decreases by 'hydrostatic distance' between the heart and the cranium. 'Normal ICP' in the horizontal position is from 5 to 15 mmHg. The limit of 'abnormal pressure' depends on pathology, and in head injury, 'elevated ICP' is said to exist at 20–25 mmHg.

Generally, the ICP has three components: (i) an arterial vascular component; (ii) a CSF circulatory component; and (iii) a venous outflow component.

The vascular component is difficult to express quantitatively. It is probably derived from the pulsation of the CBV (all waves, as heart rate-related changes in CBV and active vasogenic slow changes in CBV may play a role) and averaged by non-linear mechanisms of regulation of CBF. More generally, multiple variables such as the arterial pulsatile pressure, autoregulation and cerebral venous outflow all contribute to the vascular component.

The circulatory CSF component has been probably most widely investigated, and may be expressed using Davson's equation:

CSF circulatory component of ICP =
(resistance to CSF outflow) × (CSF formation)+
(pressure in sagittal sinus).

CSF is actively filtered from brain arterial blood, circulates along natural fluid passages and pools, and is absorbed into cerebral venous blood. Under normal conditions, without long-term fluctuations of the CBV, the production of CSF is balanced by its storage and reabsorption via the sagittal sinus:

Production of CSF = circulation of CSF
= storing of CSF
+ reabsorption of CSF

The storage of CSF is one of the fundamental mechanisms assuring favourable mechanical conditions for the CNS. Circulation of CSF, if disturbed by closing anatomical channels for CSF flow, for example due to brain oedema, may produce acute intracranial hypertension. Reabsorption of CSF fluid into the venous compartment takes place predominantly (in humans) through arachnoid granulations that penetrate the walls of the sagittal sinus. It is important to recognize that reverse transport through the arachnoid granulations is impossible, i.e. drainage ceases if the subarachoid ICP is less than sagittal sinus pressure (SSP). An alternative component of CSF drainage (in pathology) is a possible leakage into the brain parenchyma. This can be visualized on CT or MRI scans as periventricular lucency, i.e regions of hypodensity, particularly around the horns of the lateral ventricles. Monitoring of a radioactive tracer injected into the lumbar space often shows that the tracer accumulates in ventricles. This is indirect evidence of intraparenchymal CSF absorption, consistent with the clinical picture of normal pressure hydrocephalus, both idiopathic and post-injury. Periventricular CSF is probably subsequently absorbed into capillaries or passes into perivascular spaces and is transported inversely to the direction of CBF outside the cranial cavity and absorbed in lymphatic nodes. Although this mechanism helps to reduce the CSF component of ICP, it may interfere with regional CBF and probably metabolic rate in the white matter.

In addition to the net circulation at a rate equivalent to its production, CSF is also subject to pulsatile flow. Pulsatile CSF flow is observed in the aqueduct cerebri (with a stroke volume of around 40 μl) and in the cervical region of the subarachnoid space (with a stroke volume of around 500 μl). For half of the cardiac cycle, fluid flows down into the spinal subarachnoid space, and for the remaining part it flows upward. Net aqueductal CSF flow is small in comparison with a pulsatile 'void flow' (it is equivalent to around 5 μl in stroke volume, providing the heart rate is 60 strokes min^{-1}). This movement of CSF is caused by pulsatile arterial blood inflow and venous outflow. Mismatch between inflow and outflow of brain blood seen temporarily during one cardiac cycle is compensated by CSF movement. Pulsatile movement of CSF is undoubtedly associated with the pulse wave of CSF pressure, which is almost always present in recordings of ICP. The role of CSF flow and pressure pulsations is unclear but is being studied in hydrocephalus and other diseases that manifest with abnormal CSF dynamics.

The last component of ICP – venous outflow – is sometimes neglected. In fact, any factor increasing central venous pressure also increases ICP. In addition, obstruction of venous outflow from the intracranial cavity (cerebral venous sinus thrombosis, or sinus collapse due to extrinsic pressure, etc.) may increase ICP. Coupling between the ICP and pressure in bridging and cortical veins provides the basis for the definition of CPP. Another coupling mechanism between ICP and venous outflow may be associated with dynamically collapsing venous sinuses. This mechanism has been observed in idiopathic intracranial hypertension, but it may provoke intracranial hypertension in other diseases. A rise in ICP squeezes sinuses, producing a rise in sinus pressure, obstruction of cranial venous outflow, further rises in ICP, etc., in a positive-feedback loop fashion (Fig. 4.2).

Any factor that disturbs CBF or CSF circulation may provoke an increase in ICP. This may occur in the absence of CNS pathology (e.g. with jugular compression during a Queckenstedt test or an endotracheal tube tie, or with very high intrathoracic pressures) or with intracranial pathology (e.g. brain swelling, space-occupying lesions or obstruction of CSF circulation pathways).

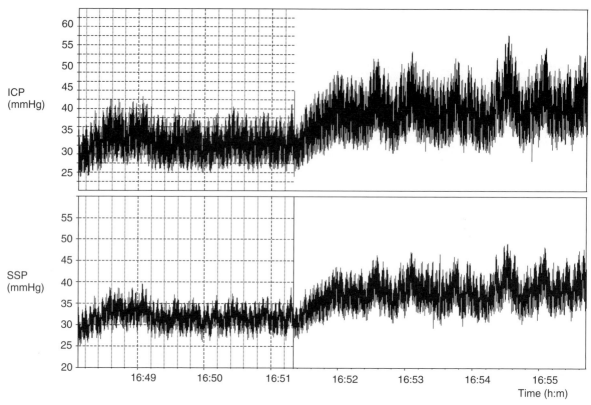

Fig. 4.2. An example of cerebrospinal fluid (CSF) pressure (intracranial pressure, ICP) and sagittal sinus pressure (SSP) recording in a patient with idiopathic intracranial hypertension. Both ICP and SSP were elevated (32 and 30 mmHg, respectively). An increase in ICP was caused by a constant rate (1 ml min⁻¹) of infusion of Hartmann's solution into the CSF space to evaluate resistance to CSF outflow. The observed rise in ICP was associated with an increase in SSP. During the infusion, slow waves in ICP and SSP were obviously associated.

Any increase in ICP may reduce CPP, reduce CBF and cause ischaemia. Ischaemia can cause a further rise in ICP due to increased cerebral oedema and further reduce CPP. This mechanism may develop into a vicious positive-feedback loop, causing irreversible brain damage. Therefore, ICP is both an important surrogate marker of injured brain and a potential cause for secondary insults.

Intracranial compliance

Intracranial compliance is a concept often associated with CSF storage. It is defined as the change of pressure (dP) of per unit as change of volume (dV) per unit. The inverse of the compliance is called elastance (dP/dV), also known as the volume–pressure response (VPR).

$$\text{Compliance} = (dV)/(dP) = 1/\text{elastance} = 1/\text{VPR}$$

Compliance decreases with increasing ICP, and the VPR or elastance increase with rising ICP. It has been demonstrated that the non-linear volume–pressure relationship could be modelled as a straight-line relationship to the logarithm of volume to pressure. This implies a monoexponential relationship between volume and pressure. This relationship has been described quantitatively by a pressure–volume index (PVI), which is the volume required to raise ICP tenfold. The PVI can be determined by rapid injection or withdrawal of fluid from the CSF space and measuring the pressure change.

In fact, cerebrospinal compliance is more complex than a single lumped parameter. Physiologically, it can be expressed as the sum of three compliances: CSF space (associated with CSF buffering capacity), arterial bed compliance and venous compliance (Fig. 4.3). Arterial compliance is controlled by active modification of a tension of arterial wall smooth muscles. This compliance is, in most circumstances, the lowest of the three components. The venous compartment has far greater compliance, and cerebral venous blood volume is an important component of cerebral buffering

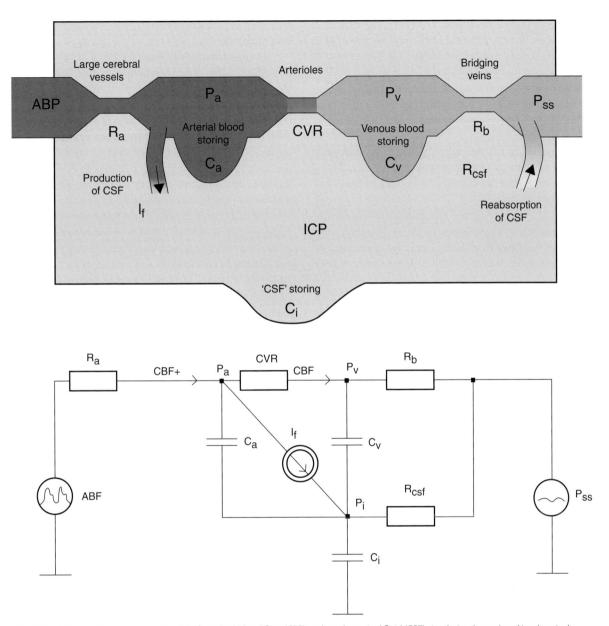

Fig. 4.3. A lumped hydrodynamic model of cerebral blood flow (CBF) and cerebrospinal fluid (CSF) circulation (upper) and its electrical equivalent (lower). Arterial blood flow is into the intracerebral space through a linear low resistance, R_a. The volume of arterial blood is stored in arterial compliance, C_a. The main cerebral resistive vessels (CVR) are where autoregulation acts. The blood then flows to the venous part of the cerebral circulation and is stored in a venous and capillary pool (C_v). R_b represents the squeezable venous structures (cortical and bridging veins). The CSF is formed from arterial blood, and flows around all structures and is absorbed (through resistance R_{csf}) back to the blood in the sagittal sinus (P_{ss}). The compliance of the CSF space (C_i) is associated with the ability of the lumbar dural sac to expand in the lumbar canal through compression of the venous plexi. From the aspect of addition of CSF (point P_i on the electrical diagram), all three compliances – arterial, venous and CSF – are connected in parallel; therefore, net intracerebral compliance can be approximated as $C_a + C_v + C_i$. P_a, cerebral arterial blood pressure in small arteries; P_v, venous blood pressure; ICP, intracranial pressure; ABP, arterial blood pressure; I_f, CSF inflow.

capacity, as cerebral venous pressure is low and approximates ICP. This buffering volume does not represent a high proportion of total cranial volume, just around 70 ml, but after exhaustion of all CSF buffering capacity (150–170 ml), venous blood volume is the next buffer. If, after head injury, we cannot see any CSF volume in the ventricles and basal cisterns on a CT scan due to brain swelling, it is not unequivocally associated with exhaustion of venous blood buffering capacity and high ICP. A further decrease in the venous blood volume reserve may result in reductions in blood flow, a phenomenon that commonly occurs at a range of CPP below the lower limit of autoregulation of CBF.

In fact, following traumatic brain injury (TBI), all three compensatory mechanisms – autoregulation of CBF, CSF compensation and venous blood compensation – may be exhausted very dynamically, almost in parallel, allowing a very short time for clinical intervention before the development of refractory intracranial hypertension.

Measurement of brain compliance is classically performed using a CSF bolus injection. However, one recent ICP monitoring device includes a distensible balloon that can be repeatedly inflated for measurement of intracranial compliance. New and less invasive techniques for compliance estimation include phase-coded MRI (which is the most accurate) and transcranial Doppler ultrasound (TCD) (probably less accurate but suitable for continuous monitoring).

Measurement techniques of intracranial pressure

In sedated patients with TBI, continuous ICP monitoring is recommended, and can only be achieved by direct invasive measurement. The indications for ICP monitoring are discussed below.

Different methods of monitoring ICP have been described. The gold standard for ICP monitoring is a catheter inserted into the lateral ventricle (usually via a small right frontal burr hole) and connected to an external pressure transducer. The reference point for the external pressure transducer is the foramen of Monro, which in practice is equated to the external auditory meatus. The advantages of ventricular catheters are the feasibility of repetitive calibration, withdrawal of CSF to treat elevated ICP and that it is a low-cost method. Disadvantages include difficulty with insertion in patients with brain swelling and small ventricles. Furthermore, the external pressure transducer needs to be moved to accommodate patient head movement so that an appropriate reference can be assured. Intraventricular catheters have infection rates between 2 and 27%, with significant attendant morbidity and mortality. Factors identified to increase the risk of external ventricular drain (EVD)-related infections are duration of catheterization, frequency of EVD manipulation (CSF sampling), insertion technique and intraventricular haemorrhage. In particular,

after intraventricular haemorrhage, the catheters may become blocked.

The most common location for ICP monitoring nowadays is the brain parenchyma using intraparenchymal probes. In these devices, a miniature strain gauge pressure sensor, a semiconductor strain gauge or fibre optic or pneumatic technology is used to transduce pressure. In the miniature strain gauge pressure sensor, ICP results in a change in resistance, and with the fibre optic, ICP results in a change in reflection of the light beam. The pneumatic system uses a catheter with an air pouch at the tip, and transmits the pressure over the catheter to the electronic hardware. The pneumatic system is able to calibrate itself repeatedly, but miniature pressure sensor and fibre-optic devices cannot be recalibrated in vivo, and a small drift of the zero reference may occur. However, this drift is generally considered negligible. The complication rate of intraparenchymal probes is very low, with infection rate or the risk of major bleeding being below 2%.

As a substitute for the intraparenchymal probes, subarachnoid, subdural and epidural probes can be used, but the accuracy of these devices is lower. In an acute setting, estimation of ICP through a lumbar drain is generally not recommended, as the accuracy is limited and brain swelling or a space-occupying lesion can cause brain herniation.

The concept of cerebral perfusion pressure

Cerebral perfusion pressure is defined as the difference between cerebral arterial pressure and pressure in the cerebral venous bed just before the outlet to the major venous sagittal sinuses, i.e. in cortical or bridging veins. Cerebral perfusion pressure is the pressure driving blood to flow through the cerebrovascular bed. As the pressure in bridging veins is difficult to measure and can be approximated by ICP, the clinical definition of CPP is:

CPP = mean arterial pressure (MAP) − mean ICP

Too low a CPP causes ischaemia, while too high a CPP causes hyperaemia. The ability of the cerebrovascular bed to autoregulate CBF depends on CPP, and there are defined upper and lower CPP limits within which such autoregulation can operate. Therefore, decreasing CPP is particularly dangerous after head injury: it both decreases the driving force for cerebral blood to flow and compromises autoregulation. Cerebral perfusion pressure-oriented therapy has been introduced to decrease the risk of ischaemia in post-injury care. The distribution of mean CPP for different outcome groups after head injury matches that of mean ICP. In patients who die, the mean CPP is significantly lower. Other outcome groups have similar CPP levels.

Intracranial pressure monitoring

The first continuous manometric monitoring of ICP was performed by Guillaume and Janny in 1951. Further studies, describing various waves of ICP, were conducted by Lundberg, who is regarded as the founder of contemporary continuous ICP monitoring.

The indications for ICP monitoring vary from centre to centre and include head injury, intracerebral haemorrhage, subarachnoid haemorrhage, hydrocephalus, ischaemic stroke, hypoxic brain injury with cerebral oedema, meningitis/encephalitis and hepatic encephalopathy. For traumatic head injury, established guidelines exist (e.g. Brain Trauma Foundation Guidelines). There is also support for the use of ICP monitoring in selected patients with intracranial haemorrhage and subarachnoid haemorrhage. While routine ICP monitoring in all patients with hemispheric stroke has no impact on management or outcome, it may be useful in selected patients with severe intracranial hypertension and/or midline shift. Similarly, it may have a role in selected patients with severe meningoencephalitis or fulminant hepatic failure. In all instances, the benefits of ICP monitoring in the detection and management of intracranial hypertension must, in each individual patient, be weighed against the clinical and economic costs of such monitoring: in addition to the cost of the devices used, the technique requires special medical and nursing expertise for device insertion and maintenance, and has associated risks of haemorrhage or infection.

In head injury, guidelines have been established and periodically updated (http://www.braintrauma.org). Patients with traumatic head injury who present with a low Glasgow Coma Score (GCS) of ≤8 and CT abnormalities such as haematomas, contusions, swelling, herniation or compressed basal cisterns should receive ICP monitoring. Also patients with a GCS of ≤8 and normal CT scan may be considered for ICP monitoring if they are >40 years and uni- or bilateral motor posturing or systolic ABP under 90 mmHg occur. These recommendations may be modified from centre to centre. Nevertheless, any diagnostic or therapeutic intervention has to be considered individually according to the patient's age, personal medical history and

assumed will. In monitored patients, thresholds for treatment are generally set at 20–25 mmHg.

Monitoring requirements and ICP treatment thresholds in other conditions with persistent high ICP, such as chronic hydrocephalus or idiopathic intracranial hypertension (also known as pseudotumour cerebri), need to be decided in context. The rise in ICP in these conditions signifies a disturbance of CSF circulation due to an increase in resistance of CSF outflow or increased cerebral venous pressure. In both diseases, overnight ICP monitoring and assessment of the cerebrovascular volume compensatory reserve through CSF infusion may add some additional diagnostic information, especially in patients who suffer under persisting or recurring symptoms after shunt insertion.

Normal ICP varies with age and body position. In the upright position, ICP is negative with an approximate mean of −4 mmHg but not exceeding −10 mmHg. Furthermore, in the absence of disease, ICP may rise during coughing, sneezing or a Valsalva manoeuvre up to 50 mmHg without noticeable neurological impairment. Therefore, it is the interaction of raised ICP with other intracranial pathology that leads to the pathological consequences, rather than elevated ICP per se.

There are a few distinctive patterns of ICP usually seen in recordings after TBI (Fig. 4.4). In head-injured patients, low and stable pressure is characterized by a low and stable mean ICP over time (around 15 mmHg) and a low pulse amplitude. This pattern can be observed during the first 6–8 h after head injury without or with minimal signs of brain swelling or a space-occupying lesion in cross-sectional imaging of the brain (Fig. 4.4a). When ICP is elevated over 20 mmHg, the pulse waveform may express vasogenic waves with a high amplitude due to reduced intracranial compliance. A further increase in ICP may lead to secondary cerebral insults that may cause cerebral oedema that again may increase ICP (Fig. 4.4b).

Various waves of ICP may be observed in clinical practice. Lundberg plateau waves (Fig. 4.4c) undoubtedly have a vasogenic origin, and the underlying model was elegantly described as a 'vasodilatory cascade' by Rosner. According to his theory, any vasodilatory stimulus produces an initially small increase in CBV. Under conditions of a weak pressure–volume compensatory reserve, this small change in CBV produces a substantial rise in ICP, leading to a decrease in CPP, further autoregulatory-induced rises in CBV, a further rise in ICP, and so on, until a point is reached where autoregulator vasodilation is maximal. At the plateau

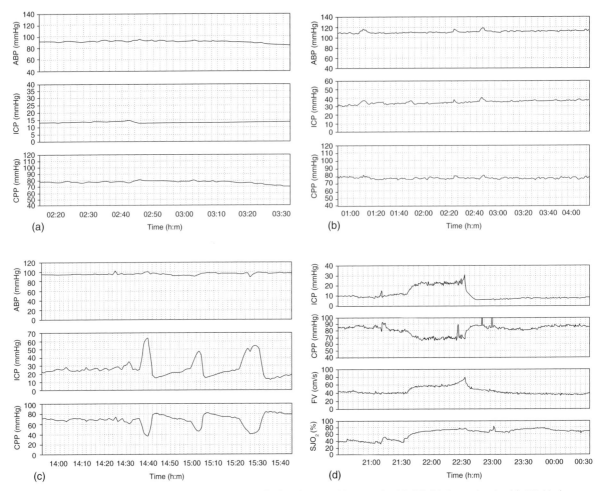

Fig. 4.4. Examples of intracranial pressure (ICP) recordings after head trauma: (a) Low and stable ICP; (b) elevated and stable ICP; (c) plateau waves of ICP; (d) elevation of ICP due to hyperaemia. ABP, arterial blood pressure; CPP, cerebral perfusion pressure; FV, blood flow velocity in the middle cerebral artery; SjO$_2$, jugular bulb saturation.

phase, both CPP and CBF are reduced (Fig. 4.4c). The plateau wave may be terminated spontaneously when a vasoconstrictory stimulus occurs and reverses the cascade to reduce ICP. Such spontaneous termination may be the consequence of a Cushing response, which elevates the MAP and reverses the vasodilation associated with autoregulation. Short-term hyperventilation or a bolus of hypertonic saline may be administered to terminate the plateau wave. Plateau waves are not associated with a worse outcome after head injury, unless they last excessively long – longer than 30 min. Therefore, active termination of long plateau waves is extremely important in the neurocritical care of TBI patients.

Another source of temporary ICP elevation may be hyperaemia. An increase in ICP is initiated as in a plateau wave by vasodilation (increase in CBV) and is maintained by a rapid increase in brain oedema. Vessels stay dilated as ICP increases and CPP decreases, but, contrary to plateau waves, CBF stays elevated (Fig. 4.4d). Finally, and most frequently, waves and irregular patterns seen in ICP monitoring are associated with transients in ABP.

It should be stressed that ICP is more than a number; it has its mean value and dynamic, variable components. Diagnostically relevant information is included in both factors. A instantaneous ICP value of 8 mmHg does not preclude the possibility that the ICP 2 min later may be 80 mmHg. Only inspection of properly monitored time trends, ideally supported by computer analysis, warning about poor compensatory reserve, autoregulation failure, etc., may help in the interpretation of ICP with confidence.

Non-invasive intracranial pressure estimation

The middle cerebral artery is a large vessel with elastic walls. It can be considered a membrane transducer able to detect changes in transmural pressure and, with knowledge of the MAP, allow computation of ICP. Unfortunately the elastic properties of the membrane are unknown and may be variable in time. Therefore, the value of the calibration coefficient and its linearity and stability in time are unknown. Nevertheless, it is known that CPP affects the shape of the blood flow velocity waveform, which can be non-invasively visualized using TCD. However, the arterial pulse waveform, heart rate, tension of arterial carbon dioxide, distal vascular resistance and age can all affect the blood flow velocity waveform and confound the estimation of ICP.

Some simple formulas have been proposed in the past to assess non-invasive CPP (nCPP) from ABP and blood flow velocity (FV) waveforms. Out of these, one particular method has reached possibly satisfactory accuracy (error <10 mmHg in >80% of measurements):

$$nCPP = (MAP \times FV_d/FV_m) + 14$$

where FV_d is diastolic blood flow velocity and FV_m is mean flow velocity.

The availability of non-invasive estimates of CPP are useful both to estimate absolute CPP and to monitor changes in CPP with time. The 95% confidence limit for estimation of CPP is 12 mmHg. Although this seems to be satisfactory for CPP, such a precision would be not good enough to estimate ICP.

Non-invasive measurement of ICP can be carried out using various methods: tympanic membrane displacement, time-of-flight ultrasound through the skull, change in skull diameter, change in blood FV in the straight sinus or analysis of the pulse waveform of TCD. The pulsatility index (PI) increases with rising ICP. Prediction of absolute ICP using PI is not accurate enough as many other factors may influence PI (arterial pulse, heart rate, arterial carbon dioxide tension ($PaCO_2$), vascular tone, proximal stenosis, spasm, etc.). Estimation of ICP can be carried out using the formula proposed by Aaslid (see Chapter 5):

$$MAP - A1/F1 \times FV_m$$

where F1 and A1 are first harmonic components of flow velocity and arterial pressure pulse waveforms, respectively, which gives a 95% confidence limit of around ±25 mmHg.

The moving-average model of transmission between ABP and ICP, modified by the relationship between ABP and FV, gives a mean absolute error of

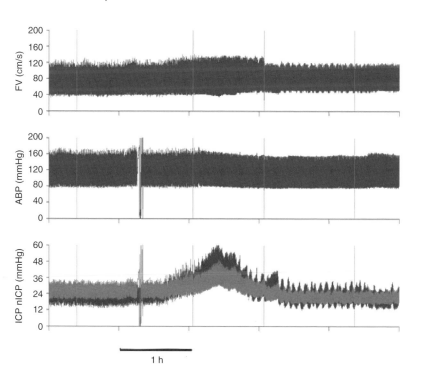

Fig. 4.5. Example of dynamic non-invasive monitoring of intracranial pressure (ICP), using arterial blood pressure (ABP) and blood flow velocity (FV) waveform. The pale grey tracing shows the non-invasive estimate, and the grey trace shows simultaneously measured ICP during transient intracranial hypertension.

around 6 mmHg (see Fig. 4.5). The method is based on analysis of a large data base of patients with homogeneous pathology undergoing full ICP, ABP and FV direct monitoring and is most probably pathology-dependent. Changes in $PaCO_2$, spasm and proximal stenosis are confounding factors.

Non-invasive ICP techniques allow a wide insight into intrahemispherical pressure gradients. As long as the CSF communicates freely between different fluid cavities within the brain, there should not be any substantial differences in regionally measured ICP. This fact has been employed to use ultrasonographic or MRI measurement of the optic nerve sheath diameter to estimate ICP. Measured 3 mm behind the globe, an optic nerve sheath diameter >6 mmHg makes intracranial hypertension highly likely, while a diameter of <5 mm makes it very unlikely.

Direct measurements of pressure in two CSF compartments are rarely performed. However, following head injury, intrahemispheric pressure gradients have been reported. There are intrahemispheric pressure gradients in non-invasive CPP associated with midline shift, side of contusion (assessed using CT) or side of craniectomy. Surprisingly, non-invasive estimates of nCPP and nICP indicate that CPP is greater on the side of the contusion or expanding brain in the case of midline shift or on the side of craniectomy. This may support the hypothesis that the interhemispheric differences in ICP are the consequence not of brain tissue volume expansion but of a vascular expansion. This hypothesis may be further supported by the fact that cerebral autoregulation is worse on the side of contusion or brain expansion. Asymmetry in nCPP and nICP correlates with worse outcome following head injury.

Intracranial pressure waveforms

Intracranial pressure waveforms include distinct periodic components: heart pulse waves, respiratory waves and quasi-periodic slow vasogenic waves (Lundberg B waves). Every waveform has its characteristic frequency (heart rate 50–180 bpm, respiratory waves 8–20 cycles min^{-1} and slow waves 0.3–3 cycles min^{-1}), and can be identified using spectral analysis. By definition, a frequency spectral analysis examines the spectral compositions and intensities of sinusoidal waveforms. The pulse and the respiratory waveform have a fundamental amplitude and several harmonic components. The amplitude of the fundamental component of the pulse waveform (AMP) is useful for the

evaluation of various indices describing cerebrospinal pressure dynamics. It correlates positively with mean ICP, a finding that can be explained by the decrease in compliance in the steep part of the volume–pressure curve, as seen in Fig. 4.1. With rising ICP, every stroke volume ejected by the heart transiently increases intracranial volume and leads to an increase in AMP. The exponential shape of the pressure–volume relationship is not the only factor influencing the magnitude of ICP pulse waves. The delay between arterial inflow and venous or CSF outflow profiles (pulsatile CSF flow through aqueduct cerebri) varies with mean ICP and hence also shapes the ICP pulse waveform. Further modulatory factors include the elastic properties of cerebral arteries, actively modulated by CPP and $PaCO_2$, and the increase in pulsatility of arterial blood inflow with rising ICP.

Morphological composition of the pulse wave and system analysis both try to describe similarities and discrepancies between the pulse waveform of arterial pressure and ICP. Some authors have proposed a classification of three distinctive 'peaks' seen during heart evolution in ICP: P1, transmitted 'passively' from systole of ABP, and P2–P3, associated with pressure–volume compensation of arterial blood inflow (Fig. 4.6). Whether such a classification has deeper physiological relevance or clinical application remains to be seen.

Respiratory waves are almost always present in ICP recordings. The pressure signal itself is complex, as both arterial and venous factors contribute to the respiratory waves seen in ICP.

All components that have a spectral representation within the frequency limits of 0.05–0.0055 Hz (20 s–3 min) can be classified as slow or Lundberg B waves and nowadays are not defined as precisely as in the original Lundberg thesis. Slow waves occur due to fluctuations of CBF that lead to changes in intracranial blood volume and hence ICP. The origin and reason for the presence of slow waves is still under debate. As slow fluctuations of pressure also occur in ABP, ICP slow waves can be interpreted as a response to ABP variations, depending on the state of cerebral autoregulation. Another theory suggests that slow waves are triggered by a 'central pacemaker' due to a cyclic demand of brain metabolites. These waveforms can also be seen in healthy subjects, but in this context they are much smaller amplitude (≤ 3 mmHg). Increases in the amplitude of these slow waves above 8 mmHg and more suggest reduced intracranial compliance and imply intracranial pathology. On the other

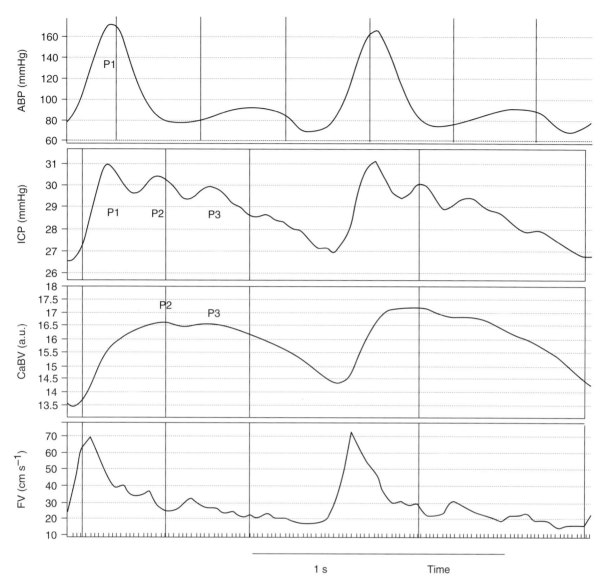

Fig. 4.6. Morphology of the pulse waveform of intracranial pressure (ICP), showing the distinctive peaks P1, P2 and P3. P1 is usually associated with systole of arterial blood pressure (ABP). Peaks P2 and P3 (delayed) are associated with blood volume transport. The arterial blood volume (CaBV) curve may be estimated by time integration of flow velocity (FV) detected with transcranial Doppler ultrasonography. Peaks P2 and P3 seem to be associated with arterial blood volume changes and the pressure–volume compensatory reserve. a.u., Arbitrary units.

hand, a complete absence of slow waves is also a bad predictor in head-injured patients.

Lundberg A waves, known as 'plateau waves', are pathological slow vasogenic waves that may lead to ICP rising above 40 and up to 80 mmHg. They dramatically reduce CPP in minutes and cause cerebral ischaemia. Plateau waves can be observed in about 25% of patients with head injury. They develop more often in younger patients and do not affect the outcome unless they last for a very long period.

Finally, Lundberg C waves occur at a rate of 4–8 min^{-1} and are of limited duration and amplitude; therefore, they are probably of little pathological significance.

Secondary indices derived from intracranial pressure

The method to calculate secondary indices from ICP waveform is based on the 'moving correlation coefficient' method. This method was developed in order to examine the degree of correlation between two factors within a time series where the number of paired observations is large. In a moving correlation window (3–10 min), time-averaged values from each factor (6–10 s) are plotted as an x–y scattergram. Calculation of the correlation coefficient, which ranges from maximal −1 (negative correlation) to maximal +1 (positive correlation), is renewed every 6–10 s or at longer intervals. The 'moving correlation coefficient' may be presented and analysed as a time-dependent variable, responding to dynamic events such as ICP increase, such as that seen in a plateau wave, or arterial hypo- and hypertension.

Pressure–volume compensatory reserve

A secondary ICP index that describes the pressure-volume curve is called RAP (correlation coefficient (R) between the amplitude of the fundamental component (A) of ICP and mean ICP (P)). This index indicates the degree of correlation between AMP and mean ICP over a defined time period (usually 3–5 min). A lack of synchronization between changes in the amplitude of the fundamental component and mean ICP indicates a RAP close to 0 and indicates a good pressure–volume compensatory reserve. In this phase, the intracranial compartment can cope with the increase in volume and produces no or very little change in ICP. The AMP varies directly with mean ICP, when the RAP increases to +1. This indicates that the focus of the pressure–volume curve shifts to the steep part. At this stage, any further increase in volume may produce a rapid increase in ICP. The RAP is usually close to +1 following head injury and subsequent brain swelling. When ICP increases further, AMP decreases and the RAP value falls below 0. This may occur when the cerebral autoregulatory capacity is exhausted and the pressure–volume relationship flattens again. In this situation, the capacity of cerebral arterioles to dilate in response to a CPP decrement is exhausted (they tend to collapse passively). Normally, a negative RAP and an ICP >20 mmHg indicates a terminal cerebrovascular disturbance with deterioration in pulse pressure transmission from the arterial bed to the intracranial compartment (Fig. 4.7). Following decompressive craniotomy, a decrease in RAP to 0 indicates recovery of the pressure–volume compensatory reserve.

Both RAP and PVI describe the pressure–volume curve, but generally there is no correlation between the two indices. Whereas PVI precisely describes the steepness of the pressure–volume curve over a defined segment, RAP indicates the focal point on the pressure–volume curve. The RAP also correlates with CBF, suggesting that severe cerebrovascular disturbance is associated with inadequate brain perfusion.

An alternative method to assess the cerebrospinal volume compensatory reserve can be done by a special system, such as the Spiegelberg brain compliance monitor. This has been developed to measure brain compliance by measuring the ICP response to a known small increase in volume by inflating and deflating the air pouch at the end of the catheter. It may act as an early warning system before decompensation, but correlation with outcome has not yet been demonstrated.

Cerebrovascular pressure reactivity

The cerebrovascular pressure reactivity index (PRx) is another ICP-derived index for assessing cerebrovascular reactions by observing the response of ICP to slow spontaneous fluctuations in ABP. In other words, cerebrovascular pressure reactivity reflects the ability of smooth muscle tone in the walls of cerebral arteries and arterioles to react to changes in transmural pressure. With increasing CPP, intact cerebrovascular pressure reactivity will lead to vasoconstriction and a reduction in CBV and hence ICP. Slow waves of ABP are almost always present and are of sufficient magnitude to provoke a vasomotor response. Taking advantage of this fact, cerebrovascular pressure reactivity can be determined continuously without manipulation of ABP by monitoring the response of ICP to these normal fluctuations in mean ABP. The PRx is determined by calculating the 'moving correlation coefficient' between time-averaged values of ICP and ABP. A positive PRx signifies a positive gradient of the regression line between the slow components of ABP and ICP, which is associated with passive behaviour of a pathological, non-reactive arterial vasculature. A negative value of PRx reflects normal reactive cerebral vessels, as ABP waves provoke inversely correlated waves of ICP.

The PRx value is an indicator of cerebral autoregulation, although these two terms should not be used synonymously as they describe slightly different concepts that operate over slightly different ranges of cerebrovascular physiology – vasodilation reaches its maximum at arterial pressures below the lower

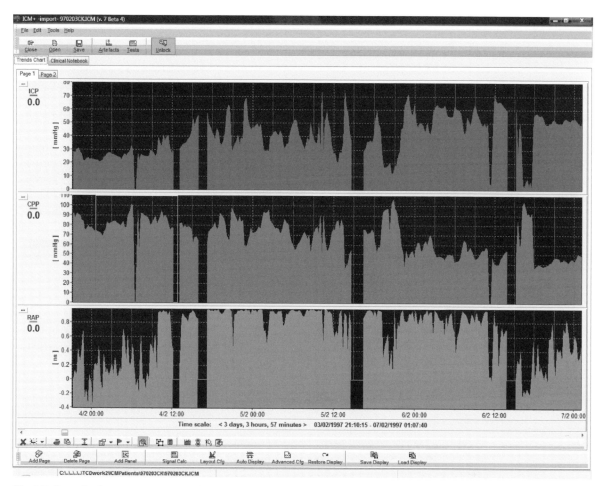

Fig. 4.7. Example of continuous recording of cerebral compensatory reserve using RAP index in a patient after traumatic brain injury: the entire period of recording covers approximately 4 days. During the initial period, even with elevation of intracranial pressure (ICP; mean 22 mmHg), RAP is low, indicating a good compensatory reserve. Later, ICP increases to 30–40 mmHg and is unstable, and RAP increases to +1, indicating a poor compensatory reserve. In the final period, ICP remains elevated, but cerebral perfusion pressure (CPP) decreases; RAP also decreases, indicating a final derangement of regulation of cerebrovascular tone. The patient died. See colour plate section.

threshold for constant CBF. However, PRx shows a good correlation with cerebral autoregulation indices assessed by TCD or positron emission tomography. It correlates also with ICP and CPP. During ICP plateau waves, PRx consistently increases from near-zero to positive values (Fig. 4.8). Similarly, during episodes of arterial hypo- or hypertension that exceed the physiological limits of autoregulation, PRx increases to positive values.

Intracranial pressure and outcome following head injury

Many studies have demonstrated the detrimental role of intracranial hypertension and dysautoregulation on outcome after head injury. An averaged ICP above 25 mmHg over the whole monitoring period increases the risk of death twofold in severe head injury. Furthermore, reductions in the amplitude of slow waves and averaged RAP and PRx are strong predictors of fatal outcome. Whereas ICP and RAP only differentiate patients with fatal outcome from those who survive at 6 months, PRx distinguishes among patients with good outcome, moderate disability, severe disability and death. The outcome impact of indices such RAP and PRx suggest that good vascular reactivity is an important element of brain homoeostasis, enabling the brain to protect itself against uncontrollable elevations in intracranial volume and hence ICP.

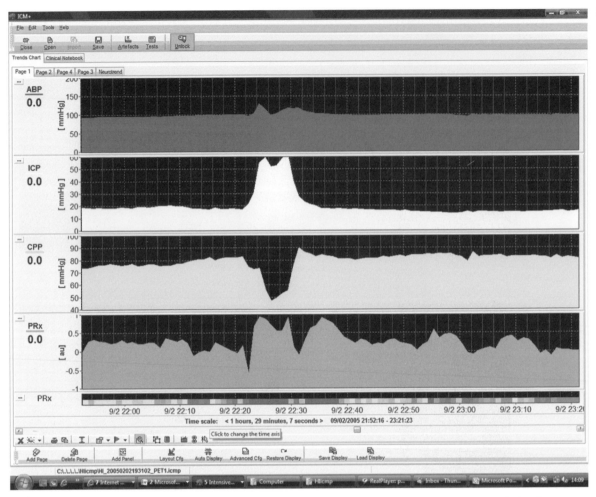

Fig. 4.8. Stable intracranial pressure (ICP) disturbed by a single plateau wave, which is associated with a decrease in cerebral perfusion pressure (CPP) and an increase in cerebrovascular pressure reactivity index (PRx), with the latter continuously monitored as a variable changing in time. On the bottom graph, green denotes good reactivity and red disturbed reactivity. Periods of disturbed reactivity extend for a period past the elevation of ICP, indicating that the ischaemic insult must have affected normal vascular tone for a longer period than the wave itself. ABP, arterial blood pressure. See colour plate section.

It is important to emphasize that mean ICP correlates strongly with both AMP and RAP. In a multivariate analysis of outcome, increased ICP and positive PRx are independent variables associated with a worse outcome. As mean CPP is an actively controlled variable in CPP-oriented protocols, it has lost its predictive power for outcome in more contemporary statistical evaluations. However, there is evidence that systemic hypotension independently increases morbidity and mortality. It is currently proposed that the critical threshold for CPP is between 50 and 60 mmHg, so management nowadays aims to keep CPP above 65–70 mmHg with judicious use of vasopressors.

Protocols: cerebral perfusion pressure (CPP)-, intracranial pressure- and 'optimal CPP'-oriented therapy

The continuous measurement of ICP is an essential modality in brain monitoring systems. After a decade of enthusiastic attempts to introduce newer modalities for brain monitoring (e.g. tissue oxygenation, microdialysis, cortical blood flow, TCD and jugular bulb oxygen saturation), ICP monitoring remains a robust clinical tool that provides the core of clinical monitoring in most critical care units. There is, however, increasing recognition of the complex and detailed information provided by the technique regarding compensatory

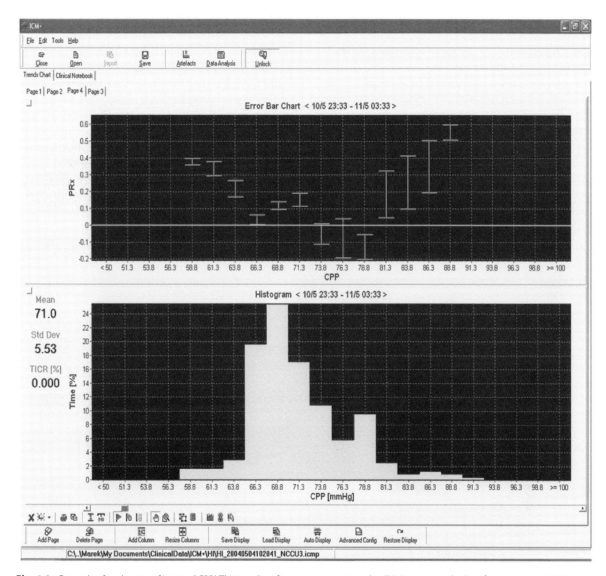

Fig. 4.9. Example of evaluation of 'optimal CPP'. This is a plot of pressure reactivity index (PRx) versus cerebral perfusion pressure (CPP) over a period of 4–6 h. The plot shows the typical U-shaped curve found in the presence of preserved autoregulation. The value of CPP associated with the lowest PRx is the 'optimal CPP'. The bottom graph shows a histogram of CPP over the same period of time. If the peak of the histogram is at the same CPP level as the bottom of the U-shaped curve in the top graph, it indicates that the current CPP is well matched to the optimal level. In this particular case, the optimal CPP was 76 and current modal CPP was 68 mmHg. According to the algorithm suggested by Steiner and colleagues, CPP should be slightly increased in the next step. See colour plate section.

mechanisms intrinsic to the brain as well as information about regulation of CBF.

The management and control of raised ICP requires its continuous monitoring. For example, most authors agree that ICP should be monitored in acute states such as head injury, poor-grade subarachnoid haemorrhage and intracerebral haematoma, and that the level of ICP can be used to titrate and select therapy. Cerebral perfusion pressure-oriented protocols and the 'Lund protocol' cannot be conducted correctly without guidance from real-time ICP recordings.

More sophisticated use of the technique recognizes that autoregulation of CBF is one of the most important mechanisms of brain protection following head injury. The relationship between PRx (or autoregulation assessed using TCD) and CPP shows a U-shaped curve (Fig. 4.9). The curve indicates that CPPs that are too low or too high are associated with autoregulation failure. Therefore, the 'optimal CPP' in which cerebral autoregulation is strongest may be identified by plotting PRx against CPP in individual cases (from the moving time window of the last few hours). Patients with a greater distance between their averaged CPP and post-hoc assessed 'optimal CPP' have worse outcomes after head trauma. An algorithm has been proposed by Steiner and colleagues to modify CPP-oriented therapy to maintain CPP close to 'optimal CPP'. However, it remains to be demonstrated prospectively whether such a strategy is able to improve outcome.

Refractory intracranial hypertension

When secondary cerebral insults lead to 'refractory intracranial hypertension', mean ICP rises above 80 mmHg as a result of brain swelling. The term 'refractory intracranial hypertension' implies that ICP increases over a few hours to very high values and leads to death of the patient unless aggressive ICP treatment is installed. This increase in ICP is commonly accompanied by a reduction in pulse amplitude and a gradual increase in ABP (the Cushing reflex). The moment of brainstem herniation through the foramen magnum is commonly marked by a rapid decrease in ABP, a rise in heart rate and a terminal decrease in the cerebral perfusion. When all pressure–volume compensatory reserves are exhausted, any further increase in intracranial volume produces fast and often fatal elevations in ICP. Decompressive craniectomy is often seen as a last resort in this setting. However, its greatest benefit may

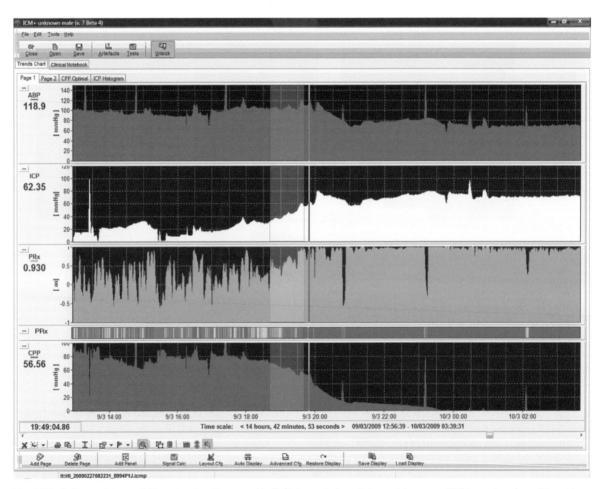

Fig. 4.10. Refractory intracranial hypertension. The second half of this graph shows intracranial pressure (ICP) increasing above 60 mmHg, while cerebral perfusion pressure (CPP) falls well below 40 mmHg. The patient died. The earlier part of the graph shows a rise in ICP from 20 to 40 mmHg, associated with a decrease in CPP below 50 mmHg. This period of progressive ICP elevation is preceded by a 60 min phase during which the pressure reactivity index (PRx) increases (note the change of colour of a bar from greenish to red within the critical period indicated by a grey background). See colour plate section.

require that the decision about surgery be undertaken well before uncontrollable elevations in ICP occur – with the intervention optimally being employed at ICP values that do not exceed 25 mmHg. However, several patients with ICP at this level will not develop refractory ICP elevations, and we need better early markers of subsequent refractory intracranial hypertension. In this context, some measures of cerebrovascular physiology may predict refractory intracranial hypertension – one being early loss of cerebrovascular reactivity (PRx) (Fig. 4.10).

Further reading

Asgeirsson, B., Grande, P. O. and Nordstrom, C. H. (1994). A new therapy of post-trauma brain oedema based on haemodynamic principles for brain volume regulation. *Intensive Care Med* **20**, 260–7.

Avezaat, C. J., van Eijndhoven, J. H. and Wyper, D. J. (1979). Cerebrospinal fluid pulse pressure and intracranial volume–pressure relationships. *J Neurol Neurosurg Psychiatry* **42**, 687–700.

Bratton, S. L., Chestnut, R. M., Ghajar, J. et al. (2007). Guidelines for the management of severe traumatic brain injury. VI. Indications for intracranial pressure monitoring. *J Neurotrauma* **24** (Suppl. 1), S37–44.

Bratton, S. L., Chestnut, R. M., Ghajar, J. et al. (2007). Guidelines for the management of severe traumatic brain injury. VII. Intracranial pressure monitoring technology. *J Neurotrauma* **24** (Suppl. 1), S45–54.

Chapman, P. H., Cosman, E. R. and Arnold, M. A. (1990) The relationship between ventricular fluid pressure and body position in normal subjects and subjects with shunts. A telemetric study. *Neurosurgery* **26**, 181–9.

Citerio, G. and Andrews, P. J. (2004) Intracranial pressure. Part two: clinical applications and technology. *Intensive Care Med* **30**, 1882–5.

Czosnyka, M. and Pickard, J. D. (2004). Monitoring and interpretation of intracranial pressure. *J Neurol Neurosurg Psychiatry* **75**, 813–21.

Davson, H., Hollingsworth, G. and Segal, M. B. (1970). The mechanism of drainage of the cerebrospinal fluid. *Brain* **93**, 665–78.

Ekstedt, J. (1978). CSF hydrodynamic studies in man. Normal hydrodynamic variables related to CSF pressure and flow. *J Neurolog Neurosyrg Psychiatry* **41**, 345–53.

Guillaume, J. and Janny, P. (1951). Manometrie intracranienne continué interest de la methode et premiers resultants. *Rev Neurol (Paris)* **84**, 131–42.

Kelly, G. (1824). Appearances observed in the dissection of two individuals; death from cold and congestion of the brain. *Trans Med Chir Sci Edinb* **1**, 84–169.

Klingelhofer, J., Conrad, B. and Benecke, R. (1988). Evaluation of intracranial pressure from transcranial Doppler studies in cerebral disease. *J Neurol* **235**, 159–62.

Lofgren, J., von Essen, C. and Zwetnow, N. N. (1973) The pressure–volume curve of the cerebrospinal fluid space in dogs. *Acta Neurol Scand* **49**, 557–74.

Lundberg, N. (1960). Continuous recording and control of ventricular fluid pressure in neurosurgical practice. *Acta Psychiatr Scand Suppl* **36**, 1–193.

Marmarou, A., Maset, A. L., Ward, J. D. et al. (1987). Contribution of CSF and vascular factors to elevation of ICP in severely head-injured patients. *J Neurosurg* **66**, 883–90.

Miller, J. D., Stanek, A. and Langfitt, T. W. (1972). Concepts of cerebral perfusion pressure and vascular compression during intracranial hypertension. *Prog Brain Res* **35**, 411–32.

Miller, J. D., Garibi, J. and Pickard, J. D. (1973). A clinical study of intracranial volume pressure relationships. *Br J Surg* **60**, 316.

Miller, J. D., Becker, D. P., Ward, J. D. et al. (1977). Significance of intracranial hypertension in severe head injury. *J Neurosurg* **47**, 503–16.

Narayan, R. K., Kishore, P. R., Becker, D. P. et al. (1982). Intracranial pressure: to monitor or not to monitor? A review of our experience with severe head injury. *J Neurosurg* **56**, 650–9.

Overgaard, J. and Tweed, W. A. (1974). Cerebral circulation after head injury. Part 1: Cerebral blood flow and its regulation after closed head injury with emphasis on clinical correlation. *J Neurosurg* **41**, 531–41.

Patel, H. C, Menon, D. K., Tebbs, S. et al. (2002). Specialist neurocritical care and outcome from head injury. *Intensive Care Med* **28**, 547–53.

Piper, I., Miller, J. D, Dearden, M., Leggate, J. R. and Robertson, I. (1990). System analysis of cerebrovascular pressure transmission: an observational study in head injured patients. *J Neurosurg* **73**, 871–80.

Rosner, M. J. and Becker, D. P. (1984). Origin and evolution of plateau waves. Experimental observations and a theoretical model. *J Neurosurg* **60**, 312–24.

Rosner, M. J., Rosner, S. D. and Johnson, A. H. (1995). Cerebral perfusion pressure: management protocol and clinical results. *J Neurosurg* **83**, 949–62.

Schmidt, B., Czosnyka, M., Raabe, A. et al. (2003). Adaptive noninvasive assessment of intracranial pressure and cerebral autoregulation. *Stroke* **34**, 84–9.

Steiner, L. A., Czosnyka, M., Piechnik, S. K. et al. (2002). Continuous monitoring of cerebrovascular pressure reactivity allows determination of optimal cerebral perfusion pressure in patients with traumatic brain injury. *Crit Care Med* **30**, 733–8.

Whitfield, P. C., Patel, H., Hutchinson, P. J. *et al.* (2001). Bifrontal decompressive craniectomy in the management of posttraumatic intracranial hypertension. *Br J Neurosurg* **15**, 500–7.

Wolfla, C. E., Luerssen, T. G., Bowman, R. M. and Putty, T. K. (1996). Brain tissue pressure gradients created by expanding frontal epidural mass lesion. *J Neurosurg* **84**, 642–7.

Zhong, J., Dujovny, M., Park, H. K. *et al.* (2003). Advances in ICP monitoring techniques. *Neurol Res* **25**, 339–50.

Chapter

5

Bedside measurements of cerebral blood flow

Amit Prakash and Basil F. Matta

Introduction

Monitoring cerebral blood flow (CBF) continues to be a long-standing challenge in the neurocritical care unit. The tight flow–metabolism coupling associated with normal brain function is often disturbed following brain injury, and alteration in blood flow not aligned to changes in metabolism may exacerbate secondary neuronal injury. Patients with traumatic brain injury (TBI) and those with subarachnoid haemorrhage (SAH) are particularly susceptible to changes in CBF as a result of reductions in cerebral perfusion pressure (CPP) due to increases in intracranial pressure (ICP), or arterial vasospasm. Although techniques like positron emission tomography (PET) provide 'snapshot' measurements of CBF, the ability to measure CBF continuously would allow early detection of cerebral ischaemic events, allowing the clinician to institute therapy rapidly, which may improve outcome. This has been one of the main drivers for the continuous search for reliable techniques for bedside CBF measurement. This chapter will outline the methods most commonly employed for the measurement and estimation of CBF in the operating theatre and in intensive care.

Kety–Schmidt method

The Kety–Schmidt method is the reference method for the measurement of global CBF, cerebral metabolic rate (CMR) and flux. It is based on Fick's principle. Briefly, this states that the amount of a substance taken up or eliminated by an organ is equal to the difference between the amount in the arterial blood and the amount in the venous blood supplying that organ, in the same time period.

Thus, for the brain:

$$QB_t = QA_t - QV_t$$

where QB_t is the quantity of tracer taken up by the brain in time t, QA_t is the quantity of tracer delivered to the brain by arterial blood in time t and QV_t is the amount of tracer removed by cerebral venous blood in time t.

The concentration of a tracer, nitrous oxide (N_2O) in this case, is measured across the cerebral circulation by withdrawing paired arterial and venous (jugular bulb catheter) blood samples, during a 10 min wash-in period. The brain tissue is fully saturated when jugular bulb and arterial blood concentrations of N_2O are almost equal.

The amount of N_2O delivered to or removed by the brain thus equals CBF multiplied by the arterial or venous concentrations, respectively. As the arterial and venous concentrations of N_2O vary with time, the equation can be rearranged as:

$$QB_t = TF \times \int (A - V) dt$$

where TF is CBF (ml min^{-1}), A is arterial N_2O concentration (ml l^{-1}) and V is venous N_2O concentration.

Thus:

$$TF = \frac{QB_t}{\int (A - V) dt}$$

CBF per gram weight of brain is then:

$$CBF = \frac{QB_t / W}{\int (A - V) dt}$$

where W is the brain weight (g) (Fig. 5.1).

Once CBF is determined, additional values such as cerebral metabolic requirement for oxygen and vascular resistance can then be derived. One of the advantages of using N_2O as the tracer is that it has a partition coefficient unaffected by varying levels of lipid and water, and therefore the measurement is unlikely to be

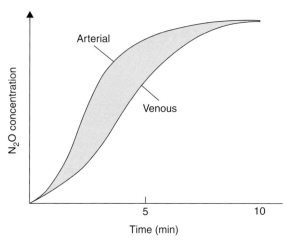

Fig. 5.1. The Kety–Schmidt technique for measuring cerebral blood flow using the freely diffusible tracer N_2O. After 10 min of N_2O inhalation, the brain is theoretically saturated and the arterial and venous concentrations of N_2O are almost equal. The shaded area between the two curves is proportional to hemispheric blood flow.

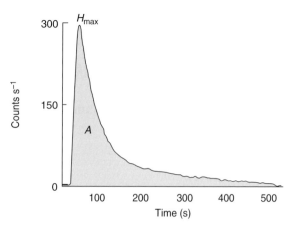

Fig. 5.2. Measurement of cerebral blood flow using intracarotid injection of ^{133}Xe. Blood flow is calculated from the maximal height (H_{max}) and integration of the area under the curve (A).

affected by age or the presence of cerebral oedema. The original Kety–Schmidt technique for measuring CBF is limited by the fact that CBF calculated by this technique represents the mean blood flow from the area of the brain (plus some extracranial tissues) draining into the particular jugular venous bulb being sampled – the ipsilateral cerebral hemisphere; hence, it often overestimates CBF. Also, CBF measurements obtained by this method are global and it is not possible to discriminate between grey and white matter or to detect changes in regional CBF.

Radioactive tracer clearance techniques

The introduction of radioisotope techniques for the measurement of CBF has allowed the progression from global CBF measurements to the two-dimensional maps of cortical blood flow. The radioactive isotope ^{133}Xe dissolved in saline is injected intra-arterially, and the clearance curve is detected using highly collimated scintillation counters placed externally over the scalp. ^{133}Xe is insoluble and passes freely through cell membranes, crosses the blood–brain barrier and is not metabolized in the body. After injection into the internal carotid artery, it is retained momentarily in brain tissue and is then released through normal venous outflow channels. Cerebral blood flow can be measured by the exponential pattern of clearance of the gas from the brain. A scintillation detector assembly consisting

of the collimator, crystal, photomultiplier tube and preamplifier is mounted on a stand that can be moved up to the patient's head. The electrical pulses generated by the detector assembly are fed through pulse height analysers and clearance curves are created. Mean blood flow through the volume of brain 'seen' by each crystal is thus:

$$\text{Flow}(\text{ml g}^{-1}\text{min}^{-1}) = \frac{\lambda(H_{max} - H_{10})}{A}$$

where λ is the brain–blood partition coefficient, H_{max} is the maximal height of the clearance curve, H_{10} is the height at 10 min and A is the area under the clearance curve (Fig. 5.2).

In humans, when clearance curves are plotted on a semi-logarithmic scale, two rates of exponential decay representing flow through grey and white matter are easily identified. Using a process termed 'exponential stripping', it is possible to isolate the individual components of blood flow (Fig. 5.3).

^{133}Xe has a low solubility in blood and is rapidly cleared from the blood, thus allowing further studies to be performed within a short period of time (approximately 30 min). An obvious advantage of this method over the Kety–Schmidt technique is the absence of repeat blood sampling. Other advantages include the ability to calculate either the 'mean' flow value from height/area under the curve analysis or more specific regional flow rates by exponential stripping. The accuracy and specificity of this method depend on the number and size of the externally placed detectors. With a

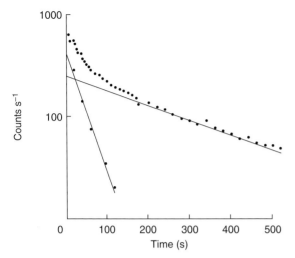

Fig. 5.3. Compartmental analysis of cerebral blood flow using a semi-logarithmic plot. The curve shows flow through grey and white matter, or fast and slow components, respectively.

larger number of detectors (up to 254 detectors have been used), it is possible to measure flow in discrete regions of the brain, such as the small changes in blood flow associated with functional brain activation.

However, this method is not without its disadvantages, which include potential inaccuracies from variations in the partition coefficient of ^{133}Xe in normal or abnormal brain tissue, and the 'look-through' artefact phenomenon, i.e. the failure to indicate areas of low or no flow because the detector can see only areas of perfused tissue.

Over the years, the method of administration of the radioactive isotope has been altered to either the less hazardous intravenous route or the non-invasive inhalation route. Both approaches use the same external detectors as with the intra-arterial approach, applying the same principles and theory. These routes of administration of xenon have reduced morbidity over the intra-arterial route, and certainly the inhalation technique is relatively non-invasive and easy to use. In addition, with advances in technology, a reduction in the size of apparatus and the use of microprocessor-based computers, equipment has become far more portable and user-friendly for application in the intensive care unit or the ward.

Nevertheless, non-invasive techniques still have significant disadvantages. As well as exposing the whole body to radiation, inhalation of radioactive xenon distorts the clearance curves because of isotope recirculation. This necessitates the measurement of end-tidal

^{133}Xe and performance of a correction computation, which accounts for this recirculation. The presence of radioactive isotope in the scalp and extracranial tissues requires a further correction before accurate estimations of CBF are possible.

Jugular venous bulb oximetry

Jugular venous bulb oximetry, first described by Meyerson and colleagues in 1927, is frequently used in the intensive care of patients with brain injury as a bedside measure of cerebral oxygen delivery and extraction and as a tool to estimate CBF. As CBF and metabolism are usually coupled, during a period of stable cerebral metabolism, CBF can be determined from the arteriovenous oxygen content difference across the cerebral circulation (AVDO$_2$). The AVDO$_2$ is calculated using the equation:

$$AVDO_2 = CaO_2 - CjO_2 = [Hb \times 1.39 \times SaO_2 + (0.003 \times PaO_2)]$$
$$-[Hb \times 1.39 \times SjO_2 + (0.003 \times PjO_2)]$$

where CaO$_2$ is the arterial oxygen content, CjO$_2$ is the jugular venous oxygen content, Hb is the haemoglobin concentration, SaO$_2$ is the arterial oxygen saturation, PaO$_2$ is the arterial partial pressure of oxygen, SjO$_2$ is the jugular venous oxygen saturation and PjO$_2$ is the jugular venous partial pressure of oxygen.

Although this method has been used in head-injured patients for estimating CBF, the technique has several limitations. The AVDO$_2$ is a global measure that cannot reliably detect regional ischaemia. Sampling from the right jugular bulb has commonly been assumed to provide the best estimate of hemispheric blood flow (the cortex is preferentially drained via the right jugular bulb), but this may not apply in all patients or conditions. Other factors that can affect the accuracy of CBF estimation using jugular bulb oximetry include contamination of jugular bulb blood with extracerebral blood, malpositioning of the catheter tip, speed of blood withdrawal from the catheter and the position of the patient's head. Therefore, for best results, radiographic confirmation of the position of the catheter tip (at the level of and just medial to the mastoid bone), withdrawal of blood at a rate of <2 ml min^{-1} and careful attention to head position are mandatory. Even with all these conditions, this method has a very high false-negative rate as it can only detect global hypoperfusion and is unlikely to be of much benefit in detecting regional ischaemia.

Jugular thermodilution technique

This technique, first used to measure coronary sinus flow, has been successfully adapted to measure CBF with reasonable accuracy. A catheter with a built-in thermistor is placed in the jugular bulb and the position of its tip confirmed radiographically. Cold fluid is infused at a constant rate, and the resulting change in temperature measured downstream gives an estimate jugular venous blood flow (Fig. 5.4).

CBF is then calculated using the equation:

$$(T_b - T_m) \times V_b \times \lambda_b \times \rho_b = (T_m - T_i) \times V_i \times \lambda_i \times \rho_i$$

$$\text{(heat lost by blood)} = \text{(heat lost by indicator)}$$

where T_b, T_i and T_m, are the temperature of blood, indicator, and a mixture of blood and indicator; V_b and V_i are the volumes (ml) of blood and indicator; λ_b and λ_i are the specific heat of blood and indicator;

and ρ_b and ρ_i are the density of blood and indicator, respectively.

If time is brought into the equation, the volumes become flows (F) and:

$$F_b = \frac{F_i \times (\lambda_i \times \rho_i) \times (T_m - T_i)}{(\lambda_b \times \rho_b) \times (T_b - T_m)}$$

If saline is used as the indicator:

$$\frac{\lambda_i \times \rho_i}{\lambda_b \times \rho_b} = \frac{1.005 \times 0.997}{1.045 \times 0.87} = 1.10$$

When a pre-set pump determines the rate of saline infused, flow can be calculated.

This technique is simple, safe, reproducible and easy to apply at the bedside. Measurements can be repeated at frequent intervals, and, as the 'indicator' is non-cumulative, there is no associated morbidity for the patient or clinician.

In addition to the limitations of jugular bulb catheters for the measurement of CBF, adequate mixing of the blood and injectate at the thermistor, accurate injectate temperature recording and heat loss from the system may also affect the accurate measurement of CBF.

Laser Doppler flowmetry

Laser Doppler flowmetry (LDF) is based on the assessment of Doppler shift of low-power laser light, which is scattered by moving red blood cells (RBCs) (Fig. 5.5).

Briefly, monochromatic laser light, with a wavelength above the maximal absorption of haemoglobin and below the maximal absorption of water (600–780 nm), is delivered to and detected from a 1 mm^3 volume of brain tissue by a flexible fibre-optic light guide. The laser light is scattered randomly by both static structures and moving tissue particles, mainly RBCs. Laser light reflected from stationary tissues remains unchanged in frequency, whereas light reflected by moving particles is both scattered and undergoes a frequency shift. Multiple scattering at various angles of incidence precludes the exact measurement of velocity of the moving RBCs; however, as the bandwidth of the Doppler shift frequencies increases linearly in proportion to the RBCs' velocities, the mean frequency shift and the power are directly proportional to the velocity and the number of moving RBCs, respectively (Fig. 5.6).

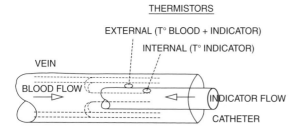

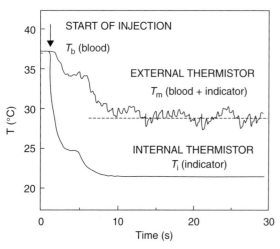

Fig. 5.4. Top: diagrammatic representation of a thermodilution catheter using two thermistors, which can be inserted in the jugular bulb for the measurement of CBF. Bottom: temperatures recorded by internal and external thermistors over a period of 30 min. (Redrawn from Melot *et al.*, 1996. *J Cereb Blood Flow Metab* **16**, 1263–70, with permission from Macmillan Publishers Ltd.)

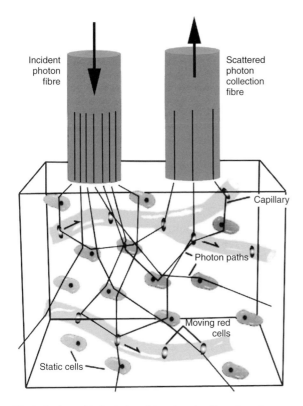

Fig. 5.5. A graphic depiction of the principle of laser Doppler flowmetry. (Redrawn with permission from Arbit, E. and DiResta, G. R., 1996. *Neurosurg Clin N Am* **7**, 741–8. © Elsevier.)

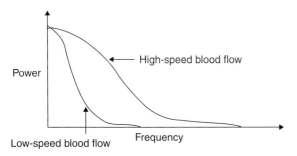

Fig. 5.6. The theory behind laser Doppler flowmetry for the measurement of CBF. Doppler frequency and power depend on the speed of red blood cells. Bandwidth broadens as red blood cells speed increases, but amplitude and shape remain constant.

As the blood cell flux is equal to the velocity of the cells multiplied by their concentration, if the concentration of the RBCs remains constant, the power of the frequency-weighted Doppler spectrum is proportional to the RBC flux through the capillary bed and hence to CBF.

Laser Doppler flowmetry produces a continuous, real-time flow output, which is linearly related to CBF. Although laser Doppler flowmetry is a fast, continuous, non-radioactive bedside monitoring of CBF that can detect changes at the cellular level, there are still many practical as well as theoretical limitations to overcome. The device is invasive, requiring insertion of the probe during operation or via a burr hole. Changes in tissue perfusion are often accompanied by changes in the tissue geometry and may affect flow measurements. Tissue density and geometry may also be altered after brain injury, and therefore site selection is critical to the accuracy of the measurements. Probes measure flow within approximately 1.5 mm of the tips; hence, the measurement area is localized and caution must be exercised in making assumptions about global CBF. A further source of false readings is the presence of arterioles and venules, which amplify laser Doppler flowmetry signals, thereby over-representing microvascular blood flow.

Thermal clearance

Thermal diffusion flowmetry is used to estimate cortical blood flow by measuring changes in a temperature gradient, which exists between two thermistors within a probe applied to the cortex. The distal thermistor (active) measures flow via heat transfer to the capillaries while the proximal thermistor (passive) measures the baseline temperature. The primary measurement technique relies on detection of the temperature gradient between the large plate generating heat and the second smaller detector plate. The difference in temperature between the two plates is inversely proportional to the thermal conductivity of the brain tissue. The temperature gradient decreases as the flow increases so that:

$$CBF = K \times (1/V - 1/V_0)$$

where CBF is cerebral (cortical) blood flow, K is a constant, V is the voltage difference between the two plates at the time of measurement and V_0 is the voltage difference at no flow.

The thermal diffusion CBF technique has many advantages in that it is simple, continuous and does not use ionizing radiation. Codman have produced an FDA-approved CBF monitor (Hemdex Cerebral Blood Flow Monitor) for continuous bedside measurement of CBF, measured in ml $(100\,\mathrm{g})^{-1}$ min^{-1}. The monitor has been evaluated for use in aneurysm repair and extracranial/intracranial bypass surgery as a modality for intraoperative CBF monitoring.

The early results with thermal diffusion flowmetry have been promising for detection of vasospasm in SAH patients and for use as a bedside monitor for changes in carbon dioxide reactivity.

Limitations encountered with this technique include inaccuracies due to sudden temperature change (e.g. irrigation, rapid infusion of fluids) and motion artefacts. Meticulous probe placement is key, as the area monitored is localized to a sphere of tissue around 4–5 mm in diameter around the probe.

Transcranial Doppler ultrasonography

Transcranial Doppler ultrasonography (TCD) introduced by Aaslid and colleagues in 1982, is a non-invasive monitor that uses a Doppler transducer to measure RBC velocity and pulsatility of blood flow in the large vessels at the base of the brain.

As TCD measures RBC velocity and not flow, changes in flow velocity (FV) only represent true changes in CBF when both the angle of insonation and the diameter of the vessel insonated remain constant. Provided these limitations are recognized, the technique can be utilized to obtain information about CBF.

Principle of transcranial Doppler

Transcranial Doppler ultrasonography is based on the Doppler principle described in 1843 by Christian Doppler. The probe emits a wave with a known frequency in the order of 2 MHz referred to as f_0 and propagation speed c towards the moving target, in this case RBCs. The echo perceived has an altered frequency, f_e, which is dependent on the velocity of the RBCs. The difference between the f_0 and f_e is the Doppler shift, f_d. The reflected wave can be a higher or lower frequency, which is termed positive or negative shift.

The FV of the RBC is calculated as:

$$FV = \frac{c \times f_d}{2 \times f_o}$$

The FV determined by TCD is dependent on the cosine of the angle of insonation, represented as:

$$FV = \frac{c \times f_d}{2 \times f_o \times \cos\theta}$$

Hence, at 0° the TCD calculated and true velocity are equal (cosine of 0° = 1). However, at 90° the calculated

FV is 0, irrespective of the actual velocity. Fortunately, with the transtemporal window most commonly used to insonate anterior middle and posterior cerebral arteries, the anatomic limitations are such that signal capture is only possible at narrow angles (<30°) minimizing the error to <15%.

The other ultrasonic windows are transorbital for the carotid siphon and suboccipital for the basilar and vertebral arteries. It should be noted that up to 8% of the population does not have an adequate acoustic window.

There is ample evidence suggesting that the diameter of the middle cerebral artery (MCA) does not change significantly with changes in arterial pressure, carbon dioxide partial pressure, or the use of anaesthetic or vasoactive agents. Hence, it is generally accepted that, during steady-state anaesthesia, changes in FV reflect corresponding changes in cortical CBF.

Practical application

The TCD system displays information as a velocity–time waveform. The peak systolic (PSV) and the end-diastolic (EDV) blood flow velocities are measured from the waveform display.

Calculated indices are described below.

Mean flow velocity

$$\text{Mean FV} = \frac{PSV + (EDV \times 2)}{3}$$

The range of normal values for adults was determined by Aaslid and colleagues.

Mean FV values >120 cm s^{-1} are generally considered abnormal. Both vasospasm and hyperaemia can lead to elevated FV. The Lindegaard ratio is an index used to distinguish between vasospasm and hyperaemia by comparing the FV of the MCA with that of the extracranial portion of the ipsilateral internal carotid artery. The ratio of FV in the MCA to that in the external carotid artery increases with the severity of vasospasm. Hence, an FV ratio of <3 is consistent with hyperaemia, while 3–6 is indicative of mild vasospasm and >6 is consistent with severe vasospasm.

Waveform pulsatility

The pulsatility of the FV waveform reflects the resistance of the more distal cerebral vasculature. The most widely used measures are:

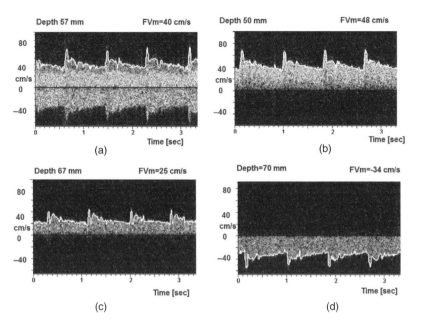

Fig. 5.7. Schematic representation of FV trace obtained from internal carotid artery bifurcation at 5.5–6.5 cm (a), the M1 segment of the middle cerebral artery at 3–6 cm (b), the posterior cerebral artery (P1) at 6–8 cm (c) and the anterior cerebral artery (A1) at 6–8 cm (d). Flow above the horizontal is towards the probe, while flow below the horizontal is away from the probe. See colour plate section.

$$\text{Pulsatility index (PI)} = \frac{\text{PSV} - \text{EDV}}{\text{MV}}$$

where MV is mean velocity, and:

$$\text{Resistance index (RI)} = \frac{\text{PSV} - \text{EDV}}{\text{PSV}}$$

An increase in these indices has been correlated with an increase in ICP within the ICP range of 5–40 mmHg (Fig. 5.7).

Clinical applications of transcranial Doppler

Subarachnoid haemorrhage

Delayed ischaemic neurological deficit (DIND) secondary to vasospasm occurs in up to 30% of patients within 3–14 days after SAH. Early detection of clinically significant vasospasm can prompt the clinician to direct therapy towards prevention of long-term ischaemic complications. Although correlations between TCD velocity and DIND has been reported by many authors, TCD velocity and CBF readings do not always correlate; moreover, intermittent TCD examinations may miss significant vasospasm. Daily TCD examinations may alert to the development of early vasospasm, especially in those sedated patients in whom assessment of neurology is not possible.

Intraoperative monitoring during carotid endarterectomy

Hypoperfusion and/or hyperperfusion may be responsible for a small number of perioperative strokes in patients undergoing carotid endarterectomy. Given that a TCD probe can be fixed without the interfering surgical field to provide a non-invasive continuous assessment of CBF, it is widely used for this procedure. Flow velocity MCA should be >40% of the preclamping value – a decrease below 15% can be used as an indication for shunt placement. Emboli are clearly audible during surgery, and waveform analysis can differentiate air from particulate emboli. Post-operatively, continuous TCD monitoring has been used to detect showers of emboli and patency problems with the graft. Furthermore, it is possible to assess cerebral autoregulation and the need for post-operative blood pressure control in order to avoid hyperaemic complications.

Traumatic brain injury

Transcranial Doppler ultrasonography can be used to provide a non-invasive assessment of ICP, cerebral autoregulation, carbon dioxide reactivity and the detection of vasospasm following TBI. Waveform pulsatility indices are known to correlate with ICP over a certain range, providing an estimation of distal cerebral resistance. The Lindegaard ratio helps differentiate vasospasm from hyperaemia, facilitating clinical management. A low FV of $<35\,\mathrm{cm\,s^{-1}}$ has been correlated with poor neurological outcome.

In TBI, loss of cerebral autoregulation or carbon dioxide reactivity has been correlated with severity of injury, and may result in worse outcome and an increase in mortality.

Brain death

In countries where confirmation of death requires demonstration of CBF, angiography is considered to be the gold standard. There have been many case reports detailing the use of TCD to confirm cerebral circulatory arrest. As CPP approaches zero, three patterns of TCD waveforms are observed: oscillating flow, small systolic spikes and no signal. It is not clear which pattern is the most sensitive or specific for diagnosing cerebral circulatory arrest. Moreover, given that 8% of the population does not have an acoustic window, the results should be interpreted with caution.

In our opinion, TCD findings should not be used in isolation, as with any clinical measurement, but more to complement other monitoring modalities available in the neurointensive care.

Further reading

Aaslid, R. (1986) The Doppler principle applied to measurement of blood flow velocities in cerebral arteries. In Aaslid, R. (ed.) *The Doppler Principle Applied to Measurement of Blood flow Velocities in Cerebral Arteries.* Vienna: Springer, pp. 22–38.

Aaslid, R., Markwalder, T. M. and Nornes, H. (1982). Noninvasive transcranial Doppler ultrasound recording of flow velocity in basal cerebral arteries. *J Neurosurg* **57**, 769–74.

Anderson, R. E. (1996). Cerebral blood flow Xenon-133. *Neurosurg Clin N Am* **7**, 703–8.

Azevedo, E., Teixeira, J., Neves, J. C. and Vaz, R. (2000). Transcranial Doppler and brain death. *Transplant Proc* **32**, 2579–81.

Bonner, R. and Nossal, R. (1981). Model for laser Doppler measurements of blood flow in tissue. *Appl Opt* **20**, 2097–107.

Cruz, J. (1993). Combined continuous monitoring of systemic and cerebral oxygenation in acute brain injury: preliminary observations. *Crit Care Med* **21**, 1225–32.

Donley, R. F., Sundt, T. M. Jr, Anderson, R. E. and Sharbrough, F. W. (1975). Blood flow measurements and the 'look-through' artifact in focal cerebral ischemia. *Stroke* **6**, 121–31.

Gibbs, E. L. and Gibbs, F. A. (1934). The cross section areas of the vessels that form the torcular and the manner in which blood is distributed to the right and the left lateral sinus. *Anat Rec* **54**, 419–26.

Gosling, R. G. and King, D. H. (1974). Arterial assessment by Doppler-shift ultrasound. *Proc R Soc Med* **67**, 447–9.

Graham, D. I. and Adams, J. H. (1971). Ischaemic brain damage in fatal head injuries. *Lancet* **1**, 265–6.

Gunn, H., Matta, B. F., Lam, A. M. and Mayberg, T. S. (1995). Accuracy of continuous jugular bulb venous oximetry during intracranial surgery. *J Neurosurg Anesthesiol* **7**, 174–7.

Ingvar, D. H. and Lassen, N. A. (1961). Quantitative determination of cerebral blood flow in man. *Lancet* **2**, 806–7.

Kirkpatrick, P. J., Czosnyka, M., Smielewski, P. and Pickard, J. D. (1994). Continuous monitoring of cortical perfusion using laser Doppler flowmetry in ventilated head injured patients. *J Neurol Neurosurg Psychiatry* **57**, 1382–8.

Lam, J. M. and Smielewski, P. (2000). Predicting delayed ischemic deficits after aneurismal subarachnoid hemorrhage using a transient hyperemic response test of cerebral autoregulation. *Neurosurgery* **47**, 819–25.

Lindegaard, K. F., Nornes, H., Bakke, S. J., Sorteberg, W. and Nakstad, P. (1988). Cerebral vasospasm after subarachnoid haemorrhage investigated by means of transcranial Doppler ultrasound. *Acta Neurochir* **42** (Supplement), 81–4.

Mapleson, W. W., Evans, D. E. and Flook, V. (1970). The variability of partition coefficients for nitrous oxide and cyclopropane in the rabbit. *Br J Anaesth* **42**, 1033–41.

Matta, B. F. and Lam, A. M. (1995). Isoflurane and desflurane do not dilate the middle cerebral artery appreciably. *Br J Anaesth* **74**, P486–7.

Matta, B. F. and Lam, A. M. (1996). The speed of blood withdrawal affects the accuracy of jugular venous bulb oxygen saturation measurements. *Anesthesiology* **86**, 806–8.

Matta, B. F., Mayberg, T. S. and Lam, A. M. (1995). The effect of halothane, isoflurane, and desflurane on cerebral blood flow velocity during propofol-induced isoelectric electroencephalogram. *Anesthesiology* **83**, 980–5.

Mayberg, T. and Lam, A. (1996). Jugular bulb oximetry for the monitoring of cerebral blood flow and metabolism. *Neurosur Clin N Am* **7**, 755–65.

Melot, C., Berre, J., Moraine, J. J. and Kahn, R. J. (1996). Estimation of cerebral blood flow at bedside by continuous jugular thermodilution. *J Cereb Blood Flow Metab* **16**, 1263–70.

Meyerson, A., Halloran, R. D. and Hirsh, H. L. (1927). Technique for obtaining blood from the internal jugular vein and carotid artery. *Arch Neurol Psychiat* **17**, 807–9.

Obrist, W. D. and Wilkinson, W. E. (1990). Regional cerebral blood flow measurements in humans by Xenon-133. *Cerebrovasc Brain Metab Rev* **2**, 283–327.

Obrist, W. D., Thompson, H. K., King, C. H. and Wang, H. S. (1967). Determination of regional cerebral blood flow by inhalation of Xenon-133. *Circ Res* **20**, 124–35.

Paulson, O. B., Cronqvist, S., Risberg, J. and Jeppesen, F. I. (1968). Regional cerebral blood flow: comparison of 8-detector and 16-detector instrumentation. *J Nucl Med* **10**, 164–73.

Richards, H. K., Czosnyka, M., Kirkpatrick, P. and Pickard, J. D. (1995). Estimation of laser Doppler flux biological zero using basilar artery flow velocity in the rabbit. *Am J Physiol* **268**, 213–17.

Rothoerl, R. D., Woertgen, C. and Brawanski, A. (2004). Hyperemia following aneurysmal subarachnoid hemorrhage: incidence, diagnosis, clinical features, and outcome. *Intensive Care Med* **30**, 1298–302.

Shepherd, A. P. and Oberg, P. A. (eds) (1990). *Laser-Doppler Blood Flowmetry*. Boston, MA: Kluwer Academic Publishers.

Soukup, J., Bramsiepe, I., Brucke, M., Sanchin, L. and Menzel, M. (2008). Evaluation of a bedside monitor of regional CBF as a measure of CO_2 reactivity in neurosurgical intensive care patients. *J Neurosurg Anesthesiol* **20**, 249–55.

Stocchetti, N., Paparella, A., Bridelli, F. *et al.* (1994). Cerebral venous oxygenation studied with bilateral samples in the internal jugular veins. *Neurosurgery* **34**, 38–44.

Taudorf, S., Berg, R. M. G, Bailey, D. M. and Moller, K. (2009). Cerebral blood flow and oxygen metabolism measured with Kety–Schmidt method using nitrous oxide. *Acta Anaesthesiol Scand* **53**, 159–67.

Vajkoczy, P. and Schomacher, M. (2007). Monitoring cerebral blood flow in Neurosurgical Intensive Care. *U S Neurolog Dis* 1–4.

Vajkoczy, P., Roth, H., Lucke, T. *et al.* (2000). Continuous monitoring of regional cerebral blood flow – experimental and clinical validation of a novel thermal diffusion microprobe. *J Neurosurg* **93**, 265–74.

Vajkoczy, P., Horn, P., Thome, C., Munch, E. and Schmiedek, P. (2003). Regional cerebral blood flow monitoring in the diagnosis of delayed ischaemia following aneurismal subarachnoid hemorrhage. *J Neurosurg* **98**, 1227–34.

Waltz, A. G., Wanek, A. R. and Anderson, R. E. (1972). Comparison of analytic methods for calculation of cerebral blood flow after intracarotid injection of Xenon-133. *J Nucl Med* **13**, 66–72.

Chapter

6

Cerebral oxygenation

Ari Ercole and Arun K. Gupta

Introduction

Maintaining the balance between cerebral metabolic supply and demand underpins much of neurocritical care and neuroanaesthetic practice. Cerebral perfusion pressure (CPP) and metabolic rate can be manipulated by a number of means, but these are not benign interventions and do not guarantee the absence of regional oxygenation deficits. A bedside technique for the quantitative, continuous measurement of cerebral oxygen supply and demand is clearly highly desirable.

Such a system should alert the clinician to the presence of regions of failing oxygenation and ideally be sensitive, specific, minimally invasive, robust and easy to use. A number of technologies aimed at detecting oxygen supply/demand imbalance have been developed of which jugular bulb oximetry is the most mature. More recently, near-infrared spectroscopy and direct brain tissue oxygen measurement have become clinically available. These techniques employ very different measurement principles and, as we shall see, all have their individual shortcomings. However, by combining them with other parameters in a synergistic, multimodal approach, some of these difficulties may be mitigated.

Jugular bulb oximetry

Percutaneous sampling and analysis of human cerebral venous blood from the jugular bulb was first described by Myerson and colleagues in 1927. Arteriovenous differences between oxygen, glucose and lactate content were later studied by Gibbs and colleagues, who proposed them as global measures of the balance between cerebral metabolic supply and demand. Since its introduction as a monitoring technique, the technology for jugular venous sampling and oximetry has been refined, most recently with the introduction of

reliable fibre-optic catheters capable of continuous oxygen saturation measurement, making the technique a routine element of multimodal monitoring in neurocritical care.

Anatomy

Deoxygenated blood from the brain is collected by the major cranial venous sinuses. The majority of this blood then drains into the left or right sigmoid sinuses. These follow a curved path in the posterior fossa, passing caudally and forwards to form an internal jugular vein (IJV) in the posterior jugular foramen on each side (Fig. 6.1). The paired inferior petrosal sinuses are an exception to this common pathway, emptying instead directly into the IJV. The occipital sinuses are of variable anatomy but typically drain into the vertebral venous plexus rather than the IJV, although this represents only a small contribution to the total blood flow when supine. The venous outflow from left and right hemispheres is mixed with approximately 30% of the IJV blood arising from the contralateral side. In most cases, one side (usually the right) is dominant, although subcortical areas tend to drain preferentially to the left. A small percentage of the blood is extracranial in origin, from anatomically variable emissary veins and the cavernous sinus.

At its origin in the posterior part of the jugular foramen, the IJV is dilated and known as the (superior) jugular bulb. Several veins carrying extracerebral blood, of which the facial vein is the most significant, empty into the IJV a few centimetres below. From its origin, the vein runs down the neck within the carotid sheath, lateral to the vagus nerve and carotid artery, where it can be conveniently cannulated. Caudally, it dilates again, forming the inferior jugular bulb before joining the subclavian vein to become the brachiocephalic vein behind the medial clavicle at the thoracic

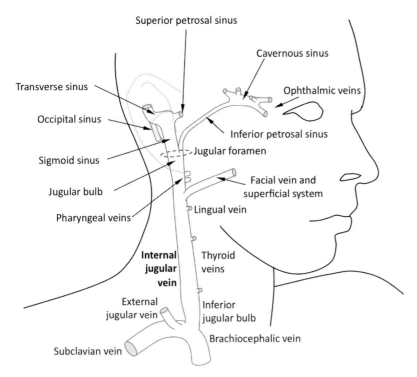

Fig. 6.1. Schematic diagram of the right jugular bulb and internal jugular vein. The majority of the cerebral venous blood drains into the superior jugular bulb either indirectly via the sigmoid sinus or directly in the case of the inferior petrosal sinus. Significant extracerebral contamination of the internal jugular venous blood occurs just below the jugular bulb, most notably from the facial vein.

inlet. The vein is related anterolaterally to the superficial cervical fascia, platysma, deep cervical fascia and sternomastoid muscle. The transverse processes of the cervical vertebrae, cervical plexus, phrenic nerve and (on the left) thoracic duct lie posteriorly to the vein. A bicuspid valve is typically found just above the inferior bulb, the central venous system cephalad being valveless.

Physiology

The brain extracts oxygen from arterial blood at a rate to supply its global metabolic requirements leaving an oxygen-poor venous effluent. The oxygen saturation of this venous blood is related to the cerebral metabolic rate for oxygen ($CMRO_2$) and cerebral blood flow (CBF) by the Fick equation:

$$CMRO_2 = CBF \times (CaO_2 - CjO_2)$$

The quantities CaO_2 and CjO_2 represent the arterial and jugular venous oxygen contents, respectively. If we rearrange this equation, it is clear that the arteriovenous oxygen difference ($AVDO_2$) is a measure of the ratio $CMRO_2/CBF$:

$$CaO_2 - CjO_2 = AVDO_2 = CMRO_2/CBF$$

In the healthy brain, flow–metabolism coupling results in the $AVDO_2$ being relatively constant in the range of 4–9 ml dl^{-1}. High values, however, suggest a situation where blood flow is low relative to metabolic requirements. Conversely, low values represent states of hyperaemia, where CBF is in relative excess.

For practical reasons, it is helpful to work with blood oxygen saturation rather than content, as this can be measured straightforwardly by optical techniques. Assuming fixed oxyhaemoglobin dissociation characteristics, the arterial and venous saturations, SaO_2 and SjO_2, are related to oxygen content and haemoglobin concentration [Hb] by:

$$CaO_2 = SaO_2 \times 1.34 \times [Hb] + 0.0031 \times PaO_2$$

$$CjO_2 = SjO_2 \times 1.34 \times [Hb] + 0.0031 \times PjO_2$$

The contribution from dissolved oxygen, given by terms involving arterial and jugular venous partial pressures of oxygen PaO_2 and PjO_2 in this equation, are small and can safely be neglected. Combining these and the two previous equations, we find that the venous oxygen saturation is equivalently given by:

$$SjO_2 = SaO_2 - \text{constant} \times CMRO_2/CBF$$

Again assuming constant arterial oxygenation, SjO_2 represents the balance between oxygen supply and demand. In health, flow–metabolism coupling maintains SjO_2 between about 55 and 75%. These values are somewhat lower than mixed venous saturations, reflecting the brain's relatively high metabolic requirements. Indeed, measured values down to 45% may be normal in health if extracerebral contamination is carefully avoided by angiography-guided catheterization of the jugular bulb.

In pathological circumstances, $CMRO_2$ and CBF may become uncoupled. In circumstances of hypoperfusion without a corresponding decrease in $CMRO_2$, the brain must extract a greater proportion of arterial oxygen, and SjO_2 will be observed to fall. However, there is a limit to how far oxygen extraction can be increased. Values of SjO_2 below 50% imply that oxygen supply may be critically low for the metabolic demand, and the brain is at risk of ischaemic injury.

Practical procedure

Jugular venous oxygenation can be measured intermittently by serial blood sampling or continuously by fibre-optic oximetry. Intermittent sampling has the advantage of low cost and additionally allows $AVDO_2$ and the arteriovenous glucose and lactate difference to be measured by oximetry, co-oximetry and blood biochemical analysis. As venous flow velocities are low, it is essential to draw the sample slowly ($<2\,ml\,min^{-1}$) to avoid contamination with extracranial blood (Fig. 6.2).

Spectrophotometric catheters measure SjO_2 continuously, avoiding the difficulties of blood sampling and also allowing more transient supply/demand

mismatch events to be detected. Two systems for continuous oximetry are available: Oximetrix (Abbott Laboratories, North Chicago, IL, USA) and Edslab II (Baxter Healthcare Corporation, Irvine, CA, USA). Both systems consist of narrow-gauge double-lumen catheters. One lumen contains transmit and receive optical fibres by means of which the SjO_2 is measured optically. The other lumen is available for blood sampling and may be continuously flushed with saline at 2–$4\,ml\,h^{-1}$ to maintain patency. The spectrophotometric determination of SjO_2 relies on the different absorption properties of oxygenated and deoxygenated haemoglobin in the red and near-infrared range. The Edslab II system alternately sends two different wavelengths down one fibre at millisecond intervals and measures the reflected light. As the absorption also depends on haemoglobin concentration, this must be entered manually into the machine. The device then calculates SjO_2 by averaging the reflection measurements over several seconds. The Oximetrix system is similar except that three different optical wavelengths are used, which obviates the need for prior determination of the haemoglobin concentration and may make it more stable under situations where this is rapidly changing.

The current generation of catheters are relatively stiffer and are thus less prone to kinking, which has been a problem in the past. Modern catheters also have an antimicrobial and antithrombotic coating to minimize the reduction in signal that occurs with fibrin deposition over the fibre end, and should require recalibration only every 24–48 h. However, inaccurate or unreliable behaviour can still be observed if the catheter abuts the vessel wall, which can be a particular

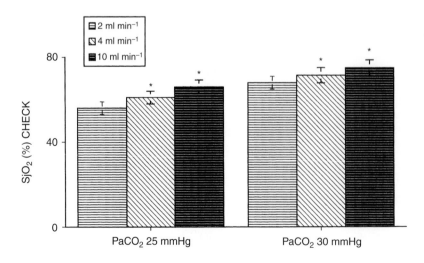

Fig. 6.2. The speed of withdrawal from jugular bulb catheters affects accuracy of readings. SjO_2 values are higher with faster rates of blood withdrawal due to contamination with extracranial blood. Optimal rate appears to be $2\,ml\,min^{-1}$.

problem if the patient's head is not in the neutral position. Despite the advances in continuous SjO_2 technology, careful blood sampling and co-oximetry remain the 'gold standard' and should be performed before instituting a change of therapy based on the continuous spectrophotometric results alone.

Placement of a jugular venous bulb catheter is a quick and safe procedure in experienced hands. Continuous oximetry catheters are introduced through an intravenous sheath, introduced by retrograde cannulation of the IJV using a Seldinger technique. The site is selected, prepared and infiltrated with local anaesthetic using a strict aseptic technique, as for conventional central venous cannulation. Ultrasound visualization, which has been demonstrated to reduce complications in central venous access, may be particularly helpful in avoiding the need for significant head-down tilt, which may otherwise have deleterious effects on intracranial pressure. Conventional anterograde central venous access may also be obtained at the same time by a second venepuncture a short distance caudal to the jugular venous catheter insertion site. In this case, both guidewires can be placed first to avoid accidentally damaging the first catheter while positioning the second line (Fig. 6.3).

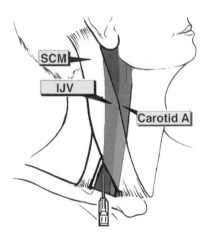

Fig. 6.3. The technique used in our unit for inserting jugular bulb catheters. The junction between the sternal and clavicular heads of the sternocleidomastoid muscle is localized and the skin is punctured under ultrasound guidance with a 16 gauge 5.25 inch Angiocath catheter (Becton and Dickinson) mounted with a 5 ml syringe. During gentle aspiration, the needle is passed in a cranial direction for 1–2 cm, at an angle of 15–20° in the sagittal plane. Once the vein is entered, the catheter is advanced over the needle until a slight elastic resistance is felt, or when the tip of the catheter is estimated to be just behind the mastoid process. SCM, sternocleidomastoid muscle; IJV, internal jugular vein; carotid A, carotid artery.

Complications are similar in frequency and nature to those seen in standard central venous access and specifically include those due to the venepuncture itself (such as carotid artery puncture and haematoma formation) and late complications (such as infection and thrombosis). A rise in intracranial pressure (ICP) is rarely if ever seen as a result of jugular venous cannulation. However, subclinical thrombosis is an ultrasound finding in up to 40% of patients with catheters after 6 days.

A number of considerations are noteworthy when choosing which side to monitor from. In health, similar saturations are usually found between the left and right sides. However, the venous drainage is variably lateralized between left and right hemispheres and even between subcortical and cortical regions. It is therefore not surprising that measurements of SjO_2 may become asymmetrical with highly focal or unilateral pathology and that this asymmetry is unpredictable from patient to patient.

The dominant side for venous drainage is generally chosen and so must first be determined. Transient manual compression of a dominant IJV leads to a greater rise in ICP compared with the non-dominant side. Alternatively, ultrasonography of internal jugular flow or CT determination of the larger jugular foramen have also been suggested. The dominant system is usually the right, and this offers an alternative pragmatic solution where better information is not available.

Catheter position is important if the measurements are to be reliable and robust. In particular, if the catheter tip is too caudal, significant error may occur as a result of admixture with extracranial blood from the facial vein: a 2 cm displacement may result in up to 10% contamination. Thus, once the catheter has been placed and secured, its position should be confirmed with an anteroposterior (AP) radiograph or appropriately penetrated lateral film. The catheter tip is usually positioned cephalad of the level of the inferior border of C1 on the lateral view. CT studies suggest that the tip is optimally placed if it is cephalad of both a line connecting the tips of the mastoid processes and of the level of the atlanto-occipital joint but caudal to the transverse plane through the level of the inferior margin of the orbit on the AP view (Fig. 6.4).

Clinical applications

Monitoring of cerebral oxygenation in critical care

Jugular venous saturation below 50% suggests a relative failure of oxygen supply compared with demand,

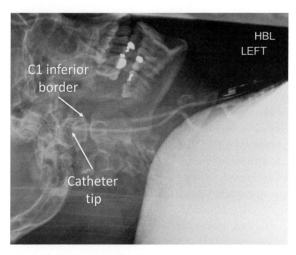

Fig. 6.4. Lateral radiograph of the cervical spine showing a jugular bulb catheter positioned with its tip cephalad to the inferior border of the first cervical (C1) vertebra.

and such episodes have been demonstrated to predict poor outcome after head injury in a dose-dependent way. Low SjO_2 is often seen in comatose patients with head injuries or subarachnoid haemorrhage, even when therapy is guided by invasive haemodynamic and ICP monitoring. Jugular venous desaturation can be observed to occur before or without changes in measured CPP. Furthermore, desaturation events are particularly common in the first days after head injury and are usually secondary to poor perfusion secondary to hypotension or hypocapnic vasoconstriction, suggesting that it might be a meaningful parameter to use when targeting cardiovascular and respiratory support in the emergency setting.

Conversely, values of SjO_2 >85% suggest a state of hyperaemia (for example secondary to hypercapnia) or failing oxygen utilization either due to a state of cellular dysoxia or due to shunting of arterial blood, which may also be associated with a poor outcome.

From the above, it would appear that jugular venous saturation measurement is a specific indicator of imbalance between oxygen supply and demand with at least prognostic significance. Unfortunately, false-positive desaturations are common. Moreover, it is by its very nature a global, hemispheric measure and thus may have poor sensitivity under certain circumstances. Focal areas of ischaemia are not reliably detected, SjO_2 remaining normal until 13% of the brain becomes ischaemic. Indeed, regions of shunt from infarcted tissue may mask the effect of surrounding ischaemic areas leading to falsely reassuring values of SjO_2.

Jugular bulb oximetry has been used to guide hyperventilation therapy in acute intracranial hypertension. Excessive hypocapnia is associated with a global reduction in CBF that may be harmful. Under such circumstances, cerebral oxygen supply falls and this should be detected as a fall in SjO_2. However, a normal SjO_2 may be falsely reassuring, as regional hypoperfusion may be present but not detected.

Jugular bulb oximetry can be used to detect disorders of both cerebral autoregulation and carbon dioxide reactivity. Assuming a constant $CMRO_2$, SjO_2 is expected to rise in response to transient increases in cerebral perfusion. Fortune and colleagues studied a group of head-injured patients and identified instances where the rise in SjO_2 due to hyperaemia persisted significantly beyond the perfusion returning to baseline, suggesting a disturbance of vasoconstriction in these cases. By measuring the response of $AVDO_2$ to blood pressure manipulation and changes in arterial carbon dioxide tension ($PaCO_2$), Sahuquillo and colleagues demonstrated that jugular venous oximetry could be used to differentiate between autoregulatory dysfunction and failed carbon dioxide reactivity, which may occur independently.

Failure of oxygen delivery, as evidenced by a fall in jugular venous oxygenation, is at best a measure of global tissue hypoxia. In failure of the aerobic metabolism, cerebral lactic acid production is increased, which can be used as an additional measure of cerebral oxygenation. If blood is sampled from the jugular bulb, an arteriovenous lactate difference (AVDL) can be determined by comparison with arterial blood. The lactate oxygen index (LOI), which relates lactate production to oxygen extraction, is calculated as:

$$LOI = -AVDL/AVDO_2$$

Patients with failing oxygen extraction typically have values of LOI >0.08. Cerebral lactate production is markedly increased in the first 24 h after head injury, with both AVDL and LOI having prognostic significance, even when oxygen extraction, derived from SaO_2 and SjO_2 measurements, remained apparently normal. It is noteworthy that the LOI implicitly depends on haemoglobin concentration (through $AVDO_2$), which may lead to falsely high values in anaemia.

Intraoperative monitoring

It has been shown that jugular venous desaturation occurs on average in 50% of patients undergoing a

Table 6.1 Factors determining jugular venous oxygen saturation

Decreased SjO$_2$ (relative hypoxia)	Increased SjO$_2$ (relative hyperaemia)
Abnormal autoregulation	**Abnormal autoregulation**
Reduced oxygen delivery	Increased oxygen delivery
• Inadequate cerebral perfusion pressure	• Increasing cerebral perfusion pressure
• Vasoconstriction/hypocapnia	• Vasodilation/hypercapnia
• Vasospasm	• Systemic hypertension
• Arterial hypoxia	• Arteriovenous malformations
• Hypotension	
• Anaemia/haemoglobinopathy	
• Sepsis	
Increased oxygen consumption	Reduced oxygen consumption
• Increasing cerebral metabolism	• Coma/sedative drugs
• Hyperthermia	• Hypothermia
• Pain/inadequate analgesia	• Cerebral infarction
• Light anaesthesia/stimulation	• Brain death
• Seizures	

variety of neurosurgical procedures (with a higher incidence in patients undergoing aneurysm repair or with intracranial haematomas). In a study by Matta *et al.* (1994), it was demonstrated that, although severe desaturation was substantially less common, such episodes of relative hypoperfusion would not have been detectable with normal monitoring alone.

Cerebral oxygenation has been studied by jugular bulb cannulation during aneurysm clipping surgery. It was demonstrated that many patients exhibit a critical threshold for mean arterial pressure below which SjO$_2$ falls. This was a more common finding in patients in which aneurysm rupture had occurred acutely, suggesting a state of altered autoregulation. However, a normal SjO$_2$ did not exclude an elevated LOI, as significant regional ischaemia may not have been detected. Furthermore, elevation of the LOI was found to be a predictor of poor short-term (although not long-term) outcome.

Cardiac surgery

Neurological injury is unfortunately not uncommon after cardiopulmonary bypass (CPB) and is believed to be a result of inadequate oxygen supply secondary to either microembolism or hypoperfusion. It seems reasonable to suppose that a measure of cerebral oxygenation such as jugular bulb oximetry might be useful in the timely detection and hopefully prevention of damaging events. A correlation between jugular venous desaturation and poor post-operative cognitive outcome has been demonstrated, as has the fact that cerebral hypoperfusion that was diagnosed by oximetry could not have been detected by conventional intraoperative parameters alone.

It has been known for some time that jugular venous saturations are typically well maintained during hypothermic CPB, even in the presence of hypotension, as CMRO$_2$ may be very much reduced compared with oxygen supply. Rewarming is, however, a much higher risk period for SjO$_2$ desaturation, particularly when normothermia is rapidly restored, whereupon oxygen consumption rises quickly in the face of a potentially disturbed cerebral autoregulation mechanism. By comparison, oxygen extraction during normothermic CPB tends to be higher, with jugular venous desaturation episodes occurring soon after establishing bypass, reflecting the effects of haemodilution or hypotension, which may, to some extent, be ameliorated by careful anaesthetic technique.

Cardiac arrest

Jugular venous saturation has been studied as a potential prognostic marker in comatose patients in which spontaneous circulation has been restored after cardiac arrest (Table 6.1). Measured SjO$_2$ is not normally low in these patients except under circumstances of cardiovascular failure when mixed venous oxygen saturation ($SmvO_2$) also falls. However, in non-survivors, a gradual increase in SjO_2 compared with $S_{mv}O_2$ is observed over the first 24 h after resuscitation, suggesting a progressive global failure of cerebral oxygen extraction. A SjO_2 becoming greater than mixed venous oxygen saturation at 24 h appears to have reasonable specificity for mortality. A ratio of SjO_2 to $S_{mv}O_2$ of >1 is similarly seen in brain death after severe head injury or intracranial haemorrhage.

Near-infrared spectroscopy

Biological tissues contain a number of light-absorbing pigments known as chromophores such as haemoglobin, myoglobin and cytochrome oxidase, which have absorption spectra that depend on their redox state. It so happens that these changes are reasonably pronounced in the near-infrared part of the electromagnetic spectrum (700–1000 nm) where absorption from skin and bone is low. Such light can thus penetrate several centimetres through scalp and skull to non-invasively probe brain tissue. By measuring optical absorption at several wavelengths, relative tissue chromophore concentrations can be inferred in real time and this forms the basis of near-infrared spectroscopy (NIRS) as a method for measuring regional cerebral oxygenation (Fig. 6.5).

Physical principles

The intensity of light passing through an ideal absorbing medium varies with the chromophore concentration and path length according to the well-known Beer–Lambert law. In principle then, it is possible to measure the concentration of a single chromophore from the optical absorption at a suitable wavelength. Where a mixture of different chromophores is present,

it is necessary to perform absorption measurements at a number of different wavelengths. As the dominant cerebral chromophores, oxygenated and deoxygenated haemoglobin (HbO_2 and HHb), have markedly different near-infrared absorption spectra, it is possible to infer the blood oxygenation status. As approximately 75% of cerebral blood is venous, NIRS oximetry gives a measure of predominantly venous oxygenation, which therefore reflects oxygen extraction.

In practice, the physics of light transport in biological tissue is more complex. Tissue is turbid so that light is attenuated not just by absorption but also by scattering. The Beer–Lambert law must be modified to include both absorption and scattering terms, as in the following equation, which complicates the interpretation of spectroscopic data:

$$\text{Optical density} = \log (I_0/I) = (\alpha \times c \times d \times B) + G$$

where I_0 is the source intensity, I is the detected light intensity, α is the absorption coefficient of the chromophore (a function of wavelength), c is the chromophore concentration, d is the distance between the source and the detector, B is the differential path length (discussed below) and G is a scattering term, which depends on optical geometry and tissue characteristics.

Although the existence of scattering introduces additional complexity, it is useful clinically, as the adult cranium has a diameter too great even for infrared light to penetrate, making direct transillumination measurements impossible. However, by measuring the intensity of the back-scattered light instead, spectroscopy can be performed in a 'reflection' mode with the light source and detector ('optodes') applied to the scalp some 4–7 cm apart.

Multiply scattered photons do not travel directly from source to detector. Instead, they migrate randomly

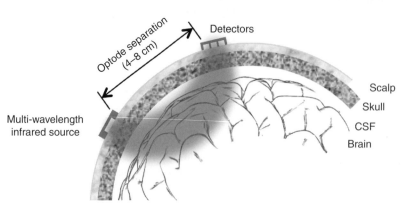

Fig. 6.5. Schematic diagram of a typical near-infrared spectroscopy system. Two optodes are applied to the scalp away from large venous sinuses. The emitter can be switched sequentially between three or four infrared light sources of different wavelengths. Scattering causes light to diffuse randomly through scalp, skull, cerebrospinal fluid and brain tissues such that what arrives at the detector has passed through a 'banana-shaped' region. The penetration depth is proportional to the optode separation. The detector consists of an array of several photodiodes with different optode separations, an arrangement that allows the scattering contribution to be estimated.

through an unknown volume of tissue before being detected, so that the actual path length is ill-defined. Therefore, an average path length must be assumed that is rather longer than the optode separation. This effective path length is given by the source–detector separation multiplied by a scaling parameter called the differential path-length factor, which must previously be estimated from experiments.

Signal contamination by unwanted optical attenuation in extracerebral tissue is an important limitation of NIRS. Even if the optodes are positioned away from large venous sinuses, the light must necessarily traverse superficial tissue such as the scalp, whose blood content and oxygenation state are not necessarily constant and which may contain other oxygen-sensitive chromophores such as myoglobin. This may seriously affect the clinical reliability of the technique as a measure of cerebral oxygenation. Optical diffusion means that effectively a 'banana-shaped' volume between optodes is sampled, the depth of penetration being related to the optode separation. Thus, if the source and detector are <4 cm apart, virtually only extracerebral tissue is sampled. Larger separations sample increasingly deep tissues, albeit at the expense of signal intensity and thus increasing noise. Even at 7 cm spacing, extracerebral contamination may be appreciable. By measuring at two different detector positions simultaneously, however, it is possible to at least approximately subtract the superficial tissue component.

It is difficult to measure absolute chromophore concentrations spectroscopically as the scattering term, G in the above equation, is unknown. However, if the scattering is constant then the above equation can be used to relate *changes* in absorption to corresponding *changes* in HbO_2 and HHb (termed ΔHbO_2 and ΔHHb, respectively) from an arbitrary baseline as the parameter G cancels out. This technique is known as differential NIRS.

More recently, a method known as spatially resolved NIRS has been described, which allows the absolute haemoglobin saturation to be measured. This technique employs a multiple-wavelength source and a probe containing several detectors at different path lengths. The scattering contribution is then estimated using photon diffusion theory. The derived ratio of HbO_2 to total Hb ($Hb + HbO_2$) is presented as a tissue oxygenation index (TOI) or regional oxygenation saturation (rSO_2), which have similar utility.

The technique of NIRS can be used as a monitor of cerebral blood volume (CBV) as this is related to total haemoglobin concentration if the haematocrit is constant. Trends in CBV from an arbitrary baseline are then simply proportional to trends in total haemoglobin signal ($\Delta HbO_2 + \Delta HHb$). Alternatively, spatially resolved NIRS can be used to calculate the tissue haemoglobin index (THI), which is a measure (in arbitrary units) of the total haemoglobin in the optically sampled region. Direct estimation of CBV itself is also possible by measuring ΔHbO_2 and ΔHHb after an artificially induced small change in arterial saturation (for example, by varying the inspired oxygen concentration).

In addition to haemoglobin species, cytochrome oxidase has a near-infrared absorbance that changes with redox state. Cytochrome oxidase has a key role in transferring electrons to the terminal electron acceptor, oxygen, within the mitochondrial respiratory chain. Cytochrome oxidase comprises four metal centres (heme a, heme b, Cu_a and Cu_b). The Cu_a centre is responsible for the infrared spectral characteristics of the molecule and is of particular interest. Its dimeric Cu–Cu form facilitates the transfer of electrons from cytochrome c to heme a. Thus, the average Cu_a redox state reflects differences in the rates of electrons arriving and leaving. This may become perturbed if oxygen supply becomes metabolically limiting. Because changes in Cu_a redox state result in changes in near-infrared absorption, in principle cytochrome oxidase NIRS offers a method for probing mitochondrial energy failure. Commercial instruments are now capable of measuring deviations of cytochrome oxidase concentrations from baseline, but such measurements remain controversial. Unfortunately, while the absorption spectra for HHb and HbO_2 are very different, reduction of cytochrome oxidase only influences absorption in a narrow absorption band. Additionally, the total contribution of Cu_a absorption to the total NIRS absorption is very small, making it difficult to separate from the haemoglobin signal.

Clinical applications

A number of studies have investigated NIRS in patients with carotid occlusive disease. Vernieri and colleagues used NIRS to measure cerebral carbon dioxide reactivity and found differences between symptomatic and asymptomatic patients. Intraoperative NIRS during carotid endarterectomy demonstrated cerebral desaturation in 50% of patients after internal carotid artery cross-clamping. Cerebral oxygen saturation has been found to correlate with transcranial Doppler blood flow, EEG and clinical evidence of ischaemia. Sensitivity and specificity vary between studies but may potentially be high: a drop in TOI >13% has been suggested as a threshold for ischaemia.

Use of NIRS to monitor patients with traumatic brain injury has shown similar changes with oxygenation status to other monitoring modalities. However, Kirkpatrick and colleagues showed that NIRS was able to detect 97% of cerebral hypoperfusion events compared with only 53% detected by jugular bulb oximetry. A small study has shown a correlation between TOI and CPP. Tissue saturation >75% was usual when CPP was > 70 mmHg. Conversely, TOI < 55% was typically associated with CPP < 70 mmHg.

The method of NIRS brain oximetry has been evaluated for preventing cerebral injury during cardiac surgery. The influence of hypothermia, alkalosis and the extracorporeal circulation on the NIRS algorithms is unclear. While episodes of cerebral desaturation correlate with poor neurological outcome, comparisons with SjO_2 monitoring have yielded mixed results. This perhaps serves to emphasize that these approaches to cerebral oxygenation measurement are fundamentally distinct and consequently may respond differently in certain circumstances.

Extracerebral signal contamination, changes in the optical properties of injured tissue and the local nature of the technique are all limitations of NIRS as a mature monitoring technology. However, its completely non-invasive nature, portability, real-time temporal resolution and relatively low cost make the technique promising.

Brain tissue oxygen measurement

The flux of oxygen through the extracellular compartment arises from a concentration gradient that is maintained by a balance between supply at the capillaries and consumption within the cells. The average extracellular oxygen tension, therefore, reflects this source–sink equilibrium as well as the nature of the diffusion barrier. Direct measurement of brain tissue oxygenation ($PbrO_2$) at the bedside is now possible with microsensors introduced directly into the cerebral parenchyma either through a bolt or tunnelled from a craniotomy site.

Technology

The LICOX sensor is a miniature electrochemical sensor based on the Clark polarographic cell. It is contained in a flexible polyethylene microcatheter and has a diameter of <1 mm with a sensitive region approximately 5 mm in length. Oxygen from brain tissue within a few millimetres from the device diffuses into the sensor cell where it accepts electrons on a charged catalytic surface generating an electric current in proportion to the dissolved oxygen tension. Temperature compensation is achieved in the most recent generation of devices by means of an integral sensor, which also allows the instrument to display brain temperature. The device does not require calibration, but results may be unreliable for the first 2 h after insertion as a result of microtrauma in the region immediately adjacent to the surface of the sensor.

Of historical interest is the NeuroTrend monitor, which was able to simultaneously measure $PbrO_2$, $PbrCO_2$ and brain tissue pH using a bundle of optical fibre sensors. While this monitor is no longer available commercially, a substantial body of research has previously been published using this technology. However, differences in probe geometry mean that absolute comparisons between LICOX and NeuroTrend $PbrO_2$ measurements should be made with caution.

Clinical practice

In health, tissue oxygen tension varies considerably with position depending on local brain activation as well as neuronal and blood vessel density. Measurements are usually made from white matter, which has lower and more stable $PbrO_2$. Sensor site selection is not a clear-cut decision, particularly where brain injury is extensive or multifocal. With focal brain lesions, two approaches are common. Measurements made in the contralateral hemisphere (or in the less-injured hemisphere) attempt to characterize the oxygenation state of non-contused brain, and such values of $PbrO_2$ correlate well with SjO_2 measurements. Alternatively, the sensor may be placed in perilesional tissue in order to directly optimize oxygenation of this 'at-risk' tissue where $PbrO_2$ is typically lower. Placement of the device within either infarcted tissue or a haematoma is clearly unhelpful.

Clinical experience to date with direct tissue oxygen sensors has mainly been accrued from patients either with severe traumatic brain injuries or undergoing cerebrovascular surgery. Measured values of $PbrO_2$ are accurate to within about 10%, and values of around 22 mmHg are typical in health. This is much lower than the oxygen tension of arterial blood, reflecting the high metabolic requirements of cerebral tissue. Thresholds for ischaemia are not yet clearly defined, but a $PbrO_2$ of <8–10 mmHg seems to indicate a high risk of ischaemia in patients with subarachnoid haemorrhage. Low values of $PbrO_2$, particularly if they are sustained, are associated with poor outcome after traumatic brain injury, and there is some evidence that brain tissue oxygen-directed therapy may improve outcome in such patients.

Similarly to jugular bulb oximetry and NIRS, measurements of $PbrO_2$ are expected to reflect supply–demand imbalances of oxygen. Comparison with positron emission tomography has demonstrated that changes in $PbrO_2$ correlate well with changes in local venous oxygen tension. However, it is also observed that the absolute value of $PbrO_2$ is consistently lower than local venous oxygen tension by an amount that varies from patient to patient. This is unsurprising as the sensor measures an average oxygen tension over a volume containing regions of oxygen supply, diffusion and consumption. For a given oxygen flux, the extracellular oxygen concentration may also be affected by tissue and endothelial oedema, which reduce the facility with which oxygen can diffuse across this barrier. Thus, brain tissue oxygen measurements are sensitive to the properties of a tissue compartment to which NIRS and jugular bulb oximetry do not have access but which may be physiologically highly relevant.

In contrast to $PbrO_2$, measured $PbrCO_2$ (40–70 mmHg) is higher than that of the arterial blood, thus providing a concentration gradient favouring the elimination of this highly diffusible metabolic product. Brain tissue pH is typically in the range of 7.05–7.25, again predictably lower than that of arterial blood. These parameters may have some prognostic significance. It seems that the risk of vasospasm is increased in patients with cerebrovascular disease if the pH is <7.0 and $PbrCO_2$ is >60 mmHg. Mortality after severe traumatic brain injury is increased in tissue acidosis when the pH is below 7.0 (Figs 6.6 and 6.7).

Conclusions

The need to maintaining a cerebral oxygen supply sufficient for the metabolic requirements is axiomatic to strategies for cerebral protection. While there is an absence of prospective evidence, it is reasonable to assume that early detection of ischaemia may improve outcome by allowing targeted instigation of corrective therapy. The techniques described aim to provide such

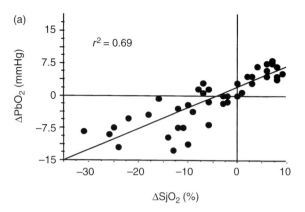
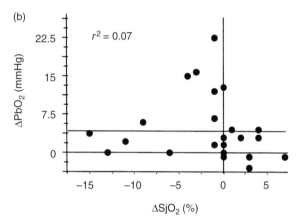

Fig. 6.6. Demonstration that the correlation between changes in jugular venous oxygen saturation (ΔSjO_2) and brain tissue oxygen pressure (ΔPbO_2) is dependent on the position of the sensor. There is good correlation when the sensor is in normal brain tissue (a) and poor correlation when the sensor is in an area of focal pathology (b). (Reproduced with permission from Valdaka et al., 1998.)

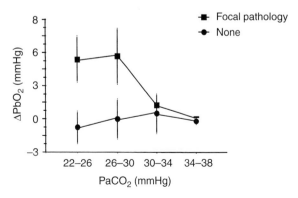

Fig. 6.7. The effect of hyperventilation on brain tissue oxygenation in areas of focal pathology and with no pathology. (Reproduced with permission from Valdaka et al., 1998.)

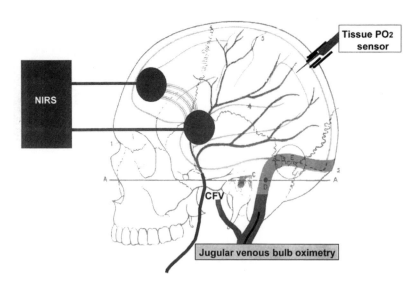

Fig. 6.8. A summary diagram showing the currently available methods for cerebral oximetry. NIRS, near-infrared spectroscopy; PO₂, oxygen pressure.

an early warning system. Although cumbersome and prone to artefact, jugular venous oximetry is the oldest technology and thus a natural benchmark against which to evaluate newer systems. However, it is prone to false positives and is a fundamentally global measure, which also limits its sensitivity. The techniques of NIRS and tissue oxygen measurement are more local probes, but there may be circumstances where this is not necessarily advantageous either: NIRS has a number of other very attractive features but is less well quantified and extracranial signal contamination is a limitation. Experience with brain tissue oxygenation microsensors is increasing and clearly these provide a very direct measurement of tissue metabolism, but their invasive nature precludes their use outside specialist neuroscience centres. To some extent, all these technologies are complementary because of the diversity in the principles and assumptions that underpin their operation. In view of all these strengths and limitations, it is the synthesis of data from multiple modalities that hopefully allows timely and targeted therapy (Fig. 6.8).

Further reading

Al-Rawi, P. G. and Kirkpatrick, P. J. (2006). Tissue oxygenation thresholds for cerebral ischemia using near-infrared spectroscopy. *Stroke* **37**, 2720–5.

Al-Rawi, P. G., Smielewski, P. and Kirkpatrick, P. J. (2001). Evaluation of a near-infrared spectrometer (NIRO300) for the detection of intracranial oxygenation changes in the adult head. *Stroke* **32**, 2492–500.

Andrews, P. J. D., Dearden, N. M. and Miller, J. D. (1991). Jugular bulb cannulation: description of a cannulation technique and a validation of a new continuous monitor. *Brit J Anaesth* **67**, 553–8.

Bankier, A. A., Fleischmann, D., Windisch, A. *et al.* (1995). Position of jugular oxygen saturation catheter in patients with head trauma: assessment by use of plain films. *Am J Roentgenol* **164**, 437–41.

Buunk, G., van der Hoeven, J. G. and Meinders, A. E. (1999). Prognostic significance of the difference between mixed venous and jugular bulb oxygen saturation in comatose patients resuscitated from a cardiac arrest. *Resuscitation* **41**, 257–62.

Charbel, F. T., Du, X., Hoffman, W. E. and Ausman, J. I. (2000). Brain tissue PO₂, PCO₂ and pH during cerebral vasospasm. *J Neurosurg* **97**, 1302–5.

Chieregato, A., Calzolari, F., Trasforini, G., Targa, L. and Latronico, N. (2003). Normal jugular bulb oxygenation saturation. *J Neurol Neurosurg Psychiatry* **74**, 784–6.

Coles, J. P., Minhas, P. S., Fryer, T. D. *et al.* (2002). Effect of hyperventilation on cerebral blood flow in traumatic head injury: clinical relevance and monitoring correlates. *Crit Care Med* **30**, 1950–9.

Coles, J. P., Fryer, T. D., Smielewski, P. *et al.* (2004). Incidence and mechanisms of cerebral ischemia in early clinical head injury. *J Cereb Blood Flow Metab*, **24**, 233–8.

Coplin, W. M., O' Keefe, G. E., Grady, M. S. *et al.* (1997). Thrombotic, infectious, and procedural complications of the jugular bulb catheter in the intensive care unit. *Neurosurgery* **41**, 101–7.

Croughwell, N. D., White, W. D., Smith, L. R. *et al.* (1995). Jugular bulb saturation and mixed venous saturation during cardiopulmonary bypass. *J Card Surg* **10** (Supplement), 503–8.

De Deyne, C., Vandekerckhove, T., Decruyenaere, J. and Colardyn, F. (1996). Analysis of abnormal jugular bulb oxygen saturation data in patients with severe head injury. *Acta Neurochi* **138**, 1409–15.

Delpy, D. T. and Cope, M. (1997). Quantification in tissue near-infrared spectroscopy. *Philos Trans R Soc Lond B Biol Sci*, **352**, 649–59.

Díaz-Regañón, G., Miñambres, E., Holanda, M. *et al.* (2002). Usefulness of venous oxygen saturation in the jugular bulb for the diagnosis of brain death: report of 118 patients. *Intensive Care Med* **28**, 1724–8.

Duncan, A., Meek, J. H., Clemence, M. *et al.* (1995). Optical pathlength measurement on adult head, calf, forearm and the head of the newborn infant using phase resolved optical spectroscopy. *Phys Med Biol* **40**, 295–304.

Dunham, C. M., Sosnowski, C., Porter, J. M., Siegal, J. and Kohli, C. (2002). Correlation of noninvasive cerebral oximetry with cerebral perfusion in the severe head injured patient: a pilot study. *J Trauma* **52**, 40–6.

Elwell, C. E., Cope, M., Edwards, A. D. *et al.* (1994). Quantification of adult cerebral hemodynamics by near-infrared spectroscopy. *J Appl Physiol* **77**, 2753–60.

Fortune, J. B., Feustel, P. J., Weigle, C. G. and Popp, A. J. (1994). Continuous measurement of jugular venous oxygen saturation in response to transient elevations of blood pressure in head-injured patients. *J Neurosurg* **80**, 461–8.

Gagnon, R. E., Macnab, A. J., Gagnon, F. A., Blackstock, D. and LeBlanc, J. G. (2002). Comparison of two spatially resolved NIRS oxygenation indices. *J Clin Monit Comput* **17**, 385–91.

Germon, T. J., Kane, N. M., Manara, A. R. and Nelson, R. J. (1994). Near-infrared spectroscopy in adults: effects of extracranial ischaemia and intracranial hypoxia on estimation of cerebral oxygenation. *Br J Anaesth* **73**, 503–6.

Gibbs, E. L., Lennox, W. G., Nims, L. F. and Gibbs, F. A. (1942). Arterial and cerebral blood. Arterial–venous differences in man. *J Biol Chem*, **144**, 325–32.

Goetting, M. G. and Preston, G. (1991). Jugular bulb catheterization does not increase intracranial pressure. *Intensive Care Med* **17**, 195–8.

Gupta, A. K., Menon, D. K., Czosnyka, M. *et al.* (1997). Non-invasive measurement of cerebral blood volume in volunteers. *Br J Anaesth* **78**, 39–43.

Gupta, A. K., Hutchinson, P. J., Al-Rawi, P. *et al.* (1999). Measurement of brain tissue oxygenation compared with jugular venous oxygen saturation for monitoring cerebral oxygenation after traumatic brain injury. *Anesth Analg* **88**, 549–53.

Gupta, A. K., Hutchinson, P. J., Fryer, T. *et al.* (2002). Measurement of brain tissue oxygenation performed using positron emission tomography to validate a novel monitoring method. *J Neurosurg* **96**, 263–8.

Gupta, A. K., Zygun, D., Johnston, A. J. *et al.* (2004). Extracellular brain pH and outcome following severe traumatic brain injury. *J Neurotrauma* **21**, 678–84.

Harris, D. N., Cowans, F. M., Wertheim, D. A. and Hamid, S. (1994). NIR in adults – effect of increasing optode separation. *Adv Exp Med Biol* **345**, 837–40.

Jones, P. A., Andrews, P. J., Midgley, S. *et al.* (1994). Measuring the burden of secondary insults in head-injured patients during intensive care. *J Neurosurg Anesthesiol* **6**, 4–14.

Kett-White, R., Hutchinson, P. J., Al-Rawi, P. G. *et al.* (2002). Adverse cerebral events detected after sub-arachnoid hemorrhage using brain oxygen and microdialysis probes. *Neurosurgery* **50**, 1213–21.

Kirkpatrick, P. J., Smielewski, P., Whitfield, P. *et al.* (1995). An observational study of near infrared spectroscopy during carotid endarterectomy. *J Neurosurg* **82**, 756–63.

Kirkpatrick, P. J., Smielewski, P., Czosnyka, M., Menon, D. K. and Pickard, J. D. (1995). Near-infrared spectroscopy use in patients with head injury. *J Neurosurg* **83**, 963–70.

Lang, E. W. and Chesnut, R. M. (1999). A lesson learned from jugular venous oximetry. *J Clin Neurosci* **6**, 70–3.

Macmillan, C. S. A., Andrews, P. J. D. and Easton, V. J. (2001). Increased jugular bulb saturation is associated with poor outcome in traumatic brain injury. *J Neurol Neurosurg Psychiatry* **70**, 101–4.

Matcher, S. J., Kirkpatrick, P., Nahid, K., Cope, M. and Delpy, D. T. (1995). Absolute quantification methods in tissue near infrared spectroscopy. *Proc SPIE* **2389**, 486–95.

Matta, B. F. and Lam, A. M. (1996). The speed of blood withdrawal affects the accuracy of jugular venous bulb oxygen saturation measurements. *Anesthesiology* **86**, 806–8.

Matta, B. F., Lam, A. M., Mayberg, T. S., Shapira, Y. and Winn, H. R. (1994). A critique of the intraoperative use of jugular venous bulb catheters during neurosurgical procedures. *Anesth Analg* **79**, 45–750.

McLeod, A. D., Igielman, F., Elwell, C., Cope, M. and Smith, M. (2003). Measuring cerebral oxygenation during normobaric hyperoxia: a comparison of tissue microprobes, near-infrared spectroscopy, and jugular venous oximetry in head injury. *Anesth Analg* **97**, 851–6.

Menon, D. K., Coles, J. P., Gupta, A. K. *et al.* (2004). Diffusion limited oxygen delivery following head injury. *Crit Care Med* **32**, 1384–90.

Metz, C., Holzschuh, M., Bein, T., Kallenbach, B. and Taeger, K. (1998). Jugular bulb monitoring of cerebral oxygen metabolism in severe head injury: accuracy of unilateral measurements. *Acta Neurochi* **71** (Supplement), 324–7.

Millar, S. A., Alston, R. P., Souter, M. J. and Andrews, P. J. D. (1999). Continuous monitoring of jugular bulb oxyhaemoglobin saturation using the Edslab dual lumen oximetry catheter during and after cardiac surgery. *Br J Anaesth* **82**, 521–4.

Moss, E., Dearden, N. M. and Berridge, J. C. (1995). Effects of changes in mean arterial pressure on SjO2 during cerebral aneurysm surgery. *Br J Anaesth*, **75**, 527–30.

Murr, R., Stummer, W., Shürer, L. and Plasek, J. (1996). Cerebral lactate production in relation to intracranial pressure, cranial computed tomography findings, and outcomes in patients with severe head injury. *Acta Neurochi* **138**, 928–37.

Myerson, A., Halloran, R. D. and Hirsch, H. L. (1927). Technique for obtaining blood from the internal jugular vein and internal carotid artery. *Arch Neurol Psychiatry* **17**, 807–8.

Nakajima, T., Kuro, M., Hayashi, Y. *et al.* (1992). Clinical evaluation of cerebral oxygen balance during cardiopulmonary bypass: on-line continuous monitoring of jugular venous oxyhemoglobin saturation. *Anesth Analg* **74**, 630–5.

Pennings, F. A., Schuurman, P. R., van den Munckhof, P. and Bouma, G. J. (2008). Brain tissue oxygen pressure monitoring in awake patients during functional neurosurgery: the assessment of normal values. *J Neurotrauma*, **25**, 1173–7.

Rigamonti, A., Scandroglio, M., Minicucci, F. *et al.* (2005). A clinical evaluation of near-infrared cerebral oximetry in the awake patient to monitor cerebral perfusion during carotid endarterectomy. *J Clin Anesth* **17**, 426–30.

Robertson, C. (1993). Desaturation episodes after severe head injury: influence on outcome. *Acta Neurochi* **59** (Supplement), 98–101.

Robertson, C. S., Narayan, R. K., Gokaslan, Z. L. *et al.* (1989). Cerebral arteriovenous oxygen difference as an estimate of cerebral blood flow in comatose patients. *J Neurosurg* **70**, 222–30.

Sahuquillo, J., Poca, M. A., Ausina, A. *et al.* (1996). Arterio-jugular differences in oxygen (AVDO2) for bedside assessment of CO_2-reactivity and autoregulation in the acute phase of severe head injury. *Acta Neurochi*, **138**, 435–44.

Schneider, G. H., Helden, A. V., Lanksch, W. R. and Unterberg, A. (1995). Continuous monitoring of jugular bulb oxygen saturation in comatose

patients – therapeutic implications. *Acta Neurochir*, **134**, 71–5.

Shaaban Ali, M., Harmer, M. and Latto, I. P. (2001). Jugular bulb oximetry during cardiac surgery. *Anaesthesia* **56**, 24–37.

Sheinberg, M., Kanter, M. J., Robertson, C. S. *et al.* (1992). Continuous monitoring of jugular venous oxygen saturation in head-injured patients. *J Neurosurg* **76**, 212–17.

Shenkin, H. A., Harmel, M. H. and Kety, S. S. (1948). Dynamic anatomy of the cerebral circulation. *Arch Neurol Psychiatry* **60**, 240–52.

Stochetti, N., Paparella, A., Bridelli, F. *et al.* (1994). Cerebral venous oxygen saturation studied with bilateral samples in the internal jugular veins. *Neurosurgery* **34**, 38–44.

Souter, M. and Andrews, P. (1996). A review of jugular venous oximetry. *Intensive Care World* **13**, 32–8.

Stiefel, M. F., Spiotta, A., Gracias, V. H. *et al.* (2005). Reduced mortality rate in patients with severe traumatic brain injury treated with brain tissue oxygen monitoring. *J Neurosurg* **103**, 805–11.

Suzuki, S., Takasaki, S., Ozaki, T. and Kobayashi, Y. (1999). A tissue oxygenation monitor using NIR spatially resolved spectroscopy. *Proc SPIE* **3597**, 582–92.

Taillefer, M.-C. and Denault, A. Y. (2005). Cerebral near-infrared spectroscopy in adult heart surgery: systematic review of its clinical efficacy. *Can J Anesthesiol* **52**, 79–87.

Valdaka, A. B., Gopinath, S. P., Constant, C. F., Usura, M. and Robertson, C. S. (1998) Relationship of brain tissue PO2 to outcome after severe head injury. *Crit Care Med* **26**, 1576–81.

van den Brink, W., van Santbrink, H., Steyerberg, E. *et al.* (2000). Brain oxygen tension in severe head injury. *Neurosurgery* **46**, 868–76.

van der Hoeven, J. G., de Konig, J., Compier, E. A. and Meinders, A. E. (1995). Early jugular bulb oxygenation monitoring in comatose patients after an out-of-hospital cardiac arrest. *Intensive Care Med* **21**, 567–72.

Vernieri, F., Tibuzzi, F., Pasqualetti, P. *et al.* (2004). Transcranial Doppler and near-infrared spectroscopy can evaluate the hemodynamic effect of carotid artery occlusion. *Stroke* **35**, 64–70.

Ward, K. R., Ivatury, R. R., Wayne Barbee, R. *et al.* (2006). Near infrared spectroscopy for evaluation of the trauma patient: a technology review. *Resuscitation* **68**, 27–44.

Brain tissue biochemistry

Arnab Ghosh and Martin Smith

Introduction

Cerebral microdialysis is a well-established laboratory tool that was introduced into clinical practice in the mid 1990s. It is now widely used as a bedside monitor of brain tissue biochemistry to identify cerebral hypoxia/ischaemia and assess cellular bioenergetics after brain injury. This chapter will review the principles of cerebral microdialysis and identify its role in detecting derangements of cerebral metabolism after brain injury. The application of cerebral microdialysis in clinical management will be discussed and its potential research applications explored.

History of microdialysis

In 1966, Bito implanted dialysis sacks filled with 6% dextran into the cerebral hemispheres of dogs. The sacks were removed 10 weeks later and the fluid that they contained was analysed for levels of amino acids. This technique was extended by Delgado, who produced a system in which a solution that perfused a 'dialytode' was made immediately accessible for analysis. However, it was the pioneering work of Ungerstedt and colleagues at the Karolinska Institute in Stockholm during the 1970s that refined and developed the microdialysis technique. This group substantially improved the design and effectiveness of the microdialysis probe and collection system and used their technique to quantify monoamine levels in neural tissue.

By 1987, a microdialysis catheter suitable for implantation in the human brain had been developed, and the first clinical study, using a stereotactically inserted probe to monitor brain tissue biochemistry in a patient with Parkinson's disease, was undertaken. Shortly afterwards, the technique was used to monitor cerebral ischaemia after brain tumour surgery and in head-injured patients. Enthusiasm from these early studies led to further modification of the technology and the subsequent development of a complete system suitable for clinical use. Commercially produced microdialysis catheters and a bedside microdialysis analyser became available in 1995 (CMA Microdialysis AB, Solna, Sweden). Microdialysis is used for a variety of clinical indications, including tissue monitoring in myocutaneous flap surgery, transplant surgery and bowel anastamoses, but its application as a monitor of the processes of brain injury during neurointensive care is of particular interest.

Principles of cerebral microdialysis

The microdialysis technique is simple and is based on the principle of diffusion of water-soluble substances through a semi-permeable membrane. A microdialysis catheter consists of a thin (0.6 mm) double-lumen probe, with parallel inlet and outlet tubes, lined at its tip with a dialysis membrane (Fig. 7.1). The catheter is inserted into biological tissue, in this case the brain, and perfused with fluid that is isotonic with the tissue interstitium. The perfusate enters the microdialysis catheter via the inlet tube and its flow rate is controlled by a precise, miniature pump. Perfusate passes along the catheter to a cylindrical tip that is covered by a semi-permeable polyamide dialysis membrane across which exchange of molecules between interstitial and perfusion fluid takes place. At the distal end of the catheter, the fluid – now the microdialysate – passes via the outlet tube to a small collecting chamber, the microvial. The microvials are removed regularly, usually every hour, and placed in a bedside microdialysis monitor where the dialysate is analysed (Fig. 7.2). Samples can also be stored for later, off-line, analysis.

Diffusion drives the passage of molecules across the dialysis membrane along their concentration gradient and, because the perfusate flows and is removed

Core Topics in Neuroanaesthesia and Neurointensive Care, eds. Basil F. Matta, David K. Menon and Martin Smith. Published by Cambridge University Press. © Cambridge University Press 2011.

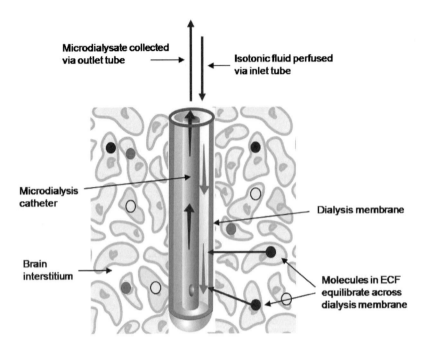

Microdialysate collected
via outlet tube

Isotonic fluid perfused
via inlet tube

Microdialysis
catheter

Dialysis membrane

Brain
interstitium

Molecules in ECF
equilibrate across
dialysis membrane

Fig. 7.1. Schematic representation of a microdialysis catheter in brain tissue. Fluid isotonic to the brain extracellular fluid (ECF) is pumped through the microdialysis catheter at a rate of 0.3 µl min^{-1}. Molecules at high concentration in the brain ECF equilibrate across the semi-permeable microdialysis membrane and can be analysed in the collected perfusate (the microdiasylate). See colour plate section. (Reproduced with permission from Tisdall and Smith, 2006. *Brit J Anaesth* **97**, 18–25.)

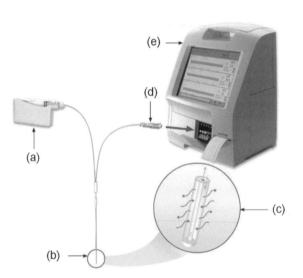

Fig. 7.2. Components of a clinical microdialysis system: (a) microdialysis pump; (b) microdialysis catheter; (c) microdialysis catheter tip showing exchange of molecules across the dialysis membrane; (d) microvial for collection of the microdialysate; (e) bedside analyser. See colour plate section. (Reproduced with permission from CMA Microdialysis AB, Solna, Sweden.)

Recovery

It is immediately apparent that, unless there is total equilibration between the perfusate and brain ECF, the concentration of a given molecule in the dialysate will be lower than its concentration in the ECF. The relationship between dialysate and ECF concentrations is termed the relative recovery and is defined as the dialysate/interstitial concentration ratio expressed as a percentage:

$$\text{Relative recovery} = \frac{[\text{dialysate}]}{[\text{ECF}]}$$

where [dialysate] is the dialysate concentration and [ECF] is the tissue interstitium concentration.

There are several important factors that determine the recovery and therefore the concentration of sampled substance in the dialysate:

1. *Membrane pore size*. The molecular weight of sampled molecules is limited by the pore size of the dialysis membrane, i.e. by its molecular weight 'cut-off' size. Catheters with molecular weight cut-off sizes of 20 kDa (CMA 70; CMA Microdialysis AB) and 100 kDa (CMA 71; CMA Microdialysis AB) are commercially available and have comparable recovery of the variables commonly measured at the bedside making them both suitable for routine clinical use. Catheters with a 100 kDa cut-off size

at a constant rate, the concentration gradient is maintained. The concentration of substances in the dialysate will depend on the balance between substrate delivery to, and uptake from, the brain extracellular fluid (ECF) but also on several other factors that are described in the following section.

also allow sampling of macromolecules such as cytokines and other proteins, and are widely used for research purposes.

2. *Membrane surface area*. Relative recovery also increases in proportion to the area of the dialysis membrane. Commercially available catheters are a standard 0.6 mm in diameter, so membrane area is determined by catheter length. Those designed for use in the brain are usually 10 mm long.

3. *Perfusate flow rate*. A lower perfusion fluid flow rate allows a greater chance for equilibration of substances across the dialysis membrane and a higher recovery. This is not a linear relationship, as the curve flattens with higher flow rates. The standard flow rate is 0.3 μl min^{-1} and this allows hourly sampling with good recovery rates, typically around 70% for commonly measured substances. Such an arrangement is generally sufficient for clinical monitoring on the neurointensive care unit, but there are circumstances, such as intraoperative monitoring, where increased temporal resolution is required. Flow rates of up to 1.0 μl min^{-1} allow more frequent sampling but at the expense of a recovery of only 30%.

4. *Diffusion speed of the substance being analysed.* The diffusion rate of a substance in the interstitial tissue varies with its molecular weight and also with the properties of the interstitium. Relative recovery therefore varies between tissues and also changes within a given tissue depending on its pathophysiological state, for example if brain oedema is present. The issues relating to diffusion rates are insignificant during routine clinical monitoring but are clearly of relevance in drug studies when microdialysis is being used to quantify pharmacokinetics.

Although microdialysis does not provide an absolute concentration of measured biochemical variables, the clinical benefits of establishing absolute tissue concentrations are limited, as it is the temporal changes in tissue biochemistry that are of importance. However, when comparing results between patients and between clinical studies, it is necessary to understand exactly what sampling methods and materials have been used in order to account for the confounding effects of different recovery rates. In clinical practice in the neurointensive care unit, the most commonly used system comprises a 10 mm catheter (0.6 mm diameter) with a 20 or 100 kDa molecular weight cut-off, perfused with commercially available perfusate solution (Perfusion Fluid CNS; CMA Microdialysis AB) at 0.3 μl min^{-1}. The combination of the relatively large dialysis membrane area and slow perfusion rate in this system provides a relative recovery of 70% for bedside measured variables.

Catheter insertion

The microdialysis catheter can be introduced under direct vision during craniotomy or via a cranial access device. The open technique allows accurate catheter placement at a particular site, but a cranial access device has the advantage of allowing the microdialysis catheter to be inserted at the bedside. A multilumen access device allows simultaneous insertion of several monitoring probes, such as those for intracranial pressure (ICP), brain tissue oxygen tension (PbrO$_2$) and microdialysis, through the same burr hole. Microdialysis catheters have a small incorporated gold tip that allows their position to be confirmed using CT (Fig. 7.3).

Catheter location

Microdialysis is a regional monitoring technique that characterizes local tissue biochemistry. Selection of the correct site for monitoring is therefore crucial. There is marked heterogeneity of metabolic and blood flow

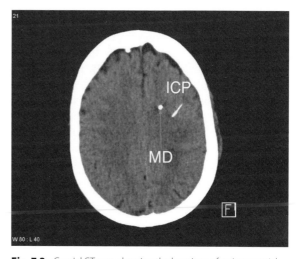

Fig. 7.3. Cranial CT scan showing the locations of an intracranial pressure monitor (ICP) and microdialysis catheter (MD). Microdialysis catheters have a small incorporated gold tip allowing their position to be clearly identified on a CT scan. See colour plate section.

disturbances in the injured brain, and many studies have shown that brain tissue at risk of secondary injury, and therefore presumably with the greatest potential for salvage, should be monitored. In 2004, a conference of clinical microdialysis experts reached a consensus on the clinical indications for microdialysis and on catheter placement. This group recommended that in traumatic brain injury (TBI), the microdialysis catheter should be located in 'at-risk' pericontusional tissue and that, if there is the option for placement of a second catheter, this should be located in 'normal' tissue. Probe placement within contusions was agreed to be of no value, as only neurochemical disturbances indicative of irreversible tissue damage are revealed. In diffuse axonal injury, the catheter should be placed in the right frontal lobe on the grounds of practicality and cortical ineloquence. In aneurysmal subarachnoid haemorrhage (SAH), the microdialysis catheter should be located where possible in the vascular territory of the parent vessel of the ruptured aneurysm, as this is the area of brain most susceptible to vasospasm-related ischaemic injury.

Another issue is whether microdialysis catheters should be placed in grey or white matter. Although there is substantial evidence that ischaemia generates differential changes in microdialysis variables in these two locations, it makes most sense to place the catheters in the metabolically active grey matter. Practically, this is of course also the most straightforward.

Perfusion fluid

The perfusate solution should be isosmolar with the tissue interstitium and contain adequate levels of cations, in particular Na^+, K^+, Ca^{2+} and Mg^{2+}, to prevent depletion from surrounding tissue. Ideally, it should also have a low protein content to facilitate high-performance liquid chromatographic analysis of the dialysate (for research indications) without the need for prior deproteinization. Suitable perfusion fluids include Ringer's solution and commercially available artificial cerebrospinal fluid (CSF) preparations (Perfusion Fluid CNS; CMA Microdialysis AB).

Bedside analysis

As catheter insertion inevitably causes some local tissue damage, markers of cellular metabolism and distress may be artificially high shortly after insertion. There is therefore a period of unreliable biochemical values for at least 1 h after insertion, and clinical

monitoring should not begin until after this 'run-in' period. There is also recent evidence confirming the presence of a local inflammatory response, demonstrated by increased levels of interleukin (IL)-1β and IL-6, after catheter insertion but the significance of this is, as yet, unknown.

Microdialysis samples are typically collected at hourly intervals at the bedside and analysed using commercially available monitors (CMA 600 or ISCUS series; CMA Microdialysis AB). These incorporate enzymatic reagents and colorimetric measurement for the analysis of glucose, pyruvate, lactate, glycerol and glutamate. The latest generation of bedside analysers, the ISCUS[flex] (CMA Microdialysis AB), was introduced in 2008. It uses similar technology to its predecessors but is substantially smaller, has batch processing capability, and permits monitoring and data display on up to eight patients simultaneously. Following bedside analysis, dialysate can be stored prior to remote off-site analysis for an infinite range of substrates using enzyme spectrophotometry and high-performance liquid chromatography.

Specially designed software allows microdialysis analysers to be interfaced with other monitoring systems so that temporal changes in physiological and biochemical data can be displayed simultaneously on most intensive care unit monitoring systems.

Complications of microdialysis

As microdialysis is an invasive technique, there is the possibility of insertion-related complications. However, these are rare. One group reported small intracerebral blood collections (<1 ml) around the catheter in 3% of 122 microdialysis catheter insertions, but these did not affect the functioning of the catheters and were clinically irrelevant. Another group, reporting microdialysis monitoring in over 400 patients, many with multiple catheter insertions, also identified no serious side effects and no episodes of catheter-related infection.

The tissue reaction to long-term microdialysis catheter placement has been studied in animals and, as in clinical studies, occasional small haemorrhages are evident around the probe within the first 2 days. By day 3, a local astrogliotic reaction with macrophage infiltration has developed, and by day 14, layers of reticulin-positive fibres surround the dialysis membrane. Similar changes in the human brain are likely to be less intense because, unlike in animal experiments, catheters are inserted under sterile conditions. In any

Table 7.1 Normal values of commonly measured biochemical markers

Microdialysate concentration	Normal value + SD[a]	Normal value + SD[b]
Glucose (mmol l^{-1})	1.7 + 0.9	2.1 + 0.2
Lactate (mmol l^{-1})	2.9 + 0.9	3.1 + 0.3
Pyruvate (µmol l^{-1})	166 + 47	151 + 12
Lactate:pyruvate ratio	23 + 4	19 + 2
Glycerol (µmol l^{-1})	82 + 44	82 + 12
Glutamate (µmol l^{-1})	16 + 16	14.0 + 3.3

[a] Reinstrup and colleagues placed microdialysis catheters in unaffected frontal lobes of patients undergoing craniotomy for benign posterior fossa lesions and quantified 'normal' values from dialysate samples collected in the post-operative period.
[b] Schulz and colleagues identified 'normal' metabolite concentrations in samples collected from microdialysis catheters sited in areas of cortex with no clinical or radiological evidence of ischaemia in patients with aneurysmal subarachnoid haemorrhage.

Table 7.2 Biochemical markers of brain injury

Microdialysis variable	Biomarker for	Comments
Low glucose	Hypoxia/ischaemia Reduced cerebral glucose supply Cerebral hyperglycolysis	Interpret in association with serum glucose concentration
Increased lactate/pyruvate ratio	Hypoxia/ischaemia Cellular redox state Reduced cerebral glucose supply Impairment of glycolytic pathway	Most reliable biomarker of hypoxia/ischaemia Independent of catheter recovery
Increased glycerol	Hypoxia/ischaemia Cell membrane degradation	Increased glycerol in brain extracellular fluid may also occur due to spillover from systemic glycerol
Increased glutamate	Hypoxia/ischaemia Excitotoxicty	Wide inter- and intrapatient variability

case, no practical effects from these minor histological changes have been demonstrated during long-term clinical monitoring.

Bedside microdialysis markers

As any molecule that is small enough to pass across the dialysis membrane can be sampled, microdialysis is a universal biosensor with many potential applications. This section will review the substances commonly analysed at the bedside. The research applications, investigating a myriad of other substances, will be considered later in this chapter.

The commercially available variables for bedside monitoring were chosen to cover aspects of cerebral energy metabolism, release of excitatory amino acids (EAAs) and cell membrane degradation (Fig. 7.4). Tentative normal values for the commonly measured variables have been described (Table 7.1) and the pathophysiological changes that can be monitored by cerebral microdialysis are summarized in Table 7.2.

Cerebral energy metabolism

Glucose, lactate and pyruvate concentrations provide information about cerebral glucose delivery and utilization, and the relative contributions of aerobic and anaerobic metabolism to cellular bioenergetics.

Under normal circumstances, glucose is the sole substrate for cerebral energy metabolism. In the cytosol, it is metabolized to pyruvate in a process that requires NAD^+ and which yields two molecules of ATP for each molecule of glucose (Fig. 7.5). Under aerobic conditions, the majority of pyruvate enters the tricarboxylic acid (TCA) cycle within the mitochondrial matrix where subsequent metabolism, through electron complex-mediated reduction of oxygen, yields another 36 molecules of ATP. During ischaemia, pyruvate

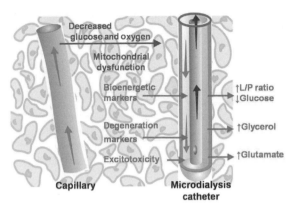

Fig. 7.4. Schematic representation of a blood capillary and microdialysis catheter in brain tissue. The concentration of substrate in the collected fluid (microdiasylate) is related to the balance between substrate delivery to, and uptake/excretion from, the brain extracellular fluid. L/P ratio, lactate to pyruvate ratio. See colour plate section. (Reproduced with permission from Tisdall and Smith, 2006. *Brit J Anaesth* **97**, 18–25.)

undergoes anaerobic metabolism to lactate outside the TCA cycle, with a low yield of ATP. Changes in aerobic and anaerobic metabolism after brain injury contribute to decreased metabolic flux through the glycolytic pathway and pose a bioenergetic threat to the injured brain.

There are no significant stores of glucose in the brain, so a continued supply is essential to sustain normal metabolic activity. Cerebral microdialysis is able to assess the balance between cerebral delivery and utilization of glucose. A low brain ECF glucose concentration can be a reflection of decreased cerebral glucose delivery because of hypoperfusion or systemic hypoglycaemia, or hyperglycolysis secondary to hypoxia/ischaemia-induced anaerobic metabolism. It is therefore important to interpret brain ECF glucose concentration within the context of systemic blood glucose levels and other monitored intracranial variables.

Lactate and pyruvate diffuse through cell membranes, and measurement of the brain ECF lactate to pyruvate (L/P) ratio reliably assesses cellular redox state, reflecting the balance between (oxidized) NAD^+ and (reduced) NADH in the mitochondrial matrix:

$$\frac{[NAD][H^+]}{[NAD]} = \frac{[Lactate] \times K_{LDH}}{[Pyruvate]}$$

where K_{LDH} is the lactate dehydrogenase equilibrium constant.

Elevation of the L/P ratio is a robust indicator of the degree of anaerobic metabolism. It increases immediately after oxygen delivery becomes inadequate and returns to normal upon reoxygenation. Bioenergetic perturbations associated with elevated L/P ratio that are unrelated to hypoxia/ischaemia have also been described and are likely to reflect impaired mitochondrial function. Thus, two types of elevated L/P ratio are described. Type 1 changes are associated with reduced ECF pyruvate and elevated lactate concentrations secondary to classic ischaemia, reflecting a redox state where the lactate dehydrogenase reaction is shifted towards lactate as a result of an inadequate supply of oxygen and glucose. The type 2 pattern occurs when reduced pyruvate is the predominant metabolic perturbation, a situation that reflects impairment of the glycolytic pathway in the presence of adequate (or reduced) glucose supply. The characteristic metabolic changes associated with regional hypoxia/ischaemia after brain injury (i.e. elevation in the L/P ratio in association with reduced brain ECF glucose) correlate with the positron emission tomography (PET)-measured oxygen extraction fraction in some studies (type 1 changes), whereas in others there is less impressive evidence of ischaemia (type 2 changes). Type 2 changes are also observed in the presence of normal $PbrO_2$, whereas brain tissue oxygenation is usually severely depressed in the type 1 pattern of L/P ratio elevation. These findings support the presence of non-ischaemic pathophysiology after brain injury and reinforce the importance of interpreting biochemical changes within the context of changes in other monitoring modalities. It has been difficult to establish a tissue hypoxic threshold for an abnormal L/P ratio, and different thresholds for abnormality, ranging from 20 to 40, are applied by different research groups.

Lactate is an unreliable sole indicator of metabolic distress after brain injury for several reasons. Brain ECF lactate levels may not rise during complete ischaemia because translocation between intra- and extracellular compartments relies on energy-dependent carrier systems. Lactate production is also dependent on a sustained supply of glucose, and this may fail during complete ischaemia. It is for this reason that attention has focused on the L/P ratio as a superior marker of ischaemia than lactate concentration alone. This has an additional advantage: as lactate and pyruvate have very similar molecular weights, the L/P ratio is independent of catheter recovery.

The lactate to glucose (L/G) ratio is also a sensitive marker of hypoxia/ischaemia and, in general,

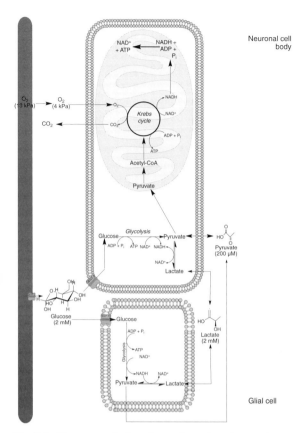

Fig. 7.5. Glucose metabolic pathways. See colour plate section.

reflects sustained lactate production driven by hypoxia/ischaemia-induced hyperglycolysis. Because of the potential role of lactate in normal cerebral metabolism, elevation of the L/G ratio might also occur because of functional adaptation processes after brain injury. Lactate was classically believed to be a metabolically inactive waste product of anaerobic metabolism, but there is increasing evidence that it is a key intermediary in normal metabolic pathways. Lactate fuels energy-requiring processes and, in this context, astrocytes are a major source of lactate production in response to glutamate released by neurons. This lactate may become a preferred fuel for neurons, in particular after traumatic or hypoxic brain injury, even during conditions of preserved aerobic glycolysis. It also seems likely that brain tissue can utilize lactate produced elsewhere in the body. Excessive glutamate-mediated neuronal activation has also been shown to increase lactate production under experimental conditions, and the L/G ratio is therefore a potential

marker of glutamate-driven metabolic impairment (see below).

Cell membrane degradation

Failure of cellular metabolism allows intracellular influx of calcium, induction of phospholipases and subsequent enzymatic degradation of cell membrane triglycerides. Free fatty acids and glycerol are released into the brain ECF, making glycerol a reliable marker of tissue hypoxia, cellular energy failure and cell death. Glycerol levels increase relatively slowly during cellular energy failure and remain elevated for some time after energy metabolism is normalized.

Cerebral microdialysate glycerol concentrations can be 'contaminated' by alterations in systemic glycerol concentration as a result of peripheral catecholamine-induced lipolysis or because of systemic administration of glycerol-containing substances. For example, substantial rises in brain ECF glycerol have been reported following administration of a glycerol enema. Simultaneous measurement of systemic glycerol levels from a reference microdialysis catheter placed in subcutaneous tissue allows improved interpretation of brain ECF glycerol levels, but this is not undertaken routinely in the clinical setting.

Excitatory amino acids

L-Glutamate is a non-essential amino acid with multiple roles within the central nervous system (CNS). It is involved in a variety of cellular metabolic pathways including energy metabolism, and mediates normal synaptic activity. Glutamate is the primary excitatory neurotransmitter: >90% of excitatory synapses are glutamatergic. Brain ischaemia leads to cell depolarization and release of glutamate, aspartate and other EAAs. Glutamate reuptake is also reduced during ischaemia. Release of EAAs is a proposed mechanism of secondary brain injury, and animal studies have demonstrated that brain ECF glutamate concentration is significantly elevated in global cerebral ischaemia. The importance of glutamate within the context of clinical microdialysis monitoring is its potential to assess the amino acid milieu of the injured brain and, as glutamate is released uncontrollably during brain injury-induced energy failure, as a marker of bioenergetic insufficiency. Changes in many brain ECF amino acid concentrations are also seen in chronic neurological conditions such as schizophrenia, Parkinson's disease and Alzheimer's disease.

Early animal experiments confirmed the severity-related release of glutamate and other EAAs after brain injury, and these findings have been replicated in human studies. There was significant interest in the measurement of glutamate in early clinical microdialysis studies of cerebral ischaemia. However, in contrast to animal studies, glutamate concentrations remain high for some days in clinical studies and this difference raises concerns about the extrapolation of animal data to the clinical situation. Because glutamate has multiple CNS roles, both physiological and pathophysiological, it is often difficult to distinguish between its neuroprotective and neurotoxic roles. This is one factor that has led to a reappraisal of the supposed key pathological role of EAAs after brain injury, and as a consequence the early enthusiasm for the microdialysis measurement of glutamate in the clinical setting of brain injury has waned.

Astrocytes convert glutamate to glutamine that is released and reconverted to glutamate in neurons. This glutamate–glutamine cycle is energy dependent and cellular energy failure after brain injury leads to a low interstitial glutamine/glutamate ratio. Several studies have identified correlations between the L/P and glutamine/glutamate ratios. Elevations in the L/P ratio combined with low pyruvate levels are associated with decreased interstitial glutamine levels, suggesting ischaemia-driven failure of astrocytic synthesis of glutamine. On the other hand, elevations in the L/P ratio with normal or high pyruvate levels are associated with increased glutamine levels, indicating the possibility of astrocytic hyperglycolysis. Thus, it appears that, in the presence of an elevated L/P ratio, the brain ECF pyruvate level might determine whether there is sufficient energy capacity for astrocytic glutamate–glutamine cycling.

Clinical applications of cerebral microdialysis

The pathophysiology of acute brain injury is complex, but two factors are of crucial importance – reduction of substrate delivery below critical thresholds and the inability of brain cells to utilize delivered oxygen and glucose because of failing cellular metabolism. There are multiple studies that have utilized the unique potential of microdialysis to enhance our understanding of the pathophysiology of brain injury. Early clinical studies focused on the relationship between biochemical markers, clinical status and other monitored variables. More recent investigations have examined the utilization of microdialysis to evaluate and guide clinical interventions, but it remains unclear whether therapy targeted to normalization or amelioration of abnormal cerebral tissue biochemistry will result in reduced mortality or improved functional outcome after brain injury. In order to maximize the clinical potential of microdialysis, biochemical changes should always be interpreted alongside other physiological variables, including intracranial and cerebral perfusion pressures, $PbrO_2$ and cardiorespiratory changes.

Analysis of the temporal profile of biochemical markers after brain injury reveals fluctuating values that presumably reflect the changing levels of regional metabolic activity and the clinical course. This changing metabolic state makes it difficult to interpret 'one-off' microdialysis measurements in isolation, and measured variables must be interpreted pragmatically in order to derive maximum utility and avoid harm from poorly directed treatment or overtreatment. To this end, the 'LTC method' has been proposed as a way of interpreting microdialysis variables in three regards:

1. The *level* of measured microdialysis variable is compared with the physiological range.
2. The *trend* of the measured variable over recent hours is reviewed.
3. A *comparison* is made between microdialysis and other physiological variables, such as ICP, cerebral perfusion pressure (CPP) and $PbrO_2$.

Traumatic brain injury

Various clinical studies have demonstrated a correlation between adverse clinical events, including high ICP, low CPP, low systemic blood pressure and systemic hypoxaemia, and abnormalities in brain ECF lactate, glycerol, EAAs, glucose and the L/P ratio after TBI.

Catheter placement in traumatic brain injury

As microdialysis is a focal monitoring technique, catheter placement is particularly important in patients with traumatic mass lesions (Fig. 7.6). In an early study of severe TBI, microdialysis variables were investigated in three areas of brain – close to focal traumatic lesions ('at-risk' tissue) and in remote and apparently healthy brain regions in the ipsilateral and contralateral hemispheres. Tissue biochemistry was normal at all times in 'normal' brain tissue, whereas all biochemical

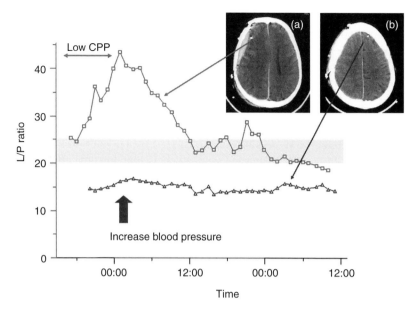

Fig. 7.6. Changes in lactate/pyruvate (L/P) ratio in 'at-risk' (a) and normal (b) brain tissue during a period of low and normal cerebral perfusion pressure (CPP). The normal range for the L/P ratio is shown by the shaded area. Note the rise in L/P ratio in the 'at-risk' tissue during a period of cerebral hypoperfusion but normal values measured by the catheter in normal brain. See colour plate section. (Modified with permission from Tisdall and Smith, 2006. *Brit J Anaesth* **97**, 18–25.)

variables, except for pyruvate but including the L/P ratio, were abnormal in the 'at-risk' tissue early after injury and slowly normalized during the first few days. In another study, microdialysis and $PbrO_2$ monitoring were undertaken in brain tissue underlying a subdural haematoma in 33 patients with severe TBI. Seventeen of the 33 patients developed delayed focal secondary injury reflected by elevation in the L/P ratio and reduced $PbrO_2$ in the 'at-risk' tissue, whereas there were no changes in global measures including jugular venous oxygen saturation, ICP and CPP. As described earlier, expert consensus guidance recommends catheter placement, whenever possible, in 'at-risk' brain tissue, as this is likely to provide the most clinically relevant information.

Identifying pathophysiological processes

Cerebral microdialysis has been used extensively to monitor pathophysioloigcal changes after TBI.

Glucose metabolism

Brain ECF glucose concentration is typically reduced after TBI. Although profound reductions may be associated with tissue ischaemia ($PbrO_2 < 1.3$ kPa), there is substantial evidence that, in some cases at least, a low brain glucose concentration may be related to regional hyperglycolysis rather than the critical supply of glucose and oxygen because of reduced perfusion. Decreased brain glucose concentration is a poor

prognostic indicator after brain injury, although the 'threshold' for abnormality is unclear. Brain ECF glucose concentrations of < 0.66 mmol l^{-1} during the first 2 days after injury have been independently associated with poor outcome after TBI.

As described previously, energy failure after TBI in the absence of vascular or tissue hypoxia is likely to be related to mitochondrial dysfunction. In one study, there was a 25% incidence of metabolic crisis after severe TBI but only a 2.4% incidence of PET-determined cerebral ischaemia in the region of interest around the microdialysis catheter. As clinical monitors such as $PbrO_2$ and jugular venous oximetry identify only ischaemia, the addition of microdialysis to the multimodal monitoring array brings additional and important information that may be used to guide clinical management.

Glycerol

Brain ECF glycerol concentration is typically elevated in the first 24 h after TBI, with the degree of elevation reflecting the severity of the primary injury. The changes may be substantial, with four- or eightfold increases reported in severe focal or global ischaemia, respectively. There follows an exponential decline in glycerol during the ensuing 72 h, with subsequent rises being associated with adverse secondary ischaemic events including intracranial hypertension, low CPP, low $PbrO_2$ and seizures. However, not all secondary insults lead to elevations in glycerol concentration and the majority of studies show little correlation between glycerol levels and outcome.

EAAs

Brain ECF glutamate levels can be 6–20 times higher than normal in the early hours after TBI. In most individuals, these persist for 12–18 h and thereafter trend downwards, but in some patients high levels remain for up to 9 days after injury. Secondary elevations in glutamate levels correlate with secondary ischaemic events, including low CPP, raised ICP and reduced cerebral blood flow. Outcome is worse in patients with high levels of dialysate EAAs and massive increases, up to 20–30 times normal, have been observed in patients with uncontrollable rises in ICP that progress to brain death.

Cerebral perfusion pressure

The impact of different levels of CPP on markers of glucose metabolism has been widely investigated. In a study in which microdialysis catheters were placed in 'at-risk' tissue adjacent to evacuated mass lesions/pericontusional areas, and in non-affected frontal ('normal') tissue, dialysate lactate concentration was higher in 'at-risk' compared with 'normal' brain tissue. Furthermore, lactate and L/P ratio increased when CPP fell below 50 mmHg in 'at-risk' tissue, suggesting that microdialysis monitoring can be used to identify the safe lower limit of CPP. However, other studies have not confirmed this relationship, suggesting that elevation in the L/P ratio can be unrelated to CPP values that are customarily considered to be adequate. These findings again reinforce the importance of using data from multiple sources to guide individualized patient management.

Intracranial pressure

Because cerebral microdialysis monitors the processes of brain injury, it has potential to detect biochemical abnormalities before changes are noted in other monitoring modalities. In a study of 25 patients with severe TBI, microdialysis variables in the presence of normal ICP were used to calculate the risk of intracranial hypertension developing within the next 3 h. An L/P ratio of >25 and glycerol >100 μmol l^{-1} were associated with a significantly higher risk of imminent intracranial hypertension (odds ratios of 9.8 and 2.2, respectively), but glutamate >12 μmol l^{-1} was not predictive. In this study, an abnormal L/P ratio predicted a subsequent rise in ICP above normal levels in 89% of cases.

The identification of biochemical impairment before the onset of intracranial hypertension provides early warning of energy crisis, potentially before irreversible tissue damage has occurred. Whether this can be exploited to bring forward the window for therapeutic intervention remains to be seen.

Glycaemic control

Hyperglycaemia has been shown in multiple studies to be associated with unfavourable outcome after brain injury. The target for systemic glucose control remains uncertain, but recent studies suggest that blood glucose should not be treated unless >10 mmol l^{-1} and that rapid changes in blood glucose concentration should be avoided. Although blood glucose concentration influences brain metabolism after TBI, brain ECF and blood glucose concentrations are not always related. Cerebral low- and high-glucose episodes can both occur independently of blood glucose concentration. Although cerebral hypoglycaemia is usually associated with markers of severe cellular distress (i.e. an increase in the L/P ratio, glutamate and glycerol), elevated brain ECF glucose often occurs as an isolated biochemical abnormality. Recent microdialysis studies suggest that cerebral glucose concentrations <1 mmol l^{-1} are likely to be detrimental because they are usually associated with increases in L/P and L/G ratios. However, there are no data confirming whether interventions targeted to increase brain glucose influence outcome.

Systemic hyperglycaemia (glucose >15 mmol l^{-1}) is widely associated with an increased L/P ratio after brain injury, but high-dose insulin to control elevated blood glucose can also be associated with an increased incidence of cerebral bioenergetic distress. A 70% reduction in brain ECF glucose concentration has been reported in patients treated with intensive insulin therapy compared with a 15% reduction in those treated with a loose insulin protocol. In one study in brain-injured patients, tight systemic glucose control (4.4–6.7 mmol l^{-1}) was associated with a greater prevalence of low cerebral glucose concentration (65 vs. 36%) and brain energy crisis (25 vs. 17%) than intermediate-level control (6.8–10.0 mmol l^{-1}). Cerebral glucose concentration was significantly lower in non-survivors than in survivors (0.46 vs. 1.04 mmol l^{-1}), and brain energy crisis was associated with significantly increased hospital mortality (adjusted odds ratio of 7.36). After adjusting for ICP and CPP, both systemic glucose concentration and insulin dose independently predicted brain energy crisis.

Temperature

Although it is well known that post-ischaemic pyrexia exacerbates neuronal damage, pyrexia-related biochemical changes after brain injury have not been well investigated in humans. In one study, increases in brain temperature from 38.0 to 39.3°C were associated with increases in ICP and PbrO$_2$ but not with changes in brain tissue biochemistry, suggesting that, as long as substrate and oxygen delivery remain adequate, hyperthermia in isolation does not induce further neurochemical disturbances.

The application of therapeutic hypothermia has been widely studied after TBI, and recent evidence suggests that moderate hypothermia might have a preferential beneficial metabolic effect in 'at-risk' brain tissue. In one study, L/P and L/G ratios and glycerol concentration were significantly decreased in perilesional tissue during hypothermia, raising the possibility that biochemical variables might provide a potential therapeutic target for induced hypothermia after brain injury.

Seizures

Non-convulsive seizures are common after TBI and result in an elevated L/P ratio, possibly reflecting a situation where seizure-induced increases in tissue energy demands are not being adequately met. Similarly, cortical spreading depolarization (CSD) is increasingly recognized as a cause of secondary brain injury and has been identified in up to 50% of patients after TBI. Recent work, using a rapid-sequence on-line microdialysis technique, has characterized the neurochemical changes associated with CSD and identified marked depletion of local glucose and elevation of lactate. The severity of the glucose depletion is proportional to the number of depolarizations, and it has been suggested that a vicious cycle is established whereby CSD leads to glucose depletion and bioenergetic distress, which in turn lead to further depolarization waves.

Aneurysmal subarachnoid haemorrhage

Cerebral microdialysis has been extensively studied in SAH and data exist to support its use in the monitoring and management of cerebral vasospasm.

Cerebral vasospasm

Cerebral microdialysis allows detection of the metabolic changes associated with vasospasm-related ischaemia. Increases in the L/P ratio, lactate, glutamate and aspartate concentrations, and reductions in glucose, have all been associated with regional ischaemia during cerebral vasospasm and correlated with clinical outcome. Biochemical disturbances peak on day 1 after ictus with the degree of change reflecting the severity of the initial haemorrhage. The biochemical abnormalities thereafter return towards normal, but secondary elevations, presumably due to vasospasm-related ischaemia, are seen in some patients between days 5 and 10. Elevated glutamate and L/P ratio are sensitive albeit non-specific predictors of acute and delayed ischaemic neurological deficit (DIND) after SAH. Patients who subsequently develop a DIND have significantly higher lactate, glutamate and L/P ratio compared with those who remain asymptomatic. Ischaemia-related biochemical abnormalities can be reversed following the institution of standard treatments for vasospasm including hypertensive–hypervolaemic–haemodilution (triple H) therapy and balloon angioplasty.

The changes in metabolite concentration associated with cerebral ischaemia often precede the onset of the clinical symptoms of vasospasm. In an interesting study in 42 patients with SAH, microdialysis variables in patients who developed a DIND were compared with those who remained asymptomatic. An ischaemic biochemical pattern, defined in this study as a >20% increase in the L/P and L/G ratios from baseline followed by a 20% increase in glycerol concentration, was identified in 17/18 patients who developed a DIND and in only 3/24 who did not. The ischaemic pattern preceded the onset of DIND in all 17 cases, and the mean delay from the peak in the L/P or L/G ratios to the occurrence of the DIND was 23 h (range 4–50 h). The full-scale ischaemic pattern (peaks in L/P and L/G ratios, followed by a peak in glycerol concentration) predicted a subsequent DIND with a sensitivity of 94% and a mean warning period of 11 h. Identification of early changes in tissue biochemistry effectively brings forward the potential treatment window for cerebral vasospasm, but this will be of clinical significance only if an efficacious therapy for cerebral vasospasm can be applied within this timescale. The increased availability of interventional treatment options, such as balloon angioplasty, suggests that this might be possible, but whether such interventions will translate into improved outcome remains to be seen.

ICP

The adverse effects of intracranial hypertension after SAH are undisputed, but the indications for ICP monitoring, or thresholds for treatment, remain unclear. Microdialysis monitoring might provide some insight into this issue. One study explored the relationship between intracranial dynamics and brain tissue energy metabolism in 182 patients with SAH. Patients were classified into two groups depending on ICP – 164 had normal ICP (<20 mmHg) and 18 high ICP (> 20 mmHg). Intracranial hypertension was a strong predictor of mortality (odds ratio of 24.6) and, throughout the entire monitoring period, the L/P ratio and glycerol were significantly increased in patients with high ICP compared with those with normal ICP, and glucose levels were significantly lower. These findings suggest that metabolism-guided, optimized ICP therapy might have the potential to minimize secondary brain injury after SAH.

Ischaemic stroke

Brain ECF lactate and glycerol concentrations, and L/P and L/G ratios, are massively elevated in acute ischaemic stroke. Surprisingly, while elevated glutamate levels have been demonstrated in several animal models, the evidence for similar elevations in the clinical setting is weak. Cerebral microdialysis has been shown to be a sensitive predictor of malignant transformation in hemispheric stroke, with elevated glycerol (>543 μmol l^{-1}) having a 100% sensitivity in one study. Conversely, glutamate levels of <46 μmol l^{-1} and an L/P ratio <50 have a negative predictive value of 99% for a malignant course. Following decompressive craniectomy, abnormal biochemical variables rapidly return towards normal as ICP falls. Microdialysis might therefore have the potential to guide neurosurgical intervention after malignant hemispheric stroke.

Prognosis

Different patterns of brain ECF biochemical change can have an impact on survival and outcome after acute brain injury, although these relationships are not fully characterized. The association in some studies between low brain ECF glucose concentration and mortality after TBI has been discussed earlier in this chapter, but the predictive value of other biochemical variables is less clear. A relationship with poor outcome for elevated EAAs, L/P ratio and glycerol has been reported, but most studies include small numbers of patients and use mortality as the only outcome measure.

The degree of disturbance in brain tissue biochemistry is clearly associated with the severity of SAH. In one study of 149 patients, cerebral metabolism was severely deranged in patients with poor-grade SAH (World Federation of Neurological Surgeons (WFNS) grades IV and V) compared with good-grade SAH (WFNS grades I–III). Significant elevations in lactate, glycerol and the L/P ratio, and non-significant rises in glutamate, were identified in the poor-grade patients. This study also found that both L/P ratio and glutamate were significant independent predictors of outcome along with the established strong predictors of outcome – age and WFNS grade.

Recent data suggest that microdialysis might be able to predict tissue outcome after neurotrauma. An interesting study found that the percentage of time that the L/P ratio was elevated higher than 40 in the first 4 days after severe head injury correlated closely with the degree of frontal lobe atrophy, but not global brain atrophy, at 6 months after injury. The predictive effect of the L/P ratio was independent of patient age, Glasgow Coma Scale score and volume of any frontal lobe contusion. This study provides preliminary evidence that metabolic crisis is associated with subsequent tissue loss, and suggests that elevation of the L/P ratio is a particularly important brain microdialysis marker in terms of determining tissue prognosis. It remains to be seen whether modification of L/P ratio through therapeutic manipulation will result in protection against long-term atrophy. However, given that the L/P ratio often remains elevated for a considerable period of time after TBI, the window of opportunity for neuroprotection might be longer than previously thought.

Future directions of clinial microdialysis

The potential applications of cerebral microdialysis continue to expand, and technological developments offer the possibility of real-time analysis.

Novel biomarkers

While the majority of early human microdialysis research has involved analytes that can easily be measured at the bedside, these represent only the tip of the iceberg in terms of the potential markers of pathology and cellular metabolic function after brain injury. Because cerebral microdialysate is a facsimile of brain ECF, containing all molecules small enough to pass through the microdialysis membrane, all pathological processes that result in changes in the ECF biochemical composition can theoretically be monitored by microdialysis.

ATP

Increased utilization of ATP results in increased formation of its breakdown products, adenosine, inosine and hypoxanthine, which can be used as markers of ischaemia and cellular metabolic dysfunction. As hypoxanthine may be an important substrate for oxygen-free radical production and a cause of further secondary brain injury, it is unsurprising that elevated levels have been associated with poor outcome following SAH. Pathological depletion of ATP stores leads to cessation of cellular function, cell membrane depolarization and massive efflux of K^+ into the ECF. Microdialysis-measured brain ECF K^+ concentration has been used as a marker of severe ischaemia, and it has been suggested that the degree of increase in ECF K^+ can be used to distinguish severe from mild-to-moderate ischaemia.

Reactive oxygen species

Reactive oxygen species (ROS) have extremely short half-lives, making their measurement in biological systems virtually impossible. However, products of enzymes that co-produce ROS can be used as indirect measures. For example, xanthine and urate are co-produced by xanthine oxidase in a reaction forming superoxide anion radicals. Increased brain ECF levels of xanthine have been demonstrated in animal models of cerebral ischaemia, as well as after human TBI.

Protein S100β

The calcium-binding astrocyte protein S100β is released during brain injury, and plasma and CSF S100β levels have been used to monitor secondary injury. Several studies have shown that it is possible to measure brain ECF S100β using microdialysis, and this might provide a more sensitive and specific monitor of secondary injurious processes than measurement in plasma or CSF. A dynamic pattern of brain ECF S100β has been observed after TBI and elevated levels associated with secondary adverse events related to ICP surges.

Nitric oxide

Nitric oxide (NO) has a biphasic effect in the CNS with important functions related to the normal regulation of cerebrovascular tone and, at higher concentrations, a deleterious effect that exacerbates secondary brain injury. Nitric oxide is a reactive molecule and is difficult to detect directly, but endogenous production can be estimated by measurement of the concentration of its downstream metabolites, nitrate and nitrite – termed NOx. Increasing NOx correlates significantly with decreasing L/P ratio and lactate and increasing glucose, suggesting that higher concentrations of NO are associated with more favourable metabolism in injured brains. Values of NOx are significantly lower in patients who die from their injury compared with those who survive – 14.3 versus 31.9 μmol in one study.

L-Arginine is the immediate precursor of NO, making measurement of cerebral L-arginine concentration of interest. In addition, glutamate, which is itself a mediator of secondary brain injury, may stimulate arginine release from glial cells. Microdialysis studies have confirmed low levels of arginine in the first 3 days after TBI, suggesting that non-availability of substrate could contribute to the observed decrease in NO levels.

Amino acids

As well as the bedside measurement of glutamate, the temporal profiles of multiple interstitial amino acids, including alanine, aspargine, glutamine, isoleucine, leucine, phenylalanine, serine and tyrosine, have been studied using microdialysis. Increases in non-transmitter amino acids have been noted in the first 2 days after SAH and might reflect an increased amino acid turnover in an attempt to repair the injured brain. Large increases (up to 1350-fold) in γ-aminobutyric acid (GABA), in association with increases in glutamate and aspartate concentrations, have also been identified during cerebral ischaemic episodes after brain injury.

N-Acetylaspartate (NAA) is a neuronal marker present at a high concentration in the CNS and is synthesized almost exclusively in the mitochondrion of neurons. Proton magnetic resonance spectroscopy has confirmed NAA depletion in several types of acute and chronic brain injury, suggesting early (<4h) impaired mitochondrial function. It is also possible to measure NAA using cerebral microdialysis, and clinical studies have confirmed that brain ECF NAA concentration is >30% lower in non-survivors than survivors after TBI. A significant non-recoverable fall in NAA is seen in non-survivors from day 4 onwards, and this is associated with a concomitant rise in L/P ratio and glycerol concentration. These findings suggest that NAA is a candidate marker for monitoring therapeutic strategies aimed at preserving mitochondrial function after brain injury.

Inflammatory markers

Cytokines are proteins that exert a broad range of physiological effects. Individual cytokines have multiple actions but, in general terms, are either pro- or anti-inflammatory. The overall inflammatory state is determined by the complex interplay between multiple cytokines. Historically, cytokines have been measured in CSF or serum, but recent developments have allowed their measurement in brain ECF by microdialysis. Techniques have been quantified for the measurement of substances such as IL-1β, IL-6 and nerve growth factor (NGF), and microdialysis cytokine studies are leading to an improved understanding of the neuroinflammatory changes after acute brain injury.

Early studies confirmed significant associations between higher levels of brain ECF IL-6, but not serum IL-6, and improved outcome after brain injury. In one study there was a significant correlation between peak ECF IL-6 levels and Glasgow Outcome Score but no association between peak IL-β or NGF and mortality. Subsequently, high levels of the whole IL-1 family of cytokines have been associated with improved outcome after TBI, and it has been suggested that this reflects a potential neuroprotective role for cytokines. Intracranial hypertension is associated with strong activation of a local (brain) and systemic inflammatory response, and microdialysis measurements of cytokine levels could play a role in the investigation of future anti-inflammatory therapies targeted at cerebral oedema.

Proteomic research

Using 100 kDa molecular weight cut-off catheters and a combination of electrophoresis and mass spectrometry, ten proteins that are not present in CSF following acute ischaemic stroke have been identified in microdialysate. More recently, metabolic distress after TBI has been shown to be associated with a differential proteome, indicating cellular destruction during the acute phase. Novel biomarkers have also been identified as early markers of symptomatic vasospasm after SAH. A study investigating a proteome-wide screening identified several isoforms of glyceraldehyde-3-phosphate dehydrogenase that were higher in patients with symptomatic vasospasm, whereas heat-shock cognate 71 kDa protein (HSP7C) isoforms were decreased. These changes in protein concentrations were detected an average of 3.8 days before the onset of symptoms. While further characterization of individual proteins

and their relevance in brain injury is awaited, this is clearly an exciting field of research with the potential to provide new insights into the pathophysiology of the injured brain.

Neuropharmacology

Microdialysis provides the technology to determine the cerebral penetration of drugs during neuropharmacological research. Examples of novel insights gained using microdialysis include the transmission of morphine, antibiotics and anti-epileptic drugs, such as phenytoin and topiramate, across the blood–brain barrier.

By altering the constituents of the perfusate, it is also possible to use a microdialysis catheter as a hyperfocal drug-delivery device. While little work has been carried out in humans, there is the potential to use microdialysis for stereotactic drug delivery to specific structural targets in the CNS. This novel approach to localized pharmacological intervention is an exciting area of research into therapeutic strategy, and animal work has already been undertaken in models of alcohol addiction and Parkinson's disease.

On-line analysis

A major drawback of commercially available microdialysis systems is the limited temporal resolution and off-line quantification of analyte concentration. This limits the clinical application of microdialysis, which is currently insensitive to brief but potentially clinically relevant perturbations in cerebral metabolism. Novel systems for real-time, on-line microdialysis have been developed and applied in animal and human studies. Although on-line microdialysis has the potential to use either enzyme-linked colorimetric or solid-state biosensors, the number of variables that can currently be analysed is limited. A commercial on-line system that will provide additional analytes is under development.

A research automated on-line method has been used to assay microdialysate samples during animal models of CSD. Perfusate at high flow rates (2 μl min^{-1}) is directed into a flow-injection system incorporating enzyme-based biosensors for glucose and lactate capable of determining metabolite concentration every 30 s. This system has also been used to allow the early detection of intraoperative ischaemia-related metabolic changes during interventions such as temporary vessel clipping during aneurysm surgery. In this situation, the technique was capable of detecting changes 9 min after intraoperative events occurred. The response time is related to probe-to-sensor tubing length, and technical advances are likely to improve the temporal resolution further.

Summary

Cerebral microdialysis brings a unique contribution to monitoring the injured brain. With its ability to create a facsimile of brain tissue ECF and characterize metabolic and biochemical changes, microdialysis is able to elucidate pathophysiological processes after brain injury and provide objective end points for clinical interventions and research. Monitoring biochemical variables also provides confidence to withhold potentially dangerous treatments in patients without evidence of brain ischaemia or metabolic distress. Microdialysis allows early recognition of cerebral hypoxia/ischaemia and bioenergetic failure, and potentially extends the time windows for therapeutic intervention.

Translating microdialysis from its well-established research role into a routine clinical tool faces substantial challenges. The sensitivity and specificity of microdialysis markers of ischaemia and bioenergetic failure are not well characterized and there are no data to confirm whether microdialysis-guided therapy can influence outcome. Future research must identify metabolically informed therapeutic strategies with the ultimate goal of developing individualized treatments aimed at minimizing secondary brain injury and improving functional outcome. Studies are also required to identify sensitive and specific biochemical predictors of outcome after brain injury. The development of a system providing rapid analysis in 'real time' is crucial to maximize the clinical applicability of the microdialysis technique.

Further reading

Bellander, B. M., Cantais, E., Enblad, P. et al. (2004). Consensus meeting on microdialysis in neurointensive care. *Intensive Care Med* **30**, 2166–9.

Belli, A., Sen, J., Petzold, A. et al. (2006). Extracellular N-acetylaspartate depletion in traumatic brain injury. *J Neurochem* **96**, 861–9.

Belli, A., Sen, J., Petzold, A. et al. (2008). Metabolic failure precedes intracranial pressure rises in traumatic brain injury: a microdialysis study. *Acta Neurochir* **150**, 461–9.

Clausen, T., Alves, O. L., Reinert, M. et al. (2005). Association between elevated brain tissue glycerol levels and poor outcome following severe traumatic brain injury. *J Neurosurg* **103**, 233–8.

Engstrom, M., Polito, A., Reinstrup, P. et al. (2005). Intracerebral microdialysis in severe brain trauma: the importance of catheter location. *J Neurosurg* **102**, 460–9.

Goodman, J. C. and Robertson, C. S. (2009). Microdialysis: is it ready for prime time? *Curr Opin Crit Care* **15**, 110–17.

Helmy, A., Carpenter, K. L. and Hutchinson, P. J. (2007). Microdialysis in the human brain and its potential role in the development and clinical assessment of drugs. *Curr Med Chem* **14**, 1525–37.

Hillered, L., Vespa, P. M. and Hovda, D. A. (2005). Translational neurochemical research in acute human brain injury: the current status and potential future for cerebral microdialysis. *J Neurotrauma* **22**, 3–41.

Hutchinson, P. J., O'Connell, M. T., Al-Rawi, P. G. et al. (2002). Increases in GABA concentrations during cerebral ischaemia: a microdialysis study of extracellular amino acids. *J Neurol Neurosurg Psychiatry* **72**, 99–105.

Hutchinson, P. J., O'Connell, M. T., Rothwell, N. J. et al. (2007). Inflammation in human brain injury: intracerebral concentrations of IL-1α, IL-1β, and their endogenous inhibitor IL-1ra. *J Neurotrauma* **24**, 1545–57.

Lakshmanan, R., Loo, J. A., Drake, T. et al. (2010). Metabolic crisis after traumatic brain injury is associated with a novel microdialysis proteome. *Neurocrit Care* **12**, 324–36.

Marcoux, J., McArthur, D. A., Miller, C. et al. (2008). Persistent metabolic crisis as measured by elevated cerebral microdialysis lactate–pyruvate ratio predicts chronic frontal lobe brain atrophy after traumatic brain injury. *Crit Care Med* **36**, 2871–7.

Maurer, M. H., Haux, D., Sakowitz, O. W., Unterberg, A. W. and Kuschinsky, W. (2007). Identification of early markers for symptomatic vasospasm in human cerebral microdialysate after subarachnoid hemorrhage: preliminary results of a proteome-wide screening. *J Cereb Blood Flow Metab* **27**, 1675–83.

Nordstrom, C. H., Reinstrup, P., Xu, W, Gärdenfors, A. and Ungerstedt, U. (2003). Assessment of the lower limit for cerebral perfusion pressure in severe head injuries by bedside monitoring of regional energy metabolism. *Anesthesiology* **98**, 809–14.

Oddo, M., Schmidt, J. M., Carrera, E. et al. (2008). Impact of tight glycemic control on cerebral glucose metabolism after severe brain injury: a microdialysis study. *Crit Care Med* **36**, 3233–8.

Peerdeman, S. M., Girbes, A. R., Polderman, K. H. and Vandertop, W. P. (2003). Changes in cerebral interstitial glycerol concentration in head-injured patients; correlation with secondary events. *Intensive Care Med* **29**, 1825–8.

Peerdeman, S. M., van Tulder, M. W. and Vandertop, W. P. (2003). Cerebral microdialysis as a monitoring method in subarachnoid hemorrhage patients, and correlation with clinical events – a systematic review. *J Neurol* **250**, 797–805.

Reinstrup, P., Stahl, N., Mellergard, P. *et al.* (2000). Intracerebral microdialysis in clinical practice: baseline values for chemical markers during wakefulness, anesthesia, and neurosurgery. *Neurosurgery* **47**, 701–9.

Samuelsson, C., Hillered, L., Zetterling, M. *et al.* (2007). Cerebral glutamine and glutamate levels in relation to compromised energy metabolism: a microdialysis study in subarachnoid hemorrhage patients. *J Cereb Blood Flow Metab* **27**, 1309–17.

Sarrafzadeh, A., Haux, D., Küchler, I., Lanksch, W. R. and Unterberg, A. W. (2004). Poor-grade aneurysmal subarachnoid hemorrhage: relationship of cerebral metabolism to outcome. *J Neurosurg* **100**, 400–6.

Schulz, M., Wang, L. P., Tange, M. and Bjerre, P. (2000). Cerebral microdialysis monitoring: determination of normal and ischemic cerebral metabolism in patients with aneurysmal subarachnoid hemorrhage. *J Neurosurg* **93**, 233–8.

Skjoth-Rasmussen, J., Schulz, M., Kristensen, S. R. and Bjerre, P. (2004). Delayed neurological deficits detected by an ischemic pattern in the extracellular cerebral metabolites in patients with aneurysmal subarachnoid hemorrhage. *J Neurosurg* **100**, 8–15.

Stocchetti, N., Protti, A., Lattuada, M. *et al.* (2005). Impact of pyrexia on neurochemistry and cerebral oxygenation after acute brain injury. *J Neurol Neurosurg Psychiatry* **76**, 1135–9.

Timofeev, I., Carpenter, K. L., Nortje, J. *et al.* (2011). Cerebral extracellular chemistry and outcome following traumatic brain injury: a microdialysis study of 223 patients. *Brain* **134**, 484–94.

Tisdall, M. M. and Smith, M. (2006). Cerebral microdialysis: research technique or clinical tool. *Br J Anaesth* **97**, 18–25.

Ungerstedt, U. (1991). Microdialysis – principles and applications for studies in animals and man. *J Intern Med* **230**, 365–73.

Vespa, P., Bergsneider, M., Hattori, N. *et al.* (2005). Metabolic crisis without brain ischemia is common after traumatic brain injury: a combined microdialysis and positron emission tomography study. *J Cereb Blood Flow Metab* **25**, 763–74.

Vespa, P. M., McArthur, D, O'Phelan, K. *et al.* (2003). Persistently low extracellular glucose correlates with poor outcome 6 months after human traumatic brain injury despite a lack of increased lactate: a microdialysis study. *J Cereb Blood Flow Metab* **23**, 865–77.

Vespa, P. M., O'Phelan, K., McArthur, D. *et al.* (2007). Pericontusional brain tissue exhibits persistent elevation of lactate/pyruvate ratio independent of cerebral perfusion pressure. *Crit Care Med* **35**, 1153–60.

Chapter

8

Neurophysiology

Dick Moberg and Sabrina G. Galloway

Introduction

Clinical neurophysiology encompasses a variety of diagnostic tests including EEG, nerve conduction studies, electromyography, evoked potentials and polysomnography. This chapter will describe the tests that are most widely used for monitoring during neuroanaesthesia and neurocritical care, specifically, EEG, somatosensory evoked potentials, brainstem auditory evoked potentials, motor evoked potentials and electromyography (EMG). Other techniques, such as electrocorticography and specialized evoked potential monitoring, are covered elsewhere in this book and Further reading section at the end of this chapter.

The two main uses for neurophysiological monitoring are to guide therapy and detect problems. For example, EEG monitoring can be used to guide seizure management and assess the level of consciousness during anaesthesia, while EEG and evoked potentials (EPs) are widely used to detect cerebral or spinal cord ischaemia, respectively, during surgery and allow intervention before permanent damage ensues. The central nervous system (CNS) is the most fragile organ system of the body and damage to it results in the highest cost of continued care for the patient, his or her family and society. Thus, preventing CNS damage is of the utmost importance during neuroanaesthesia and neurocritical care, and neurophysiological monitoring has a key role to play in its prevention. Because of the complex nature of the brain and spinal cord, and the complexity of monitoring technology, neurophysiological monitoring is not universally performed. However, innovations in the field of neurophysiological monitoring continue, and it is likely that it will soon become as straightforward

and accurate as monitoring vital signs. In the meantime, there are some regional standards of care that prescribe neuromonitoring in certain situations, whereas in other areas it is for the clinician to determine in which individual cases the application of this technology will yield the greatest benefit.

Physiological basis of EEG and evoked potentials

In order to appreciate their capabilities and limitations, it is crucial to understand relevant neuroanatomy and neurophysiology prior to using EEG and EPs for monitoring. Interpretation of EEG is based largely on the recognition of patterns as well as changes from a baseline, and as it is difficult, if not impossible, to correlate specific EEG patterns and even gross EEG changes with cellular and subcellular events, a detailed background in classical neurophysiology is not necessary to interpret straightforward EEG abnormalities. As EPs have stronger anatomical and physiological correlates than EEG, a basic knowledge of neurophysiology and neuroanatomy aids their interpretation. The physiology presented in this chapter is therefore limited to topics that will assist in performing effective neuromonitoring using EEG and EPs. The reader is directed towards more comprehensive coverage in other chapters of this text or in general neurophysiology textbooks for more detailed information about specific topics.

Origin of EEG and its use in monitoring

EEG originates from the synchronous firing of a large number of neurons in the surface layers of the cortex. This cortical origin of the signal is relevant to monitoring, as focal problems deeper in the brain are generally

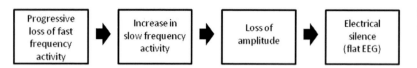

Fig. 8.1. Changes in the EEG waveform due to sustained cerebral ischaemia.

not seen in the EEG. In general terms, the EEG can be used to monitor:

1. Electrical alterations that are represented on the cortex such as seizures and other pathophysiological patterns, e.g. cortical spreading depression.
2. Global cerebral ischaemia.
3. Focal cerebral ischaemia, provided it is cortical and there are recording electrodes over the ischaemic area.
4. Drug effects, provided they act on the EEG.

Blood supply to the brain and implications for monitoring

Blood is supplied to the brain via the two internal carotid arteries and the two vertebral arteries that join to form the basilar artery. These feed into the circle of Willis, which is a 'traffic rotary' from which arteries branch out to supply various parts of the brain. This arterial architecture ensures collateral flow to the brain in case one or two of the main supplying arteries become occluded. Although the system seems simple, the pearls for monitoring often lie in the anatomical variations and pathological changes seen in individuals. For example, in an anatomically perfect world, clamping one carotid artery during a carotid endarterectomy would not produce any cerebrovascular changes because of the collateral circulation from the other vessels. Anatomical variations in the circle of Willis, however, are well known and occur in about 65% of the population, and the presence of plaque in one carotid bifurcation is also a good indicator that there will be plaque in the other. Thus, using EEG to monitor the adequacy of cerebral circulation during a carotid clamp can yield results that are unexpected from the simple model of the cerebral circulation. In one study of over 300 endarterectomies, changes in the EEG during carotid cross-clamping were seen in the ipsilateral hemisphere, the contralateral hemisphere, in both hemispheres and in neither, illustrating the dependency on individual anatomy. A case

was reported in the 1980s where the EEG monitor was connected (fortunately) prior to intubation. When the anaesthetist tilted the head back for intubation, the EEG pattern surprisingly indicated ischaemia, and this change correlated with the degree of head tilt. Subsequently, it was found that this patient had a high-degree carotid stenosis as well as vertebrobasilar insufficiency, and tilting the head therefore reduced blood flow to the brain to a level identifiable in the EEG. Such undetected variations in anatomy and pathology make it difficult to predict which individuals will benefit from CNS monitoring and provide a compelling rationale for monitoring on a routine basis.

Ischaemic patterns and thresholds

The EEG waveform progresses through a classic change in morphology with increasing cerebral ischaemia (Fig. 8.1), and it is important to be able to recognize this pattern. Increasing doses of some drugs show similar effects on the EEG, and it is therefore important to interpret all neurophysiological monitoring within the context of the individual patient.

Changes in the EEG and EPs at decreasing levels of cerebral blood flow are shown in Fig. 8.2. At a reduced level of blood flow, and as time progresses, the brain enters a state where cellular function is altered and a period of reversible cell damage is followed by an irreversible state of cell death. The goal of monitoring is to detect the altered function early enough so that intervention can be undertaken before permanent damage occurs. This is the basis of using EEG and EPs as monitoring tools for cerebral and spinal cord ischaemia.

A natural question is how much time one has to intervene after the onset of electrophysiological changes but before irreversible tissue damage has occurred. There are no markers on the timescale in Fig. 8.2 specifically because the time to irreversibility depends on so many factors. For example, cooling and certain drugs prolong the time until irreversible cellular changes occur and prior pathology can shorten it.

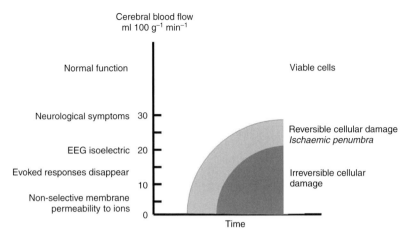

Cerebral blood flow
ml 100 g⁻¹ min⁻¹

Fig. 8.2. The basis of using EEG and evoked potentials for detection of central nervous system ischaemia. Reductions in cerebral blood flow are associated with typical changes in EEG and evoked potentials (left side of figure). As blood flow is reduced, and as time progresses, cerebral cellular function is altered and a period of reversible cell damage is followed by an irreversible state of cell death (right side of figure).

Normal function

Viable cells

Neurological symptoms   30

Reversible cellular damage
Ischaemic penumbra

EEG isoelectric   20

Evoked responses disappear

Irreversible cellular
damage
10

Non-selective membrane
permeability to ions   0

Time

Anatomy and physiology relevant to evoked potentials

The measurement of EPs involves stimulating a neural structure (nerve or brain) and recording the response at a distant location (brain or muscle) to evaluate the functioning of the intervening pathway. Thus, knowledge of specific pathways is important when using EPs for monitoring, and these are described below.

One of the main uses for EPs is in monitoring the spinal cord for ischaemia, particularly during surgery. The blood supply to the cord is via the anterior and posterior spinal arteries, which are in turn fed by larger arteries at various points outside the spine. There are two points of relevance for spinal cord monitoring:

1. Although there is collateralization between the anterior and posterior spinal arteries, it is possible for ischaemia to develop in the anterior motor pathways without effects seen in the posterior sensory pathways. Monitoring both pathways (using motor and somatosensory EPs) is therefore recommended.
2. The mid-thoracic region has the fewest feeder arteries and is a watershed area at risk during low perfusion states.

Understanding the anatomy as well as the surgical procedures that can compromise the spinal cord is therefore important for effective monitoring. For example, spinal cord injury may occur during spine surgery because of ischaemia secondary to spinal distraction and disruption of perforating radicular

vessels or because of direct trauma during placement of pedicle screws or resection of an intrinsic spinal cord lesion. The spinal cord is also at risk during abdominal aortic aneurysm repair when the aorta is cross-clamped. Perfusion to the cord can be compromised resulting in a repaired aneurysm but a paralysed patient.

EEG

EEG is mainly used as a diagnostic procedure during which brain electrical activity is recorded using electrodes placed on the scalp. It is a fundamental test in clinical neurophysiology and has been used since the 1930s to diagnose a wide range of disorders. Prior to the 1980s, EEG was used to locate abnormal areas in the brain's cortex including tumours and regions of ischaemia, but the advent of CT and MRI largely rendered these indications redundant. Currently, the main indications for EEG are in the diagnosis and management of epilepsy, sleep studies and neuromonitoring. The intraoperative and critical care applications of the last are the focus of this section.

To help understand the EEG, comparison to the more familiar ECG will be made throughout this section. Like ECG, there are two steps to performing an EEG study – a technical component that produces an EEG recording and an interpretation component that determines the clinical significance of the recording. These components are generally performed by different staff members. A third component, processed EEG, which aids in the interpretation especially during neuromonitoring, can be added.

Technical aspects of EEG recording

It is important to follow all the steps for producing an EEG in order to record high-quality data. The seemingly random nature of the EEG can make certain artefacts hard to distinguish from the real signal, leading to incorrect interpretation. Further details can be found in more comprehensive EEG texts or in texts targeted to the technologist or monitoring personnel.

The steps for producing an EEG recording include:

1. Determination of the scalp locations for the electrodes.
2. Selection and application of the electrodes.
3. Connection of the electrodes to the amplifier to produce a recording montage.
4. Adjustment of the amplification and filtering.
5. Checking for artefacts and minimizing if present.
6. Displaying the EEG in the desired format.

Electrode locations

As with ECG, a distinction is made between diagnostic and monitoring applications of EEG in the number of electrodes used. In surgery and critical care, the ECG is usually monitored with a reduced number of leads compared with a 12-lead diagnostic study. The same is true for EEG in that fewer electrodes are normally used during neuromonitoring compared with diagnostic studies. Also similar to ECG, the EEG signal is different depending on where the electrodes are placed. For this reason, an international standard for electrode placement has been developed for both ECG and EEG to maintain consistency in recordings within a single patient and between patients.

The International 10–20 System of electrode placement is the reference standard for EEG electrodes (Fig. 8.3). The '10–20' refers to percentages of distance along a grid that is measured on the head and provides a method that places electrodes in the same relative location on heads of different sizes.

The terminology describing electrode position consists of paired letters and numbers. The letters indicate the area of the cortex: frontal-polar (Fp), frontal (F), central (C), parietal (P), occipital (O), auricular (A) and temporal (T). The numbers increase with the distance from the midline, with odd numbers on the left hemisphere and even numbers on the right. Midline sagittal electrodes are designated with a 'z' for zero instead of a number. For example, F3 is an electrode over the frontal area on the left side at 'position 3'

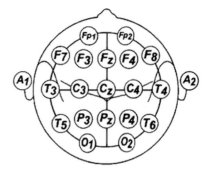

Fig. 8.3. The International 10–20 System for EEG electrode placement.

out from the midline. The '3' is not an absolute number but is determined by the measured grid and the percentage distance along the grid. It is useful to note the symmetrical electrodes, as symmetry is an important characteristic of the EEG. Note, for example, that F4 is the corresponding and symmetrical position to F3 but on the right hemisphere. Exceptions to the numbering rule are the temporal lobe numbers, which increase from anterior to posterior.

Selecting and applying the electrodes

There are a variety of electrode types and application methods, each with advantages and disadvantages (Table 8.1). For monitoring, the most commonly used electrodes are gold cups that are applied to the head with collodion glue. Such electrodes can stay in place for several days. Needle electrodes are discouraged for routine diagnostic use because of the risk of infection, but they remain widely used during monitoring where a quick application is desired, or in patients with sensitive skin, such as neonates. Recently, MRI-compatible electrodes have been developed, which do not require removal during imaging studies.

Connecting the electrodes to the amplifier – the montage

Similar to the ECG, a channel of EEG (a waveform on the EEG display) is recorded by an amplifier that measures the difference between two electrode locations. A channel is named by the pair of electrodes used. Thus, F3–C3 is the measured difference between the scalp potentials located at F3 and C3 (see Fig. 8.3). Pairs of electrodes are selected for recording depending on the purpose of the monitoring. The particular selection of electrode pairs and the way that they are connected to the amplifier box is referred to as a montage. There are

Table 8.1 Electrode types and application methods during EEG recording.

Electrode type and application	Advantages	Disadvantages
Cup – collodion	Will stay on head for several days. Good for long-term recordings	Labour-intensive. Not as easy to remove as paste
Cup – paste	Paste is quicker to apply than collodion	Paste does not last as long as collodion. Not good for long-term recordings
Needle	Quick and easy to apply	Risk of infection if not properly applied

two basic types of montages, referential and bipolar. A referential montage measures the difference between each active electrode and a common reference electrode. Examples of electrode pairs (channels on the display) in a referential montage would be F3–Ref, F4–Ref, C3–Ref, C4–Ref, etc. In a bipolar montage, two scalp electrodes, generally adjacent to each other, become the pair and they are usually linked as 'chains'. For example, F3–C3, C3–P3, P3–O1 would be one such chain on the left side. Although there are standard montages depending on the type of patient (neonate or adult), and on the purpose of the monitoring, variations are commonly applied.

Amplification and filtering

EEG amplifiers must deal with a wide range of signal input varying from a few microvolts for recordings of activity during electrocerebral silence or brain death, up to 500 µV or more during seizure activity. All modern EEG monitors use similar amplifier circuitry and, in general, the user need not be concerned with amplifier characteristics or with calibration.

With digital EEG equipment, the signal is generally amplified with little filtering to produce a wide band of frequencies. Software-based filters can then be set by the user to extract the required frequency band. A low filter typically reduces frequencies in the 0.5–1.0 Hz range and a high filter in the 30–70 Hz range. A notch filter reduces the activity in a narrow frequency band and is used to eliminate 50 or 60 Hz mains interference. For monitoring applications, filters help to reduce noise in the EEG signal, which is much greater during surgery and in the critical care unit than in the relative electrical calm of the neurophysiology laboratory. For monitoring, a filter range of 1–30 Hz is generally acceptable.

Artefacts and electrode impedance – obtaining a reliable signal

An important and sometimes challenging step in EEG monitoring is the recognition and elimination of artefacts. Unlike most other physiology variables where there is a recognizable pattern (e.g. blood pressure waveforms, ECG), the EEG can appear quite random and artefacts can be difficult to distinguish from the actual EEG.

The first step in ensuring a quality signal is to check the electrode impedance, which is a measure of how well an electrode is attached to the skin, as a loose contact can act like an antenna and introduce noise into a channel. All EEG monitors provide a function that checks electrode impedances and some do this continuously. A warning is displayed if electrode impedance is unacceptably high. Other types of common artefacts are listed in Table 8.2. Less frequent sources of artefact are more elusive and the ability to identify and eliminate them only comes with considerable experience in this field.

Displaying the EEG

Due to the number of EEG channels that are displayed, it is customary to arrange them on the monitor to aid their interpretation. There are no standards for arranging EEG channels, and both the montage and channel display are sometimes determined by personal preference. However, one custom is to display left-hemisphere channels on the top and right-hemisphere channels on the bottom (or vice versa) so that asymmetries can be visualized more easily. Other arrangements pair corresponding electrodes from each side together, for example paring F3–C3 with F4–C4. For each channel, the display on an EEG machine shows the source of the channel (electrode pair), the amplification and filter settings. The timescale for all channels is shown at the bottom of the display.

Interpreting the EEG

To a novice, the normal EEG exhibits a series of seemingly random patterns. Interpreting the EEG in a diagnostic study consists of describing these patterns using a common set of descriptors and, because of its complexity,

Table 8.2 EEG artefacts and how to minimize them

Artefact	Description	Comments
Line frequency	Line (mains) frequency interference is seen as a high-frequency signal (60 Hz in North America, 50 Hz in Europe) superimposed on the EEG. It causes the signal to look fuzzy and thick	If seen in all channels, this external artefact is most likely generated by nearby equipment such as a ventilator. Improper grounding of the patient and/or EEG instrument may increase the possibility of seeing this artefact. Make sure the ground electrode is properly attached to the patient and has acceptable impedance. If the line frequency artefact does not occur in all channels, it is most probably due to imbalanced or high impedances
Electrode pop	Electrical artefacts, commonly known as 'pops', can appear as spikes in an electrode pair or channel. They are caused by the build-up of electrical charge under electrodes poorly attached to the scalp, which then suddenly discharge. These artefacts can be mistaken for epileptic spikes	Pressing down on the problem electrode(s) to help restore normal impedance should eliminate this artefact. If the artefact persists, it may be necessary to reapply the problem electrode(s)
High-frequency ventilator artefact	It is possible for a high-frequency ventilator to cause vibrations throughout the body of a newborn and also the attached electrodes. Depending on the frequency of the ventilator, a rhythmic artefact from approximately 4 to 12 Hz can appear in the EEG, and can superficially resemble a seizure	As this artefact occurs in the typical EEG frequency range (0.5–30 Hz), it cannot be filtered out. If recognized, be sure not to misinterpret it as epileptiform or other neurological activity
Eye movement interference	Eyelid movement and eye movement create artefacts in the frontal leads of all EEG recordings. The eyeball has an electrical potential, which is positive in the front (at the cornea) and negative in the back (at the retina). This corneoretinal potential creates a high-voltage source for an electrical field to occur. When the eyes blink, this voltage field is slower and higher voltage than the average EEG. Eye movements are not seen in patients that are anaesthetized or comatose	Eye movements are normal physiological potentials. They should only appear in EEG channels containing a frontal electrode (e.g. Fp1 or Fp2), and should not be mistaken for epileptic spikes

EEG interpretation is performed by specifically trained clinicians. The reader is referred to general textbooks on EEG as well as EEG atlases for more information on interpreting routine diagnostic EEG studies.

In monitoring applications, the concept of a 'normal' EEG is relatively unimportant, as the patients are usually anaesthetized, sedated or in a coma and these states change the EEG. Thus, during monitoring, the objective is largely to identify changes from a baseline and for this a reduced number of descriptors are used.

EEG descriptors for monitoring

The basic descriptors for monitoring are amplitude, frequency, symmetry, and patterns (Fig. 8.4).

Amplitude is measured quantitatively in microvolts but is generally reported as low or high compared with normal, or with a prior baseline. In monitoring, it is difficult to provide a normal amplitude range, as many drugs affect the amplitude. A reduction in EEG amplitude can indicate cerebral ischaemia and a continuous 'flat' EEG (below 2 µV) is used in some criteria for brain death.

Frequency is measured in hertz (cycles s^{-1}) and is generally reported as slow or fast activity. There are four classical frequency bands, delta (<4 Hz), theta (4–8 Hz), alpha (8–13 Hz) and beta (13–30 Hz), that identify various physiological and behavioural states. Although these are often used to describe monitored EEG, the

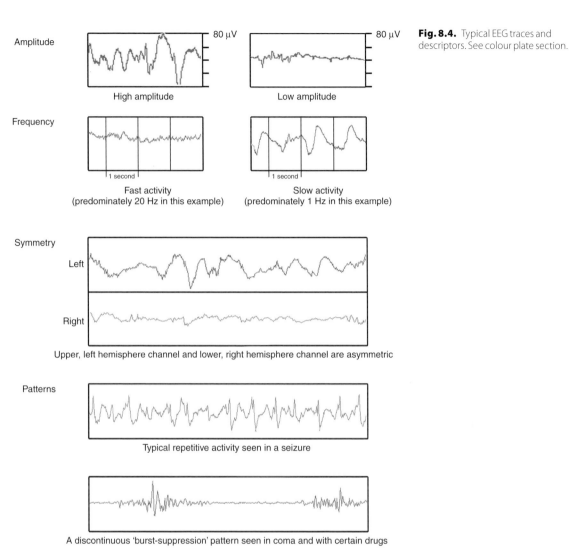

Fig. 8.4. Typical EEG traces and descriptors. See colour plate section.

connotations associated with them during diagnostic procedures (e.g. alpha is eyes closed and relaxed) do not hold for monitoring, as drugs, stages of consciousness and various pathologies alter the frequency of the EEG. During monitoring, frequency changes are therefore usually described in general terms such as generalized slowing, focal slowing, etc. For example, a sudden slowing of the EEG (not correlated to drug administration) generally indicates cerebral ischaemia.

Symmetry of the EEG from side to side can be assessed visually or by computer processing and is used to detect unilateral problems, which are usually cerebrovascular in origin. EEG patterns, such as those associated with seizures and changes in continuity (Fig. 8.4), can provide diagnostic clues during monitoring. For example, certain seizures, particularly non-convulsive status epilepticus (NCSE), can only be detected by EEG monitoring. Continuity of the EEG can change in several situations. A discontinuous EEG consists of alternating periods of low amplitude and regular amplitude and occurs normally at a specific gestational age during the maturation of the neonatal EEG. At other ages, it is referred to as a burst-suppression pattern (Fig. 8.4) and is either pathological or induced by drugs such as high-dose barbiturates or propofol.

When performing EEG monitoring during surgical procedures, the most common clinically significant change is that due to cerebral ischaemia (described above). In critical care, abnormal EEG patterns,

Table 8.3 Abnormal EEG patterns seen in neurointensive care

Condition	Use of EEG monitoring
Status epilepticus	Non-convulsive status epilepticus (NCSE) frequently occurs following acute brain injury and is often missed or diagnosed late as it can alter consciousness and behaviour and be mistaken for other causes. The longer the diagnosis is delayed, the harder it is to treat and the higher the rate of mortality. Monitoring by EEG is the only way to positively diagnose NCSE
Focal cerebral ischaemia	Focal and hemispheric cerebral ischaemia can result from a number of pathological processes: 25–40% of patients with vasospasm due to subarachnoid haemorrhage suffer symptomatic ischaemia and detecting the ischaemia with EEG can provide an early warning of deterioration. The CT scan is often normal in acute stroke, but the EEG changes within minutes following ischaemia. In the emergency department, EEG may be useful in differentiating stroke patients from those with symptoms that may mimic stroke. This is particularly important given the short window for use of thrombolytic therapies
Coma	Several EEG patterns are useful in the prognosis of coma. The lack of sleep–wake cycles, a monotonous, non-changing EEG and the lack of reactivity of the EEG are all indications of a poor prognosis from coma. The lack of sleep–wake cycles, however, can be caused by other factors and this should not be used as the sole predictor of coma outcome
Acute severe head trauma	The use of EEG in the management of head trauma is still being explored and will probably play a greater role with the increased use of multimodality monitoring systems that integrate EEG metrics with other physiology. For now, EEG is used in several ancillary ways. It can assess the level of barbiturate-induced coma by monitoring the duration of the interburst interval in the burst-suppression pattern that is seen. Seizures, including NCSE, are a frequent complication of head trauma, and EEG can be used to monitor the effectiveness of the anti-epileptic drugs. Focal EEG slowing can be seen in a new or enlarging mass lesion, and this observation can help substantiate the decision to transport the patient for imaging studies

including seizure activity, are seen frequently, and their detection and recognition can play a significant role in the management of the patient as well as in the determination of prognosis. Table 8.3 lists conditions where abnormal EEG patterns yield important information for patient management on the neurointensive care unit.

Effects of anaesthesia and cooling on EEG

The EEG is a very sensitive but not very specific measurement, and one of the challenges of EEG monitoring is to determine the cause of any change. Most of the drugs used during anaesthesia and sedation result in changes in the EEG. This is both good and bad. It is bad because drug-induced EEG changes can mimic an ischaemic event, although this problem can be minimized by interpreting the EEG alongside knowledge of what drugs are being administered and, if possible, by withholding the administration of drugs during critical monitoring periods such as carotid artery clamping. Additionally, drug effects are almost always global, whereas focal or hemispheric changes are usually indicative of an ischaemic origin. The effect of

anaesthetic drugs on the EEG also has a good side. This characteristic has spawned several decades of research into an EEG-based measure of the depth of anaesthesia and resulted in a series of commercially available products.

Cooling also produces changes in the EEG but only at lower temperatures. Periodic complexes appear in the EEG after cooling to about 30°C, burst suppression at around 25°C and electrocerebral silence at 18°C. Thus, the EEG should not be altered during mild hypothermia (33°C), which is used therapeutically following cardiac arrest, but cooling during deep hypothermic circulatory arrest can produce electrocerebral silence.

Continuous EEG and computer processing

When the field of EEG transitioned from paper to digital recording in the late 1980s and early 1990s, longer-term monitoring became practical. The digital display and storage of EEG data solved the problems inherent with paper recordings but created another problem, i.e. that of having to review longer periods of EEG recording to detect clinically significant events.

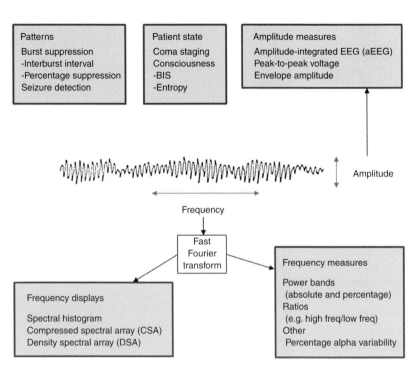

Fig. 8.5. EEG displays and derived measurements to aid in long-term monitoring. BIS, bispectral index.

Patterns
Burst suppression
-Interburst interval
-Percentage suppression
Seizure detection

Patient state
Coma staging
Consciousness
-BIS
-Entropy

Amplitude measures
Amplitude-integrated EEG (aEEG)
Peak-to-peak voltage
Envelope amplitude

Amplitude

Frequency

Fast Fourier transform

Frequency displays
Spectral histogram
Compressed spectral array (CSA)
Density spectral array (DSA)

Frequency measures
Power bands
(absolute and percentage)
Ratios
(e.g. high freq/low freq)
Other
Percentage alpha variability

The solution to this has similarities to ECG monitoring, in which measurements such as heart rate can be derived and trended to detect changes. Alarms are sounded when set heart rate limits are breached, or on the recognition of specific patterns, such as arrhythmias. In a similar manner, the entire EEG does not have to be watched on a minute-by-minute basis, but a set of measurements and alternative displays can be derived from the EEG to help visualize changes over time. Like cardiac arrhythmia detection, patterns in the EEG, such as seizure activity and levels of consciousness, can be detected automatically. A variety of methods to process and display the EEG have been developed and these are summarized in Fig. 8.5. They can be classified as measures of amplitude, frequency, patterns and patient state.

Amplitude measures

One of the earliest monitors of processed EEG was the cerebral function monitor, developed in the UK in the late 1960s. This processed the EEG into a highly compressed display of average amplitude, which later became known as the amplitude-integrated EEG (aEEG). Although initially developed for use in anaesthesia, it became widely applied in neonatology because of its simplicity and the ability of non-EEG specialists to identify basic patterns. When used together with

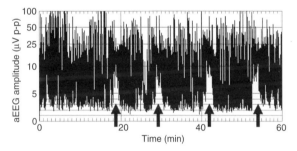

Fig. 8.6. Example of amplitude-integrated EEG (aEEG) from a neonate with repetitive seizures. The arrows point to segments where the lower margin of the aEEG is elevated – this is characteristic of seizures.

other processed measurements, and alongside the raw EEG as a reference, the aEEG is a very useful tool for identifying long-term changes in amplitude as well as patterns such as burst suppression and certain kinds of seizures. It remains an optional display format on many commercial EEG systems today. Figure 8.6 shows an example of the aEEG from a neonate with repetitive seizures.

Other measures of amplitude include the peak-to-peak voltage and envelope amplitude. Peak-to-peak voltage is defined as the difference between the maximum and minimum EEG voltage over a specific period, usually 1–2 s. Envelope amplitude is an estimate of the 'envelope' of the EEG signal and can be processed in various ways to provide a more robust amplitude estimate than simply computing peak-to-peak voltages.

Measures of frequency

Most EEG monitors can analyse the frequency content of successive segments of multichannel EEG in real time. This is commonly accomplished by a computer algorithm called a fast Fourier transform (FFT). The resulting spectra are histograms of the power at each frequency (usually between 0 and 30 Hz) present in the EEG segment. Using these histograms, it is possible, for example, to quantify the amount of EEG slowing by examining the power in the delta band (0 to <4 Hz). As the EEG amplitude is proportional to the power, these spectral histograms can be used to monitor both amplitude and frequency changes.

Monitoring applications require the ability to see changes over time, and for this reason a variety of methods have been developed to view successive spectra in a time-compressed manner. The two most widely used methods are the compressed spectral array (CSA) and the density spectral array (DSA). The CSA display plots the newest spectrum in front of the last, shifted slightly down the time axis and hiding parts of the last spectrum as if the new one was opaque, i.e. the lines from the last spectrum that would be hidden by the newer one are erased. In this manner, a three-dimensional 'mountain range' effect is created and this can be used to follow the predominant EEG frequency (Fig. 8.7). The DSA uses a colour map to indicate the amount of power in a particular frequency band. Thus, for monitoring, one can follow the bands of colours to see if the EEG is slowing, or if certain patterns are present. For example, burst suppression and certain types of seizure show up nicely in the DSA display. An advantage of the DSA is that it can be formatted to display left to right along a more conventional horizontal time axis, so changes can be correlated with trends in other physiological changes (Fig. 8.7).

The CSA and DSA displays have proven to be good at producing recognizable patterns that correlate with a variety of events such as ischaemia, certain types of seizures and changes in drug levels. However, with the goal of obtaining more quantifiable metrics, parameters have been derived from the EEG spectra that can be correlated with other measurements. The more common ones are shown in Table 8.4 and the most notable is the spectral edge frequency (SEF).

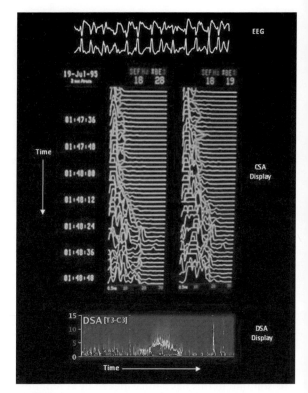

Fig. 8.7. EEG, compressed spectral array (CSA) and density spectral array (DSA) displays showing a seizure. A segment of the raw EEG during the seizure shown at the top and the spectral edge frequency (described in Table 8.4) is plotted on top of the CSA. At the bottom of the figure, a horizontal DSA display shows a seizure as the bright coloured area in the centre of the DSA. See colour plate section.

Detection of EEG patterns

For years, the Holy Grail of EEG analysis has been to develop methods for automatic interpretation, but this has not yet been achieved in reality. The major effort is to recognize and classify features that appear spatially in the set of recorded channels on the scalp and which change over time.

Most effort has been put into the automatic detection of seizure activity. This has been quite successful for epilepsy monitoring but less so for monitoring in critical care, most probably because of the variability in the background EEG related to drug effects and the underlying pathology. Several recent attempts at producing seizure detection methods specific for neonates have produced encouraging results, but, as the neonatal and adult EEG is quite different, adult-based algorithms have generally failed.

Recognition of simpler EEG patterns has been more successful. The automatic recognition and quantification of burst suppression is available commercially

Table 8.4 Measurements derived from the EEG spectrum

Measurement	Description
Spectral edge frequency (SEF)	The SEF denotes the highest 'significant' frequency in the EEG spectrum. It is calculated by noting the frequency below which lies X% of the power in that segment's spectrum. Commonly 95–97% is used in the calculation. The SEF has been used to indicate cerebral ischaemia, as one of the hallmarks of such an insult is the dropout of high EEG frequencies followed by slowing of the EEG. The SEF was widely investigated as an indication of the depth of anaesthesia but has been replaced by more powerful measurements such as bispectral index
Peak power frequency (PPF)	The PPF indicates the peak power in the spectrum and can be used to follow the predominant frequency of an EEG over long periods of time
Total power (TP)	The TP is the sum of the power for all frequencies in the histogram. It is proportional to the amplitude so that a decrease in this measurement indicates decreasing amplitude
Power bands	The power in specific frequency bands can be calculated and trended. Most systems allow the calculation to be performed as an absolute power or a relative power (percentage of the total power). For example, the percentage delta (0.5–3.5 Hz) band will increase during slowing of the EEG, which could be an indication of cerebral ischaemia
Ratios	Ratios of power bands have also been calculated. A common one is the ratio of high frequencies to low frequencies, which increases the dynamic range of a metric for cerebral ischaemia from that of just observing the percentage of delta activity (as the high frequencies tend to approach zero during cerebral ischaemia)
Percentage alpha variability (PAV)	The PAV was developed because EEG from patients with good outcomes from brain injury have large variability, whereas those with poor outcomes generally do not. The PAV looks at the variability in the alpha band and trends this over time

from several manufacturers. The quantification comes in the form of two metrics – an interburst interval (the time between bursts, in seconds) and the percentage suppression (the percentage of 'flattened' EEG, usually in a 1 or 2 min EEG segment).

Measures of patient state

To simplify the EEG further into clinically relevant metrics, work has been done over the past few decades to correlate parameters derived from the EEG with various patient states. Some of the earlier work used EEG to classify stages of coma, in particular that of metabolic origin (e.g. hepatic failure), as specific EEG patterns are seen in this state.

One derived measurement, the bispectral index (BIS), is perhaps the most widely validated and successful EEG-based variable yet developed. It has been correlated with depth of anaesthesia or, more precisely, the level of consciousness or hypnosis in anaesthetized patients. Early work in this area focused on one measurement (such as the SEF) that worked well with certain anaesthetic drugs but not others. The BIS integrates multiple derived metrics from the EEG (fast

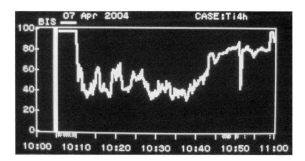

Fig. 8.8. A bispectral index (BIS) recording. Note the induction of, maintenance and recovery from anaesthesia.

activity, slowing, burst suppression, the EEG bispectrum, etc.) using a discriminate function to produce a unitless metric, the BIS. It is suggested that anaesthesia be adjusted to maintain BIS in the range of 45–60 which is deep enough to reduce the incidence of awareness and light enough to minimize post-operative side effects. Figure 8.8 shows BIS recorded during a routine colonoscopy, with induction, maintenance and recovery stages clearly visible.

Other monitors of the depth of anaesthesia have been developed. One, called Entropy, separates the metric into two components – one that assesses background activity and one that measures the reactive component, which may be correlated with analgesia.

Evoked potentials

Evoked potentials are the electrical response from the nervous system to an external stimulus. They can be used in diagnostic and monitoring settings and evaluate conduction along, and therefore the integrity of, neural pathways. They are used during intracranial and spine surgery to guide the surgeon by identifying reversible changes and allowing intervention (or cessation of a surgical intervention) before permanent neurological injury occurs. They are used less in critical care because of the technological challenges related to long-term EP monitoring. There are two types of EPs – sensory and motor. Somatosensory evoked potentials (SSEPs) monitor the integrity of sensory pathways, including peripheral nerves, and motor evoked potentials (MEPs) the motor pathways.

Technical aspects of evoked potential recording

Recording EPs is technically more challenging than EEG and is best performed by those with experience. This particularly applies during complex spine surgery where multiple types of EP are often used simultaneously and in association with other monitoring techniques.

Recorded SSEPs from the scalp have very small amplitude (a few microvolts) and are buried by the EEG, which has much greater amplitude (tens of microvolts or more). However, it is possible to extract the EP signal from the EEG, as it is time-locked to the stimulus whereas the EEG is random. Multiple stimuli are applied rapidly (hundreds, sometimes a thousand or more) and the cortical responses from a fixed time segment (e.g. 0–120 ms) following the stimuli are averaged together. The random EEG averages out at each time point following the stimulus, whereas the peaks and troughs of the evoked response build in amplitude with each average. At the end of the repetitive simulations, the average of all the time segments produces the displayed EP. As artefacts and other conditions can affect the recorded responses, two or more responses (completed averages in the case of SSEPs) must be obtained and superimposed to demonstrate repeatability of the waveform components before the response is

interpreted. In the MEP, the response is from the muscle and is much larger and therefore requires only one stimulus and no averaging.

Diagnostic EPs are evaluated on the basis of their latency and amplitudes of the waveform peaks and troughs compared with a normal control group. In the operating theatre, EPs are compared with initial baselines for evaluation of neural transmission.

Sensory evoked potentials

Sensory EPs deliver a sensory stimulus and record the response at the brain and at various points along the neural pathway. They are named according to the type of sensory stimulus that is applied to generate the EP – SSEPs, auditory evoked potentials (AEPs) and visual evoked potentials (VEPs). Of these, only the AEPs and SSEPs are routine monitoring tools. Additionally, the early responses from an auditory stimulus originate in the brainstem and are called brainstem auditory evoked potentials (BAEPs) or the equivalent brainstem auditory evoked response (BAER).

Brainstem auditory evoked responses

The stimulus used to measure a BAER is a broad band click delivered via earphones or tubephones (a tube that connects the click generator to the ear) at a fixed rate and intensity. This stimulus includes a wide range of audiological frequencies and may be delivered as a negative pressure (rarefaction), a positive pressure (condensation) or a combination of both negative and positive (alternating) clicks of varying intensities. Although it is recommended that click intensity is acoustically calibrated in 'decibels peak-equivalent sound pressure level' (dbSPL), in practice the delivered stimulus intensity is usually 70 dB above the average hearing threshold of a group of normal young adults tested by the same laboratory under conditions identical to those used for recording BAERs. This is known as dB hearing level (dbHL). Contralateral white noise is delivered to eliminate cross-hearing. The short duration, 100 μs stimulus is delivered at a rate of 8–19 clicks s^{-1}.

For monitoring applications, BAEPs are recorded using 75–2500 Hz bandpass filters to eliminate signal artefacts from 50–60 Hz contamination. Because of the small amplitude of BAERs, it is usually necessary to measure 1000–2000 averages to obtain an adequate response. The waveforms for the identification of the BAERs are generated within 10 ms after stimulation. However, a 15–20 ms time window is usually applied, as this allows for conduction delays due to physical or pathological

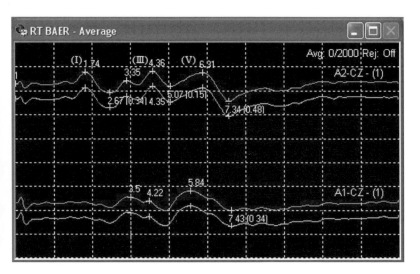

Fig. 8.9. Right brainstem auditory evoked response (BAER) recorded from ipsilateral A2–Cz and contralateral A1–Cz in a propofol-sedated patient. Waves I, III and V from the ipsilateral (to the stimulus) side are shown. See colour plate section.

conditions including wax in the external ear canal, fluid in the middle ear, structural abnormalities in the brainstem or delays due to reduced cerebral perfusion pressure or sensorineural hearing loss. It should be noted that when tubephones are used, there is an inherent 0.9 ms delay in the response because of the length of the tubing.

BAER waveforms

As the name suggests, the components of the BAER waveform are generated by the acoustic nerve and nuclei located in the brainstem. If the time window is extended to 100 ms, the mid-latency auditory evoked potentials (MLAPs) are also recorded. Although not useful in conventional monitoring applications, they have been widely studied (and commercialized) as a measure of the depth of anaesthesia.

In normal subjects, five waveforms (labelled I–V) are recorded from a scalp electrode at Cz referenced to A1 or A2 (Fig. 8.9). Waves I and II are generated in the peripheral portion of the VIIIth cranial nerve in the internal acoustic canal. Wave III is the by-product of multiple generators both from the ipsilateral lateral surface of the brainstem and the contralateral cochlear nucleus. Contemporary studies suggest that wave IV most probably originates from the contralateral superior olivary complex and wave V from the contralateral midbrain by the lateral lemniscus where it terminates in the inferior colliculus. As wave V is from the contralateral side of the brainstem, recording from contralateral electrodes generally yields a larger amplitude and better-defined response. As with all EPs, the expected latencies and amplitudes of waveform peaks in the BAER are based on recordings from normal controls (Table 8.5).

Somatosensory evoked potentials

Somatosensory evoked potentials are used most commonly to monitor the adequacy of spinal cord function during spine surgery. Peripheral nerves are stimulated in the arms or legs, depending on the procedure, and recordings are made from the scalp. Changes in the latency and/or amplitude of the response can indicate dysfunction in the neural pathway being monitored.

Stimulation for SSEP recordings consists of a 200–300 µs constant current electrical stimulus repeated at a rate of 4–7 s^{-1} and applied via a pair of skin electrodes or subdermal needles placed over the relevant nerve. Stimulus intensity is variable but, for operating theatre and intensive care unit (ICU) applications, should be supra-maximal, meaning that a visual twitch should be seen in the hand or foot. For monitoring the spinal cord, the stimulus is applied to the posterior tibial nerve at the ankle or the peroneal nerve at the knee. The resulting responses are often called lower-extremity SSEPs. For monitoring the cortical tracts, such as during carotid endarterectomy, the stimulus is applied to the median or ulnar nerves at the wrist and the resulting responses are called upper-extremity SSEPs.

Scalp electrode placements for recording SSEPs follow the International 10–20 electrode placement system but with some modifications. Waveforms are recorded from the primary cortical somatosensory cortex using scalp locations approximately 2 cm posterior to Cz (Cpz), left C3 (Cp3) and right C4 (Cp4) for lower- and upper-extremity SSEPs. Non-cephalic locations are also recorded as controls to ensure that the stimulus is working and to allow calculation of

Table 8.5 Expected wave latencies and interpeak times for the normal brainstem auditory evoked response (BAER)

(a) BAER waves and latencies

Wave	Mean (ms)	Range (ms)
Wave I	1.62	1.26–1.98
Wave II	2.80	2.23–3.37
Wave III	3.75	3.24–4.26
Wave IV	4.84	4.15–5.53
Wave IV/V	5.27	4.61–5.93
Wave V	5.62	4.93–6.31

(b) BAER interpeak times

Waves	Times (ms)
I–III	2.63
I–IV/V	4.32
I–V (age <60)	Female: <4.60 Male: <4.65

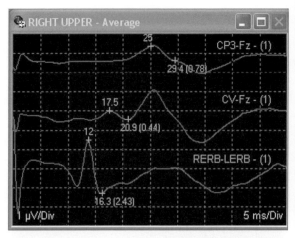

Fig. 8.10. Right upper-extremity somatosensory evoked potential (SSEP) recorded from Erb's point, C5 cervical spine and the left somatosensory cortex in a propofol-sedated patient. Note that the peripheral response (at the brachial plexus recorded at Erb's point) is delayed to 12 ms instead of the normal 9 ms. This delay shifts the subsequent peaks out by 3 ms and is most probably due to a peripheral neuropathy, but could also be due to a very long arm or a cold arm. See colour plate section.

conduction times. For lower-extremity SSEPs, recordings are made over the cervical spine at the level of the second or fifth cervical vertebra and from the popliteal fossa if not used for stimulation. For upper-extremity SSEPs, recordings are made from Erb's point over the brachial plexus. Using bandpass filters from 30 to 1500 Hz, averages are recorded over an analysis time of 50–120 ms for upper- and lower-extremity studies. By convention, SSEP peaks are designated with a capital P or N referring to a positive or negative peak, followed by a number that indicates approximate latency of the peak, e.g. N20.

Upper-extremity SSEPs

Figure 8.10 shows an example of a typical upper-extremity SSEP study. The waveform recorded over Erb's point is generated from the brachial plexus and in normal subjects appears at approximately 9 ms (referred to as N9). The next waveform is recorded from the dorsal neck (N13–14) reflecting post-synaptic activity in the cervical cord. The scalp-recorded wave at 18 ms (N18) is generated in the thalamus or thalamocortical radiations and can be seen best in awake cooperative patients. The N20 and P22 waveforms, occurring at 20 and 22 ms, are of cortical origin. Of interest in the ICU is the central conduction time (CCT), which is calculated between the N13/14 and N20 waveforms. This is generally 5–8 ms in the normal adult and is increased during cerebral ischaemia or encephalopathy.

Lower-extremity SSEPs

The initial response that passes through the cauda equina and lower spinal cord is referred to as the lumbar potential (LP). Additional recording sites can be added anywhere along the pathway to the brain. The waveform recorded from the cervical spine at about 30 ms (N30) after stimulation of the posterior tibial nerve is generated in the nucleus gracilis and that from the scalp at about 37 ms (P37) in the primary somatosensory cortex (Fig. 8.11).

Interpreting SSEPs

Somatosensory evoked potentials are sensitive to lesions of the medial lemniscus in the dorsal columns and generally are not affected by isolated involvement of the spinothalamic tract. Abnormalities are defined by prolongation of the interpeak latencies compared with normal controls or a difference of >1 ms from baseline in an individual patient. For example, a prolongation of latency between Erb's point and N13–14 suggests a lesion located between the proximal portions of the brachial plexus and the dorsal columns. As with other EPs, an abnormal SSEP finding indicates an anatomic lesion that disrupts the normal physiological mechanism of that system rather than a specific disease process. It is also important to understand that the responses (waveform peaks) of SSEPs are volume conducted through the body. Thus, if there is nerve damage along the specific pathway to the brain, earlier

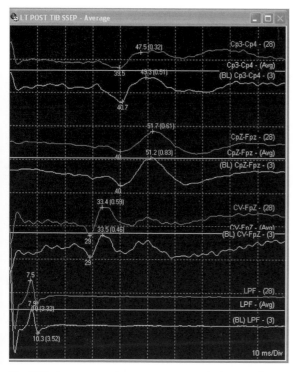

Fig. 8.11. Lower-extremity somatosensory evoked potential (SSEP), showing a peripheral response recorded from the popliteal fossa, a subcortical response recorded at the cervical spine and a cortical response recorded at the somatosensory cortex in a propofol-sedated patient. See colour plate section.

waveform responses are still seen because they are conducted through the body, albeit not by the nerve pathway. Surgical events that cause changes in baseline from the SSEP amplitudes include, most specifically, vascular insufficiency, blint trauma, traction, and compression, all of which should be investigated from other technical, systemic or anaesthetic factors.

Motor evoked potentials

Motor evoked potential measurement involves stimulation of the relevant area of brain cortex, following which the response travels to specific muscles where it is recorded as a compound muscle action potential (CMAP). There are two types of brain stimuli that can be used – electrical and magnetic. In transcranial electrical MEP (TceMEP) monitoring, the brain is stimulated electrically via scalp electrodes, whereas in transcranial magnetic stimulation, coils placed on the scalp are energized and emit a magnetic flux that stimulates the cortex. Transcranial magnetic stimulation is used most commonly in diagnostic applications including depression, migraine and a variety of other

neurological disorders, whereas TceMEPs are increasingly used in monitoring applications.

Transcranial electrical motor evoked potentials

Transcranial electrical MEPs are used during surgery to assess corticospinal tract function during procedures that place the spinal cord at risk. They can also be used to assess motor function in comatose or sedated ICU patients following motor vehicle accidents or other trauma.

Recording of TceMEPs uses anodal stimulation between the C1 and C2 scalp locations. Short-duration (50 μs), high-frequency (intersample interval of 2–5 ms) multipulse (4–7 pulses) trains are delivered to the scalp surface to elicit a reproducible TceMEP. The voltages required to elicit TceMEPs range from 200 to 600 V and, because of the risk of jaw contraction during stimulation, bilateral bite blocks should be placed between the upper and lower teeth to prevent tongue lacerations during recording. Following cortical stimulation, a CMAP can be recorded on the contralateral limbs to the anodal stimulation. Bilateral recording sites include the triceps, biceps and abductor pollicis brevis in the arms, the tibialis anterior and medial gastrocnemius in the legs and the abductor hallucis in the foot. If the suspected injury is below the cervical level, TceMEPs of the upper extremities act as a control for the lower extremities.

Transcranial electrical MEPs are complex polyphasic recordings elicited from muscles targeted to the clinical condition, with amplitudes ranging from 50 to 1000 μV (Fig. 8.12). Recordings should be made in the absence of neuromuscular blockade.

Application and interpretation of evoked potentials

Multimodal neurophysiological monitoring, using SSEPs and MEPs from upper and/or lower limbs as appropriate, and EMG (see below), is recommended during complex spine surgery because no single method can sufficiently cover the complex functions of the spinal cord. Motor evoked potentials are more sensitive to spinal cord ischaemia than SSEPs and correlate better with motor function after spine surgery. Cortical SSEPs may also be used to monitor cerebral ischaemia during intracranial and carotid endarterectomy surgery. Criteria for the interpretation of MEPs in the ICU have not been established, although the presence or absence of CMAP following TceMEP can be used to assess corticospinal tract function.

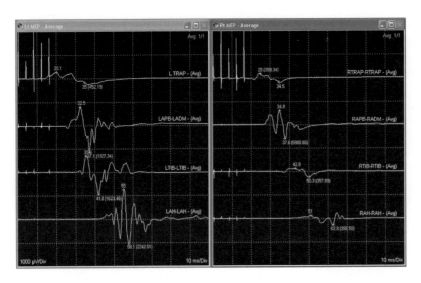

Fig. 8.12. Transcranial electrical motor evoked potentials (TceMEPs), recorded from left and right target muscles – the trapezius (TRAP) and abductor pollicis brevis (APB) in the upper extremities, tibialis anterior (TIB) in the lower extremities and abductor hallucis (AH) in the feet. See colour plate section.

Factors affecting evoked potential monitoring

The choice of anaesthetic agents and other drugs is critical if EP monitoring is to be used during surgery. Volatile anaesthetics cause a dose-dependent decrease in EP amplitude and an increase in latency and should be avoided. Most intravenous anaesthetic agents have a considerably smaller effect and can be used during monitoring. In particular, a combination of propofol and opioid is effective in maximizing EP amplitude, latency and stability. Transcranial electrical MEPs are most reliable with a train of four (TOF) equal to 4/4 twitches recorded from the target muscle group; thus, the use of neuromuscular blocking agents is contraindicated when recording MEPs. The TceMEP response amplitudes are also reduced with mean arterial pressure below 60 mmHg and anaesthetic depth sufficient to cause a burst-suppression pattern on EEG or BIS of <30.

Electromyography

Electromyography is a technique used to evaluate the electrical activity in muscle fibres. Two types of EMG monitoring are commonly used – recording spontaneous electrical activity and recording responses generated by stimulation of motor nerves.

Physiology of electromyography

The motor unit comprises a motor nerve and all the muscles fibres that it innervates. It acts as a single functional unit with all the fibres contracting synchronously. Each muscle fibre produces an action potential, and the summation of the individual potentials within the motor unit is the motor unit action potential (MUAP). The electrophysiological activity from multiple motor units is the signal evaluated during EMG recording.

Motor unit action potentials can be monophasic, biphasic or polyphasic with amplitudes between $100\,\mu V$ and $2\,mV$ and durations varying from 2 to 10 ms. Pathological states affect the duration and amplitude of the MUAP and typically result in polyphasic morphology. In general, myopathies lead to a decrease in duration and amplitude of MUAPs, whereas neuropathies cause an increase in duration and amplitude (up to 10 mV). Healthy resting muscle has no electrical activity, although placement of a needle recording electrode may result in MUAPs of short duration and low amplitude. In muscle pathology (either primary or secondary due to denervation), the response to needle insertion is prolonged and there are also polymorphous patterns of spontaneous activity including fibrillation potentials, positive sharp waves, fasciculation potentials and myotonic firing.

Recording the electromyogram

Electromyogram equipment consists of recording electrodes, a pre-amplifier (usually placed close to the patient to minimize electrical interference), an amplifier and a display system (often visual and audio). Needle electrodes inserted into the muscle (or group of muscles) to be tested are most commonly used, but surface electrodes have limited value and should not be used. The MUAPs are of sufficient amplitude relative to background electrical activity such that, unlike in SSEP monitoring, averaging is not required. This means that a response is immediately available to inform clinical decision-making.

Recording of spontaneous activity can be performed continuously, but techniques using intentional stimulation of the motor nerve are non-continuous. As nerve stimulation results in motor activity and possible patient movement, such techniques must be carefully incorporated into the surgical procedure.

Electromyography in intraoperative monitoring

The EMG is used in a variety of neurosurgical procedures, including posterior fossa and spinal surgery, to provide a continuous assessment of cranial and peripheral motor nerves and spinal nerve roots. Pairs of needle electrodes are placed into or near the muscle(s) of interest and, if the supplying nerve is touched or stretched during surgery, EMG activity will be detected. Mild nerve irritation leads to transient EMG discharges, while more serious stretching or irritation may produce sustained activity. However, transection of the nerve may not provoke an EMG response. Direct stimulation can be used to locate the nerve of interest or to assess its integrity. Small monopolar or bipolar electrodes are applied directly to the nerve and the EMG response from single or multiple stimuli of low-intensity current (0.5–5 mA) of short duration (0.5–1.0 ms) are recorded in the target muscle(s). The EMG responses recorded during nerve stimulation are known as CMAPs. During intraoperative monitoring, real-time acoustic feedback of EMG activity is provided to the surgeon.

Electromyography is more resistant than SSEPs and MEPs to the depressant effects of anaesthetic agents and other physiological variables such as blood pressure and temperature. Although an appropriate response can be recorded with 75% suppression of baseline CMAPs, neuromuscular blockade is generally avoided because small-amplitude EMG responses from nerve irritation can be difficult to detect in damaged or poorly functioning nerves. Under such circumstances, even controlled neuromuscular blockade can render CMAPs totally unrecordable.

Monitoring cranial nerves
All cranial nerves with a motor component (III, IV, V, VII, IX, X, XI and XII) can be monitored using EMG, but VIIth nerve monitoring is most common. Because

the facial nerve is often intertwined within brainstem tumours, VIIth nerve monitoring is considered by many to be a standard of care during vestibular schwannoma surgery. It is also commonly used during other operations at the cerebellopontine angle. During VIIth nerve monitoring, the ipsilateral orbicularis oculi and oris muscles are used for EMG recording.

Monitoring spinal nerve roots
Electromyography can be used to identify peripheral nerves and spinal nerve roots and detect their functional continuity, and to monitor intact nerves/roots to minimize the risk of inadvertent surgical injury. Depending on the site of surgery, EMG monitoring of muscles of the upper or lower limbs can be used when there is a risk of nerve root damage during spinal surgery. As radiculopathy is more common than myelopathy after thoracolumbar surgery, lower-limb EMG is recommended in addition to SSEPs during procedures in these regions. Spontaneous EMG in the relevant muscle is recorded by paired subdermal needle electrodes and, in addition, stimulated EMG can be used to confirm accurate placement of pedicle screws by stimulation of the screw or screw hole with a monopolar electrode. Because bone cortex has a higher resistance to current flow than soft tissue, generation of an EMG response by a low threshold of stimulus indicates a breach in the bone and screw misplacement.

Another important application of intraoperative EMG is for monitoring the nerve roots of the cauda equina, as damage to the sacral nerves will result in post-operative sphincter disturbance. This technique is particularly useful in surgery for spinal dysraphism or conus tumours when recordings from stimulation can differentiate nerve roots from other structures. For example, the stimulation threshold for filum terminale fibres is more than 100 times higher than that for motor nerves.

Electromyography in the intensive care unit

Electromyography recording is a crucial component of the diagnostic strategy of critical care-acquired neuromuscular weakness (see Chapter 26). However, differentiation between critical illness myopathy (CIM) and polyneuropathy (CIP) is extremely difficult if not impossible using standard EMG techniques. Critical illness myopathy can be diagnosed by abnormal EMG during voluntary contraction in conscious and cooperative patients but has limited applicability in critically ill patients who are often unable to cooperate with the investigation. In uncooperative patients, direct muscle stimulation (DMS) can be used to differentiate between CIP and CIM. In CIP, there is a reduced or absent CMAP on motor nerve stimulation but a normal response with DMS, whereas the CMAP is reduced or absent after both motor nerve and DMS in CIM. Stimulating and recording electrodes must be placed in the muscle distal to the end-plate zone and DMS is therefore technically difficult.

Further reading

Chan, M., Gin, T. and Goh, K. Y. (2004). Interventional neurophysiologic monitoring. *Curr Opin Anaesthesiol* **17**, 389–96.

Chiappa, K. H. (1979). Results of electroencephalographic monitoring during 367 carotid endarterectomies. Use of a dedicated minicomputer. *Stroke* **10**, 381–8.

Deletis, V. and Sala, F. (2008). Intraoperative neurophysiological monitoring of the spinal cord during spinal cord and spine surgery: a review focus on the corticospinal tracts. *Clin Neurophysiol* **119**, 248–64.

Ebersole, J. and Pedley, T. (2003). *Current Practice of Clinical Electroencephalography*, 3rd edn. Baltimore, MD: Lippincott Williams & Wilkins.

Guerit, J., Amantini, A., Amodio, P. *et al.* (2009). Consensus on the use of neurophysiological tests in the intensive care unit (ICU): electroencephalogram (EEG), evoked potentials (EP), and electroneuromyography (ENMG). *Neurophysiol Clin* **39**, 71–83.

Hellstrom-Westas, L., Rosen, I. and de Vries, L. (2008). *An Atlas of Amplitude-integrated EEGs in the Newborn*, 2nd edn. London: Informa Healthcare.

Hirsch, L. and Brenner, R. (2010). *Atlas of EEG in Critical Care*. New York: Wiley.

Jordan, K. G. (1993). Continuous EEG and evoked potential monitoring in the neuroscience intensive care unit. *J Clin Neurophysiol* **10**, 445–75.

Kelleher, M. O., Tan, G., Sarjeant, R. and Fehlings, M. G. (2008). Predictive value of intraoperative neurophysiological monitoring during cervical spine surgery: a prospective analysis of 1055 consecutive cases. *J Neurosurg Spine* **8**, 215–21.

Misulis, K. E. and Head, T. C. (2003). *Essentials of Clinical Neurophysiology*, 3rd edn. Boston, MA: Butterworth-Heinemann.

Niedermeyer, E. and Lopes da Silva, F. (2004). *Electroencephalography: Basic Principles, Clinical Applications, and Related Fields*, 5th edn. Baltimore, MD: Lippincott Williams & Wilkins.

Rampil, I. J. (1998). A primer for EEG signal processing in anesthesia. *Anesthesiology* **89**, 980–1002.

Scheuer, M. (2002). Continuous monitoring in the intensive care unit. *Epilepsia* **43** (Suppl. 3), 114–27.

Stecker, M. M., Cheung, A. T., Pochettino, A. *et al.* (2001). Deep hypothermic circulatory arrest: I. Effects of cooling on electroencephalogram and evoked potentials. *Ann Thorac Surg* **71**, 14–21.

Vespa, P. M., Boscardin, W. J., Hovda, D. A. *et al.* (2002). Early and persistent impaired percent alpha variability on continuous electroencephalography monitoring as predictive of poor outcome after traumatic brain injury. *J Neurosurg* **97**, 84–92.

Guidelines and technical standards

Guideline 1: Minimum technical requirements for performing clinical electroencephalography (2006). *J Clin Neurophysiol* **23**, 86–91.

Guideline 2: Minimum technical standards for pediatric electroencephalography (2006). *J Clin Neurophysiol* **23**, 92–6.

Guideline 3: Minimum technical standards for EEG recording in suspected cerebral death (2006). *J Clin Neurophysiol* **23**, 97–104.

Guideline 9A: Guidelines on evoked potentials (2006). *J Clin Neurophysiol* **23**, 125–37.

Guideline 9C: Guidelines on short-latency auditory evoked potentials (2006). *J Clin Neurophysiol* **23**, 157–67.

Guideline 9D: Guidelines on short-latency somatosensory evoked potentials (2006). *J Clin Neurophysiol* **23**, 168–79.

Guideline 11A: Recommended standards for neurophysiologic intraoperative monitoring – principles (2009). American Clinical Neurophysiology Society. Available at http://www.acns.org/pdfs/Guideline%2011A.pdf.

Guideline 11B: Recommended standards for intraoperative monitoring of somatosensory evoked potentials (2009). American Clinical Neurophysiology Society. Available at http://www.acns.org/pdfs/Guideline%2011B.pdf.

Guideline 11C: Recommended standards for intraoperative monitoring of auditory evoked potentials (2009). American Clinical Neurophysiology Society. Available at http://www.acns.org/pdfs/Guideline%2011C.pdf.

Chapter

9

Multimodality monitoring

Nino Stocchetti and Luca Longhi

Definition and purpose of multimodality monitoring

Patients with acute brain damage are unstable and may deteriorate: one in three patients with traumatic brain injury (TBI) shows such clinical deterioration. Deterioration is dangerous, sometimes life-threatening, and is associated with worse long-term outcomes. For brain protection, it is essential to capture early signs of worsening and, where possible, the warning signals that precede it. This is the reason why monitoring (the repeated and consistent measurement of biological variables) is so crucial. In deeply sedated patients, instrumental monitoring can become the predominant source of information, but clinical observation (at least considering the pupils' diameter and light reactivity) coupled with imaging such as a CT scan or nuclear magnetic resonance remain essentials.

Very rarely in neurointensive care is a single parameter measured in isolation: current practice recommends the simultaneous acquisition of multiple data. The simple concept of cerebral perfusion pressure (CPP), for instance, incorporates intracranial pressure (ICP) and mean arterial pressure (MAP). All available commercial monitors, moreover, offer multiple parameters to be registered and displayed simultaneously. Intracranial disturbances are better treated when their causes are identified, and the most productive way of achieving this goal is performed by integrating multiple sources of information. Any ICP rise, for instance, can be better understood, and treated, when possible causes, such as fever, hyponatraemia or hypercapnia, are identified. This requires that multiple parameters are recorded and considered simultaneously. Therefore, monitoring is usually multimodal.

The concept of multimodality monitoring refers more to the purpose and to the level of integration than to the number of tools assembled. Interestingly, in a pioneer paper by Gaab and colleagues in 1986 describing multimodality monitoring for neurointensive care, two computers were used (the processing power of a single CPU was not adequate) to allow the desired data integration.

Multimodality monitoring can be defined as a system where several sources of information are put together, analysed and processed to achieve a comprehensive picture of the patient's status.

The concept is not new, and has been used in intensive care units (ICUs) for > 30 years, in parallel with the development of more sophisticated computers.

The purposes of multimodality monitoring mimic the aims of monitoring:

- To continuously measure relevant biological variables.
- To verify the effects of treatment.
- To identify trends in the clinical evolution of disease.
- To contribute to the assessment of prognosis.

Additionally, multimodality monitoring may indicate associations between parameters and may contribute to clinical research.

Sources of information for multimodality monitoring

Many parameters can be included in a multimodality monitoring system, and the type and number of their combination is theoretically endless. A substantial component of multimodality monitoring should be systemic parameters concerning oxygenation and perfusion, such as arterial oxygen saturation, ECG, arterial pressure, etc. When, at an international meeting, Professor J. D. Miller (a neurosurgeon among the founders of neurointensive care) was asked to rank the parameters that should be measured together with ICP, he answered 'arterial pressure and pulse oximetry'. In this chapter, we assume that good data concerning adequate oxygen delivery (DO_2) to the organs and maintenance of homeostasis are already part of routine ICU monitoring, and we concentrate on tools focused on the brain.

Cerebral global monitors

Intracranial pressure

Intracranial pressure is defined as the pressure required in a needle placed in the cerebrospinal space to prevent the escape of cerebrospinal fluid (CSF). It is synonymous with CSF pressure. In the setting of brain trauma, it has been shown that there is an association between poor outcomes and the proportion of time spent with an ICP of >20 mmHg, which is a suggested threshold for treatment. Intracranial hypertension is the result of processes leading to increased intracranial volume. Two mechanisms of brain damage are associated with intracranial hypertension.

Firstly, in the presence of mass lesions, the ICP is not uniform within the central nervous system, and pressure gradients develop between different compartments leading to tissue compression, distortion and herniations. In the presence of a mass lesion located in the temporal lobe, herniations have also been documented with an ICP of <20 mmHg, suggesting that numerical data should be integrated with clinical information (i.e. development of a new dilated pupil). Secondly, raised ICP may reduce CPP (see below), and the resulting reductions in perfusion may result in regional or global ischaemia.

While there are no studies that prove that ICP monitoring per se improves the outcome of patients with acute brain damage, in modern neurointensive care units it is well accepted that ICP should be monitored in all salvageable comatose patients with an abnormal CT scan. Clinical and radiological tools alone are inaccurate methods to document raised ICP, and might lead to an underestimation and undertreatment of the problem. In some centres, ICP is also monitored in patients undergoing elective resection of brain tumours, particularly in complex cases when post-operative complications such as haemorrhage or swelling are likely to occur.

Cerebral perfusion pressure

Cerebral perfusion pressure is calculated as the difference between MAP and ICP, and represents the driving force for cerebral blood flow (CBF). In order to allow accurate calculation of CPP, transducers measuring ICP and MAP should be zeroed at the level of the foramen of Monro, the external landmark for which is the level of the external acoustic meatus.

Pressure autoregulation ensures a constant CBF within a CPP range from about 50 to 150 mmHg – outside these limits, CBF is passively dependent on CPP. In the hypertensive patient, the autoregulatory curve is shifted upwards, suggesting that higher pressures are required to ensure an adequate CBF. The vasodilator response to arterial hypotension may trigger rises in ICP; in contrast, vasoconstrictive responses to increases in blood pressure reduce cerebral blood volume, and have led to the suggestion that MAP elevations are a potential therapy for episodes of intracranial hypertension. Following TBI, up to 30% of patients show defective autoregulation. As autoregulatory capacity varies among patients and, over time, within patients, the ability to monitor it continuously at the bedside offers advantages. The pressure reactivity index (PRx) is the moving linear correlation coefficient between MAP and ICP. In patients with preserved autoregulation, increases in MAP trigger autoregulatory vasoconstriction, while reductions in MAP trigger autoregulatory cerebral vasodilation. Consequently, a negative PRx implies preserved autoregulation, while positive PRx values imply pressure passive behaviour of the cerebral circulation and is seen when autoregulation is absent. Assessment of autoregulation may be useful for setting an appropriate CPP for a given patient. To date, the recent *Guidelines for the Management of Severe Traumatic Brain Injury* suggest that CPP should be in the range of 50–70 mmHg and that those patients with intact autoregulation might tolerate higher CPP values.

Additionally, in cases of focal ischaemia, autoregulation might be lost and therefore regional CBF may become pressure-dependent. This physiological context provides the rationale for raising MAP to increase regional CBF in patients with vasospasm-associated cerebral ischaemia. Indeed, the majority of patients admitted to neurointensive care units are characterized by heterogeneous diseases (e.g. TBI, cerebrovascular diseases, brain tumours), in which different areas of the brain might require different perfusion pressures to overcome regionally increased vascular resistance and to ensure adequate DO_2. Ideally, we should be able to combine monitoring tools to assess both global and regional adequacy of perfusion and set

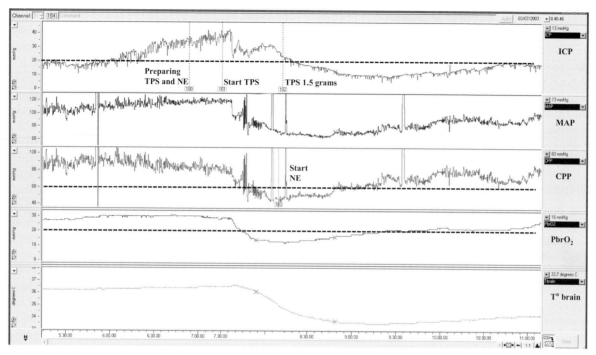

Fig. 9.1. Chart showing the changes in ICP, CPP, brain tissue oxygen tension (PbrO$_2$) and brain temperature (measured in the vicinity of a hypodense lesion) during barbiturate induction for the treatment of raised ICP. Thiopental effectively lowered ICP but induced a CPP reduction and an associated regional brain hypoxia that was corrected using norepinephrine. In this patient, these data showed the CPP threshold required to ensure an adequate brain oxygenation in a vulnerable area of the brain. TPS, thiopental; NE, norepinephrine. See colour plate section.

the CPP accordingly to an individualized approach. As patients with supranormal CPP obtained with aggressive volume resuscitation and vasopressor therapy are at increased risk of cardiorespiratory complications, it is also important to identify clinical priorities in individual patients and to balance the physiological requirements of the brain with the potential harm of aggressive therapy (Fig. 9.1).

Jugular venous oxygen saturation

The global adequacy of cerebral DO$_2$ can be assessed by measuring jugular bulb oxygen saturation (SjO$_2$) and calculating the arterio-jugular oxygen difference (AjDO$_2$)

$$(AjDO_2) = [(SaO_2 - SjO_2) \times Hb \times 1.34] + [(PaO_2 - PjO_2 \, mmHg) \times 0.003]$$

where SaO$_2$ is the arterial oxygen saturation, Hb is the haemoglobin concentration (g dl^{-1}), and PaO$_2$ and PjO$_2$ are arterial and jugular bulb partial pressures of oxygen, respectively. The SjO$_2$ represents the balance between cerebral metabolic rate of oxygen (CMRO$_2$) and cerebral DO$_2$. Normal values of SjO$_2$ are in the range

55–70%. In cases in which cerebral DO$_2$ is insufficient for cerebral metabolic needs, the brain extracts more oxygen and therefore lowers SjO$_2$. Values of SjO$_2$ below 50% represent global ischaemia, and their occurrence has been associated with unfavourable outcome following TBI. The AjDO$_2$ represents the balance between CMRO$_2$ and CBF; normal values are around 6 ml dl^{-1}; values >9 ml dl^{-1} are indicative of inadequate CBF with increased oxygen extraction, and values < 4 ml dl^{-1} are indicative of decreased oxygen extraction with relative hyperaemia. Comatose TBI patients show a mean AjDO$_2$ of 4.2 ± 1.3 ml dl^{-1}, with higher values on day 1 and progressive decreases thereafter. Patients with better outcomes show significantly higher values than those seen in patients who die or who survive in a vegetative or severely disabled state 6 months post-injury, presumably because low values indicate that the brain is unable to extract and use oxygen (because of either infarction or severe mitochondrial dysfunction).

Monitoring of SjO$_2$ should be used to guide hyperventilation therapy, which is commonly used to reduce ICP by producing hypocapnic vasoconstriction. We suggest cannulating the internal jugular vein of the more damaged hemisphere in patients with predominant focal injury; in contrast, the dominant internal jugular vein should be cannulated in patients with diffuse injury, as this is more representative of the whole brain. The position of the catheter should be checked on anteroposterior and lateral skull radiographs, with the tip at the level of C1–C2. We do not cannulate the internal jugular vein on the side of an arteriovenous malformation or decompressive craniectomy because data are unreliable due to the shunt effect.

Electrical monitoring

The brain normally produces low-voltage electrical activity. This can be measured via an EEG, which is ordinarily recorded from the scalp with small surface electrodes. Potential applications of EEG monitoring in neurointensive care are covered in Chapters 8 and 27, but include the diagnosis of non-convulsive status epilepticus, titration of barbiturates/propofol infusions to achieve burst suppression during the treatment of status epilepticus, diagnosis of new ischaemia in patients with subarachnoid haemorrhage (SAH) at risk of vasospasm, aiding outcome prediction (spontaneous burst suppression, or alpha/theta pattern coma are associated with unfavourable outcome) or helping to confirm brain death. However, interpretation of EEG information requires special expertise, because several ICU-related artefacts originating from infusions pumps, mechanical ventilators and heating blankets may produce appearances that suggest seizure activity. Evoked potentials have a more limited role in neurointensive care: the median nerve somatosensory evoked potential (SSEP) is most used. Stimulation of the medial nerve produces impulses that can be recorded at the cortex (barbiturate infusion does not affect the recordings). Recently it has been proposed that the bilateral absence of a cortical response to median nerve stimulation recorded on days 1–3 or later after cardiopulmonary resuscitation accurately predicts a poor outcome in patients with post-anoxic encephalopathy.

Brain temperature

There is a physiological relationship between brain metabolism and temperature. Hypothermia has been shown to be neuroprotective in several models of acute brain injury and has been recommended for post-cardiac arrest care by several guidelines. However, to date, it is unclear whether hypothermia can improve outcome following TBI and stroke, despite a solid mechanistic rationale, robust pre-clinical data and promising data showing that hypothermia is effective in controlling intracranial hypertension. In contrast, hyperthermia occurs frequently in patients with TBI and stroke and is associated with a worse outcome. Consequently, there is a general consensus that fever should be treated aggressively in patients with acute brain damage, with the goal of reaching and maintaining normothermia. Brain temperature can be measured using parenchymal or ventricular sensors coupled to ICP monitoring probes. Studies of the relationship between brain and core temperature in neurocritical care patients show that, on average, brain temperature exceeds core temperature by 0.3°C. Notably, this gradient increased during febrile episodes, which were also associated with raised ICP, suggesting that during the phases in which temperature exerts its major detrimental effects, core measurements underestimate the actual brain temperature. As temperature appears to be an important modulator of brain damage and a potential target for treatment, it would be advisable to measure it within the brain. Contraindications to brain temperature monitoring are similar to those for ICP monitoring.

Monitors of cerebral blood flow

Transcranial Doppler ultrasonography

Transcranial Doppler ultrasonography (TCD) is a non-invasive tool to evaluate the large intracranial arteries at the bedside. It can provide information on arterial patency, ICP, pressure autoregulation and vasoreactivity, and can be used as a confirmatory test supporting the clinical diagnosis of brain death. Its major application is the monitoring of vasospasm in patients following SAH, particularly in the basal segments of the intracranial arteries, such as the middle cerebral artery (MCA): a sudden increase in flow velocity exceeding $50 \, \text{cm s}^{-1}$, or an isolated flow velocity reading between 120 and $200 \, \text{cm s}^{-1}$ coupled with a Lindegaard ratio >3–6 (ratio between velocity of the MCA and extracranial internal carotid artery) are associated with vasospasm. The ranges for absolute flow velocity and Lindegaard ratio underline the fact that this is not an absolute diagnosis – the higher the velocity and Lindegaard ratio, the higher the specificity of the finding. However, a comparison of TCD flow velocity measurements with quantitative measurements of CBF using xenon-enhanced CT in comatose/sedated patients following SAH suggests that high flow velocities do not uniformly denote ischaemia.

Laser Doppler flowmetry and thermal diffusion flowmetry

Regional CBF can be measured invasively using laser Doppler flowmetry (LDF) and thermal diffusion flowmetry (TDF). Laser Doppler flowmetry provides qualitative CBF information on a small volume of tissue (typically $1\,mm^3$) and allows rapid detection of regional perfusion changes. However, the data are not expressed in $ml\,(100\,g)^{-1}\,min^{-1}$ but in relative percentage changes, and can be influenced by haemodilution and various artefacts (patient movement or displacement). These issues limit its applicability in neurointensive care patients. In contrast to LDF, TDF provides real-time, quantitative regional CBF values that have been validated when compared with those obtained using a xenon-enhanced CT scan. Thermal diffusion flowmetry provides information on 25–$30\,mm^3$ of brain tissue, and might be specifically indicated in comatose patients following SAH at risk of vasospasm where it has been shown to be more reliable when compared with transcranial ultrasonography.

Monitors of the adequacy of cerebral oxygen delivery

Brain tissue oxygen tension

Regional cerebral oxygenation can be measured continuously using a probe containing a miniaturized Clark-type electrode placed in the brain parenchyma. Brain tissue oxygen tension ($PbrO_2$) represents a balance between cerebral DO_2 and its consumption, measured in a few mm^3 of tissue containing extracellular fluid, capillaries, cells and axons. The $PbrO_2$ is influenced by PaO_2 and CBF. Normal values change at different depths from the cortical surface, reflecting the capillary density of the sampled tissue (in the range 20–$45\,mmHg$). Suggested thresholds for regional brain hypoxia are in the range 10–$20\,mmHg$, but more work is needed to determine the threshold and duration of brain hypoxia associated with irreversible histological damage. When compared with the gold standard (the end-capillary oxygen tension measured using positron emission tomography), $PbrO_2$ was different but showed similar changes following physiological perturbations known to affect CBF, suggesting that $PbrO_2$ is an adequate indicator of changes in regional oxygenation that occurs in patients. Regional brain hypoxia occurs following severe TBI, both in pericontusional tissue and in normal-appearing tissue, even when CPP and SjO_2 are normal. As there is an association between the degree and duration of brain hypoxia and unfavourable outcome following TBI, normal $PbrO_2$ is emerging as a therapeutic target for patients with acute brain injury. Potential applications for monitoring of $PbrO_2$ in patients with SAH and/or intracerebral haemorrhage includes intraoperative monitoring for diagnosis of vascular occlusion, diagnosis of vasospasm-associated cerebral ischaemia and response to its treatment, and monitoring of the tissue compressed by a haematoma. Despite the advantages of $PbrO_2$ monitoring, it remains unclear whether $PbrO_2$-oriented therapy can improve outcome, and which is the most appropriate means of normalizing a pathologically reduced $PbrO_2$ (CPP augmentation, increases in the fraction of inspired oxygen (FiO_2) or transfusion).

Cerebral microdialysis

Microdialysis allows the measurement of neurochemistry using a perfusion pump and a small two-lumen probe inserted into the brain parenchyma. The probe has a semi-permeable membrane with a molecular cut-off ranging from 20 to $100\,kDa$ and contains a gold tip, which makes it visible on CT scans. The biophysical principle of microdialysis is that molecules below the cut-off size of the membrane diffuse from the extracellular space to the perfusion fluid and vice versa along a concentration gradient. The recovery of an individual molecule is defined as the ratio between the concentration of the molecules collected in the perfusion fluid and the true extracellular concentration. The length of the probe and perfusion velocity affect recovery: at the commonly used $0.3\,\mu l\,min^{-1}$, the recovery is about 70%. The most commonly investigated markers using microdialysis have been metabolic markers such as glucose, lactate and pyruvate, and the lactate/pyruvate ratio, which is independent of recovery rate and considered the best indicator of the cerebral redox state. Microdialysis has also been used to monitor extracellular concentrations of neurotransmitters such as glutamate and γ-aminobutyric acid (GABA), and markers of cellular damage such as glycerol. As a research tool, microdialysis allows measurement of molecules participating in secondary processes of injury and recovery such as cytokines and neurotrophic factors, and quantitation of drugs concentration in the brain extracellular compartment. An additional potential neuropharmacological application is 'reverse microdialysis' to deliver drugs into the brain, bypassing the blood–brain barrier. In neurointensive care, microdialysis has contributed to the understanding of brain metabolism following TBI, and has been tested as a tool to diagnose vasospasm-associated ischaemia following SAH. However, although the technique has been widely used as a research tool, microdialysis is currently performed as a part of clinical management protocols in only a minority of centres worldwide, as it requires dedicated personnel and expertise.

Practical considerations regarding regional cerebral blood flow, brain tissue oxygen tension monitoring and microdialysis

For the location of probes, it is well known that data obtained from normal-appearing tissue (usually right frontal subcortical white matter) and pericontusional tissue are very different. Consequently, the location of probes is a key issue for appropriate interpretation of these monitoring tools and for integrating their data with the clinical status and other monitoring modalities. Two recent consensus conferences have recommended that the location should be individualized for each patient.

Following TBI, it has been suggested that target sites should be selected based on the following considerations:

- Probes should be sited in vulnerable and potentially salvageable tissue such as the pericontusional tissue (never the core of the contusion) and tissue underlying a subdural haematoma.
- Eloquent locations should be avoided.
- When structurally normal tissue is monitored, probes should be placed in the subcortical white matter of the more injured hemisphere.

Following SAH, it has been suggested that target sites should be in the cortex within the expected distribution area of the parent artery of the aneurysm, which is at highest risk for developing delayed ischaemia.

While the literature reports a very low rate of complications (haemorrhage/infections) with these probes, several caveats need to be considered in their use. Firstly, their invasiveness means that insertion should be avoided in the presence of haemostatic abnormalities (thrombocytopaenia or coagulopathy); secondly, that the data obtained are from small volumes of tissue (which may sometimes be unrepresentative of the wider brain); and finally, that the technology is relatively fragile.

Integration of multimodality monitoring data – potential and pitfalls

Multimodality monitoring integrates multiple sources of information in a number of possible combinations. These combinations reflect local expertise, equipment availability and the clinical interest of a specific research group. Usually, ICP and CPP are incorporated as core data, while other techniques may vary considerably. Miller, in 1994, published a system aimed at monitoring perfusion and oxygenation in both the systemic and cerebral circulation of trauma patients. This system included arterial pressure, ICP, body temperature, SjO_2 and TCD. Similar systems, with the addition of $PbrO_2$, have been used subsequently. An essential component of multimodality monitoring is the description of events, artefacts and human interventions, such as physical and pharmacological treatments. Without comments, notes and remarks, a meaningful interpretation of a stream of thousands of data points per day is both cumbersome and unrewarding. This has been shown by Signorini, who reported approximately 13,000 comments added to the raw data at the time of collection. The inclusion of such comments lead to substantial differences, in some cases nearly 50%, between validated and unvalidated data on the quantity of secondary insult observed.

However, the combination of multiple monitoring modalities does not guarantee per se the detection of all relevant events, as shown in a case report by Andrews and colleagues in 1996 in which, despite the accurate measurement of SjO_2, AjD lactate, evoked potentials, CPP, TCD and systemic haemodynamics, a cerebral infarction was missed.

Concordant versus discordant data, and clinical interpretation

When multiple parameters are acquired simultaneously, the meaning of every single measure may change in relation to other data. The preliminary requirement is that all data are reliable and artefacts or errors have been excluded. Once only meaningful data have been filtered, the interplay among variables becomes challenging.

When different monitoring techniques explore the same anatomical areas, or the same physiological event, consistent changes in multiple monitored variables add credence to the finding. In contrast, when a

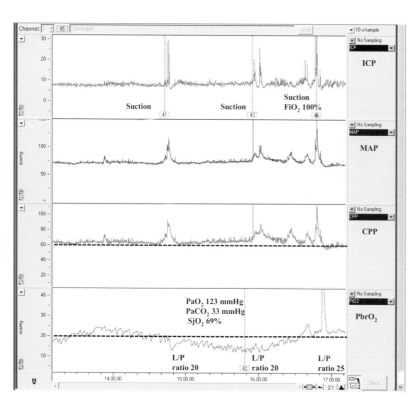

Fig. 9.2. Chart showing the occurrence of an episode of transient regional brain hypoxia (brain tissue oxygen tension ($PbrO_2$) measured in normal-appearing tissue) with no apparent cause and with spontaneous resolution. Cerebral perfusion pressure was stable and remained above the threshold of 60 mmHg, arterial partial pressure of oxygen (PaO_2)was adequate and $PaCO_2$ was in the range of mild hyperventilation. Jugular bulb oxygen saturation (SjO_2) was normal. The episode was followed by an increase in lactate/pyruvate (L/P) ratio measured in the corresponding area from 20 to 25. At follow-up CT scan, no ischaemic changes were observed in the monitored area. These data highlight the complexity of understanding the pathophysiology of regional oxygenation and integrating it with other physiological variables. FiO_2, fraction of inspired oxygen. See colour plate section.

single parameter in a multimodality monitoring dataset provides discordant information, caution needs to be exercised, as the risk of malfunction or other causes of unreliable data in the single discordant modality is high.

However, in other contexts, discordant data may imply complex pathophysiology, rather than technical problems (Fig. 9.2). Measures of cerebral oxygenation, such as SjO_2 and $PbrO_2$ for instance, can have parallel trends or may diverge, depending on the $PbrO_2$ probe location and on the mechanisms involved. In the case of a drop in cerebral perfusion leading to global cerebral hypoxia, it is likely that both parameters will follow a trend in the same direction. However, where focal ischaemia develops, this may be detected when it is in an area monitored by a tissue probe but produce no change in jugular saturation, which averages the venous drainage from the whole brain.

An extreme example of dissociation between these two variables is determined by brain death. When cerebral perfusion ceases, tissue oxygenation drops to zero, while jugular saturation rises, as no more flow can derive from the brain and only extracerebral blood can be sampled from the jugular bulb.

In some cases, as when a risk of vasospasm exists, additional parameters are used in order to detect focal disturbances unlikely to be reflected in more general monitoring techniques. In 60 patients affected by SAH, hourly microdialysis samples were correlated with TCD and angiography, and revealed characteristic metabolic changes that occurred during vasospasm in 13 of 15 patients with symptomatic vasospasm.

Finally, some techniques, such as microdialysis, have been employed using several probes in order to explore different parts of the brain, specifically 'hunting' for discordant but informative data that separately characterizes, for example, the pericontusional penumbra and normal-appearing brain tissue. Up to three microdialysis probes have been inserted in each TBI patient, aiming at contused versus unaffected areas of the brain. However, despite the very low rate of complications reported with invasive monitoring, there is no clinical evidence that supports the consistent use of more than a single probe in each patient, except in the rigorously controlled context of research studies.

The interpretation of concordant versus discordant data underlines a fundamental component of multimodality monitoring, which is clinically meaningful interpretation. The transformation of a mass of data into useful information, and the use of this information for the benefit of patients, demands a substantial exercise of human effort, in a context that is still very far from a robotic form of intensive care, even if robots have been used for assisting the physician duties.

Computer-aided multimodal monitoring

In every ICU, enormous quantities of data can be captured from each patient and, depending on the number of monitoring modalities employed and the rate of data acquisition, thousands to many millions of data points can be generated by a single monitored patient. These considerations suggest an obvious role for computers in managing, integrating, analysing and displaying such data.

Commercial bedside data management packages are available, but several research groups have set up their own system, with specific aims and tools.

Each system has pros and cons, but a pre-requisite is that the data need to be filtered. Every time a patient is moved to a CT scan and the lines are disconnected, or every time the ventricular catheter is opened for CSF withdrawal, artefactual data can be recorded. The importance of textual data for assisting in the interpretation has already been mentioned. Some publications suggest that a computerized system, which included ICP monitoring as part of a multimodal approach, offers advantages over traditional nursing techniques. The necessity of dedicated software and hardware increases the complexity of clinical work, mainly for the nurses and other members of the ICU staff, who have to be trained to use the monitoring systems.

Computers can be used not only for data recording and analysis but also for discovering new relationships among the data itself. This has been shown in children and adults. Finally, the integrated view of physiology that computers derive from multimodal monitoring can provide important indicators for clinical management and decision-making, as already demonstrated in anaesthesia.

Cost–benefit analysis of multimodal monitoring

Multimodality monitoring has been around for over two decades, and it is tempting to try to undertake cost–benefit analysis of this approach to patient management. Experts involved in the development and use of advanced systems tend to be positive and claim that each system provides advantages for patient care. However, on the 'cost' side, the total cost of any system is likely to be high, because of the initial investment and the human work implied in maintaining and implementing it. In fact, technology is advancing, new 'toys' are on the horizon and a conclusive statement about the utility (or otherwise) of multimodality monitoring may be premature. With the actual rate of progress in imaging, it is likely that future systems will incorporate continuous data (traditional monitoring) and information produced by both structural and functional imaging. However, even as things stand, multimodality monitoring has improved our detection and interpretation of pathophysiology at the bedside, and is increasingly seen as a basis for selecting and implementing therapies. It is now an integral part of neurointensive care and has moved from the limited research domain to use in routine clinical management.

Further reading

Andrews, P. J., Murugavel, S. and Deehan, S. (1996). Conventional multimodality monitoring failure to detect ischemic cerebral blood flow. *J Neurosurg Anesthesiol* **8**, 220–6.

Andrews, P. J., Citerio, G., Longhi, L. *et al.* (2008). NICEM consensus on neurological monitoring in acute neurological disease. *Intensive Care Med* **34**, 1362–70.

Bellander, B. M., Cantais, E. and Enblad, P. (2004). Consensus meeting on microdialysis in neurointensive care. *Intensive Care Med* **30**, 2166–9.

Bouma, G. J. and Muizelaar, J. P. (1990). Relationship between cardiac output and cerebral blood flow in patients with intact and with impaired autoregulation. *J Neurosurg* **73**, 368–74.

Chieregato, A., Sabia, G., Tanfani, A. *et al.* (2006). Xenon-CT and transcranial Doppler in poor-grade or complicated aneurysmatic subarachnoid hemorrhage patients undergoing aggressive management of intracranial hypertension. *Intensive Care Med* **32**, 1143–50.

Claassen, J., Hirsch, L. J., Kreiter, K. T. *et al.* (2004). Quantitative continuous EEG for detecting delayed cerebral ischemia in patients with poor-grade subarachnoid hemorrhage. *Clin Neurophysiol* **115**, 2699–710.

Gaab, M., Ottens, M., Busche, F., Moleer, G. and Trost, H. A. (1986). Routine computerized neuromonitoring. In Miller, J.D. and Teasdale, G. M., eds., *ICP VI*. Berlin: Springer Verlag, pp. 240–7.

Gopinath, S. P., Robertson, C. S., Contant, C. F. *et al.* (1994). Jugular venous desaturation and outcome after head injury. *J Neurol Neurosurg Psychiatry* **57**, 717–23.

Greer, D. M., Funk, S. E., Reaven, N. L., Ouzounelli, M. and Uman, G. C. (2008). Impact of fever on outcome in patients with stroke and neurologic injury: a comprehensive meta-analysis. *Stroke* **39**, 3029–35.

Gupta, A. K., Hutchinson, P. J., Fryer, T. *et al.* (2002). Measurement of brain tissue oxygenation performed using positron emission tomography scanning to validate a novel monitoring method. *J Neurosurg* **96**, 263–8.

Hillered, L., Vespa, P. M. and Hovda, D. A. (2005). Translational neurochemical research in acute human brain injury: the current status and potential future for cerebral microdialysis. *J Neurotrauma* **22**, 3–41.

Hutchinson, P. J., O'Connell, M. T., Al-Rawi, P. G. *et al.* (2000). Clinical cerebral microdialysis: a methodological study. *J Neurosurg* **93**, 37–43.

Jones, P. A., Minns, R. A., Lo, T. Y. *et al.* (2003). Graphical display of variability and inter-relationships of pressure signals in children with traumatic brain injury. *Physiol Meas* **24**, 201–11.

Longhi, L., Pagan, F., Valeriani, V. *et al.* (2007). Monitoring brain tissue oxygen tension in brain-injured patients reveals hypoxic episodes in normal-appearing and in peri-focal tissue. *Intensive Care Med* **33**, 2136–42.

Miller, J. D., Piper, I. R. and Jones, P. A. (1994). Integrated multimodality monitoring in the neurosurgical intensive care unit. *Neurosurg Clin N Am* **5**, 661–70.

Neumar, R. W., Nolan, J. P., Adrie, C. *et al.* (2008). Post-cardiac arrest syndrome: epidemiology, pathophysiology, treatment, and prognostication. A consensus statement from the International Liaison Committee on Resuscitation (American Heart Association, Australian and New Zealand Council on Resuscitation, European Resuscitation Council, Heart and Stroke Foundation of Canada, InterAmerican Heart Foundation, Resuscitation Council of Asia, and the Resuscitation Council of Southern Africa); the American Heart Association Emergency Cardiovascular Care Committee; the Council on Cardiovascular Surgery and Anesthesia; the Council on Cardiopulmonary, Perioperative, and Critical Care; the Council on Clinical Cardiology; and the Stroke Council. *Circulation* **118**, 2452–83.

Nordstrom, C. H., Reinstrup, P., Xu, W., Gardenfors, A. and Ungerstedt, U. (2003). Assessment of the lower limit for cerebral perfusion pressure in severe head injuries by bedside monitoring of regional energy metabolism. *Anesthesiology* **98**, 805–7.

Nortje, J. and Gupta, A. K. (2006). The role of tissue oxygen monitoring in patients with acute brain injury. *Br J Anaesth* **97**, 95–106.

Polderman, K. H. (2008). Induced hypothermia and fever control for prevention and treatment of neurological injuries. *Lancet* **371**, 1955–69.

Rossi, S., Zanier, E. R., Mauri, I., Columbo, A. and Stocchetti, N. (2001). Brain temperature, body core temperature, and intracranial pressure in acute cerebral damage. *J Neurol Neurosurg Psychiatry* **71**, 448–54.

Signorini, D. F., Piper, I. R., Jones, P. A. and Howells, T. P. (1997). Importance of textual data in multimodality monitoring. *Crit Care Med* **25**, 2048–50.

Sloan, M. A., Alexandrov, A. V., Tegeler, C. H. *et al.* (2004). Assessment: transcranial Doppler ultrasonography: report of the Therapeutics and Technology Assessment Subcommittee of the American Academy of Neurology. *Neurology* **62**, 1468–81.

Steiner, L. A, Coles, J. P., Johnston, A. J. *et al.* (2003). Assessment of cerebrovascular autoregulation in head-injured patients: a validation study. *Stroke* **34**, 2404–9.

Stocchetti, N., Penny, K. I., Dearden, M. *et al.* (2001). Intensive care management of head-injured patients in Europe: a survey from the European brain injury consortium. *Intensive Care Med* **27**, 400–6.

Stocchetti, N., Canavesi, K., Magnoni, S. *et al.* (2004). Arterio-jugular difference of oxygen content and outcome after head injury. *Anesth Analg* **99**, 230–4.

Stocchetti, N., Zanier, E. R., Nicolini, R. *et al.* (2005). Oxygen and carbon dioxide in the cerebral circulation during progression to brain death. *Anesthesiology* **103**, 957–961.

Unterberg, A. W., Sakowitz, O. W., Sarrafzadeh, A. S., Benndorf, G. and Lanksch, W. R. (2001). Role of bedside microdialysis in the diagnosis of cerebral vasospasm following aneurysmal subarachnoid hemorrhage. *J Neurosurg* **94**, 740–9.

Vajkoczy, P., Horn, P., Thome, C., Munch, E. and Schmiedek, P. (2003). Regional cerebral blood flow monitoring in the diagnosis of delayed ischemia following aneurysmal subarachnoid hemorrhage. *J Neurosurg* **98**, 1227–34.

van den Brink, W. A., van Santbrink, H., Steyerberg, E. W. *et al.* (2000). Brain oxygen tension in severe head injury. *Neurosurgery* **46**, 868–76.

Wijdicks, E. F., Hijdra, A., Young, G. B. *et al.* (2006). Practice parameter: prediction of outcome in comatose survivors after cardiopulmonary resuscitation (an evidence-based review): report of the Quality Standards Subcommittee of the American Academy of Neurology. *Neurology* **67**, 203–10.

Chapter

10

Imaging

Jonathan P. Coles and David K. Menon

Introduction

Imaging is central to how we define the cause and extent of neurological injury, manage acute patients and attempt to predict functional outcome. Despite improvements in how we use such data to improve clinical management, patients continue to suffer an enormous burden of physical disability and neurocognitive deficits. The costs of such chronic illness are high in terms of the acute hospital and long-term healthcare, as well as the impact on the individual and society as a whole. Advances in neuroimaging techniques may allow the development of new treatments and refinement of existing therapies aimed at ameliorating such neuronal injury and improving functional outcome for patients. This chapter will discuss the role of structural imaging using CT and MRI, conventional angiography and CT angiography, and physiological imaging using CT perfusion, [131]Xenon CT, MRI and magnetic resonance spectroscopy (MRS), single-photon emission computed tomography (SPECT) and positron emission tomography (PET) in the assessment, management and prediction of outcome following neurological injury.

Imaging modalities

Structural imaging

CT

CT has replaced the use of plain skull radiographs and is routinely used to assess all patients with acute neurological injury and trauma to the brain who require admission and observation within hospital. Such imaging provides early assessment of the extent of injury and can be obtained quickly using modern multidetector high-resolution scanners, which are generally available. Patients admitted via emergency

departments within major centres and peripheral hospitals can be transferred to the radiology suite and images reviewed online or transferred electronically for specialist review. The short imaging time and ease of acquisition is of considerable benefit in agitated patients and those who present with severe trauma or critical illness. Image slices that are degraded by motion artefact can easily be repeated. In addition, imaging data can also be acquired at the bedside within the critical care and theatre environments (Fig. 10.1).

Development and validation of rules for evaluation of trauma patients with head CT guide the most efficient use of the technique. Indeed, the adoption of guidelines developed by The National Institute for Health and Clinical Excellence (NICE) in the UK has changed the way CT is used.

Following head injury, these guidelines state that a CT scan should be obtained if any of the following is present:

- Glasgow Coma Score <13 at any point since the injury.
- GCS equal to 13 or 14 at 2 h after the injury.
- Suspected open or depressed skull fracture.
- Any sign of basal skull fracture.
- Post-traumatic seizure.
- Focal neurological deficit.
- More than one episode of vomiting.
- Amnesia for >30 min of events before impact.

Imaging data can be visualized using brain or bone contrast windows and reconstructed into three-dimensional CT datasets in order to demonstrate bony injury (Fig. 10.2) and intracranial pathology. Imaging demonstrates the differences between normal and abnormal brain in terms of the degree of X-ray attenuation. A blood clot, which has a high degree of X-ray attenuation, appears as a hyperdense or white area, while

Core Topics in Neuroanaesthesia and Neurointensive Care, eds. Basil F. Matta, David K. Menon and Martin Smith. Published by Cambridge University Press. © Cambridge University Press 2011.

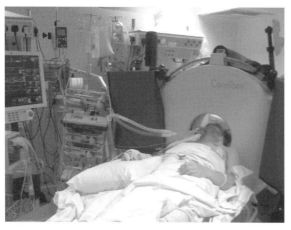

Fig. 10.1. Bedside CT. This patient sustained severe brain, chest and orthopaedic injuries following a road traffic accident. Using the CereTom mobile CT scanner (NeuroLogica Corporation, Danvers, MA, USA), imaging was obtained at the bedside without the need to transfer the patient to the radiology suite. See colour plate section.

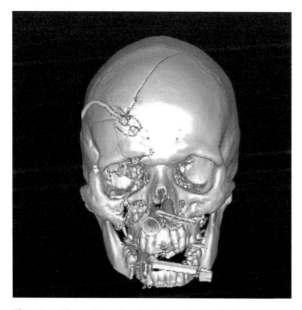

Fig. 10.2. Three-dimensional CT reconstruction. This patient sustained injury following a road traffic accident. The reconstruction allowed operative planning of the cranial and facial fractures.

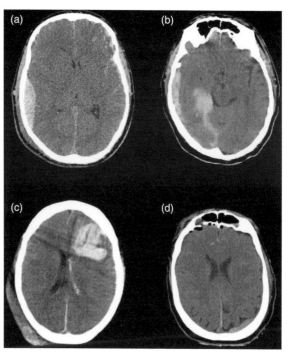

Fig. 10.3. CT imaging of space-occupying lesions. (a) Right extradural haematoma. Bleeding has occurred within the potential epidural space and is usually associated with a fracture. The expanding lesion has resulted in compression of the ipsilateral ventricle but no midline shift. In addition, there is a contrecoup with evidence of haemorrhagic contusion within the left fronto-temporal cortex. (b) Right subdural haematoma. Bleeding occurs between the arachnoid and inner meningeal layer of the dura. There is also subdural blood tracking along the tentorium. (c) Large left intracerebral haemorrhage with extension into the lateral ventricle secondary to brain contusion. There is compression of the ipsilateral ventricle and midline shift. (d) Facial fractures involving the frontal sinus. These are associated with frontal haemorrhagic contusions and intracranial air. There is also a left occipital subdural haematoma but no midline shift.

oedematous or ischaemic regions with increased water content and lower electron density appear dark due to reduced attenuation. Acute CT is useful in identifying those individuals in whom deterioration is as a result of a mass lesion and can demonstrate extradural, subdural or intracranial haemorrhage and midline shift (Fig. 10.3), or subarachnoid haemorrhage (SAH) and ventricular abnormality (Fig. 10.4). The ease of access and speed of data acquisition ensures that, where appropriate, patients benefit from early surgical management which has been shown to improve outcome.

Within many trauma centres, multislice CT has replaced plain radiographs of the spine as a screening tool for patients at high risk of spinal injury. In fact, as many trauma patients undergo whole-body CT imaging in order to assess the effects of trauma on the thoraco-abdominal compartments, it has become routine to reformat the data and review bony windows of the entire spine. This is clearly an advantage in patients with depressed consciousness and haemodynamic instability, where clinical assessment is limited, and repeated trips to the radiology department are to be

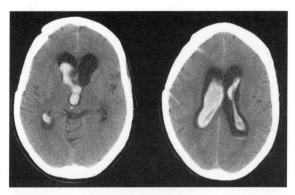

Fig. 10.4. CT imaging of subarachnoid haemorrhage and ventriculomegaly. These images are taken from two levels in the same patient. There is extensive intraventricular blood within the lateral and third ventricles. The ventricular system is generally enlarged and the brain parenchymal is compressed, with loss of the normal appearance of the brain sulci and gyri. This patient may benefit from placement of an external ventricular drain in order to remove cerebrospinal fluid and control intracranial pressure.

avoided. CT is able to provide rapid assessment of whether the spine is fractured, whether the fracture is unstable, and whether the spine is properly aligned (Fig. 10.5). In fact, fractures of the spine are more clearly demonstrated with CT compared with MRI.

CT imaging is also undertaken following the injection of iodinated contrast in order to demonstrate abnormal regions of brain where disruption of the blood–brain barrier results in tissue uptake of contrast. The resulting change in image intensity results from a change in X-ray attenuation and appears as a region of increased density or whiteness. Such changes are typical of regions of the brain infiltrated by tumour or severe infection (Fig. 10.6). Contrast-enhanced CT imaging is also used to produce CT angiography and perfusion imaging, which are discussed later in this chapter. An important consideration with all such techniques is the risk of contrast-induced nephropathy in patients with pre-existing renal impairment or who have additional risk factors such as diabetes or who are receiving other medications that are potentially nephrotoxic. Recent articles have reviewed the management of such patients and suggest that, where the administration of iodinated contrast is essential, patients should be kept well hydrated and receive prophylactic N-acetyl cysteine.

Despite its usefulness, CT imaging is limited by beam-hardening effects, which can partially obscure the posterior fossa, temporal and frontal regions, and the vertebral canal. In addition, the resolution of CT

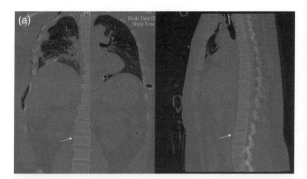
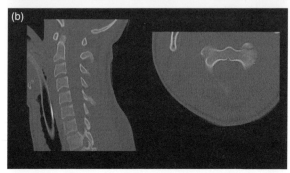

Fig. 10.5. Spinal imaging using CT. (a) Coronal and sagittal views of a thoracolumbar spine following a road traffic accident. There is a fracture of the body of the first lumbar vertebrae (arrow), but the vertebral bodies remain aligned. (b) Sagittal and axial views of the cervical spine following trauma. A vertebral fracture is clearly visualized on the axial image.

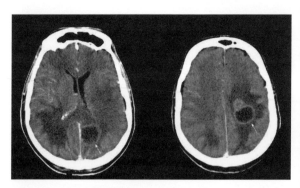

Fig. 10.6. CT imaging of intracranial sepsis. Imaging following administration of intravenous iodinated contrast. The slices shown demonstrate two circular cavities of low attenuation circumscribed by a rim of increased signal intensity (arrow), and surrounding this is a region of tissue that appears dark or hypodense. These represent intracranial abscesses with tissue enhancement following the administration of contrast within the abscess wall, and cerebral oedema within the surrounding brain tissue.

imaging is limited, and this can result in partial volume errors. Partial volume errors occur when a region of abnormal tissue has one or more dimensions that are smaller than the resolution of the acquired data. This can mean that haemorrhage or other evidence of intra-cranial or spinal pathology may remain undetected. Such issues are of particular concern within the brain-stem and spinal cord where a small area of pathology can result in devastating injury but also in patients who exhibit evidence of traumatic axonal injury (TAI) following trauma, global hypoxia and hypoperfusion, and in patients with disease processes that predomin-antly affect white-matter regions. Diffuse axonal injury is a frequent finding following traumatic brain injury accounting for up to 50% of trauma patients. Such injury is thought to result from rotational shear-strain deformation throughout the brain, as occurs with the rapid deceleration of road traffic accidents. The regions of the brain that are commonly injured include the grey–white matter interface, corpus callosum and deep white matter, periventricular and hippocampal areas, and the brainstem. Such regions are best visualized using MRI, and patients increasingly undergo acute MRI following trauma to the central nervous system.

MRI

Despite the advantages of MRI in terms of delineating the extent and severity of neurological injury, the MRI suite is not immediately accessible and has numerous hazards, which dictate that CT remains the modality of choice in the acute phase. MRI data are produced using powerful static magnetic fields and intermittent oscillating radiofrequency electromagnetic fields that elicit signals from the nuclei of certain atoms. Magnetic field strengths are measured in units termed Tesla (T). One T equals 10,000 Gauss (G). The magnetic field strength at the surface of the Earth is 0.5–1.5 G. Field strengths used in clinical MRI range from 1 to 3 T and tend to be based on cryogenic superconducting mag-nets, which are maintained at −273°C by immersion in liquid helium. Although access to the MRI suite has been improved through the provision of inte-grated monitoring and anaesthetic equipment suitable for patients with critical illness, all patients, staff and equipment must be verified to be safe prior to trans-fer, and contraindications prevent imaging in some cases. Firstly, although the available data support the safety of exposure to magnetic fields, there is currently an attempt to minimize unnecessary exposure to high magnetic fields, based on general safety principles. Indeed, most MRI scanning rooms have slave patient monitor screens installed outside the room, so that patient studies can be supervised from outside the 5 G line and away from the most intense noise produced

by gradient fields. Articles in the press detailing inci-dents involving patients, equipment and personnel underline the importance of safe practice within an MRI suite (http://www.nytimes.com/2005/08/19/health/19magnet.html), and have prompted reviews of MRI safety and the provision of anaesthetic services. The following highlight some important concerns:

- *Projectile risks from ferromagnetic objects.* Ferromagnetic objects such as oxygen cylinders, identification badges and paging devices can become dangerous projectiles and should not be taken into the MRI suite unless they are known to be safe.
- *Implanted devices.* These may be affected because they are ferromagnetic and move in the magnetic field. Such movement may be disastrous if the implant is large or in a critical location (e.g. intra-ocular foreign bodies and cerebral aneurysm clips). Patients with an intracranial aneurysm clip should not be imaged using MRI unless the clip has been documented to be non-ferromagnetic or the patient has already been imaged at the same field strength with no problems. Even non-ferromagnetic implants can result in significant image distortion or cause local burns as their temperature is increased in the presence of radiofrequency currents. Fatalities have been reported in patients with cardiac pacemakers. The magnetic field causes the reed switch on pacemakers to stick and revert to fixed rate mode where delivery of a pacing spike on the upstroke of a T wave can result in an R-on-T phenomenon and trigger ventricular fibrillation. MRI is contraindicated in the presence of pacemakers and other implanted electronic devices, unless it is known with absolute certainty that it will function safely. In the event of doubt, implants should be tested with a powerful hand-held magnet and checked against the manufacturer's specifications. MRI units usually have a comprehensive checklist for patients and staff to complete in order to exclude the presence of implants.
- *Monitoring devices.* In addition to the above hazards, monitoring devices may dysfunction as a consequence of exposure to magnetic fields. Leads from such devices present a particular hazard, as induced currents may result in burns. Simple precautions can help to ensure safety. These include: removing unnecessary equipment,

keeping monitoring equipment as far away from the examination area as possible, checking that the insulation on all monitoring wires is intact, not crossing cables or forming large-diameter loops of wire, and separating all cables from the skin using padding. Devices are described as 'MR safe' when they do not represent a risk to the patient, and 'MR compatible' when they also continue to function in the MR environment without degrading imaging.

- *Contrast.* Gadopentetate dimeglumine (Gd-DTPA, Magnevist'), the most commonly used MR contrast agent, has an excellent safety record. Gd-chelates are rapidly cleared by the kidney, but in the presence of impaired kidney function, such clearance is hampered and the release of free gadolinium can result in nephrogenic systemic fibrosis. These contrast agents are therefore contraindicated in patients with impaired renal function.

- *Cryogens and quenches.*The helium contained in cryogenic magnets can boil off ('quench') rapidly when the temperature rises. This dilutes room oxygen and the cold vapour gives frostbite and burns.

While integrated monitoring systems based on technology developed for the MRI environment are currently widely available, even MR-compatible devices should be used with special attention to ensure their safe application. Other monitoring problems include ECG distortion. Changes occur in early T waves and late ST segments that mimic hyperkalaemia or pericarditis and radiofrequency currents produce ECG artefacts. Intracranial pressure (ICP) can be measured accurately via a ventriculostomy. Several intraparenchymal sensors are MR safe, but not MR compatible.

Recent interest has focused on interventional MRI, which uses continuing or episodic imaging of the patient in the course of surgical procedures on the brain. This allows surgeons to avoid critical structures and ensure that surgical resection of tumours is complete. Some authors make the distinction between 'interventional' MRI, where the surgery continues during imaging and all surgical equipment has to be MR compatible, and 'intraventional' MRI, where surgery is periodically halted to allow imaging with a movable magnet after MR-incompatible surgical equipment has been removed. This distinction is of no consequence for anaesthesia, as anaesthetic drug delivery and patient monitoring need to continue uninterrupted with both approaches.

Despite the above concerns, many centres are increasingly using MRI in the acute setting. MRI is more sensitive at detecting white-matter abnormalities than CT, particularly following head injury. In addition, gradient echo and fluid attenuation inversion recovery (FLAIR) MRI sequences demonstrate high sensitivity for TAI and may help predict outcome. Differences in imaging contrast within both normal and injured neural tissue are dependent on the particular MRI sequence employed. Fluid attenuation inversion recovery sequences generate images in which areas of tissue T2 prolongation are bright, while the normal cerebrospinal fluid signal is nulled and appears dark. This allows the detection of periventricular and superficial cortical lesions. Gradient echo MRI is sensitive to changes in magnetic susceptibility, which results in lesions of low intensity following haemorrhage within the tissue due to local magnetic field inhomogeneities caused by the paramagnetic properties of haemosiderin. Susceptibility-weighted imaging is a new MR sequence that is exquisitely sensitive to blood products in the brain. By employing a variety of different MR sequences, the extent of injury can be demonstrated with high resolution across the whole central nervous system (Fig. 10.7). The extent of such injury has implications for functional outcome and it would clearly be beneficial if imaging data could be used to predict the quality of survival following head injury. Although imaging findings based on CT and MRI data can predict survival following head injury, they do not provide sufficient information to allow accurate prediction of functional outcome. Indeed, although patients with lesions within the deep white matter and brainstem are more likely to suffer a poor outcome, a consistent relationship based on the assessment of CT and MRI data remains elusive.

The spinal cord is best visualized using MRI as it provides better resolution, particularly within the confined environment of the spinal canal where beam-hardening effects, limited resolution and poor soft tissue contrast can limit the usefulness of CT (Fig. 10.8). Using the additional information provided by a variety of different imaging sequences, MRI can demonstrate evidence of spinal injury or extra-axial pathology such as intravertebral disc herniation and epidural haematoma (Fig. 10.9). MRI is also useful in the assessment of potential ligamentous injury of the spine, and may reduce the need for flexion/extension radiographs.

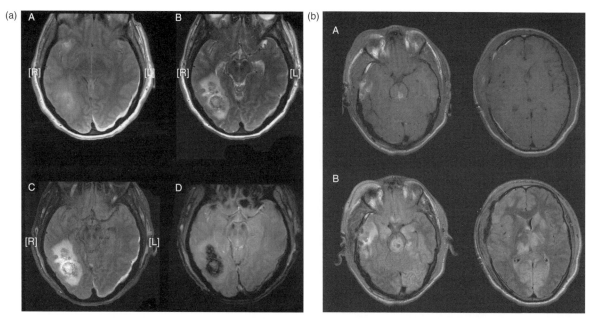

Fig. 10.7. MRI following head injury. (a) Images from a patient who sustained a severe head injury following a road traffic accident. (A) T1-weighted; (B) T2-weighted; (C) fluid-attenuated inversion recovery (FLAIR); (D) gradient echo sequences. (A) and (B) demonstrate regions of high signal intensity within the right inferior frontal and posterior temporal lobes, and a thin left subdural haemorrhage. These abnormalities are more clearly defined in (C) as the cerebral spinal fluid signal has been nulled. In (D), the large left posterior temporal lesion has a haemorrhagic component as there is signal loss within this region. (b) Two axial slices from a patient who sustained a severe head injury following an assault and underwent right frontal decompressive craniectomy and evacuation of a subdural haematoma for management of raised intracranial pressure. (A) T1-weighted; (B) FLAIR. The images in (A) demonstrate a high signal to the left of the midline within the midbrain and also within the right temporal cortex. These are consistent with haemorrhage and correspond to the regions of low signal intensity shown in (B). There are also multiple regions of high signal intensity shown in (B) within the inferior temporal, medial parietal and right superior frontal lobes. However, the most prominent lesions are within the basal ganglia, thalami, midbrain and occipital lobes. These findings suggest diffuse injury across the brain.

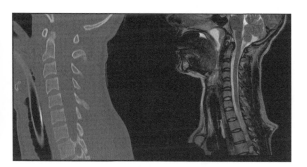

Fig. 10.8. Comparison of CT and MRI of the cervical spine. Sagittal reconstruction of CT (left panel) and T2-weighted MRI data of a patient following a fall from a horse. There is a communited minimally displaced fracture through the anterolateral portion of the second cervical vertebrae, which is not well demonstrated on these views. Both images demonstrate the normal alignment of the cervical spine, but the MRI data show better contrast for the tissue within the spinal canal, intravertebral discs, dura and spinal ligaments.

Although MRI can demonstrate injury to spinal ligaments in the absence of bony injury, stability of the spine is a dynamic concept and a complete assessment may require clinical examination when possible.

Angiography

Imaging of structure using CT and MR does not allow delineation of the adequacy of blood flow through the cerebral vessels and the subsequent venous drainage. Digital subtraction angiography (DSA) is the gold standard technique used to obtain such data but requires cannulation of a large arterial vessel, such as the femoral artery, and the passage of a catheter under continuous X-ray screening through the vascular system to within the brain. Images are acquired following injection of contrast within the intracranial segments of the internal carotid and vertebral arteries on each side of the brain. Image processing allows the non-vascular structures to be subtracted from the final images and thereby allows improved delineation of vascular anatomy. Such techniques can be used to diagnose disorders of the brain vasculature such as cerebral aneurysm, arteriovenous malformations, arterial and venous thrombosis, and arterial dissection (Fig. 10.10). More recently, CT and MR angiography (CTA and MRA, respectively) have emerged as (a)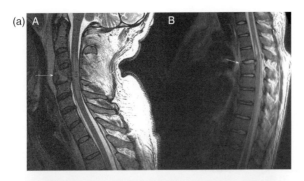

(b)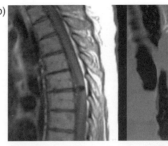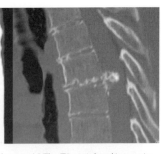

(c)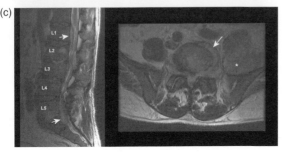

Fig. 10.9. MRI of the cervical spine. (a) The T2-weighted image in (A) is from a patient who sustained a fracture of the cervical spine following a road traffic accident. There is cord swelling and oedema between the third and sixth cervical vertebrae with heterogeneous signal changes consistent with haemorrhagic contusion. The fourth cervical vertebra is fractured (arrow) and there is high signal within the C4/5 disc consistent with disruption of the disc space. There is no epidural haematoma or disc herniation. In (B), the patient sustained a fracture of the fifth thoracic vertebra following a road traffic accident. There is minor loss of alignment (arrow), slight widening of the interspinous distance posteriorly and disruption of the T5/6 disc space suggesting ligamentous injury. There is also soft tissue swelling or disc extrusion into the epidural space posterior to the disc space (arrow). There is signal change consistent with contusion within the spinal cord extending from the third to sixth thoracic vertebrae. (b) T1-weighted MRI (left panel) and CT image (right panel) from a patient with a thoracic disc prolapse between the fifth and sixth thoracic vertebrae. The intervertebral disc is calcified, and on MRI appears as a region of low signal intensity that markedly indents the thecal sac. (c) T2-weighted MRIs in sagittal (left panel) and axial format (right panel) in a patient with an epidural abscess, osteomyelitis and a pelvic abscess. There is high signal within all the lumbar vertebrae secondary to diffuse bone oedema, and high signal within the L5/S1 and L2/3 discs. There is epidural fluid across the whole lumbosacral region, but this is most prominent behind L1/2 and L5/S1 where it is associated with thecal narrowing (arrows). The axial image demonstrates a left paraspinal collection (arrow), which extends into the epidural space and is associated with a pelvic collection, which is displacing the psoas muscle anteriorly (*).

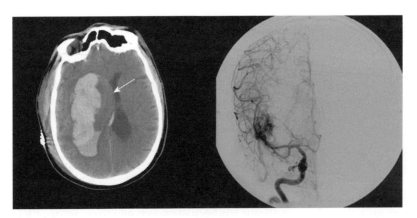

Fig. 10.10. Digital subtraction angiography. The CT image (left panel) demonstrates a large intracerebral haematoma extending into the lateral ventricle. The right lateral ventricle is effaced and there is subfalcine herniation of the innermost part of the frontal lobe under the falx cerebri and across to the left (arrow). The cerebral angiogram (right panel) shows that there is an arteriovenous malformation underlying this haemorrhage involving branches of the right middle cerebral artery.

less invasive, more rapid alternatives to DSA as they do not require arterial cannulation but rely on the intravenous administration of contrast agent followed by sequential imaging (Fig. 10.11). Although both techniques are roughly equivalent, CTA is more readily available, is less sensitive to motion artefacts and is less dependent on haemodynamic effects than MRA. As such, CTA provides easy access to diagnostic imaging of vascular anatomy, which can be obtained at the same time as baseline acute structural imaging with CT in those patients found to have evidence of intracranial haemorrhage and/or ischaemia. Where data are inconclusive or non-diagnostic, patients can still undergo digital angiography.

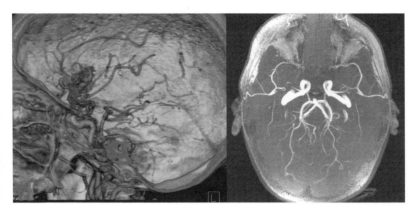

Fig. 10.11. CT and magnetic resonance angiography (MRA). The image in the left panel is from the same patient as shown in Fig. 10.10 and demonstrates the arteriovenous malformation within the region of the right Sylvian fissure. Further investigation using formal angiography was undertaken to delineate the arterial supply and venous drainage of the lesion. The image in the right panel was obtained using MRA and demonstrates a normal-appearing cerebral circulation. See colour plate section.

As well as patients presenting with acute neurological deficits secondary to cerebral ischaemic insults such as stroke, trauma to the brain and spine can lead to damage to the cerebral vasculature and result in cerebral ischaemia and infarction. Traumatic vascular injury is commonly associated with basal skull fracture, neck trauma or penetrating head injury. Such injuries can result in cerebral ischaemia within the affected vascular territory, and early assessment using digital angiography, CTA or MRA is essential, as prompt repair of treatable causes may prevent infarction and poor outcome.

Imaging the penumbra – 'tissue at risk' following acute cerebral ischaemia

Although structural imaging enables early diagnosis, directs initial management and helps to predict eventual outcome, imaging of cerebral perfusion and metabolism is desirable. It can define the early pathophysiological processes responsible for neuronal injury, direct appropriate therapy and assess its efficacy, and potentially direct the design and implementation of future therapeutic interventions aimed at reversing or preventing neuronal injury. Such concerns are particularly relevant following ischaemic stroke where imaging of tissue at risk is used to determine which patients will benefit from early thrombolysis. Following an acute ischaemic insult, tissue function is impaired. At this stage, the dysfunction is reversible, but failure to restore adequate perfusion will result in tissue necrosis and permanent functional deficit. Outcome is therefore dependent on the prompt restoration of tissue perfusion via spontaneous or therapeutic thrombolysis within the territory of the dependent vessel, or the adequacy of residual perfusion within the feeding vessel and collateral

circulation. This results in variable tissue outcomes. Experiments in models of ischaemia suggest that brain function is critically dependent on this residual blood flow, with failure of electrical activity occurring at $15–20\,\mathrm{ml}\,(100\,\mathrm{g})^{-1}\,\mathrm{min}^{-1}$, and failure of energy metabolism at $10\,\mathrm{ml}\,(100\,\mathrm{g})^{-1}\,\mathrm{min}^{-1}$. Brain tissue at risk of irreversible damage is classically described as the 'ischaemic penumbra' and exists between these perfusion thresholds. Such penumbral tissue borders the more densely ischaemic centre, in which energy failure and ion pump failure have already developed. The description of this region of brain tissue as 'penumbra' is analogous to the half-shaded zone around the centre of a complete solar eclipse (Fig. 10.12).

Unfortunately, the concept of an ischaemic penumbra is not static but is dynamic and constantly changing. In fact, the development of irreversible damage and cell death is critically dependent on three factors: the level of residual blood flow, the duration of ischaemia and the individual susceptibility of neurons. At flow levels close to the threshold of membrane failure, the tolerated ischaemic period is short. As residual blood flow increases towards the upper defining threshold for penumbra ($\sim 20\,\mathrm{ml}\,(100\,\mathrm{g})^{-1}\,\mathrm{min}^{-1}$), the length of time that neural tissue can tolerate ischaemia but still recover increases progressively. In practice, tissue plasminogen activator has been employed effectively within 3 h of symptom onset. However, many patients present outside this narrow time window, and evidence suggests that patients may still have salvageable brain for as long as 48 h post-ictus. Therefore, imaging of the penumbra may be relevant in selecting patients for thrombolytic therapy at later time points. Furthermore, evidence suggests that ischaemia is relevant to other pathological states such as head injury and intracerebral haemorrhage and SAH.

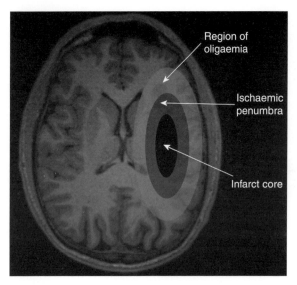

Region of
oligaemia

Ischaemic
penumbra

Infarct core

Fig. 10.12. Schematic demonstrating the ischaemic penumbra: ischaemic core of infarcted tissue (black), penumbral region of ischaemic brain tissue at high risk of cerebral infarction (purple) and the surrounding region of oligaemia (pink) above the threshold for cerebral injury following an acute vascular occlusion. See colour plate section.

Several imaging techniques are available that can measure aspects of brain physiology, including cerebral blood flow (CBF) and metabolism. Xenon-enhanced computerized tomography, CT perfusion and SPECT provide measurements of cerebral perfusion, while PET, MRI and MRS are able to assess both perfusion and cerebral metabolism. These imaging modalities are helpful in defining evidence of tissue injury, cerebral ischaemia and the penumbra, and predicting outcome.

CT perfusion

The development of high-speed helical CT scanners and the availability of image reconstruction software have allowed this technique to become clinically available. CT perfusion involves sequential acquisition of axial data during the intravenous administration of iodinated contrast material. As the change in CT enhancement (measured in Hounsfield units, HU) is proportional to the concentration of contrast, perfusion is calculated from the time course of contrast enhancement profiles for each pixel in relation to the profile of arterial contrast enhancement (the arterial input function). Based on the central volume theorem, CT perfusion is able to provide parametric images of cerebral blood volume (CBV), mean transit time (MTT), CBF and CTA alongside structural data. It is

a widely accessible, cost-effective, rapid and accurate technique that can provide a means for directing therapy and predicting outcome following ischaemic stroke and head injury, and assessing cerebral vasospasm following SAH (Fig. 10.13). A typical protocol allows acquisition of two 10 mm slices of data covering a region of interest within the brain, at the cost of an estimated radiation burden of 1.2 mSv. More recent CT systems provide multislice capability with whole-brain coverage.

Following ischaemic stroke, baseline structural imaging using CT has limited utility in demonstrating acute ischaemia. In fact, acutely hypoperfused regions of the brain at risk of infarction often appear normal. Using CT perfusion, areas of the brain with $CBV < 2\,ml\,(100\,ml)^{-1}$ are associated with infarct core, while the surrounding brain with reduced blood flow and an increase in the relative MTT >145% of the contralateral hemisphere is representative of brain at risk of infarction. CT perfusion is often combined with CTA in patients who require assessment for cerebral ischaemia and consideration of whether thrombolysis is appropriate. Despite its usefulness, CT perfusion may not be sufficient to accurately define the volume of brain at risk of ischaemic injury. The number and location of selected brain slices is limited due to radiation exposure, and repeat imaging following a therapeutic intervention is limited by the volume of contrast agent that can safely be administered. Whole-brain coverage is now possible and will clearly become more available through the development of imaging technology and as image-processing techniques improve. However, it is more difficult to image the posterior circulation using CT due to limited spatial resolution, imaging artefacts and radiation exposure to the orbits. These disadvantages are negated with MRI-based techniques as there is no ionizing radiation and image resolution is better.

Xenon-enhanced CT

This technique uses stable non-radioactive [131]Xe, which is a radio-opaque, highly lipid-soluble, diffusible indicator capable of crossing the blood–brain barrier. It provides a measure of tissue perfusion, with quantification based on a modification of the Fick principle. Data are acquired during inhalation of a gas mixture containing 28% [131]Xe and oxygen. Acquisition of a baseline structural scan without xenon inhalation is followed by serial scans at regular intervals after beginning xenon inhalation. Typically, up to six slices of data are acquired over 4.5 min, with

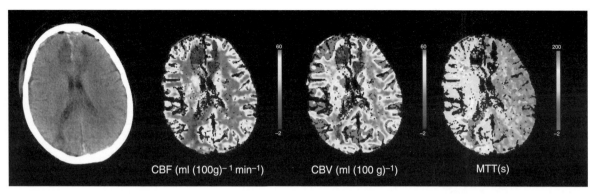

Fig. 10.13. Assessment of cerebral blood flow (CBF) using CT perfusion. This patient suffered a subarachnoid haemorrhage secondary to an anterior communicating artery aneurysm. The plain CT image on the left demonstrates hypodensity within the medial aspects of the frontal cortex in both hemispheres and also within the right occipital cortex. These areas have very low CBF and cerebral blood volume (CBV) suggestive of established infarction. In addition, there is a generalized reduction in CBF across the right hemisphere with an increase in CBV suggestive of cerebral ischaemia secondary to arterial vasospasm. This reduction of perfusion is most noticeable on the mean transit time (MTT) image, which clearly shows the delay in perfusion across the whole right hemisphere. See colour plate section.

a further 10 min for data processing. Alveolar xenon concentration is measured by end-tidal sampling and is assumed to be equal to arterial concentration. The degree of tissue enhancement of CT images is calculated and relates to an increase in the tissue ^{131}Xe concentration, which is proportional to the blood flow. Movement artefacts can be troublesome in patients due to the known sedative effects of xenon. However, such problems have been lessened by the gradual reduction in the concentration of xenon required and are irrelevant where patients are already sedated and mechanically ventilated. Although xenon can induce CBF increases of up to 30% and increase ICP, the available data suggest that both flow and ICP data are not affected adversely during the short-term inhalation of xenon required for CBF imaging using this technique. Xenon-enhanced CT provides rapid access to both structural and quantitative CBF data using equipment that is readily available. The technique has been employed in acute stroke in order to decide which patients should receive acute thrombolysis. In addition, studies can be repeated within a short period of time, allowing assessment of clinical therapy, such as thrombolysis following stroke, and hyperventilation, cerebral perfusion pressure (CPP) augmentation or hypertonic saline following trauma and SAH. Such data have been used to demonstrate early hypoperfusion consistent with ischaemia following head injury and predict cerebral infarction, raised ICP secondary to hyperperfusion and abnormal carbon dioxide reactivity and autoregulation. Despite these advantages, quantitative CBF studies

can be difficult to perform in patients with associated pulmonary pathology as the technique is based on the assumption that the end-tidal xenon concentration is identical to the arterial concentration.

Single-photon emission CT and positron emission tomography

Single-photon emission CT uses conventional gamma-emitting nuclear medicine isotopes with multiple detectors to generate tomographic images. ^{133}Xe and technetium-99m hexamethyl propylamine oxime (^{99}Tc-HMPAO) have commonly been employed to investigate blood flow within the brain. Single-photon emission CT is a relatively simple and inexpensive technique that can be used to assess cerebral perfusion, but the images produced are of relatively low resolution and are generally non-quantitative. Regions of the brain with a reduction of tracer signal compared with the contralateral hemisphere of >70% are suggestive of infarction, while a region of 40–70% suggests ischaemic brain consistent with penumbra.

Positron emission tomography measures the accumulation of positron-emitting radioisotopes within the brain. These positron-emitting isotopes can be administered via the intravenous or inhalational route, and for studies of the brain ^{15}O is used to measure CBF, CBV, cerebral metabolic rate of oxygen metabolism ($CMRO_2$) and oxygen extraction fraction (OEF), while 18-fluorodeoxyglucose (^{18}FDG) is used to measure cerebral glucose metabolism (CMRglu). The emitted positrons are annihilated in a collision with an electron resulting in the release of energy in

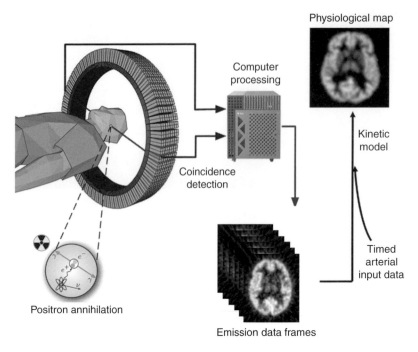

Physiological map

Computer
processing

Kinetic
model

Coincidence
detection

Timed
arterial
input data

Positron annihilation

Emission data frames

Fig. 10.14. Positron emission tomography (PET). The use of positron-emitting isotopes, incorporated into biological tracers, has enabled in vivo studies of human physiology in health and disease. These positron-emitting isotopes decay by emitting a positron, which is the positively charged anti-particle of the electron. The positron travels a short distance in tissue before it annihilates with an electron and causes the simultaneous release of two photons perpendicular to each other. As the photons are emitted simultaneously, *coincidence detection* occurs for each event through a cylindrical array of detectors. The large datasets acquired in PET require powerful computers to perform the data corrections and image reconstruction in a feasible timescale. The emission frames from the PET scanner and the arterial blood radioactivity data can be used to calculate absolute physiological parameters using appropriate kinetic models. See colour plate section.

the form of two photons (gamma rays) released at an angle of 180° to each other. This annihilation energy can be detected externally using coincidence detectors, and the region of each reaction localized within the object by computer algorithms (Fig. 10.14). Following acute stroke, PET imaging is viewed as the gold standard technique for defining the incidence, temporal pattern and outcome of the ischaemic penumbra. More recent studies have utilized the hypoxia ligand [^{18}F]fluoromisonidazole ([^{18}F]FMISO) and the neuronal receptor ligand [^{11}C]flumazenil ([^{11}C] FMZ) in order to define the characteristics and temporal pattern of ischaemic penumbra and infarct core using PET.

Positron emission tomography has also been used successfully to investigate changes in physiology following head injury. Some studies have demonstrated that early reductions in cerebral perfusion can result in cerebral ischaemia that is associated with poor outcome, despite optimal management of ICP, CPP and ventilation (Fig. 10.15). However, other PET studies have failed to find conclusive evidence of cerebral ischaemia. Indeed, brain-injured patients commonly demonstrate evidence of global hypometabolism and metabolic stress, which fail to recover in patients who have a poor outcome. Positron emission tomography studies can be repeated and used to assess changes

in physiology with commonly applied therapeutic manoeuvres, such as hyperventilation and CPP augmentation. Such studies have helped to demonstrate that the efficacy of such therapies should be determined by measurement of cerebral perfusion and metabolism within individual patients and across the injured brain (Fig. 10.16). Blood flow and metabolism vary dramatically across the traumatized brain and different regions may require different therapeutic approaches. While this is obviously not possible using global therapeutic manoeuvres, it is clear that the effect of common therapeutic interventions should be measured and only continued where benefit is demonstrated.

While several PET studies have sought to define thresholds for tissue viability and ischaemia following ischaemic stroke and head injury, a recent review by Bandera and colleagues (2006) highlights the difficulties with such published thresholds. Although brain regions with dramatic reductions in CBF are clearly incapable of surviving, patients also demonstrate functional cognitive deficits in regions without clear evidence of structural injury. One possible cause for such findings is that a region that appears structurally intact may have suffered patchy neuronal injury, which results in selective neuronal loss and functional deficit. Early PET studies of CBF and metabolism clearly help

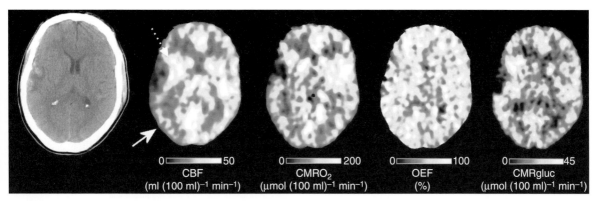

Fig. 10.15. Positron emission tomography (PET) imaging of regional metabolism following head injury. X-ray CT, PET cerebral blood flow (CBF), oxygen metabolism ($CMRO_2$), oxygen extraction fraction (OEF) and glucose metabolism (CMRglu) images obtained following early head injury. Note the right temporal haemorrhagic contusion with surrounding rim of hypodensity on the X-ray CT. The lesion core reflects infarcted brain with no or very low CBF. The pericontusional cerebral hemisphere displays variable pathophysiology. Immediately adjacent to the lesion core (dotted arrow), CBF is increased, $CMRO_2$ and OEF variable but glucose metabolism increased, while the right parietal occipital cortex (white arrow) demonstrates a decrease in CBF and $CMRO_2$ with an increase in OEF and variable glucose metabolism suggestive of regional cerebral ischaemia. The increase in CMRglu implies a switch to non-oxidative metabolism of glucose in order to meet underlying metabolic needs. See colour plate section.

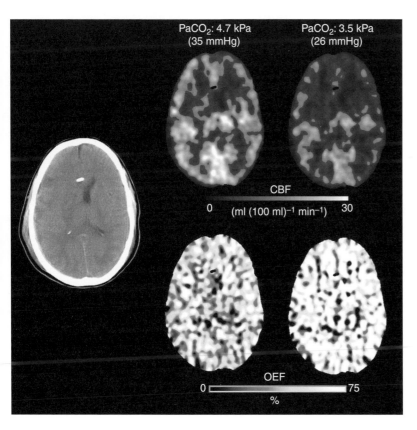

Fig. 10.16. Assessment of the efficacy of acute hyperventilation using positron emission tomography (PET) imaging. Structural CT following early head injury demonstrates a thin right subdural haematoma with underlying cerebral contusion, swollen hemisphere with effacement of the ipsilateral ventricle and midline shift. Greyscale PET cerebral blood flow (CBF) images were obtained at relative normocapnia (left panel) and hypocapnia (right panel). Voxels with a CBF <15 ml $(100 ml)^{-1}$ min^{-1} are picked out in red. Baseline intracranial pressure (ICP) was 21 mmHg and supports the use of hyperventilation to lower arterial carbon dioxide tension ($PaCO_2$) and improve ICP control. Hyperventilation did result in a reduction in ICP to 17 mmHg, but, in this individual, led to a substantial increase in the volume of hypoperfused brain. The PET oxygen extraction fraction (OEF) images show that the effect of the reduction in perfusion is a dramatic increase in OEF to levels consistent with cerebral ischaemia. See colour plate section.

to predict outcome, but further studies using markers of such selective neuronal injury, such as MRS and flumazenil PET, may improve the predictive power of such thresholds following head injury.

Although PET is clearly capable of defining many complex aspects of cerebral physiology and pathophysiology, it is a research tool that is relatively expensive and not universally available.

Magnetic resonance techniques

Blood flow can be measured using two different measurement techniques. Perfusion MRI uses rapid sequential susceptibility-weighted imaging after injection of a bolus of MRI contrast medium (typically Gd-DTPA) that induces a change in intravascular magnetic susceptibility to produce images of MTT, and relative CBF and CBV. Another MR technique uses an endogenous diffusible tracer to measure CBF by applying MR pulses to tag inflowing water protons. In this 'arterial spin labelling' approach, the changes in the amplitude of the MRI signal are used to construct quantitative images of cerebral perfusion. These techniques are now being successfully applied to clinical settings, although there are concerns regarding absolute quantification.

Diffusion-weighted MRI (DWI) images the microscopic movement of water using powerful gradient coils that undergo rapid switching in polarity on either side of a 180° excitation pulse. The random motion of diffusion leads to phase shifts and signal loss, while regions with decreased motion show little or no signal loss and appear relatively bright on DWI images. Where images are acquired with a range of diffusion weightings, maps of apparent diffusion coefficient (ADC) can be calculated. Broadly speaking, lesions that appear hyperintense on DWI images have a low ADC, and vice versa. Early hyperintensity on DWI images (with a corresponding low intensity on ADC maps) occurs following acute ischaemia and is associated with the movement of water into the intracellular compartment where it is relatively restricted (cytotoxic oedema), and represents the earliest imaging finding in ischaemia. In comparison, brain regions with vasogenic oedema and an increase in extracellular water content demonstrate an increased diffusion and therefore show reduced signal on DWI images and appear bright on ADC maps. A region demonstrating an acute decrease on ADC maps is assumed to have suffered irreversible injury (core), while the presence of reduced perfusion but normal diffusion is representative of tissue at risk of ischaemic injury (ischaemic penumbra). For these reasons a so-called perfusion/diffusion mismatch has been used to diagnose early cerebral ischaemia and direct therapy. In addition, measurements of water diffusion vary across the brain depending on the direction in which the tissue is examined. Due to the structure of white-matter fibre tracts, water diffusion will appear less restricted *along* fibre tracts compared with perpendicular to the fibre tract. The directionality of diffusion is called anisotropy and is measured by diffusion tensor imaging

(DTI) (Fig. 10.17). Such data are useful in delineating the extent of brain injury following both stroke and head injury. Indeed, evidence suggests that disruption of white-matter tracts has important implications for cognitive recovery.

Magnetic resonance spectroscopy is a non-invasive imaging technique that allows the investigation of biochemical pathology within the brain. Although both proton (^{1}H-MRS) and phosphorus (^{31}P-MRS)

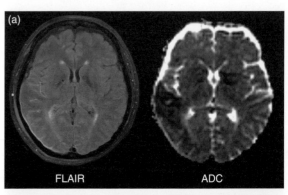

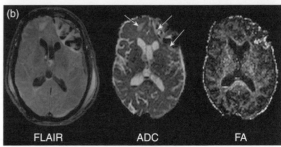

Fig. 10.17. MR diffusion tensor imaging. (a) Images from a patient who sustained a severe head injury and base of skull fracture following a road traffic accident. The fluid attenuated inversion recovery (FLAIR) image appears unremarkable except for a thin collection of subdural fluid and loss of volume within the underlying right temporoparietal cortex. The apparent diffusion coefficient (ADC) image demonstrates hypodensity in the right temporoparietal region suggesting cytotoxic oedema secondary to ischaemia. This patient sustained injury to the right internal carotid artery secondary to basal skull fracture.(b) Images obtained following acute severe head injury. The FLAIR image demonstrates frontal contusions of mixed intensity. The areas of darker intensity represent haemorrhage and the surrounding brighter regions are consistent with tissue oedema. In addition, the ventricular spaces are distended and there is a fluid level (blood) in the posterior horn of the right lateral ventricle.The ADC image in the region of the frontal contusions is composed of tissue with mixed diffusion signal. The core of the haemorrhagic contusion is necrotic tissue with no signal, while the bright areas of increased diffusion are consistent with vasogenic oedema (arrows). The fractional anisotropy (FA) image demonstrates high signal consistent with white matter, with reduced signal within the frontal regions consistent with disruption of the white-matter tracts. (Images courtesy of V. Newcombe, Wolfson Brain Imaging Centre, University of Cambridge, UK.)

spectroscopy are frequently used to study cerebral metabolism and ischaemia, ^{1}H-MRS is the prominent technique in humans. ^{1}H-MRS provides data on several biologically relevant molecules, including lactate, N-acetyl aspartate (NAA), total creatine (creatine and phosphocreatine), glutamate/glutamine and choline. Increased lactate suggests deranged energy metabolism and is consistent with cerebral ischaemia but may also represent mitochondrial dysfunction. N-Acetyl aspartate is located primarily within neurons, and a reduction in NAA can be indicative of neuronal death or dysfunction. Although MRS is not used routinely to assess patients with neurological disease, it can provide useful data concerning regional metabolism, which can be used to diagnose and treat a wide range of disorders. Following head injury, a decrease in NAA has been found and, while this may represent neuronal loss, it may also be the consequence of mitochondrial dysfunction and/or metabolic depression. Although it is clear that MRS can provide important information regarding the metabolic state and potential viability of ischaemic brain tissue, at present there are limitations to the technique. MRS imaging has been hampered by limited coverage of the brain, poor spatial resolution and the necessity for long imaging times. More recent developments of the technique provide multivoxel coverage of the whole brain with a spatial resolution of ~1 cm^3 and absolute quantification of metabolites. Indeed, MR spectroscopy has been shown to be clinically useful and promises to become widely available, as it can readily be implemented on existing MRI machines.

Functional MRI (fMRI) can be used to measure neural activation by the measurement of changes in blood oxygenation using the blood oxygen level-dependent (BOLD) technique, which is sensitive to local changes in the magnetic field induced by the presence of deoxygenated haemoglobin. This technique uses a rapid MRI sequence capable of demonstrating change after performance of a particular cognitive task aimed at inducing activation within a region of the brain. Neural activation results in an increase in regional blood flow and influx of oxygenated blood, which causes a decrease in the level of deoxygenated haemoglobin. Such techniques have been used in the assessment of patients recovering from brain injury, and patient lesions can be mapped to functional deficits. However, the BOLD technique does not measure neural activity directly, and disease processes may alter the relationship between local blood flow and neural activity. Therefore, fMRI data can be difficult to interpret in disease states. These investigations should be conducted with care to ensure that any possible confounding effects are characterized and their effects minimized. Functional MRI has also been used to assess patients who appear to be in a vegetative state following brain injury and can demonstrate that some patients may remain cognitively aware and capable of some degree of recovery. Although such positive findings have clear implications for predicting outcome following brain injury, a negative response in a particular cognitive task does not confirm that a patient is, or will remain, in a persistent vegetative state. Despite this, the technique has significant implications for the assessment of patients recovering from various forms of brain injury that appear to be in a vegetative, minimally conscious or locked-in state.

Magnetic resonance has become an extremely useful clinical tool in patients with neurological disease. It combines the ability to image perfusion, the status of tissue (DWI and MRS), vascular patency (MRA) and white-matter tracts (DTI) across the whole brain with high-resolution structural imaging. This thorough assessment of the derangements induced by a variety of disease mechanisms can be used to determine diagnosis, the likely response to therapeutic intervention and the degree of eventual functional recovery.

Conclusions

Imaging is an important clinical tool used in the management of patients with neurological disease. Rapid assessment using CT allows early diagnosis and ensures that those patients who require urgent medical or surgical intervention receive such care at the earliest opportunity. Access to high-field MRI is improving, and patients benefit from its greater spatial resolution and ability to combine imaging of structure with function across the brain. Several techniques are currently available that provide functional imaging of CBF and metabolism. Although such techniques provide 'snap shots' of physiology, they can be used to select patients for curative procedures, such as thrombolysis. In addition, such data can be repeated and used to assess the impact of therapeutic interventions. Perfusion imaging based on CT techniques (xenon-enhanced CT and CT perfusion) can easily be implemented in most hospital centres and provide quantitative perfusion data in addition to structural images. Positron emission tomography imaging provides unparalleled insights into cerebral physiology and pathophysiology but is not widely available and is primarily a research tool. Future developments of imaging technology and processing techniques should improve our understanding of the pathophysiology of disease, benefit patient management and enable prediction of functional outcome.

Acknowledgements

The research studies published by Dr Coles and Professor Menon were supported by the Medical Research Council, a Technology Foresight from the UK Government and by a Royal College of Anaesthetists/British Journal of Anaesthesia project grant. Dr Coles is currently funded by the Cambridge NIHR Biomedical Research Centre and has previously received Research Training Fellowships from the Addenbrooke's Charities, the Wellcome Foundation, Beverley and Raymond Sackler studentship, and an Academy of Medical Sciences and Health Foundation Clinician Scientist Fellowship.

Further reading

Anon. (2002). *Provision of Anaesthetic Services in Magnetic Resonance Units.* London: Association of Anaesthetists of Great Britain and Ireland.

Anon. (2005). What's new in MR safety: the latest on the safe use of equipment in the magnetic resonance environment. *Health Devices* **34**, 333–49.

Ashikaga, R., Araki, Y. and Ishida, O. (1997). MRI of head injury using FLAIR. *Neuroradiology* **39**, 239–42.

Astrup, J., Siesjo, B. K. and Symon, L. (1981). Thresholds in cerebral ischemia – the ischemic penumbra. *Stroke* **12**, 723–5.

Bandera, E., Botteri, M., Minelli, C. *et al.* (2006). Cerebral blood flow threshold of ischemic penumbra and infarct core in acute ischemic stroke: a systematic review. *Stroke* **37**, 1334–9.

Barker, P. B. (2005). Fundamentals of MR spectroscopy. In Gillard, J. H., Waldman, A. D. and Barker, P. B., eds., *Clinical MR Neuroimaging.* Cambridge: Cambridge University Press, pp. 7–26.

Baron, J. (1999). Mapping the ischaemic penumbra with PET: implications for acute stroke treatment. *Cerebrovasc Dis* **9**, 193–201.

Baron, J. C. (2005). Stroke research in the modern era: images versus dogmas. *Cerebrovasc Dis* **20**, 154–63.

Baron, J. C., Frackowiak, R. S., Herholz, K. *et al.* (1989). Use of PET methods for measurement of cerebral energy metabolism and hemodynamics in cerebrovascular disease. *J Cereb Blood Flow Metab* **9**, 723–42.

Bergsneider, M., Hovda, D. A., Lee, S. M. *et al.* (2000). Dissociation of cerebral glucose metabolism and level of consciousness during the period of metabolic depression following human traumatic brain injury. *J Neurotrauma* **17**, 389–401.

Bouma, G. J., Muizelaar, J. P., Stringer, W. A. *et al.* (1992). Ultra-early evaluation of regional cerebral blood flow in severely head-injured patients using xenon-enhanced computerized tomography. *J Neurosurg* **77**, 360–8.

Brooks, W. M., Friedman, S. D. and Gasparovic, C. (2001). Magnetic resonance spectroscopy in traumatic brain injury. *J Head Trauma Rehabil* **16**, 149–64.

Calamante, F., Thomas, D. L., Pell, G. S., Wiersma, J. and Turner, R. (1999). Measuring cerebral blood flow using magnetic resonance imaging techniques. *J Cereb Blood Flow Metab* **19**, 701–35.

Carpentier, A., Galanaud, D., Puybasset, L. *et al.* (2006). Early morphologic and spectroscopic magnetic resonance in severe traumatic brain injuries can detect "invisible brain stem damage" and predict "vegetative states". *J Neurotrauma* **23**, 674–85.

Coles, J. P. (2006). Imaging of cerebral blood flow and metabolism. *Curr Opin Anaesthesiol* **19**, 473–80.

Coles, J. P., Minhas, P. S., Fryer, T. D. *et al.* (2002). Effect of hyperventilation on cerebral blood flow in traumatic head injury: clinical relevance and monitoring correlates. *Crit Care Med* **30**, 1950–9.

Coles, J. P., Fryer, T. D., Smielewski, P. *et al.* (2004). Incidence and mechanisms of cerebral ischemia in early clinical head injury. *J Cereb Blood Flow Metab* **24**, 202–11.

Coles, J. P., Steiner, L. A., Johnston, A. J. *et al.* (2004). Does induced hypertension reduce cerebral ischaemia within the traumatized human brain? *Brain* **127**, 2479–90.

Coles, J. P., Cunningham, A. S., Salvador, R. *et al.* (2009). Early metabolic characteristics of lesion and nonlesion tissue after head injury. *J Cereb Blood Flow Metab* **29**, 965–75.

Cunningham, A. S., Salvador, R., Coles, J. P. *et al.* (2005). Physiological thresholds for irreversible tissue damage in contusional regions following traumatic brain injury. *Brain* **128**, 1931–42.

Davis, S. M., Donnan, G. A., Butcher, K. S. and Parsons, M. (2005). Selection of thrombolytic therapy beyond 3 h using magnetic resonance imaging. *Curr Opin Neurol* **18**, 47–52.

Diringer, M. N., Videen, T. O., Yundt, K. *et al.* (2002). Regional cerebrovascular and metabolic effects of hyperventilation after severe traumatic brain injury. *J Neurosurg* **96**, 103–8.

Donnan, G. A., Baron, J. C., Ma, H. and Davis, S. M. (2009). Penumbral selection of patients for trials of acute stroke therapy. *Lancet Neurol* **8**, 261–9.

Drayer, B. P., Wolfson, S. K., Reinmuth, O. M. *et al.* (1978). Xenon enhanced CT for analysis of cerebral integrity, perfusion, and blood flow. *Stroke* **9**, 123–30.

Easton, J. D., Saver, J. L., Albers, G. W. *et al.* (2009). Definition and evaluation of transient ischaemic attack: a scientific statement for healthcare professionals from the American Heart Association/American Stroke Association Stroke Council; Council on Cardiovascular Surgery and Anesthesia; Council on Cardiovascular Radiology and Intervention; Council on Cardiovascular Nursing; and the Interdisciplinary Council on Peripheral Vascular Disease. *Stroke* **40**, 2276–93.

Ebinger, M., De Silva, D. A., Christensen, S. *et al.* (2009). Imaging the penumbra – strategies to detect tissue at risk after ischemic stroke. *J Clin Neurosci* **16**, 178–87.

Ewing, J. R., Cao, Y., Knight, R. A. and Fenstermacher, J. D. (2005). Arterial spin labeling: validity testing and comparison studies. *J Magn Reson Imaging* **22**, 737–40.

Garnett, M. R., Blamire, A. M., Corkill, R. G. *et al.* (2000). Early proton magnetic resonance spectroscopy in normal-appearing brain correlates with outcome in patients following traumatic brain injury. *Brain* **123**, 2046–54.

Garnett, M. R., Cadoux-Hudson, T. A. and Styles, P. (2001). How useful is magnetic resonance imaging in predicting severity and outcome in traumatic brain injury? *Curr Opin Neurol* **14**, 753–7.

Goldfarb, S., McCullough P. A., McDermott, J. and Gay, S. B. (2009). Contrast-induced acute kidney injury: specialty-specific protocols for interventional radiology, diagnostic computed tomography radiology, and interventional cardiology. *Mayo Clin Proc* **84**, 170–9.

Guadagno, J. V., Calautti, C. and Baron, J. C. (2003). Progress in imaging stroke: emerging clinical applications. *Br Med Bull* **65**, 145–57.

Hammoud, D. A. and Wasserman, B. A. (2002). Diffuse axonal injuries: pathophysiology and imaging. *Neuroimaging Clin N Am* **12**, 205–16.

Hassan, Z., Smith, M., Littlewood, S. *et al.* (2005). Head injuries: a study evaluating the impact of the NICE head injury guidelines. *Emerg Med J* **22**, 845–9.

Heiss, W. D. (2000). Ischemic penumbra: evidence from functional imaging in man. *J Cereb Blood Flow Metab* **20**, 1276–93.

Heiss, W. D. and Rosner, G. (1983). Functional recovery of cortical neurons as related to degree and duration of ischemia. *Ann Neurol* **14**, 294–301.

Heiss, W. D., Kracht, L. W., Thiel, A., Grond, M. and Pawlik, G. (2001). Penumbral probability thresholds of cortical flumazenil binding and blood flow predicting tissue outcome in patients with cerebral ischaemia. *Brain* **124**, 20–9.

Heiss, W. D., Sobesky, J. and Hesselmann, V. (2004). Identifying thresholds for penumbra and irreversible tissue damage. *Stroke* **35**(11 Suppl 1): 2671–4

Iannetti, G. D. and Wise, R. G. (2007). BOLD functional MRI in disease and pharmacological studies: room for improvement? *Magn Reson Imaging* **25**, 978–88.

Kampfl, A., Schmutzhard, E., Franz, G. *et al.* (1998). Prediction of recovery from post-traumatic vegetative state with cerebral magnetic-resonance imaging. *Lancet* **351**, 1763–7.

Kety, S. S. and Schmidt, C. F. (1945). The determination of cerebral blood flow in man by the use of nitrous oxide in low concentrations. *Am J Physiol* **143**, 53–6.

Lammertse, D., Dungan, D., Dreisbach, J. *et al.* (2007). Neuroimaging in traumatic spinal cord injury: an evidence-based review for clinical practice and research. *J Spinal Cord Med* **30**, 205–14.

Latchaw, R. E., Yonas, H., Hunter, G. J. *et al.* (2003). Guidelines and recommendations for perfusion imaging in cerebral ischaemia: a scientific statement for healthcare professionals by the writing group on perfusion imaging, from the Council on Cardiovascular Radiology of the American Heart Association. *Stroke* **34**, 1084–104.

Laureys, S., Owen, A. M. and Schiff, N. D. (2004). Brain function in coma, vegetative state, and related disorders. *Lancet Neurol* **3**, 537–46.

Lee, B. and Newberg, A. (2005). Neuroimaging in traumatic brain imaging. *NeuroRx* **2**, 372–83.

Lin, A., Ross, B. D., Harris, K. and Wong, W. (2005). Efficacy of proton magnetic resonance spectroscopy in neurological diagnosis and neurotherapeutic decision making. *NeuroRx* **2**, 197–214.

Liu, A. Y., Maldjian, J. A., Bagley, L. J., Sinson, G. P. and Grossman, R. I. (1999). Traumatic brain injury: diffusion-weighted MR imaging findings. *AJNR Am J Neuroradiol* **20**, 1636–41.

Mannion, R. J., Cross, J., Bradley, P. *et al.* (2007). Mechanism-based MRI classification of traumatic brainstem injury and its relationship to outcome. *J Neurotrauma* **24**, 128–35.

Markus, R., Reutens, D. C., Kazui, S. *et al.* (2003). Topography and temporal evolution of hypoxic viable tissue identified by 18F-fluoromisonidazole positron emission tomography in humans after ischemic stroke. *Stroke* **34**, 2646–52.

Marmarou, A., Signoretti, S., Fatouros, P., Aygok, G. A. and Bullock, R. (2005). Mitochondrial injury measured by proton magnetic resonance spectroscopy in severe head trauma patients. *Acta Neurochir Suppl* **95**,149–51.

McLaughlin, M. R. and Marion, D. W. (1996). Cerebral blood flow and vasoresponsivity within and around cerebral contusions. *J Neurosurg* **85**, 871–6.

Menon, D. K., Coles, J. P., Gupta, A. K. *et al.* (2004). Diffusion limited oxygen delivery following head injury. *Crit Care Med* **32**, 1384–90.

Miles, K. A. (2004). Brain perfusion: computed tomography applications. *Neuroradiology* **46** (Suppl. 2), 194–200.

Munari, M., Zucchetta, P., Carollo, C. *et al.* (2005). Confirmatory tests in the diagnosis of brain death: comparison between SPECT and contrast angiography. *Crit Care Med* **33**, 2068–73.

National Institute for Clinical Excellence (2003). *Head Injury: Triage, Assessment, Investigation and Early Management of Head Injury in Infants, Children and Adults*. NICE clinical guideline.

Newcombe, V. F., Hawkes, R. C., Harding, S. G. *et al.* (2008). Potential heating caused by intraparenchymal intracranial pressure transducers in a 3-tesla magnetic resonance imaging system using a body radiofrequency resonator: assessment of the Codman MicroSensor Transducer. *J Neurosurg* **109**, 159–64.

Nguyen-Huynh, M. N., Wintermark, M., English, J. *et al.* (2008). How accurate is CT angiography in evaluating intracranial atherosclerotic disease? *Stroke* **39**, 1184–8.

Owen, A. M., Coleman, M. R., Boly, M. *et al.* (2006). Detecting awareness in the vegetative state. *Science* **313**, 1402.

Pannek, K., Chalk, J. B., Finnigan, S. and Rose, S. E. (2009). Dynamic corticospinal white matter connectivity changes during stroke recovery: a diffusion tensor probabilistic tractography study. *J Magn Reson Imaging* **29**, 529–36.

Peden, C. J., Menon, D. K., Hall, A. S., Sargentoni, J. and Whitwam, J. G. (1992). Magnetic resonance for the anaesthetist. Part II: anaesthesia and monitoring in MR units. *Anaesthesia* **47**, 508–17.

Pierallini, A., Pantano, P., Fantozzi, L. M. *et al.* (2000). Correlation between MRI findings and long-term outcome in patients with severe brain trauma. *Neuroradiology* **42**, 860–7.

Powers, W. J., Grubb, R. L. Jr, Baker, R. P., Mintun, M. A. and Raichle, M. E. (1985). Regional cerebral blood flow and metabolism in reversible ischemia due to vasospasm. Determination by positron emission tomography. *J Neurosurg* **62**, 539–46.

Prabhakaran, V., Raman, S. P., Grunwald, M. R. *et al.* (2007). Neural substrates of word generation during stroke recovery: the influence of cortical hypoperfusion. *Behav Neurol* **18**, 45–52

Provenzale, J. (2007). MR imaging of spinal trauma. *Emerg Radiol* **13**, 289–97

Rubin, G., Firlik, A. D., Pindzola, R. R., Levy, E. I. and Yonas, H. (1999). The effect of reperfusion therapy on cerebral blood flow in acute stroke. *J Stroke Cerebrovasc Dis* **8**, 9–16.

Rubin, G., Firlik, A. D., Levy, E. I., Pindzola, R. R. and Yonas, H. (1999). Xenon-enhanced computed tomography cerebral blood flow measurements in acute cerebral ischemia: Review of 56 cases. *J Stroke Cerebrovasc Dis* **8**, 404–11.

Salmond, C. H., Menon, D. K., Chatfield, D. A. *et al.* (2006). Diffusion tensor imaging in chronic head injury survivors: correlations with learning and memory indices. *Neuroimage* **29**, 117–24.

Scharf, J., Brockmann, M. A., Daffertshofer, M. *et al.* (2006). Improvement of sensitivity and interrater reliability to detect acute stroke by dynamic perfusion computed tomography and computed tomography angiography. *J Comput Assist Tomogr* **30**, 105–10.

Seelig, J. M., Becker, D. P., Miller, J. D. *et al.* (1981). Traumatic acute subdural hematoma: major mortality reduction in comatose patients treated within four hours. *N Engl J Med* **304**, 1511–8.

Shutter, L., Tong, K. A., Lee, A. and Holshouser, B. A. (2006). Prognostic role of proton magnetic resonance spectroscopy in acute traumatic brain injury. *J Head Trauma Rehabil* **21**, 334–49.

Sidaros, A., Engberg, A. W., Sidaros, K. *et al.* (2008). Diffusion tensor imaging during recovery from severe traumatic brain injury and relation to clinical outcome: a longitudinal study. *Brain* **131**, 559–72.

Stengel, A., Neumann-Haefelin, T., Singer, O. C. *et al.* (2004). Multiple spin–echo spectroscopic imaging for rapid quantitative assessment of *N*-acetylaspartate and lactate in acute stroke. *Magn Reson Med* **52**, 228–38.

Stringer, W. A., Hasso, A. N., Thompson, J. R., Hinshaw, D. B. and Jordan, K. G. (1993). Hyperventilation-induced cerebral ischemia in patients with acute brain lesions: demonstration by xenon-enhanced CT. *AJNR Am J Neuroradiol* **14**, 475–84.

van Laar, P. J., van der Grond, J. and Hendrikse, J. (2008). Brain perfusion territory imaging: methods and clinical applications of selective arterial spin-labeling MR imaging. *Radiology* **246**, 354–64

Vandenberghe, R. and Gillebert, C. R. (2009). Parcellation of parietal cortex: convergence between lesion-symptom mapping and mapping of the intact functioning brain. *Behav Brain Res* **199**, 171–82.

Vespa, P., Bergsneider, M., Hattori, N. *et al.* (2005). Metabolic crisis without brain ischemia is common after traumatic brain injury: a combined microdialysis and positron emission tomography study. *J Cereb Blood Flow Metab* **25**, 763–74.

von Oettingen, G., Bergholt, B., Ostergaard, L. *et al.* (2000). Xenon CT cerebral blood flow in patients with head injury: influence of pulmonary trauma on the input function. *Neuroradiology* **42**, 168–73.

Ward, N. S. and Frackowiak, R. S. (2006). The functional anatomy of cerebral reorganisation after focal brain injury. *J Physiol Paris* **99**, 425–36.

Wardlaw, J. M., Easton, V. J. and Statham, P. (2002). Which CT features help predict outcome after head injury? *J Neurol Neurosurg Psychiatry* **72**, 188–92; discussion 51.

Wilde, E. A., Chu, Z., Bigler, E. D. *et al.* (2006). Diffusion tensor imaging in the corpus callosum in children after moderate to severe traumatic brain injury. *J Neurotrauma* **23**, 1412–26.

Wintermark, M., Thiran, J. P., Maeder, P., Schnyder, P. and Meuli, R. (2001). Simultaneous measurement of regional cerebral blood flow by perfusion CT and stable xenon CT: a validation study. *AJNR Am J Neuroradiol* **22**, 905–14.

Wintermark, M., Ko, N. U., Smith, W. S. *et al.* (2006). Vasospasm after subarachnoid hemorrhage: utility of perfusion CT and CT angiography on diagnosis and management. *AJNR Am J Neuroradiol* **27**, 26–34.

Chapter

11

General considerations in neuroanaesthesia

Armagan Dagal and Arthur M. Lam

Patient assessment

The risk of morbidity/mortality exists with any surgical/anaesthetic procedure, but the risk to the central nervous system may be compounded in a patient undergoing a major neurosurgical procedure. The patient may be placed at risk because of his or her neurological condition, or the inherent risk of the surgical procedure, and in many cases both. The purpose of the pre-operative assessment includes the identification of modifiable risk factors, optimization of the patient's condition, explanation of the risks and formulating the best possible anaesthetic plan for the patient. Other benefits may include improved safety of perioperative care, optimal resource utilization and patient satisfaction.

A neuroanaesthesiologist's objectives for pre-anaesthetic evaluation can be summarized as follows:

1. Develop a rapport with the patient and their immediate family in order to minimize their anxiety and maximize cooperation.
2. Complete a review of medical, surgical and anaesthetic history, allergies and current medications, thus establishing a baseline profile.
3. Review relevant personal, family and social history.
4. Perform a general physical examination, recording of vital signs and examination of individual systems, in particular the central nervous and cardiopulmonary systems.
5. Interpret relevant laboratory data and arrange for further investigations and consultations if deemed necessary.
6. Optimize the patient's physiological condition.
7. Stratify the patient's morbidity and mortality risk based on the considerations above.
8. Discuss anaesthetic techniques, procedures, associated risks and benefits with the patient.
9. Plan and explain post-operative management, including pain control and the possible need for post-operative mechanical ventilation.
10. Document informed consent for the proposed anaesthetic technique and procedures.

The pre-anaesthetic evaluation ideally should be conducted during a visit to the pre-operative anaesthesia clinics. The consensus of the ASA Task Force on pre-anaesthesia evaluation is that an initial assessment should be performed prior to the day of surgery for patients with high severity of disease and/or scheduled for major surgery. Patients undergoing procedures with medium or low surgical invasiveness may be assessed on or before the day of surgery. In emergent cases, a focused pre-anaesthetic examination can be conducted and should at least include an assessment of the neurological status, airway, lungs and heart, with documentation of vital signs.

Anaesthesiologists ideally run these clinics with the assistance of trained nursing staff, to improve operating room efficiency and minimize unexpected delays and cancellations due to inadequate patient preparation. Careful triage based on a patient's history can help avoid unnecessary assessment of low-risk patients and ensure that necessary assessments for higher-risk patients are completed before the day of surgery.

For a smooth transition from patient referral to surgical intervention, dynamic communication between neurosurgeons, anaesthesiologists, the pre-anaesthesia clinic, neurophysiologists and the laboratory is essential.

General pre-anaesthetic evaluation

The American Society of Anesthesiologists (ASA) classification is a universally accepted system used for stratification of the patient's pre-existing health status

Core Topics in Neuroanaesthesia and Neurointensive Care, eds. Basil F. Matta, David K. Menon and Martin Smith. Published by Cambridge University Press. © Cambridge University Press 2011.

Table 11.1 American Society of Anesthesiologists (ASA) classification of physical status

ASA physical status	Disease state
1	A normal healthy patient
2	A patient with mild systemic disease
3	A patient with severe systemic disease
4	A patient with severe systemic disease that is a constant threat to life
5	A moribund patient who is not expected to survive without the operation
6	A declared brain-dead patient whose organs are being removed for donor purposes

(Table 11.1). Although it does not take into account the surgical risk, age, etc. and is not primarily designed for outcome prediction, it has been found to correlate well with perioperative morbidity and mortality. In fact, ASA physical status 3–5 has been found to independently predict perioperative cardiovascular complications in intracranial surgical patients, and is also a risk factor for perioperative mortality.

History and physical examination

Medical history

The following should be determined:

1. History of the primary disease for which surgical procedure is planned.
2. General medical history.
3. Surgical and anaesthesia-related history (in particular with airway management, intensive care unit (ICU) admissions, adverse reactions, intravenous access, post-operative pain and nausea/vomiting, etc.).
4. Current medications (anticonvulsant therapy is associated with increased resistance to non-depolarizing muscle relaxants and consideration for increased dosage requirements; steroid administration might be associated with hyperglycaemia and adrenal suppression) and allergies.
5. Social history (smoking, alcohol, recreational drug use).
6. Relevant family medical history and social/religious background (e.g. Jehovah's witness).

General physical examination

The general physical examination should focus on the patient's level of consciousness, degree of neurological impairment, mental status, nutrition and vital parameters for baseline. Patients with malignant tumours and those with high cervical lesions may be emaciated with significantly reduced muscle mass. On the other hand, obesity may coexist in many patients. Obese individuals have an increased likelihood of associated diabetes, hypertension, coronary artery disease, restrictive lung disease, sleep apnoea and gastro-oesophageal reflux. Obesity also increases the risk of difficult tracheal intubation and alters the pharmacological response profile to anaesthetic agents.

The incidence of altered fluid and electrolyte status is higher in neurosurgical patients compared with the general surgical population. Impaired consciousness leading to diminished intake of fluids, vomiting and the use of diuretics and contrast agents all contribute to the imbalance. Correction of significant dehydration and electrolyte derangements before induction of anaesthesia can prevent post-induction hypotension and cardiac instability in such patients.

Major blood loss is a possibility in surgery for intracranial aneurysms, arteriovenous malformations, vascular tumours and craniosynostoses. Pre-anaesthetic assessment should include investigation for pre-existing anaemia and aim to correct it pre-operatively or arrange for intraoperative transfusion on a case-by-case basis.

While the primary neurosurgical problem (e.g. cervical spine instability necessitating halo fixation) may be responsible for potential difficulties in intubation and airway management, inadequate management of the airway may adversely affect the neurological outcome. Routine manoeuvres used for airway management may worsen spinal instability in patients with cervical lesions and may lead to increased intracranial pressure (ICP) potentially with cerebral ischaemia. Hence, the patient's airway should be assessed carefully for ease of ventilation and difficulty in tracheal intubation. Mallampati score, thyromental distance, presence of overbite or underbite and neck flexion/extension collectively provide an estimate of the risk of difficult intubation. Special attention should be accorded to patients with recent supratentorial craniotomy in whom the mouth opening may be significantly reduced secondary to ankylosis of the temporomandibular joint, acromegalic patients undergoing pituitary surgery and patients with cervical spine lesions.

Assessment of system functions

Neurological system

Focused neurological assessment and careful documentation allow the establishment of baseline status and facilitate anaesthetic planning, as well as anticipation of potential perioperative complications. Patients with a depressed level of consciousness are likely to require reduced amounts of anaesthetic agents for induction, are more likely to have a slow post-operative emergence and may need post-operative mechanical ventilation. Patients with previous motor deficits may develop exacerbation of focal neurological signs after sedative doses of benzodiazepines and narcotics. The presence of brainstem lesions and/or lower cranial nerve dysfunction predisposes the patients to an increased risk of aspiration post-operatively. Finally, patients with pre-existing motor deficits or a ruptured cerebral aneurysm may develop a life-threatening hyperkalaemia secondary to succinylcholine administration, although these appear to be very uncommon. Elevated ICP can often result in symptoms of headache, nausea and vomiting, but can also lead to olfactory nerve dysfunction with a loss of sense of smell. Unilateral uncal herniation would result in a dilated unresponsive ipsilateral pupil, which should be distinguished from incidental anisocoria, or a unilateral third-nerve palsy resulting from compression by a space-occupying lesion. The field of vision may be significantly limited in patients with pituitary and other suprasellar tumours and should be documented for post-operative comparison. Dysfunction of the trigeminal nerve and facial nerve may interfere with mask ventilation and tracheal intubation. A patient with a damaged vagus nerve may present with a hoarse voice secondary to vocal cord paralysis and may be at increased risk of airway obstruction.

Respiratory system

The risk of perioperative respiratory complications is increased in the presence of pre-existing obstructive or restrictive pulmonary disease. Patients presenting with a history of pulmonary disease require an assessment of their baseline status to address any element of potential reversibility. Smoking is a common important risk factor for both cardiovascular and pulmonary disease and is associated with a threefold increase in perioperative morbidity. Cessation of smoking for 6–8 weeks is recommended for reactivation of mucociliary clearance, but cessation as little as for 24 h can reduce the carboxyhaemoglobin levels and improve oxygenation. The presence of reactive airway disease indicates an increased risk of bronchospasm with airway manipulation, tracheal extubation and an increased risk of coughing and laryngospasm during emergence.

In patients with symptomatic obstructive pulmonary disease, pre-operative pulmonary function testing including flow-volume loops before and after bronchodilators, and arterial blood gas sampling allow assessment of reversibility and determination of optimal preparation. An abnormally high arterial carbon dioxide tension ($PaCO_2$) or low PaO_2 pre-operatively is predictive of post-operative respiratory complications. Some patients with sleep apnoea might be using continuous positive airway pressure devices at home, and it is important to ensure that the same device is available post-operatively.

Patients with decreased levels of consciousness or lower cranial nerve dysfunction due to intracranial pathology or those having a high spinal cord lesion may have pre-existing lung atelectasis, which puts them at increased risk of post-operative mechanical ventilation. Aspiration pneumonitis and/or superimposed pneumonia can also occur.

In their systematic review of pre-operative pulmonary risk stratification for non-cardiothoracic surgery for the American College of Physicians in 2006, Smetana and colleagues found good evidence to support the following patient-related risk factors as predictive of post-operative pulmonary complications: advanced age, ASA class II or greater, functional dependence, chronic obstructive pulmonary disease (COPD) and congestive heart failure. They also found fair evidence indicating increased risk due to impaired sensorium, abnormal findings on chest examination, cigarette use, alcohol use and weight loss. Perioperative risk may be increased if asthma is poorly controlled.

Important procedure-related risk factors include neurosurgery, emergency surgery and prolonged surgery. The value of pre-operative testing to estimate pulmonary risk is controversial. While an abnormal chest radiograph does indicate an increased risk of post-operative pulmonary complications and spirometry may provide some risk stratification, among potential laboratory tests to stratify risk, a serum albumin level $<35\,\mathrm{g\,l^{-1}}$ is the most powerful predictor.

Cardiovascular system

The overall cardiac risk of a patient undergoing a noncardiac procedure has traditionally been assessed using the Goldman index. This has now been replaced by the more user-friendly Revised Cardiac Risk Index where the presence of three or more of the following factors is associated with a cardiac morbidity score of 9%: (i) high-risk surgery; (ii) a history of ischaemic heart disease; (iii) a history of congestive heart failure; (iv) a history of cerebrovascular disease; (v) pre-operative treatment with insulin; and (vi) a pre-operative serum creatinine level $>2.0\,\mathrm{mg\,dl^{-1}}$.

Hypertension is a common pre-existing medical condition and these patients often have reduced plasma volume, making them more susceptible to the systemic vasodilatory effects of anaesthetic agents, resulting in cardiovascular instability and labile blood pressure intraoperatively. Moreover, in chronic untreated or poorly treated hypertensive patients, increased cerebrovascular resistance causes a right shift of the cerebral blood flow (CBF) autoregulatory curve, resulting in poor tolerance to acute hypotension. However, adaptive hypertensive changes in CBF autoregulation may be reversible with adequate control of blood pressure. With the exception of angiotensin-converting enzyme (ACE) inhibitors and β-blockers, which should be discontinued for 24 h, patients should continue on their usual hypertensive medications right up to the time of surgery. Patients with evidence of myocardial ischaemia or infarction are at increased risk of post-operative myocardial infarction, congestive heart failure, malignant arrhythmias and death. Mannitol must be used carefully and judiciously or not at all in the presence of left ventricular failure.

In general, pre-operative tests are recommended only if the information obtained will result in a change in the surgical procedure performed, a change in medical therapy or monitoring during or after surgery, or a postponement of surgery until the cardiac condition can be improved or stabilized. A cardiologist consultation should be sought if deemed necessary and if surgical circumstances allow.

The American College of Cardiology/American Heart Association (ACC/AHA) 2007 guidelines helps to grade clinical risk factors as major, intermediate and minor. The presence of one or more of the major risk factors (active cardiac conditions) mandates intensive management and may require delay or cancellation of surgery unless the surgery is emergent. These include the following:

- Unstable coronary syndromes (e.g. unstable or severe angina).
- Decompensated heart failure.
- Significant arrhythmias (e.g. high-grade atrioventricular block, supraventricular arrhythmias with uncontrolled ventricular rate, symptomatic ventricular arrhythmias/bradycardia).
- Severe valvular disease (severe aortic stenosis or symptomatic mitral stenosis).

Intermediate-risk factors include:

- A history of ischaemic heart disease.
- A history of compensated or prior heart failure.
- A history of cerebrovascular disease.
- Diabetes mellitus.
- Renal insufficiency.

A history of myocardial infarction (MI) or abnormal Q waves by ECG is listed as a clinical risk factor, whereas an acute MI (defined as at least one documented MI 7 days or fewer before the examination) or recent MI (>7 days but ≤1 month before the examination) with evidence of important ischaemic risk by clinical symptoms or non-invasive study is an active cardiac condition. Although there are no adequate clinical trials on which to base firm recommendations, it appears reasonable to wait 4–6 weeks after an MI to perform elective surgery.

Minor predictors are recognized markers for cardiovascular disease that have not been proven to increase perioperative risk independently, for example, advanced age (>70 years), abnormal ECG (left ventricular hypertrophy, left bundle branch block, ST-T abnormalities), rhythm other than sinus and uncontrolled systemic hypertension.

The guidelines recommend the following stepwise approach to perioperative cardiac assessment for non-cardiac surgery:

- *Step 1: need for emergency non-cardiac surgery.* Further cardiac assessment or treatment not warranted and patient may proceed to the emergency surgery with perioperative surveillance and post-operative risk stratification and risk factor management. The cardiologist may provide recommendations for perioperative medical management and surveillance.
- *Step 2: patients with active cardiac conditions.* The presence of unstable coronary disease, decompensated heart failure, severe arrhythmia or severe valvular heart disease warrants evaluation and treatment following ACC/AHA guidelines with cancellation or delay of surgery until the cardiac problem has been clarified and treated appropriately. However, depending on the results of investigations and cardiac interventions and the risk of delaying surgery, it may be appropriate to proceed to the planned surgery with maximal medical therapy.
- *Step 3: patients undergoing low-risk surgery.* Interventions based on cardiovascular testing in stable patients rarely result in a change in management, and it is appropriate to proceed with the planned surgical procedure in these patients.
- *Step 4: patients with good functional capacity, without symptoms.* Functional status is a reliable predictor for perioperative and long-term cardiac events. In highly functional asymptomatic patients, management will rarely be changed based on the results of any further cardiovascular testing. It is therefore appropriate to proceed with the planned surgery. In patients with known cardiovascular disease or at least one clinical risk factor (ischaemic heart disease, compensated or prior heart failure, diabetes mellitus, renal insufficiency or cerebrovascular disease), perioperative heart rate control with β-blockade is considered appropriate. However, results from the Perioperative Ischemic Evaluation Study (POISE) trial indicated that the reduced cardiac morbidity with perioperative β-blocker therapy in patients not previously on β-blockers is achieved at the expense of increased stroke rate and an overall increased in mortality (see below).
- *Step 5: symptomatic patients and patients with poor or unknown functional capacity.* In this scenario, the presence of clinical risk factors determines the need for further evaluation. It is appropriate to proceed with the planned surgery, and no further

change in management is indicated if the patient has no clinical risk factors. If the patient has one or two clinical risk factors, then it is reasonable to either proceed with the planned surgery, with consideration of β-blockade for heart rate control, or undertake cardiac testing if it will change the management. In patients with three or more clinical risk factors, the surgery-specific cardiac risk is important, which in turn is related to the degree of haemodynamic cardiac stress (alterations in heart rate, blood pressure, vascular volume, pain, bleeding, clotting tendencies, oxygenation, neurohumoral activation, etc.) associated with the surgery. In patients undergoing intermediate-risk surgery (including head and neck surgery and carotid endarterectomy), there are insufficient data to determine the best strategy.

The stunned (stressed) myocardium

There is a known association between ECG changes, troponin leak and left ventricular dysfunction for acute intracranial disease including subarachnoid haemorrhage (SAH) and traumatic brain injury. This is related to the intense catecholamine and sympathetic surge occurring at the time of the ictus. Particularly in patients with SAH, this can lead to severe ventricular dysfunction and pulmonary oedema (neurogenic shock). An elevated troponin level $\geq 10\,\mu g\;l^{-1}$ is associated with a worse outcome in these patients. Pre-operative trans-thoracic or transoesophageal echocardiography is indicated under these circumstances. Ventricular dysfunction associated with SAH typically exhibits a pattern of global hypokinesia with apical sparing, although the pattern of Tako-Tsubo cardiomyopathy has also been reported.

Gastrointestinal system

Patients at risk of aspiration include those with full stomachs, delayed gastric emptying, bowel obstruction, and gastro-oesophageal reflux. Patients with cranial nerve dysfunction as well as those with a decreased level of consciousness are also at risk. In these patients, rapid sequence induction should be considered.

Renal system

Patients with kidney disease may have autonomic neuropathy, encephalopathy, fluid retention (congestive heart failure, pleural effusion, ascites) and yet intravascular volume depletion, hypertension, metabolic acidosis, electrolyte imbalances (hyperkalaemia, hyponatraemia, hypocalcaemia), anaemia and delayed gastric emptying, among other manifestations. Haematocrit, serum electrolytes, coagulation studies, blood urea nitrogen and creatinine measurements are advisable. A chest X-ray and arterial blood gas analysis might be required in patients with breathlessness, and an ECG should be examined for signs of hyperkalaemia or hypocalcaemia as well as ischaemia and conduction blocks. Pre-operative drug therapy should be carefully reviewed for drugs with significant renal elimination.

Intravascular volume depletion, contrast dye injections, aminoglycoside antibiotics, ACE inhibitors, and non-steroidal anti-inflammatory drugs (NSAIDs) are risk factors for an acute deterioration in renal function and must be avoided. Volume status is often difficult to assess and may necessitate invasive monitoring. Neuromuscular blocking agents not dependent on renal function for their elimination should be selected. Mannitol is contraindicated in anuric patients.

Haematological system

Post-operative intracranial haemorrhage is a potentially lethal catastrophe. Thus, any bleeding tendency should be investigated thoroughly and corrected pre-operatively. Aspirin should be stopped for 1 week before intracranial surgery. This decision may have to be modified in patients suffering from transient ischaemic attacks, when the risk of discontinuation may exceed those of the benefits.

Endocrine system

Hyperglycaemia is associated with hyperosmolarity, infection and poor wound healing and may worsen neurological outcome following an episode of cerebral ischaemia. Hypoglycaemia is also detrimental because the brain depends on glucose for its energy supply. Close monitoring of glucose perioperatively is therefore essential and treatment with insulin is often required, but sulfonylureas and metformin should not be used for 24–48 h before surgery because of their long half-lives. The perioperative morbidity of diabetic patients is related to pre-operative end-organ damage. Significant myocardial ischaemia may be present despite a negative history (silent myocardial ischaemia). Diabetic autonomic neuropathy may predispose patients to cardiovascular instability and even sudden cardiac death. Furthermore, autonomic dysfunction contributes to gastroparesis. Chronic hyperglycaemia can lead to glycosylation of tissue proteins and a stiff-joint syndrome. Temporomandibular joint and cervical spine mobility should be assessed carefully to anticipate difficult intubations.

Glucocorticoid excess (Cushing's syndrome) is characterized by muscle wasting and weakness, osteoporosis, truncal obesity, abdominal striae, glucose intolerance, hypertension and mental status changes. Patients with Cushing's syndrome tend to be volume overloaded and have hypokalaemic metabolic alkalosis resulting from the mineralocorticoid activity of glucocorticoids, which should be corrected pre-operatively. Patients with osteoporosis are at risk for fractures during positioning, whereas pre-operative weakness may indicate an increased sensitivity to neuromuscular blocking agents. On the other hand, acute adrenal insufficiency can be triggered in steroid-dependent patients who do not receive supplemental doses during the perioperative period.

Patients with hyper/hypothyroidism may present for neurosurgical illness. Ideally, all elective surgical procedures should be undertaken when the patient is treated euthyroid. However, mild to moderate hypothyroidism is not an absolute contraindication to surgery. Anti-thyroid medications and β-adrenergic antagonists are continued through the morning of surgery in hyperthyroid patients and thyroid hormone supplements in hypothyroid patients (although most thyroid preparations have long half-lives). If emergency surgery must proceed in a hyperthyroid patient, the hyperdynamic circulation can be controlled by titration of esmolol infusion. The possibility of associated myopathies and myasthenia gravis should be considered in hyperthyroid patients. Hypothyroid patients, on the other hand, are very prone to drug-induced respiratory depression and usually do not require much pre-operative sedation. Other potential problems with hypothyroidism include hypoglycaemia, anaemia, hyponatraemia, difficult intubation because of a large tongue, delayed gastric emptying, hypothermia from a low basal metabolic rate and slow emergence.

Laboratory investigations

The current literature does not provide sound evidence for clinical benefits or harms of routine or selected pre-operative testing. According to the ASA Task Force on pre-anaesthesia evaluation, pre-operative tests may be ordered, required or performed selectively on the basis of clinical characteristics for the purposes of guiding or optimizing perioperative patient management. An ECG may be indicated for patients with known cardiovascular risk factors or for patients with risk factors identified in the course of a pre-anaesthesia evaluation. A chest radiograph may be required in smokers and in patients with recent upper respiratory infection, chronic obstructive pulmonary disease and cardiac disease. A full blood count, serum glucose and electrolytes, and coagulation studies are indicated in most neurosurgical patients while blood levels of phenytoin may sometimes be required. For all intracranial procedures, blood should be typed and cross-matched, and for minor neurosurgical procedures, blood should at least be grouped and saved. Hormone assays are often ordered in patients with endocrinopathies. Pregnancy testing may be considered for all female patients of childbearing age. The ASA Task Force suggests that test results obtained within 6 months of surgery are generally acceptable if the patient's medical history has not changed substantially, or when test results may play a role in the selection of a specific anaesthetic technique.

Induction and maintenance of anaesthesia

Pre-medication and induction

Pre-medication should be given sparingly to neurosurgical patients, and only when truly indicated, as in a very anxious patient. The reasons are multiple: (i) benzodiazepines are long-acting agents that may interfere with the prompt assessment of neurological status at the end of the case; (ii) in patients who have had a previous stroke, narcotics and benzodiazepines given in sedative doses can unmask focal neurological signs; and (iii) in patients with elevated ICP or decreased intracranial compliance, respiratory depression with a consequent increase in $PaCO_2$ can lead to increase in ICP and compromise cerebral perfusion.

All patients undergoing major neurosurgical procedures should have adequate intravenous access. However, for most elective cases, only a smaller-bore intravenous catheter is necessary for induction. Better access can be established after the patient is anaesthetized. The sequence of induction is, to a certain extent, dependent on the patient's neurological status and the underlying disease. In patients with normal airways and without increased ICP (e.g. patients with a pituitary adenoma or an unruptured aneurysm), induction can proceed in a conventional manner with an intravenous agent such as propofol or thiopental, followed by a non-depolarizing muscle relaxant such as rocuronium

or vecuronium. Succinylcholine can be used, and its effect on ICP is trivial, although in rare cases of severe head injury and SAH, hyperkalaemia has been reported. However, anaesthetic management in most major neurosurgical cases necessitates the placement of invasive monitoring and meticulous positioning, all of which would be facilitated by the presence of neuromuscular blockade. When indicated, adjuncts such as lidocaine (1.5 mg kg^{-1}) and esmolol (500 μg kg^{-1}) can alleviate the haemodynamic response to laryngoscopy. For patients with elevated ICP, opiates should be administered simultaneously with the induction agent but not before, to minimize respiration depression and carbon dioxide retention. In patients with a ruptured aneurysm, it may be prudent to institute invasive arterial monitoring before induction of anaesthesia so systemic blood pressure can be watched closely and drugs titrated more judiciously.

Choice of anaesthetic agents

Neurosurgical patients may have one or more impaired homeostatic mechanisms. Thus, cerebral metabolism is depressed in a patient with an altered level of consciousness, ICP may be elevated, flow–metabolism coupling may be lost, autoregulation may be impaired and the blood–brain barrier may be disrupted. Except in severe injury, carbon dioxide reactivity is usually preserved.

Anaesthetic agents affect cerebral physiology in multiple ways (Table 11.2). Intravenous anaesthetic agents, including thiopental and propofol are indirect cerebral vasoconstrictors, reducing cerebral metabolic rate (CMR) coupled with corresponding reduction of CBF. Both autoregulation and carbon dioxide reactivity are preserved. Ketamine is a weak non-competitive *N*-methyl-D-aspartate (NMDA) antagonist that has sympathomimetic properties. Its cerebral effects are complex and are partly dependent on the action of other concurrently administered drugs. For example, concurrent administration of benzodiazapines or inhalation anaesthetics would eliminate any cerebral stimulatory or vasodilatory actions. Etomidate decreases the CMR, CBF and ICP. At the same time, because of minimal cardiovascular effects, cerebral perfusion pressure (CPP) is well maintained. Although changes on EEG resemble those associated with barbiturates, etomidate enhances somatosensory evoked potentials (SSEPs) and causes less reduction of motor evoked potential (MEP) amplitudes than thiopental or

Table 11.2 Cerebral effects of commonly used anaesthetic agents

Anaesthetic agents	CBF	CMR	CO$_2$ reactivity	Autoregulation	Seizure potential	Compatibility with SSEP	Compatibility with MEP
Thiopental	↓	↓	Preserved	−	−	+	+
Propofol	↓	↓	Preserved	−	−/?	+	+
Etomidate	↓	↓	Preserved	−	−	+/↑	+
Ketamine	↑	−/↑	Preserved	?	?	+/↑	+
Isoflurane	−/↑	↓	Preserved	Dose related ↓	−	Dose related ↓	−
Sevoflurane	−/↓	↓	Preserved	−	+	Dose related ↓	−
Desflurane	−/↑	↓	Preserved	Dose related ↓	−	Dose related ↓	−
Nitrous oxide	↑	↑	Preserved	−/↓	−	−	−

Data are based on studies in normal individuals. The interactive effects between neurological disease and agents are unknown. +/↑, unaffected or augmented.
CBF, cerebral blood flow; CMR, cerebral metabolic rate; SSEP, somatosensory evoked potential; MEP, motor evoked potential.

propofol. However, it may reduce brain tissue oxygen tension.

Dexmedetomidine is a highly selective α_2-adreno-receptor agonist, which provides sedation without causing respiratory depression, does not interfere with electrophysiological mapping and provides haemodynamic stability. It has been found to be particularly useful for implantation of deep brain stimulators in patients with Parkinson's disease and for the awake craniotomies, when sophisticated neurological testing is required. CMR–CBF coupling is preserved during dexmedetomidine administration in human volunteers.

The cerebral effects of inhaled anaesthetics appear to be twofold: they are generally intrinsic cerebral vasodilators, but their vasodilatory actions are partly opposed by flow–metabolism coupling-mediated vasoconstriction secondary to reduction of CMR. The overall effect is unchanged flow during low-dose inhalation anaesthesia but increased flow during high doses. With the exception of sevoflurane, which appears to preserve cerebral autoregulation at all clinically relevant doses, other inhalational agents impair cerebral autoregulation in a dose-dependent manner.

Opioids can precipitate chest wall rigidity, resulting in increased ICP either directly, or indirectly from hypercapnia secondary to respiratory depression if ventilation is poorly controlled. In patients with decreased intracranial compliance, systemic hypotension can also lead to a secondary increase in ICP from compensatory vasodilation. There is no evidence of direct opiate-mediated cerebral vasodilatory action.

Muscle relaxants generally have negligible or clinically insignificant effects on ICP, although tracheal intubation itself may cause intracranial hypertension, which may be attenuated by pre-treatment with esmolol, lidocaine and/or opioids.

Relative to inhalation agents, intravenous agents tend to result in more vasoconstriction, although carbon dioxide reactivity is maintained with both. Consequently propofol infusion is the preferred maintenance anaesthetic of many neuroanaesthesiologists. However, there are no outcome studies to suggest the superiority of one group over the other. The use of nitrous oxide (N$_2$O), however, has been reported to be associated with increased incidence of delayed ischaemic neurological deficits following aneurysm surgery for SAH and may be an important consideration.

For maintenance anaesthesia, the technique and agents may be dictated by the utilization of electrophysiological monitoring (see below). When evoked potential monitoring is not being used, either an intravenous or an inhalation agent can be used. Intravenous agents cause more profound cerebral vasoconstriction than inhalation agents; thus, total intravenous anaesthesia (TIVA) is the preferred technique when maximal brain relaxation is desired. On the other hand, low-solubility inhalation agents allow rapid wash-out and therefore prompt emergence for patients where brain relaxation is not an issue. Among inhalation agents, sevoflurane and desflurane allow the quickest recovery. Desflurane can be associated with sympathetic activation as well as dose-related impairment of cerebral autoregulation, whereas sevoflurane can cause seizure activity, particularly in the subcortical regions of the brain. Nitrous oxide causes cerebral excitation and an increase in CBF, and perhaps should be avoided during neurosurgical anaesthesia. Moreover, N_2O has a profoundly depressive effect on amplitude of both SSEPs and MEPs and should always be avoided when electrophysiological monitoring is undertaken. However, there is an absence of outcome data to ascertain the negative impact of N_2O, with the exception of the increase in the incidence of delayed ischaemic neurological deficits mentioned above. When MEP monitoring is used, muscle relaxants should be omitted from the anaesthetic regimen, although some centres use subparalytic doses of muscle relaxants, which allow monitoring of the MEP but at reduced amplitudes. The optimal anaesthetic regimen is total intravenous anaesthesia using infusion of propofol and remifentanil or fentanyl, and omitting muscle relaxants beyond those used for tracheal intubation. Intravenous dexmedetomidine infusion may be a useful adjunct, allowing sparing of both propofol and remifentanil. Bradycardia and hypotension are theoretical side effects, but they are seldom seen clinically.

Airway management

With a few exceptions, airway assessment for neurosurgical patients is similar to the general population. This was covered in the pre-operative assessment. The unique aspects include: (i) patients with an ankylosed temporomandibular joint from previous surgery; (ii) patients with unstable cervical spine fractures, or in halo-apparatus; and (iii) patients with elevated ICP and a difficult airway, or at risk of aspiration. Other practical considerations for major intracranial procedures include the following: (i) if there is lack of access to the airway during the case, the airway must be well secured; (ii) a soft bite-block should be used, and is mandatory when MEP monitoring is being used; (iii) for positions that do not maintain neutral positions of head and neck, the use of a reinforced tube should be considered. Patients with a normal airway can be approached in the conventional manner using direct laryngoscopy after induction of anaesthesia. With patients at risk of aspiration, it is prudent to perform rapid sequence induction, irrespective of any underlying ICP issue. Either succinylcholine at 1.5 mg kg^{-1} or rocuronium at 1.2 mg kg^{-1} would provide adequate

muscle relaxation allowing tracheal intubation in 60 s. Adjuncts such as lidocaine or esmolol can blunt the haemodynamic and cerebral response to laryngoscopy. In patients with difficult airways, the use of video laryngoscopy or fibre-optic laryngoscopy is indicated. Depending on the patient's ventilatory status, awake intubation may be necessary. Dexmedetomidine infusion is a useful adjunct in these cases, allowing sedation without respiratory depression, while controlling systemic haemodynamics.

Intraoperative considerations

Position and ventilation management

For most supratentorial lesions, the patients are placed supine, with or without turning the head (Fig. 11.1). The risk of malpositioning causing venous obstruction is generally insignificant in this position. With posterior fossa surgery, however, the use of the lateral or park-bench position (Fig. 11.2) may result in potential venous obstruction, and careful inspection of the head and neck must be performed before draping. The sternocleidomastoid muscle must not be tense to palpation and there should be enough clearance between the chin and the chest. The placement of a retrograde jugular bulb catheter can aid in the diagnosis of potential venous obstruction. In all cases, the extremities and bony prominences must be carefully padded after placement of pneumatic sequential compression devices on the lower extremities. The seated position provides a good anatomical approach and excellent

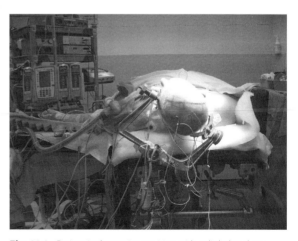

Fig. 11.1. Patient in the supine position with a slight head-up tilt. All pressure points are adequately padded and the eyes are protected. See colour plate section.

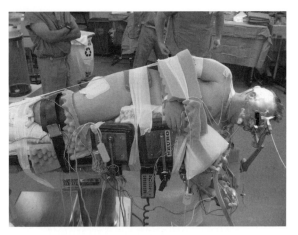

Fig. 11.2. This photograph shows a patient in the park-bench position. Once the patient is draped, the airway is not easily accessible. Therefore, securing the endotracheal tube and ensuring that the neck vessels are not obstructed is of paramount importance. See colour plate section.

surgical conditions for midline posterior fossa lesions but is now rarely utilized because of the risk of venous air embolism. Its use necessitates the placement of a pre-cordial Doppler and central venous catheter for retrieval of air should embolism occur. The placement of the central venous catheter can be guided with ECG waveform or transoesophageal echocardiography. Spontaneous ventilation was used as a monitor of brainstem function in the past, but with the advent of sophisticated electrophysiological monitoring and the use of intravenous anaesthesia, this mode of ventilation is no longer relevant to neurosurgical anaesthesia. With controlled ventilation, mild to moderate hypocapnia can be used to improve brain conditions by reducing CBF and cerebral blood volume. In the absence of either global (jugular venous oxygenation saturation) or local (brain tissue pO_2) monitoring, it is prudent not to allow $PaCO_2$ to be <30 mmHg.

Fluid and electrolyte management

Because of the presence of the blood–brain barrier, the movement of water in and out of the brain is largely governed by the osmolality of the blood, and the most important contributor to serum osmolality is the sodium ion. Thus, hyponatraemia would promote cerebral oedema, while hypernatraemia will have the opposite effect. Hyperglycaemia, when uncontrolled and excessive, can also result in elevated serum osmolality, as with urea in renal failure. Thus, electrolytes and glucose should be monitored closely intraoperatively.

In general, only isotonic or slightly hypertonic solutions containing no glucose should be given intraoperatively. Thus, Plasmalyte® or Normosol® solutions or normal saline are appropriate but not lactated Ringer's solution. Mannitol is given routinely for brain relaxation in intracranial procedures (see below). Hypertonic saline (3%) is equally efficacious and is associated with less dehydration and electrolyte disturbance. With high-dose mannitol (2 g kg^{-1}), hyperkalaemia can occur and should be monitored. In many intracranial procedures, particularly those involving surgery near the pituitary gland, intraoperative diabetes insipidus (DI) can occur insidiously or precipitously. With the concurrent administration of mannitol, the diagnosis can sometimes be difficult. Simultaneous measurement of serum and urine osmolality and electrolytes will aid the diagnosis. Should frank DI develop, it is necessary to administer intravenous 1-deamino-8-D-arginine vasopressin (DDAVP) intraoperatively, at a dose range of 1–5 µg, and titrated to effect.

As the movement of water in and out of the brain is governed only by the relative osmotic gradient across the blood–brain barrier, the concept of deliberate dehydration to limit the development of brain oedema is no longer valid or current. Neurosurgical patients should be maintained normovolaemic, and fluid depletion from osmotic diuresis should be promptly replaced. Fluid administration can be facilitated by examining systolic variation in blood pressure with the respiratory cycle, which correlates with fluid responsiveness, or monitoring of central venous pressure.

Brain relaxation therapy

To provide optimal surgical conditions and to reduce retractor ischaemic brain injury, the brain must be relaxed. This can be achieved by optimizing all three intracranial compartments: brain mass, blood volume and cerebrospinal fluid (CSF). Thus, mannitol or hypertonic saline is given to reduce brain mass, mild hyperventilation is instituted to reduce blood volume, aided by good positioning for optimal venous drainage, and ventriculostomy or a lumbar subarachnoid drain is often placed for CSF drainage. All three approaches can result in complications or undesirable side effects that the anaesthesiologist must be aware of. Mannitol can cause a triphasic response in systemic haemodynamics, with an initial decrease in blood pressure due to a decrease in systemic vascular resistance, followed by an expansion of intravascular volume, which may result in hypertension or pulmonary congestion in patients with poor ventricular function, and finally with dehydration with ongoing osmotic diuresis. Hyperventilation is efficacious and quick in onset with reduction of blood volume. However, overzealous hypocapnia can result in cerebral ischaemia, and the effects are not sustainable. Ventriculostomy can cause haemorrhage and infection, whereas lumbar spinal drainage can result in the development of post-operative central herniation syndrome, a diagnosis that can be missed without a high index of suspicion.

Monitoring

Systemic monitoring

In all patients undergoing major neurosurgical procedures (e.g. craniotomy for tumours or aneurysms), invasive direct arterial blood pressure monitoring is mandatory. Not only does it allow continuous blood pressure monitoring, it also provides access for blood sampling for blood gases and electrolytes. Routine central venous pressure monitoring is more controversial, but the advent of ultrasound guidance has significantly minimized any risk associated with its placement. Pulmonary artery catheters are seldom indicated. In patients where monitoring of cardiac output is desirable, methods based on the use of intra-arterial contour waveform analysis such as the LiDCO or PiCCO may be indicated. In some specialized neurosurgical centres, monitoring of jugular venous oxygen saturation using a retrograde jugular bulb catheter is routine. The theoretical risk of venous occlusion from placement of internal jugular catheters is exceedingly low.

Monitoring metabolic rate and blood flow in the brain

As indicated above, the placement of a retrograde jugular bulb catheter allows frequent assessment of the venous oxygen saturation, which reflects the balance between supply and demand of oxygen flux to the brain. Thus, a low jugular venous oxygen saturation (SjO_2) indicates that there is inadequate blood supply and vice versa. Paradoxically, very high SjO_2 may indicate an infarcted brain, which can no longer utilize oxygen. Intraoperative CBF can be estimated with thermodilution, laser Doppler or transcranial Doppler, none of which is currently practical for routine management. More recently, intraoperative optical imaging using indocyanine green angiography

has been introduced into clinical practice, obviating the need for conventional intraoperative angiography for aneurysm clipping.

Monitoring electrophysiological measurements in the brain

Monitoring of SSEPs and MEPs is now used routinely in intracranial procedures in many centres. For posterior fossa procedures where the cranial nerves may be involved (e.g. acoustic neuroma), Vth, VIIth, VIIIth, Xth, XIth and XIIth cranial nerve functions can also be monitored using electromyography. Although it makes logical sense that monitoring these modalities should improve patient safety and reduce the risk of neurological deficits, their functional utility has never been established with a randomized controlled trial. However, it is now a standard of care in many centres and can no longer be subjected to studies. While SSEP can be recorded during low-dose inhalation anaesthesia and facilitated by neuromuscular blockade, MEP is best recorded during total intravenous anaesthesia without the use of any neuromuscular blocking agents. Maintaining an adequate 'depth of anaesthesia' may be challenging in these cases, and some type of brain function monitoring such as the bispectral index (BIS) may be useful. Brainstem auditory evoked potential is relatively robust and can be recorded during high-dose inhalation anaesthetics. EEG has limited use in monitoring of usual intracranial procedures but may be useful for carotid endarterectomy, and corticography is essential for epilepsy surgery to locate the focus of epileptic discharge. Special electrophysiological monitoring is also required for functional neurosurgery for movement disorders. These low-voltage electrical potentials are profoundly affected by anaesthetic or sedative agents, and patients often have to undergo these procedures fully awake. Dexmedetomidine may be a useful adjunct for these cases.

Use of vasoactive agents and β-blockers

In the absence of specific brain monitoring modalities for feedback, whether metabolic or electrophysiological, anaesthesiologists have to use systemic surrogates to infer the well-being of the brain. Thus, it is important to maintain adequate cerebral perfusion by supporting systemic blood pressure when necessary, and to avoid excessive hypocapnia. It is important to remember that CPP is normally the difference between mean arterial blood pressure and ICP, but once the bone flap is raised, it is the difference between mean arterial blood pressure and jugular venous or central venous pressure. The importance of adequate blood pressure is further underscored by the fact that cerebral autoregulation may be impaired by neurological pathology, and the lower limit of autoregulation varies widely among normal individuals. It is generally prudent to maintain CPP at a minimum of 60 mmHg, and the choice of vasopressors does not seem to be as important. Either phenylephrine or norepinephrine can be used. It is important to titrate in a low-dose infusion and to avoid boluses as a sudden surge in blood pressure might do more harm than good. To lower blood pressure, labetalol is generally a good choice. Alternatively, good control can be achieved by increasing the infusion rate of remifentanil and/or propofol.

Perioperative use of β-blockers

Previous recommendations regarding the use of β-blockers during the perioperative period in patients with cardiac disease are no longer supported by evidence after the publication of the POISE trial and the recent meta-analysis by Bangalore and colleagues in 2008. These recent publications revealed that perioperative β-blocker therapy, despite reducing the incidence of perioperative non-fatal myocardial infarction, increases the incidence of perioperative stroke, clinically relevant hypotension and bradycardia with no significant reduction in overall and cardiovascular mortality. Recently, in 2009, the American College of Cardiology Foundation (ACCF) and AHA published a focused update on perioperative β-blockade. The report highlighted the evidence regarding continuation of a β-blocker in patients already taking the drug as class I. In addition, class IIa recommendations exist for patients with inducible ischaemia, coronary artery disease or multiple clinical risk factors who are undergoing vascular (i.e. high-risk) surgery and for patients with coronary artery disease or multiple clinical risk factors who are undergoing intermediate-risk surgery. Initiation of therapy, particularly in lower-risk groups, requires careful consideration of the risk:benefit ratio for an individual patient. Treatment should be started well before a planned procedure, with careful titration perioperatively to achieve adequate heart rate control while avoiding frank bradycardia or hypotension intraoperatively. In light of the current evidence, routine administration of perioperative β-blockers, particularly in higher fixed-dose regimens begun on the day of surgery, cannot be advocated. However, there should be no hesitatation in using β-blockers for intraoperative heart rate control in patients with cardiac risk factors. Ongoing and future studies in this area should continue to address limitations in our evidence base on this subject and provide further guidance regarding this important topic.

Adjuncts for brain protection

Intraoperative brain protection for high-risk cerebrovascular surgical procedures remains an elusive goal. The only proven method takes the form of 'physiological protection', with maintenance of adequate cerebral perfusion pressure, oxygen flux and delivery. Hypothermia, although efficacious in experimental cerebral ischaemia as well as in global anoxia following cardiac arrest in humans, has failed to demonstrate a protective effect in cerebral aneurysm surgery. However, it may be beneficial in cases where temporary occlusion of a major feeding artery exceeds 20 min. Similarly, there is no demonstrable protective effect from metabolic suppression with thiopental or etomidate. For occlusion time >20 min during normothermia, again there is a suggestion of beneficial effect. As the risk:benefit ratio is favourable, it is difficult to argue against its use. Thus, despite the lack of evidentiary outcome data, pharmacological metabolic protection using thiopental or propofol to effect burst suppression during the ischaemic period remains a prevalent clinical practice. However, the potential benefits would be lost if systemic hypotension ensues, further compromising collateral circulation. Thiopental at 5–10 mg kg^{-1} or propofol at 2–5 mg kg^{-1} titrated in slowly over 5 min will generally result in a burst-suppression pattern in EEG. Maintenance infusion would be required to maintain this pattern.

Intensive glucose control

Critical illness and surgically induced trauma result in altered carbohydrate metabolism, which results in insulin resistance. Hyperglycaemia ensues, even in patients who do not have pre-exiting diabetes mellitus. Previously conducted studies favouring the tight glucose control in ICUs were recently challenged by the Normoglycaemia in Intensive Care Evaluation–Survival Using Glucose Algorithm Regulation (NICE-SUGAR) trial. This large multicentre trial revealed an increased rate of mortality in the tight glucose control (TGC) group compared with the conventional treatment group. The TGC patients had higher hypoglycaemic episodes. Excess deaths were predominantly cardiovascular in origin. The study did not show any other outcome differences between the groups (length of ICU stay, length of hospital stay, number of days on mechanical ventilation, rate of positive blood cultures and red cell transfusion). The most recent meta-analysis by Griesdale and colleagues in 2009 indicated that TGC significantly increases the risk of hypoglycaemia and provides no overall mortality benefit among critically ill patients. In subgroup analysis, they concluded that TGC might be beneficial to patients admitted to a surgical ICU. Currently, in our institution, we aim to treat the neurosurgical patients with blood glucose levels ≥ 140 mg dl^{-1} with insulin infusion protocols during intra/post-operative periods. Clearly, this topic requires further large trials before definitive recommendations can be made.

Anaemia and blood transfusion

Many neurosurgical procedures are associated with significant risk of blood loss. It is known that near-normal haemoglobin levels are associated with better outcomes in general. Unfortunately, maintaining these levels through transfusion of banked, allogeneic red blood cells appears to be associated with poorer outcome.

Autologous pre-donation, erythropoietic support, acute normovolaemic haemodilution, intraoperative cell salvage, induced hypotension and the use of pharmacological agents such as tranexamic acid in addition to meticulous surgical haemostasis have all been associated with modest reductions in allogeneic blood transfusion rates during intracranial surgery. However, such practice has not been widespread, as the benefits are marginal.

Monitoring modalities such as brain tissue oxygen tension, near-infrared spectroscopy and jugular bulb catheter sampling can be used to monitor the regional or global oxygenation, and may help to determine transfusion needs. Their effectiveness in patient outcome, however, remains to be proven. Currently available evidence supports a haemoglobin threshold level of 8.0–9.0 g dl^{-1}. In the context of ongoing bleeding, lower levels (e.g. 7.0 g dl^{-1}) may result in brief periods of profound anaemia, which appear to be linked with inadequate brain perfusion.

Emergence

Emergence management of neurosurgical patients is dictated by multiple factors: (i) the pre-existing neurological condition; (ii) the likelihood of intraoperative stroke, as indicated clinically or by electrophysiological monitoring; (iii) the location of the lesion (an infratentorial lesion is more apt to be managed with delayed extubation); (iv) the duration of the procedure and position of the patient (a patient in the park-bench or prone position for a long period of time is more likely to have swelling of the upper airway); (v) brain conditions at the end of the surgical procedure; (vi) the need for tight haemodynamic control (e.g. after arteriovenous malformation resection with evidence or high risk of normal perfusion pressure breakthrough syndrome); and (vii) the amount of anaesthetic used and the anticipated duration of action (e.g. after prolonged burst-suppression therapy with thiopental infusion). The clinical decision to wake up the patient and extubate the trachea in the operating room must therefore be individualized and take all these factors into consideration, as well as balancing the risks and the benefits. In general, if the patient is in good condition pre-operatively and the surgical procedure is uneventful, attempts should be made to wake the patient up in the operating room, thus allowing prompt neurological examination. 'Deep extubation' is generally not appropriate for neurosurgical patients because of the associated respiratory depression and carbon dioxide retention and the need for prompt neurological examination. For the same reasons, long-acting opiates are seldom indicated towards the end of the surgical procedure. To reduce the incidence of coughing and bucking, intravenous lidocaine at 1.5 mg kg^{-1} is a useful adjunct. The associated central nervous depression is transient and potentially beneficial, allowing the washout of inhalation anaesthetic during this period.

Patients planned for delayed extubation because of aforementioned factors should be taken directly to the neurointensive care unit. In many centres, it is considered prudent to obtain an immediate post-operative CT scan to rule out remediable surgical complications.

Summary

Although the general principles of anaesthetic management are the same, patients undergoing different surgical procedures for different pathological conditions can have vastly different anaesthetic and monitoring requirements. The successful intraoperative management of these challenging patients requires a basic understanding of the pathophysiology and surgical demand of the procedure, all of which start with a thorough pre-operative evaluation and preparation of the patient. This methodical approach results in improved safety of perioperative care, optimal resource utilization and patient satisfaction.

Further reading

American Society of Anesthesiologists Task Force on Preanesthesia Evaluation (2002). Practice advisory for preanesthesia evaluation. *Anesthesiology* **96**, 485–96.

Arozullah, A. M., Conde, M. V. and Lawrence, V. A. (2003). Preoperative evaluation for postoperative pulmonary complications. *Med Clin North Am* **87**, 153–73.

Bangalore, S., Wetterslev, J., Pranesh, S. *et al.* (2008). Perioperative beta blockers in patients having non-cardiac surgery: a meta-analysis. *Lancet* **372**, 1962–76.

Candiotti, K., Sharma, S. and Shankar, R. (2009). Obesity, obstructive sleep apnoea, and diabetes mellitus: anaesthetic implications. *Br J Anaesth* **103** (Suppl. 1), 23–30.

Dagal, A. and Lam, A. M. (2009). Cerebral autoregulation and anesthesia. *Curr Opin Anaesthesiol* **22**, 547–52.

Devereaux, P. J., Yang, H., Yusuf, S. *et al.* (2008). Effects of extended-release metoprolol succinate in patients undergoing non-cardiac surgery (POISE trial): a randomised controlled trial. *Lancet* **371**, 1839–47.

Drummond, J. C. (1997). The lower limit of autoregulation: time to revise our thinking? *Anesthesiology* **86**, 1431–3.

Drummond, J. C., Dao, A. V., Roth, D. M. *et al.* (2008). Effect of dexmedetomidine on cerebral blood flow velocity, cerebral metabolic rate, and carbon dioxide response in normal humans. *Anesthesiology* **108**, 225–32.

Eng, C., Lam, A. M., Mayberg, T. S., Lee, C. and Mathisen, T. (1992). The influence of propofol with and without nitrous oxide on cerebral blood flow velocity and CO_2 reactivity in humans. *Anesthesiology* **77**, 872–9.

Ferreyra, G., Long, Y. and Ranieri, V. M. (2009). Respiratory complications after major surgery. *Curr Opin Crit Care* **15**, 342–8.

Finfer, S., Chittock, D. R., Su, S. Y. *et al.* (2009). Intensive versus conventional glucose control in critically ill patients. *N Engl J Med* **360**, 1283–97.

Fleischmann, K. E., Beckman, J. A., Buller, C. E. *et al.* (2009). 2009 ACCF/AHA focused update on perioperative beta blockade. *J Am Coll Cardiol* **54**, 2102–28.

Fleisher, L. A., Beckman, J. A., Brown, K. A. *et al.* (2008). ACC/AHA 2007 guidelines on perioperative cardiovascular evaluation and care for non-cardiac surgery: executive summary: a report of the American College of Cardiology/American Heart Association Task Force on Practice Guidelines (Writing Committee to Revise the 2002 Guidelines on Perioperative Cardiovascular Evaluation for Noncardiac Surgery). *Anesth Analg* **106**, 685–712.

Griesdale, D. E., de Souza, R. J., van Dam, R. M. *et al.* (2009). Intensive insulin therapy and mortality among critically ill patients: a meta-analysis including NICE-SUGAR study data. *CMAJ* **180**, 821–7.

Gronert, G. A. (2009). Succinylcholine-induced hyperkalemia and beyond. 1975. *Anesthesiology* **111**, 1372–7.

Hanel, F., Werner, C., von Knobelsdorff, G. and Schulte am Esch, J. (1997). The effects of fentanyl and sufentanil on cerebral hemodynamics. *J Neurosurg Anesthesiol* **9**, 223–7.

Hindman, B. J., Bayman, E. O., Pfisterer, W. K., Torner, J. C. and Todd, M. M. (2010). No association between intraoperative hypothermia or supplemental protective drug and neurologic outcomes in patients undergoing temporary clipping during cerebral aneurysm surgery: findings from the Intraoperative Hypothermia for Aneurysm Surgery Trial. *Anesthesiology* **112**, 86–101.

Johnson, R. G., Arozullah, A. M., Neumayer, L. *et al.* (2007). Multivariable predictors of postoperative respiratory failure after general and vascular surgery: results from the patient safety in surgery study. *J Am Coll Surg* **204**, 1188–98.

Korinth, M. C. (2006). Low-dose aspirin before intracranial surgery – results of a survey among neurosurgeons in Germany. *Acta Neurochir (Wien)* **148**, 1189–96; discussion 1196.

La Colla, L., Albertin, A., La Colla, G. and Mangano, A. (2007). Faster wash-out and recovery for desflurane vs sevoflurane in morbidly obese patients when no premedication is used. *Br J Anaesth* **99**, 353–8.

Mack, P. F., Perrine, K., Kobylarz, E., Schwartz, T. H. and Lien, C. A. (2004). Dexmedetomidine and neurocognitive testing in awake craniotomy. *J Neurosurg Anesthesiol* **16**, 20–5.

Matta, B. F., Mayberg, T. S. and Lam, A. M. (1995). Direct cerebrovasodilatory effects of halothane, isoflurane, and desflurane during propofol-induced isoelectric electroencephalogram in humans. *Anesthesiology* **83**, 980–5; discussion 27A.

McEwen, J. and Huttunen, K. H. (2009). Transfusion practice in neuroanaesthesia. *Curr Opin Anaesthesiol* **22**, 566–71.

Oddo, M., Milby, A., Chen, I. *et al.* (2009). Hemoglobin concentration and cerebral metabolism in patients with aneurysmal subarachnoid hemorrhage. *Stroke* **40**, 1275–81.

Pasternak, J. J., McGregor, D. G., Lanier, W. L. *et al.* (2009). Effect of nitrous oxide use on long-term neurologic and neuropsychological outcome in patients who received temporary proximal artery occlusion during cerebral aneurysm clipping surgery. *Anesthesiology* **110**, 563–73.

Priebe, H. J. (2009). Influence of beta-blockers on the outcome of at risk patients. *Minerva Anestesiol* **75**, 319–23.

Rozet, I., Vavilala, M. S., Lindley, A. M. *et al.* (2006). Cerebral autoregulation and CO$_2$ reactivity in anterior and posterior cerebral circulation during sevoflurane anesthesia. *Anesth Analg* **102**, 560–4.

Rozet, I., Muangman, S., Vavilala, M. S. *et al.* (2006). Clinical experience with dexmedetomidine for implantation of deep brain stimulators in Parkinson's disease. *Anesth Analg* **103**, 1224–8.

Smetana, G. W., Lawrence, V. A. and Cornell, J. E. (2006). Preoperative pulmonary risk stratification for noncardiothoracic surgery: systematic review for the American College of Physicians. *Ann Intern Med* **144**, 581–95.

Strandgaard, S. and Paulson, O. B. (1989). Cerebral blood flow and its pathophysiology in hypertension. *Am J Hypertens* **2**, 486–92.

Strebel, S., Lam, A. M., Matta, B. *et al.* (1995). Dynamic and static cerebral autoregulation during isoflurane, desflurane, and propofol anesthesia. *Anesthesiology* **83**, 66–76.

Summors, A. C., Gupta, A. K. and Matta, B. F. (1999). Dynamic cerebral autoregulation during sevoflurane anesthesia: a comparison with isoflurane. *Anesth Analg* **88**, 341–5.

Thal, G. D., Szabo, M. D., Lopez-Bresnahan, M. and Crosby, G. (1996). Exacerbation or unmasking of focal neurologic deficits by sedatives. *Anesthesiology* **85**, 21–5; discussion 29A–30A.

Werner, C., Kochs, E., Bause, H., Hoffman, W. E. and Schulte am Esch, J. (1995). Effects of sufentanil on cerebral hemodynamics and intracranial pressure in patients with brain injury. *Anesthesiology* **83**, 721–6.

Chapter

12

Anaesthesia for supratentorial surgery

Judith Dinsmore

Introduction

Space-occupying lesions such as tumours, intracranial haematomas and abscesses are the most common indications for supratentorial surgery. Anaesthesia management is directed towards the provision of optimal operative conditions, haemodynamic stability, facilitation of electrophysiological monitoring and provision of a rapid, high-quality recovery. Emergence is as important as induction during neuroanaesthesia and this is of particular relevance during 'awake' craniotomy techniques. Despite research and advances in pharmacology and monitoring, many controversies remain regarding optimal clinical practice. An understanding of neurophysiology and neuropharmacology, as well as careful attention to the basic principles of neuroanaesthesia, is crucial for optimal patient outcome. The knowledge and expertise of the anaesthetist directly influences outcome during neurosurgical procedures.

Intracranial tumours

Intracranial tumours may be divided into primary and secondary tumours.

Primary brain tumours

Primary brain tumours comprise a mixed group of neoplasms originating from brain tissue and the meninges, with the degree of malignancy ranging from benign to aggressive. Each tumour type has its own biology, treatment and prognosis, but even those that are histologically benign may prove lethal because of their location and ability to invade locally.

Although primary brain tumours account for only 2% of all malignancies in adults, with an incidence in the UK of 7 per 100,000 of the population, poor survival for many tumour types results in a disproportionate number of years of life lost compared with other cancers. Tumours can occur at any age, although there is a small incidence peak before the age of 10 years and then a steady rise from 30 years onwards. The incidence appears to flatten or fall off after 75 years of age, but this may be artefactual as a result of fewer investigations and lower detection rates in the elderly. There are also geographical and ethnic variations in brain tumour incidence, with higher rates reported in more developed countries.

The classification of primary brain tumours is complex, and the 2007 World Health Organization classification identifies more than 130 tumour types. Tumours are classified according to their predominant cell type and graded depending on the presence or absence of standard pathological features (Table 12.1). Four malignancy grades are recognized, with grade I tumours being the biologically least aggressive and grade IV the most aggressive. However, even relatively benign tumours may become more malignant with time. Gliomas and meningiomas are the most common primary brain tumours in adults, with pilocytic astrocytomas, ependymomas and medulloblastomas being the most common in children. Supratentorial tumours are most common in adults and arise in frontal, temporal and parietal lobes, whereas infratentorial tumours are more common in children.

Gliomas

Glioma is a broad term describing tumours arising from the supportive tissue or glia of the brain. There are three types of glial cells that can give rise to tumours – astrocytes, oligodendrocytes and ependymal cells. Occasionally tumours display a mixture of these different cell types. Gliomas tend to be located in the cerebral hemispheres and are more common in men. Astrocytic tumours account for 39% of all primary brain tumours

---

Core Topics in Neuroanaesthesia and Neurointensive Care, eds. Basil F. Matta, David K. Menon and Martin Smith. Published by Cambridge University Press. © Cambridge University Press 2011.

Table 12.1. A simplified classification of brain tumours and their frequency

Tumour type	Percentage of total
Tumours of neuroepithelial tissue	
• Astrocytomas	
◦ Diffuse astrocytic tumour	6%
◦ Anaplastic astrocytic	7%
◦ Glioblastoma	25%
• Oligodendrogliomas	3%
• Ependymoma	2%
• Choroid plexus tumours	0.5%
• Primitive neuroectodermal tumour	3%
Meningiomas	26%
Tumours of cranial nerves	
• Acoustic neuroma	6%
Pituitary tumours	11%
Craniopharyngioma	1%
Haemangioblastoma	1%
Miscellaneous: chordoma, colloid cysts, pineal tumours, dermoid	8%

and include pilocytic or diffuse astrocytomas (grades 1 and II), anaplastic astrocytomas (grade III) and glioblastomas (grade IV). Grade II astrocytic tumours have an average survival of 7 years, anaplastic astrocytomas 3–4 years and glioblastomas only 9–11 months. The clinical implications of tumour grading therefore make accurate histological diagnosis crucial.

Grade II astrocytomas have a peak incidence between 25 and 50 years of age and usually present with epilepsy or a late-onset focal neurological deficit. Glioblastomas (grade IV) are the most common and comprise about 20% of primary brain tumours. They occur most commonly in the 45–70 year age group and often present with signs of raised intracranial pressure (ICP) and rapidly progressive neurological deficit. There is often a short clinical history and prognosis is very poor. Radiotherapy alone makes little difference but, in combination with chemotherapy, may increase survival by some months. Oligodendrogliomas also tend to occur in the cerebral hemispheres but are uncommon. They are classified as grade II but can recur at the primary site and produce cerebrospinal fluid (CSF) seedlings in 5% of cases.

Meningiomas

Meningiomas are usually solitary lobulated tumours arising from the arachnoid and attached to the dura. Symptomatic meningiomas represent about 25% of all primary brain tumours and occur most commonly in the middle-aged and elderly. Their higher incidence in females and tendency to manifest during pregnancy suggest oestrogen and progesterone dependency. Patients with neurofibromatosis type 2 (NF2) and some other non-NF2 familial syndromes may develop multiple meningiomas. Previous exposure to ionizing radiation is also a well-recognized predisposing factor.

Meningiomas are graded I (benign) to III (sarcomatous), although the vast majority (80%) are of low malignancy. They generally expand, displace adjacent brain structures and do not invade, although there is a high rate of local recurrence. Up to 90% are supratentorial, often located between (parasagittal meningiomas) or over (convexity meningiomas) the cerebral hemispheres. Meningiomas present with a variety of symptoms depending on their location. Frontal tumours usually present late when they are quite large, whereas tentorial meningiomas present early because of brainstem compression. Meningiomas are often very vascular.

Other primary brain tumours

Ependymomas arise at ependymomal surfaces and may occur anywhere in the ventricular system or spinal cord. They account for about 2–3% of primary brain tumours and can develop at all ages. Along with colloid cysts, choroid plexus tumours and tumours of the ventricular system, ependymomas often present with obstructive hydrocephalus. Pineal tumours are very rare and also present with hydrocephalus. Other primary brain tumours include pituitary tumours, nerve sheath tumours, medulloblastomas and embryonic or primitive tumours.

Secondary brain tumours

Secondary, or metastatic, brain tumours are four times more common than primary tumours. The cancers most frequently metastasizing to the brain are lung, breast, kidney, colon, thyroid and melanoma. Treatment options include surgical excision, radiotherapy, chemotherapy or a combination. Removal of a solitary metastasis is usually worthwhile and chemotherapy is particularly useful in certain types of metastasis such as germinoma.

Pre-operative assessment

The aim of pre-operative assessment is to identify potential anaesthetic problems and coexisting medical conditions, quantify risk and plan perioperative care. The assessment of the neurosurgical patient is identical to that of other patient groups but must additionally include a complete neurological assessment. A baseline neurological examination should be undertaken in all patients, and any deficit or history of seizures documented. Special attention must be paid to the identification of raised ICP as care must then be taken to avoid any factors that might worsen intracranial hypertension perioperatively. A history of headache and vomiting, or the presence of papilloedema, suggests raised ICP. The patient's level of consciousness should be determined along with any evidence of airway compromise, including an assessment of the gag reflex. A depressed level of consciousness and/or an impaired cough or gag reflex increases the risk of sputum retention and aspiration pneumonitis. Hypoventilation may result in basal pulmonary collapse and consolidation that can lead to hypoxia and/or hypercapnia, worsened brain swelling and neurological deterioration.

Possible primary sites of metastatic tumours should be identified. This may already be known and previous surgery, chemotherapy or radiotherapy may affect the anaesthetic management plan. Primary sources for cerebral abscesses include middle ear, paranasal sinuses or dental infection, while haematogenous spread can occur from chronic infective lung disease or subacute bacterial endocarditis (SBE). Multiple abscesses occur in immunosuppressed patients and causes should be identified.

Any coexisting medical problems should be optimized prior to surgery. This is particularly important for respiratory or cardiovascular disease. In hypertensive patients, the limits of autoregulation of cerebral blood flow (CBF) are altered and patients are more at risk of cerebral ischaemia during perioperative hypotension. Intraoperative hypertension may increase the risk of brain swelling, bleeding and post-operative haematoma.

The planned operative procedure, including the surgical approach, patient position, tumour vascularity and any anticipated difficulties, should be discussed with the neurosurgeon. The pre-operative assessment also provides an opportunity to explain and discuss the proposed anaesthetic management plan with the patient and to confirm consent.

Drug history

Current and previous drug history should be reviewed. Tumour-related raised ICP with reactive oedema is often treated with dexamethasone. Patients may require prophylactic or therapeutic anticonvulsants, and plasma levels should be checked prior to surgery. Most routine medication, especially antihypertensive agents, should be continued up to and including the day of surgery. Antiplatelet agents are increasingly used in the management of all types of atherosclerotic disease or for primary prevention of cardiovascular morbidity and present particular problems in the neurosurgical patient. Aspirin and clopidogrel should ideally be stopped 7 days prior to surgery. However, in patients with drug-eluting coronary stents, the risks of stopping antiplatelet therapy may outweigh the potential benefits, and individual cases should be discussed with the neurosurgeon and cardiologist. Specialist haematological advice should be sought if patients taking anticoagulant or antiplatelet medication require emergency surgery.

Investigations

A full blood count, clotting screen, blood glucose, and urea and electrolytes should be checked. Fluid and electrolyte abnormalities occur commonly in neurosurgical patients as a result of intracranial pathology, the use of mannitol or as a consequence of vomiting and should be corrected prior to elective surgery. Plasma glucose concentration may be raised as a result of pre-operative steroids. The potential intraoperative risk of bleeding should be assessed based on tumour type and location. In general, a cross-match of 2 units of blood is sufficient for most craniotomies, but large meningiomas may be associated with significant blood loss and 4–6 units may be required. An ECG and chest X-ray should be undertaken if indicated. Review of neuroimaging is mandatory in all patients to confirm tumour size, evidence of midline shift, the extent of oedema, degree of hydrocephalus and enhancement with contrast.

Pre-medication

Pre-operative medication that produces sedation should be avoided, especially in patients with depressed levels of consciousness. However, for many patients, the prospect of intracranial surgery is frightening, and benzodiazepines can safely be prescribed to alert patients who need anxiolysis.

Principles of general anaesthesia

Neuroanaesthesia is a specialty where the knowledge and skill of the anaesthetist affects both the operative field and ultimate outcome for the patient. The basic principles of neuroanaesthesia are more important than the individual choice of anaesthetic agents and can be summarized as follows:

- Maintenance of cerebral perfusion and oxygenation.
- Provision of optimal operative conditions by manipulation of ICP.
- Rapid, smooth awakening allowing early neurological assessment.

Collaboration between the neuroanaesthetist and neurosurgeon is essential. Optimal operating conditions are a slack brain that facilitates surgical access and reduces the need for retraction of brain tissue, thereby lowering the potential for local cerebral ischaemia and post-operative oedema. Consequently the anaesthetist must understand the mechanisms underlying the control of ICP and the effects of anaesthetic agents or techniques on ICP.

Intracranial physiology

The skull is of fixed volume and consequently any changes in the volume of its contents (brain, blood and CSF) will be reflected by changes in ICP (see Chapters 1 and 2). Initially, compensatory mechanisms reduce the effect of any intracranial space-occupying lesion on ICP. These include a reduction in intracranial blood volume, displacement of CSF into the spinal canal and increased absorption of CSF. However, these mechanisms become exhausted as a lesion grows and, at that stage, further increases in its volume will lead to progressive rises in ICP. When intracranial compliance is compromised, small increases in arterial blood pressure may also produce large increases in ICP because of changes in CBF. Other factors affecting CBF, and therefore ICP, include hypercapnia, hypoxia, increases in cerebral venous pressure and cerebral vasodilation. The location, size and type of the intracranial mass will also influence the ability of the brain to compensate. For example, an acute cerebral haematoma, which develops quickly, allows little time for compensation, whereas a slowly expanding tumour may have little effect on ICP. Significant increases in ICP result in distortion of the intracranial contents and ultimately lead to two catastrophic events – cerebral ischaemia and brain herniation. The anaesthetist must take great care to select appropriate anaesthetic agents, minimize any factors that might increase ICP and maximize therapeutic options that reduce ICP.

Anaesthetic agents

There have been many studies comparing individual anaesthetic agents during neurosurgical procedures, but it has not been possible to demonstrate consistent or clinically relevant benefits of one agent over another.

Volatile agents

Volatile agents remain popular among neuroanaesthetists, and numerous studies have described their differential effects on cerebral haemodynamics and ICP. They have a direct vasodilatory effect on cerebrovascular smooth muscle and an indirect (constrictive) effect via reduction in cerebral metabolic rate (CMR). The end result on CBF reflects the balance between these two opposing effects. As the concentration of volatile agent is increased, vasodilation occurs and there will be a marked increase in CBF. All volatile agents increase ICP, although hyperventilation and adjuvant agents may modify these effects. Halothane is the most potent vasodilator and should be avoided. In studies comparing equipotent doses of isoflurane, sevoflurane and desflurane at normocapnia, CBF and ICP were greatest with desflurane and least with sevoflurane. Although more large-scale studies are needed, sevoflurane appears to be the most suitable volatile agent for neuroanaesthesia as it has the least effect on CBF and ICP and, at concentrations below 1.0–1.2%, does not adversely affect cerebral autoregulation. Enflurane should be avoided because it can produce spike and wave EEG complexes.

Nitrous oxide

The detrimental effects of nitrous oxide (N_2O) are well documented. It is a neurostimulant and, when administered alone, increases CBF, CMR and ICP. However, these effects are difficult to translate into clinical practice where they are attenuated by other agents and by moderate hyperventilation. Although N_2O has been used for countless anaesthetics and it is difficult to demonstrate adverse clinical outcome, many believe that it has no place in modern neuroanaesthetic practice.

Intravenous agents

Intravenous agents such as propofol and thiopental have many theoretical advantages and reduce both

CBF and CMR. The reduction in CMR is proportional to the depth of anaesthesia and continues until cerebral electrical activity is abolished. Intravenous agents also reduce ICP and preserve cerebral autoregulation and carbon dioxide vascular reactivity. Positron emission tomography (PET) studies in healthy subjects demonstrate that propofol reduces CBF more than sevoflurane at equipotent doses, so neurosurgical patients anaesthetized with propofol have a lower ICP than those anaesthetized with sevoflurane. However, propofol has a greater potential than sevoflurane to decrease cerebral perfusion pressure (CPP) and care must be taken to maintain systemic blood pressure during propofol anaesthesia.

Ketamine increases CMR, CBF and ICP, although the last may be attenuated by moderate hypocapnia and adjuvant agents. It has potential neuroprotective effects because of its antagonist action at the N-methyl-D-aspartate (NMDA) receptor, and its role in neuroanaesthesia is being re-evaluated.

Neuromuscular blocking drugs

Non-depolarizing muscle relaxants do not cross the blood–brain barrier (BBB) and have no effect on cerebral haemodynamics. Suxamethonium causes a small rise in ICP as a consequence of muscle fasciculation and hypertension, but this effect is transient and clinically irrelevant. Securing the airway and avoidance of hypoxia and hypercapnia take priority, and suxamethonium should be used to facilitate airway control if clinically indicated.

Opioids

The cerebral haemodynamic and metabolic effects of opioids have been studied extensively but with conflicting results. At clinically relevant doses during controlled ventilation, opioids have little effect on CBF or cerebral autoregulation. Large doses of fentanyl and remifentanil reduce CMR and decrease CBF but also reduce systemic blood pressure. Alfentanil may increase ICP under certain circumstances, but this effect is probably limited during controlled ventilation. Remifentanil is increasingly popular during neuroanaesthesia as it provides titratable analgesia and a rapid smooth recovery. It is rapidly metabolized by plasma and tissue esterases and has a very short-context sensitive half-life (3–5 min). This ensures reliable elimination whatever the duration of infusion and makes it particularly suitable for neurosurgical procedures, including 'awake' craniotomy. It is often used

as a target-controlled infusion in combination with propofol. Morphine is often used for post-operative analgesia and also has negligible effects on cerebral haemodynamics. It may, however, cause hypoventilation if given in inappropriate doses.

Intraoperative control of intracranial pressure

High ICP at the start of surgery is an independent risk factor for intraoperative brain swelling and this outweighs any effects of anaesthetic agents. Various manoeuvres and therapeutic agents may be used to decrease ICP and optimize cerebral physiology during surgery.

Glucocorticoids

Dexamethasone is prescribed routinely to patients with brain tumours and is effective in reducing peri-tumour oedema. It must be administered pre-operatively as its onset of action is slow. Relief of headache and improvement in neurological status usually occur within 12–36 h of initiating treatment. Clinical improvement can occur before the reduction in ICP, possibly due to partial restoration of the BBB. Even a single dose of dexamathasone can significantly increase blood glucose concentration in non-diabetic patients. This may increase the risk of infection and, in the setting of cerebral ischaemia, will exacerbate the extent of cerebral injury and worsen neurological outcome.

Osmotic agents

Osmotic agents are effective in reducing ICP in a variety of intraoperative indications. Mannitol is a low-molecular-weight six-carbon sugar that is an osmotic diuretic and free-radical scavenger. It is usually given in doses of 0.25–1.0 g kg^{-1} over 15–30 min. Its beneficial effects on ICP are seen within 10–15 min, with maximum effect occurring at 1–2 h. It increases blood osmolality relative to that of the brain and draws water from the brain extracellular fluid (ECF) into the vascular compartment. It is this reduction in brain ECF that causes the reduction in ICP. As mannitol relies on an intact BBB to exert its osmotic effect, disruption of the BBB may result in entry of mannitol into the brain and worsen brain swelling. Mannitol decreases cerebrovascular resistance and blood viscosity, thereby increasing blood flow to ischaemic areas of the brain. It also causes vasodilation via relaxation of vascular smooth muscle, an effect that is dependent on dose and rate of administration. This can lead to transient increases in cerebral blood volume and ICP while simultaneously decreasing systemic blood pressure, and brings a risk of decreased cerebral perfusion that can be minimized by slow administration. Prolonged use of mannitol may lead to dehydration and electrolyte disturbances. Mannitol-associated renal failure is a risk if serum osmolality increases >320 mOsmol l^{-1}.

Hypertonic saline reduces ICP in patients with refractory intracranial hypertension and may be a useful alternative to mannitol in those who need reduction of brain bulk in the presence of maintained intravascular volume. Hypertonic saline has several potential adverse effects and, although the optimal osmolar load is undetermined, it is often given as a 7.5% solution in a dose of 2 ml kg^{-1}.

Diuretics

Loop diuretics such as furosemide reduce ICP via their diuretic action and also by decreasing CSF production. The ICP effects of loop diuretics occur in the absence of changes in serum osmolality or CBF, but they are not as effective as mannitol in reducing ICP. Furosemide in combination with mannitol is more effective than mannitol alone but at the cost of increased risk of dehydration and electrolyte disturbance.

Removal of cerebrospinal fluid

Draining CSF from the ventricles or the lumbar subarachnoid space decreases ICP. Lumbar drains are usually inserted after induction of anaesthesia and are useful where surgical exposure is difficult such as during clipping of cerebral aneurysms or pituitary surgery. The lumbar drain should not be opened until the bone flap has been lifted.

General anaesthesia

Induction

Anaesthesia is usually induced with an intravenous agent such as propofol or thiopental plus an opiate. Induction should be smooth with a stable haemodynamic profile and no coughing or straining. A non-depolarizing muscle relaxant is used to facilitate tracheal intubation and a peripheral nerve stimulator should be used to confirm that muscle relaxation is complete before laryngoscopy. Attenuation of the hypertensive response to laryngoscopy can be achieved with remifentanil, an additional bolus of induction agent

or with other agents such as lidocaine (1.5 mg kg^{-1}), or β-blockers (labetalol or esmolol). In emergency situations, or if the patient has been vomiting, a rapid sequence induction may be indicated. Traditionally, a cuffed reinforced endotracheal tube is used. This should be securely taped rather than tied in position, as ties may cause venous obstruction. The eyes should be covered and protected.

Monitoring

Standard monitoring for intracranial surgery includes ECG, oxygen saturation (SpO_2), end-tidal carbon dioxide, temperature and invasive arterial blood pressure monitoring. End-tidal carbon dioxide often correlates poorly with the arterial carbon dioxide tension ($PaCO_2$), especially in patients with pulmonary disease, so arterial blood gases should be used for calibration. Central venous pressure monitoring should be considered during surgery for vascular tumours and to guide fluid replacement in patients with pre-operative cardiovascular instability. Central venous access is often obtained via the antecubital fossa, although the femoral and internal jugular routes are equally acceptable. A urinary catheter is necessary for long procedures or if mannitol is to be used. Temperature monitoring should be used for all patients and a hot-air warming blanket applied to maintain normothermia. There has been much interest in the role of hypothermia as a neuroprotective strategy, but there is no evidence to support its routine use during neurosurgical procedures. Hyperthermia must be avoided.

Neurological monitoring is used to detect changes in cerebral haemodynamics, oxygenation and neuronal function. Many new monitoring tools are available although none is yet validated as a standard of care. The anaesthetic technique must be modified if intraoperative electrophysiological monitoring is used (see Chapter 8). The bispectral index (BIS) and spectral entropy have been used to assess depth of anaesthesia with mixed success in neuroanaesthesia.

Positioning

Patient position is determined by the requirements of surgical access and the effects on ICP and brain swelling. Most supratentorial surgery is conducted with the patient supine and the head partially rotated. Extreme neck flexion or rotation should be avoided as it can impair venous return and increase ICP. If the head must be turned, a sandbag or alternative support placed under the shoulders reduces the adverse effects on ICP. A 10° reverse Trendelenburg tilt has also been shown to reduce ICP without adverse effects on CPP. The patient's head may be placed on a doughnut-type cushion or horseshoe headrest, or secured using a skull pin fixator. The application of the pin fixator can produce a hypertensive response and this should be attenuated using a bolus of induction agent, opiate or local anaesthetic infiltration of the pin sites. The lateral position is used for temporoparietal approaches.

Before surgical draping, the position of the endotracheal tube should be confirmed, the patient's pressure areas padded, and the eyes and accessibility of intravenous lines checked. Neurosurgical procedures have a high risk of incorrect site surgery because of complex patient positioning, difficulty in interpretation of scans and cross-lateralization of clinical signs. The operative procedure and patient details should therefore be carefully confirmed and documented prior to the start of surgery.

Thromboembolic prophylaxis

Because neurosurgical procedures are often prolonged and the brain is a rich source of thromboplastin (an activator of the coagulation cascade), patients are at risk of venous thromboembolism (VTE). Graduated compression stockings and intermittent calf compression should be used in all patients. Many neurosurgeons are reluctant to use low-molecular-weight heparin in the early post-operative period because of the potential increased risk of bleeding. However, this risk is low, and patients with additional risk factors for VTE should be started on low-molecular-weight heparin within the first 24 h after surgery.

Maintenance of anaesthesia

Following comprehensive checks, the surgeon may infiltrate the scalp with a local anaesthetic solution containing epinephrine to provide analgesia and improve haemostasis. This may result in transient hypotension that is not seen when epinephrine is omitted, and it is thought that this effect is related to β_2-adrenergic receptor agonism by epinephrine.

As studies have failed to show significant differences in outcome between different anaesthetic agents, the anaesthetic technique is an individual choice determined by the particular procedure and patient. The most popular techniques in the UK are either sevoflurane or propofol infusion, supplemented with remifentanil. The requirement for further doses of muscle relaxant post-intubation is virtually eliminated when remifentanil is used. If another opioid is chosen, muscle relaxation should be maintained throughout the procedure to prevent movement and aid ventilation. Ventilation is adjusted to maintain normocapnia ($PaCO_2$ 4.0–4.5 kPa). Although moderate hyperventilation has been shown to improve operating conditions during craniotomy for supratentorial tumours, it is unclear whether the risks of hyperventilation-induced ischaemia outweigh its potential benefits on surgical access.

Major fluctuations in blood pressure should be prevented by anticipating and treating episodes of painful stimulation. Hypertension can result in a rise in ICP and cerebral oedema. Modest hypotension may improve the surgical field in some circumstances, but this should never be at the expense of impaired cerebral perfusion. Blood pressure should be returned to preoperative values before closure of the dura to ensure adequate haemostasis.

Despite a meticulous anaesthetic technique, operating conditions are sometimes poor and various manoeuvres and pharmacological agents are available to reduce intraoperative brain swelling. These are summarized in Table 12.2.

Fluid management

Intravenous fluids should be chosen and used with care. Traditionally, neurosurgical patients were fluid restricted, but this is rarely, if ever, useful in reducing ICP and, because it results in hypovolaemia, hypotension, and electrolyte and acid-base disturbances, fluid restriction is no longer recommended. The goals of perioperative fluid management are normovolaemia, normotension and normoglycaemia. In patients with an intact BBB, fluid flux is determined by osmolality rather than oncotic pressure. Compound sodium lactate is effectively hypo-osmolar (effective osmolality 250 mOsm l^{-1}) as a result of aggregation of sodium ions. Sodium chloride (0.9%) is the crystalloid of choice as it is slightly hyper-osmolar compared with serum (300 compared with 285 mOsm l^{-1}). However, large volumes of sodium chloride may cause a hyperchloraemic metabolic acidosis, and alternating bags of sodium chloride and compound sodium lactate have been recommended. Blood loss should be replaced with colloid and blood products to maintain a haemoglobin level >8 g dl^{-1}. Glucose-containing solutions

Table 12.2 Intraoperative brain swelling checklist

Check	Manoeuvre
Patient position	Reverse Trendelenburg position
	Avoid excessive head rotation
	No abdominal compression
Anaesthesia	Adequate depth of anaesthesia
	Good muscle relaxation
	Consider bolus of thiopental or propofol
	Change to total intravenous anaesthesia?
Blood pressure	Avoid hypertension
Ventilation	No hypoxia
	Hypocarbia ($PaCO_2$ 4.0–4.5 kPa)
Drugs	Avoid cerebral vasodilating drugs
Steroids	Dexamethasone 8–12 mg for tumours
Diuretics	Mannitol 0.25–0.5 g kg^{-1}
	Furosemide 0.25–0.5 mg kg^{-1}

should be avoided because, after glucose metabolism, the residual free water may worsen cerebral oedema. Furthermore, hyperglycaemia exacerbates cerebral ischaemic damage.

Emergence and extubation

Closure of a craniotomy may take some time and is often painful. In addition, the application of head bandages may result in head movement and irritation from the endotracheal tube. Anaesthesia should therefore be maintained to prevent hypertension, coughing or premature movement until all procedures have been completed. If remifentanil has been used intraoperatively, additional analgesia, such as intravenous morphine, should be given at least 30 min before the end of surgery to provide adequate analgesia into the recovery period. The majority of neurosurgical patients are extubated at the end of the procedure (even after prolonged surgery) to allow early neurological assessment. Patients may be extubated 'deep' or 'awake' and there is no evidence that one method is superior to the other. Whatever approach is taken, extubation should be smooth without coughing or straining.

Emergence from anaesthesia is associated with haemodynamic and ICP responses. These should be anticipated and treated because post-operative hypertension is associated with the development of

intracranial haematomas. Various strategies are used to attenuate the cardiovascular responses to emergence and extubation, including β-blockers, intravenous lidocaine (1–2 mg kg^{-1}) and 4% lidocaine within the cuff of the endotracheal tube. It has been suggested that remifentanil may be associated with an increased incidence of post-operative hypertension, but this can be minimized by effective transitional analgesia. The α_2 agonist dexmedetomidine provides good haemodynamic stability during intracranial tumour surgery and is effective at attenuating the response to extubation and emergence from anaesthesia.

Post-operative ventilation and ICP monitoring should be considered in patients who were severely obtunded pre-operatively and in those with major intraoperative bleeding or acute brain swelling.

Recovery

A rapid recovery allows prompt neurological assessment and detection of complications that require immediate intervention. Although new short-acting agents have made this achievable, no study has demonstrated relevant differences in speed or quality of recovery between volatile and total intravenous anaesthetic techniques. In one study, remifentanil was compared with alfentanil, fentanyl and sufentanil in patients undergoing craniotomy for tumour and, although there were no significant differences in haemodynamic or respiratory variables, there was a reduced time to eye opening and earlier return of cognitive function in patients receiving remifentanil.

Early minor post-operative complications are relatively common and include nausea, vomiting, shivering, and respiratory and cardiovascular disturbance. The biggest worry is neurological deterioration due to brain swelling or intracranial bleeding, and patients should be managed in a high-dependency area at least for the first 4–6 h when the risk of complications is greatest. The majority should then be able to return to a neurosurgical ward, although continued monitoring of neurological status is essential.

Pain, nausea and vomiting

There have been several reviews of post-operative pain in neurosurgical patients, but no large-scale studies have quantified effective treatments and side effects. Codeine-based analgesia is often inadequate as is paracetamol in isolation. Morphine is safe and effective in reducing pain scores, although it is associated with an increased incidence of nausea, vomiting and urinary retention. It can be administered via intravenous or intramuscular routes or via a patient-controlled analgesia device. Tramadol and oxycodone have both been used with success after craniotomy and may have a more favourable side-effect profile than conventional opioid analgesia. Although the use of non-steroidal anti-inflammatory drugs (NSAIDs) remains controversial because of the potential risk of bleeding, they reduce opioid requirements and are used by many neuroanaesthetists. Scalp infiltration with local anaesthetic decreases post-operative pain scores and morphine consumption in the recovery room. Regular multimodal analgesia is most successful after neurosurgical procedures.

Nausea and vomiting are common after craniotomy despite the widespread use of dexamethasone and other anti-emetics. Women and patients who have had a lumbar drain or a CSF leak are particularly at risk. Ondansetron, droperidol and dexamethasone each reduce the risk of nausea and vomiting by around 25%, and metoclopramide and scopolamine have also been used with some success. There is no convincing evidence favouring one anti-emetic agent over another and it is often necessary to administer multiple drugs, particularly in high-risk patients.

Specific considerations during supratentorial surgery

The basic principles of neuroanaesthesia apply to all procedures, but specific conditions bring particular challenges.

Intracerebral tumour surgery

The management of brain tumours is changing. Smaller craniotomies, intraoperative imaging, stereotactic interventions and endoscopic procedures increase surgical precision and minimize trauma to normal tissues, allowing quicker recovery, reduced morbidity and shorter hospital stays. Day-case intracranial tumour biopsy is safe and feasible but is not yet common practice. Management of brain tumours is now multidisciplinary with neurosurgeons, neuroradiologists and oncologists discussing each case and contributing to the management plan. Surgery is indicated for diagnosis, to reduce tumour bulk and to manage raised ICP. The general approach is to remove the maximum amount of tumour without producing a neurological deficit. Surgery is usually performed under general anaesthesia, but tumours within or adjacent to eloquent areas of brain may require intraoperative neurological assessment and an 'awake' technique (see below).

Meningioma surgery

The management of meningiomas merits additional discussion because they are often large, highly vascular tumours in difficult locations. Although predominantly benign, they have a high rate of local recurrence so radical excision is the usual surgical goal. This can make for long and technically demanding operations. There is often significant peri-tumour oedema and, in association with a large tumour, this leaves little intracranial space and brings a high risk of increased ICP. Intraoperative blood loss can be large and may be reduced by pre-operative tumour embolization. Rapid blood loss most often occurs during removal of the bone flap, especially with large tumours. Several large-bore cannulae are essential and, in addition to standard monitoring techniques, central venous pressure and urinary output monitoring should be undertaken. Several units of cross-matched blood, a rapid transfusion system and a blood warmer should be available from the start of surgery. Disseminated intravascular coagulation may develop perioperatively and clotting indices should be monitored.

Cerebral infections

Cerebral infections such as empyema or cranial abscess may develop as a result of direct spread from an adjacent area or because of haematogenous spread from a distant location. Intracranial infections are uncommon and account for only 1–2% of intracranial space-occupying lesions in the UK but up to 8% in developing countries. In most cases, the infection is spread from adjacent sites such as the middle ear (to the temporal lobe) or paranasal sinuses (to the frontal lobe). Penetrating trauma is the cause in about 7% of cases and usually results in solitary abscesses. Haematogenous spread from sources including dental abscesses, chronic pulmonary sepsis or SBE occurs in around 25% of cases. Abscesses from haematogenous spread most commonly occur in supratentorial regions and are often multiple, especially in immunocompromised patients. The causative organisms vary but can usually be predicted from the site of origin (Table 12.3). More than one organism is often implicated, but the cause of the intracranial infection is unknown in 10–37% of patients.

Table 12.3 Causes of intracerebral abscesses and common infecting organisms

Cause	Organism
Local causes	
• Otitis media or mastoiditis	*Streptococcus* *Pseudomonas*
• Acute sinusitis	*Streptococcus* *Haemophilus influenzae* *Bacteroides* sp.
• Penetrating head wounds	*Staphylococcus aureus* *Streptococcus* *Clostridium*
• Post-operative wound infection	*Staphylococcus epidermidis* *Staphylococcus aureus* *Pseudomonas*
Remote causes	
• Congenital heart disease	Microaerophilic amd aerobic streptococci
• Subacute bacterial endocarditis	*Streptococcus viridans* *Staphylococcus aureus* *Enterococcus*
• Brochiectasis	Coliforms
• Lung/liver abscess	*Nocardia*
• Dental caries	*Bacteroides* *Streptococci* *Actinomyces*
• Immuno-suppression	Toxoplasmosis *Nocardia* Tuberculosis Fungal Cysticercosis
• Patient from a developing country	*Echinococcus* Tuberculosis

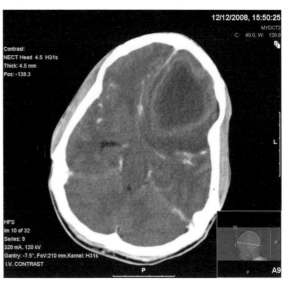

Fig. 12.1. CT scan showing an intracerebral abscess. Note the central necrotic area, the ring enhancement and surrounding area of cerebral oedema.

The clinical manifestations of intracranial infection depend on the size and location of the abscess. Symptoms usually develop over 2–3 weeks, although onset is more rapid in immunocompromised patients. Headache is often the first symptom, usually accompanied by vomiting, drowsiness or seizures. Focal neurological signs or an altered level of consciousness develop in up to 60% of patients. Fever is often present, but its absence does not exclude the diagnosis of intracranial sepsis, and many of the typical symptoms and signs of an inflammatory response are uncommon at the time of presentation. There may, however, be symptoms and signs related to the primary infective source, such as a history of ear ache, sinusitis or cardiac murmurs. Additional investigations should include chest and skull X-rays to identify pulmonary, sinus and mastoid infection, and blood cultures and echocardiogram in suspected SBE. MRI or CT scanning will confirm the diagnosis and characteristically reveals an enhancing lesion with a central necrotic area and surrounding, often intense, cerebral oedema (Fig. 12.1). Radiologically, it can sometimes be difficult to distinguish an abscess from a tumour, but abscesses classically have a smoother outline.

Isolated abscesses are best treated with a combination of surgical drainage and antibiotic therapy, but deep-seated or multiple abscesses are usually managed with antibiotics alone. Antibiotic choice should be made in consultation with medical microbiologists and guided by sensitivities from specimens taken during surgery. Abscesses can be drained via a burr hole or craniotomy, sometimes in conjunction with surgical evacuation of the primary infection site. Corticosteroids are highly effective in reducing peri-abscess oedema but may decrease the penetration of antibiotics into the abscess. Prophylactic anticonvulsants should be considered because seizures occur in up to 40% of patients with supratentorial abscesses.

Intracranial haematoma

An intracranial haematoma may be extradural, subdural or intracerebral and usually occurs as a result of trauma or rupture of an aneurysm or arteriovenous malformation (AVM). Spontaneous, usually hypertension-related, intracerebral haemorrhage is also common. The effects on neurological status and ICP depend on the speed at which the haematoma develops and its location. The anaesthetic management of neurovascular surgery and head injury is discussed in detail in Chapters 13 and 21, respectively, and only important principles are outlined here.

Extradural haematoma

Although extradural haematomas (EDHs) are relatively uncommon, they are important because they can be rapidly fatal. Except in children, an EDH is almost always associated with a skull fracture. The thin temporal bone anterior to the ear fractures relatively easily and this may rupture the underlying middle meningeal artery and result in a compact haematoma between the periostial layer of the dura and the inner table of the skull. The CT scan shows a characteristic biconvex haematoma. The classic sequence of events after an EDH is immediate loss of consciousness followed by partial recovery – the so-called lucid interval. Secondary loss of consciousness ensues as the haematoma expands a few hours after injury. However, only one-third of patients have this classic history, and EDHs are an important cause of late clinical deterioration. Pupillary dilation, hypertension and bradycardia develop as a result of increasing ICP and, if untreated, uncal herniation and brain stem compression follow. Extradural haematoma is a surgical emergency and urgent evacuation is required.

Many patients will have a markedly reduced or deteriorating Glasgow Coma Scale score and most will arrive in the neurosurgical unit already intubated and ventilated. Rapidly deteriorating patients may be transferred straight to the operating theatre, by-passing the neurointensive care unit or anaesthetic room. Traumatic haematomas are often associated with other injuries, including cervical spine injury, and life-threatening injuries require intervention or resuscitation prior to evacuation of the EDH. Induction of anaesthesia should be smooth and particular care given to maintenance of CPP and prevention of further rises in ICP. There may be a temporary, sometimes severe, fall in systemic blood pressure following surgical decompression, but this can usually be managed with a combination of fluids and vasopressors. However, to minimize this effect, pre-operative hypertension should not be treated unless it is excessive. Cross-matched blood should be available

in theatre. Patients should be transferred to the intensive care unit afterwards for further management (see Chapter 21).

Subdural haematoma

Subdural haematoma (SDH) is more common than EDH and occurs as a result of bleeding from communicating veins in the less restricted subdural space. The most common cause is trauma, although this can be minor and unnoticed, particularly in the elderly. Spontaneous SDH may occur but is rare. Acute SDH develops rapidly and presents with headache, drowsiness and confusion, and sometimes with early loss of consciousness. Acute SDHs require prompt evacuation, ideally within 4 h. Chronic SDH usually occurs in the elderly because cerebral atrophy places communicating veins under tension and allows them to rupture easily as a result of minor trauma. There is also more space for blood to accumulate and thus their presentation is delayed. As the haematoma develops, its contents alter, becoming osmotically active and slowly expanding. Presentation is insidious, with headache or a chronic confusional state, often developing over several days.

Pre-operative management should include a thorough medical assessment as the patients are often elderly and frail with multiple medical problems. Many are taking antiplatelet medication or anticoagulants, often for cardiac arrhythmias or prosthetic heart valves. Routine blood tests and a clotting screen should be performed and drugs should be stopped and anticoagulation reversed following haematological advice. Many chonic SDHs can be evacuated via a burr hole and often under local anaesthetic, although larger haematomas require a craniotomy.

Awake craniotomy

Awake craniotomy allows the intraoperative assessment of a patient's neurological status and the identification of safe resection margins during epilepsy surgery and excision of space-occupying lesions in eloquent (speech and motor) cortex, as well as the accurate localization of electrodes for deep brain stimulation. Awake testing allows maximal resection with minimal neurological deficit, allowing patients who were previously deemed inoperable to benefit from surgery. The anaesthetic techniques for awake craniotomy have evolved in parallel with the surgical techniques, although significant challenges remain. The goals are to provide adequate analgesia and sedation, a safe airway, haemodynamic stability, optimal operating conditions and an alert, cooperative patient during intraoperative neurological assessment. Various techniques have been described but they fall into three main categories:

1. Local anaesthesia.
2. Conscious sedation.
3. Asleep–awake–asleep (AAA) technique ± airway instrumentation.

The key to success is careful patient selection, an anaesthetic plan tailored to the individual case and meticulous attention to detail. The neurosurgeon and neuroanaesthetist should both be experienced in awake craniotomy and familiar with the particular technique chosen. Operative aims should be discussed beforehand and likely problems anticipated. The anaesthetist needs to be aware of the expected duration of surgery and the awake testing period, as well as the modality to be tested intraoperatively. Patients should be assessed carefully and any pre-existing neurological deficit documented. A full explanation of what is involved should be provided to the patient who must understand exactly what is expected of them and be able to lie still for the duration of the procedure. Coexisting medical problems should be optimized and routine medication continued, including on the day of surgery. Anticonvulsant prophylaxis, dexamethasone and either ranitidine or omeprazole should be prescribed. The only absolute contraindication to awake craniotomy is an uncooperative patient, but relative contraindications include morbid obesity, gastro-oesophageal reflux, a difficult airway and highly vascular tumours. These all increase the risk of perioperative complications and must be weighed against the benefits of the awake procedure.

Anaesthetic technique

The choice of technique depends on the individual case, the patient's age and any associated comorbidity. Routine monitoring used in craniotomy under general anaesthesia is also indicated for awake surgery. Surgical drapes are taped out of the way to allow easy access to the patient's face and to facilitate communication during intraoperative testing (Fig. 12.2). Padding of pressure areas and a calm relaxed atmosphere in theatre are essential to minimize patient discomfort and anxiety. A warming blanket helps prevent shivering and urinary catheterization should be avoided if possible. Anti-emetic prophylaxis must be given to all patients and a loading dose of paracetamol provides useful additional analgesia.

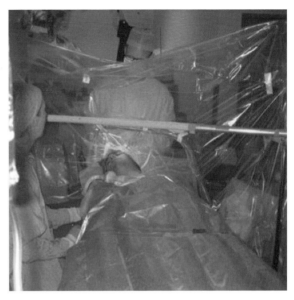

Fig. 12.2. Operating theatre arrangements for awake craniotomy. Note that the surgical drapes are placed to allow the anaesthetist access to the patient's airway and face for intraoperative testing and airway management. See colour plate section.

Local anaesthetic

Whichever technique is chosen, effective local anaesthesia is essential. This can be provided by field infiltration of the incision and pins sites or by individual nerve blockade, usually with long-acting agents such as bupivacaine or ropivacaine (± lidocaine for speed of onset) with epinephrine at 1:200,000. A large volume of local anaesthetic is required and this carries a risk of toxicity in patients who are already prone to seizures. Doses must therefore be calculated carefully. Awake craniotomy under local anaesthesia alone eliminates the hazards of excessive sedation and respiratory depression, particularly in the elderly who are sensitive to sedative agents. Burr hole procedures or small craniotomies are well tolerated under local anaesthesia, but many patients will not tolerate long, often uncomfortable procedures without sedation.

Sedation

The addition of sedation makes a craniotomy more acceptable for many patients. Historically, midazolam, fentanyl and droperidol were the agents commonly used, but propofol is now the most popular agent. It provides controllable sedation, rapid and smooth recovery and minimal residual interference with electrocorticographic recordings after it is stopped. It is often used in combination with remifentanil. Dexmedetomidine is becoming increasingly popular, especially for implantation of deep brain stimulators, as it provides readily titratable sedation, analgesia and sympatholysis without respiratory depression. It can be used as a sole agent (0.3–$0.6\,\mu g\,kg^{-1}\,h^{-1}$), an adjunct to other agents (0.01–$1.0\,\mu g\,kg^{-1}\,h^{-1}$) or as a rescue agent.

Whatever drugs are chosen, sedation can be notoriously difficult to control in the context of awake craniotomy, and respiratory depression and airway compromise are feared complications. These occur most commonly during sedation with propofol in combination with remifentanil, and in patients who are obese. Complications are less common in experienced hands. Neuroleptanalgesia has a lower incidence of respiratory depression when compared with propofol sedation but a higher incidence of seizures, nausea and vomiting. Although dexmedetomidine sedates without respiratory depression, sedative synergism is reported with midazolam.

Asleep–awake–asleep

The AAA technique, with or without airway intervention, is increasingly popular. Many agents have been used, but propofol and remifentanil are most popular. These are titrated against patient response, haemodynamic variables and in some cases guided by BIS monitoring. The remifentanil infusion is reduced to 0.005–$0.01\,\mu g\,kg^{-1}\,min^{-1}$ (1–$2\,ng\,ml^{-1}$) and propofol stopped to allow awake testing. Using this technique, the patient is awake only for the period of intraoperative testing and discomfort is thereby minimized. In addition, haemodynamic and respiratory variables are easier to control, providing optimal operative conditions for the majority of the procedure. However, the AAA technique without airway instrumentation is associated with respiratory complications, and there is some concern that time to wake up may be prolonged when compared with sedation techniques. Remifentanil significantly reduces propofol requirements, allowing a median wake-up time of 9 min when the two agents are used together.

Airway management

With any sedation technique, there is the risk of hypoventilation or airway obstruction. Poor patient positioning may contribute to airway complications and limit access in an emergency. There must always be a plan for securing the airway in an emergency. Airway adjuncts range from a nasopharyngeal airway to an endotracheal tube, although the laryngeal mask airway

Table 12.4 Complications of awake craniotomy

System	Complication
Respiratory	Airway obstruction
	Respiratory depression
Cardiovascular	Hypotension
	Hypertension
Neurological	Seizures
	Neurological deficit
	Brain swelling
Other	Pain
	Nausea and vomiting
	Local anaesthetic toxicity
	Excessive sedation/uncooperative patient
	Air embolism

(LMA) is popular for AAA techniques. It is easy to insert and remove, well tolerated at lighter planes of anaesthesia and allows ventilation to be controlled during the asleep phase. Non-invasive positive pressure ventilation (biphasic positive airway pressure and proportional assist ventilation) via an LMA has been used with some success during awake craniotomy.

Complications

Overall, awake craniotomy is safe and well tolerated, but many complications have been described (Table 12.4). Several studies have reviewed complication rates but, because of differences in case mix and anaesthetic techniques, the reported incidences vary widely and no definitive conclusions can be drawn. Fortunately, catastrophic complications are very rare.

Post-operative care

Post-operatively, patients should be managed in a high-dependency area for 4–6 h. Awake craniotomy is a very cost-effective procedure because it is associated with a lower requirement for high-dependency care and a shorter hospital stay. Some centres have now started to perform awake craniotomy as a day-case procedure.

Epilepsy surgery

Epilepsy is a chronic neurological disorder characterized by paroxysmal seizures as a result of excessive neuronal discharge. It is the second most common neurological disorder after stroke and the most prevalent involving all age groups. Epilepsy affects 1 in 200 of the population. With modern anticonvulsant medication, seizure control is effective in around 70% of patients, but, in the remainder, seizures are uncontrolled or controlled only at the cost of intolerable side effects from medication. Most patients who have not responded to three anticonvulsant agents (either separately or in combination) do not ultimately respond to pharmacotherapy. This group of patients is responsible for >75% of the healthcare costs of epilepsy in the UK because of their frequent admission to hospital, accidental injuries, psychological, social and vocational impairment, and sudden unexplained death. For many patients with medically refractory epilepsy, surgical intervention offers a real chance for a reduction in seizure frequency or even a cure. However, only a small proportion of potential surgical candidates are currently referred for surgery.

Surgery may be considered as definitive or palliative. Definitive surgery brings a significant chance of producing a seizure-free patient or a 70–90% chance of improvement in seizure severity. Palliative procedures aim to decrease seizure frequency but rarely result in seizure freedom. In general, definitive surgery involves the physical removal of seizure-producing cortex, e.g. resection of small seizure-producing tumours, vascular abnormalities, cortical malformations or mesial temporal sclerosis. The role of palliative surgery is to disrupt the pathways involved in seizure production and propagation, or to disrupt seizures with the use of electrical stimulation. Anterior temporal resection is the most common procedure for temporal lobe epilepsy and is associated with better seizure control and improved quality of life than medical therapy alone. Other procedures for more complex epilepsy syndromes include corpus callosotomy, modified hemispherectomy, multiple subpial transection surgery and vagal nerve stimulation.

Classification of epilepsy

The classification of seizure type and specific epilepsy syndromes is complex but necessary for treatment planning. Seizures are typically classified into two main groups – generalized or partial. Classic generalized seizures result from simultaneous involvement of both cerebral hemispheres and can be subdivided into inhibitory or petit mal (atonic, absence) and excitatory or grand mal (tonic, clonic, myoclonic). Partial or focal seizures are confined to a localized part of the brain and a simple partial seizure implies no alteration

in consciousness. If seizures spread to multiple regions of the brain and alter consciousness, they are classified as complex partial seizures.

Pre-surgical work-up

Decisions to proceed with epilepsy surgery are made by a multidisciplinary team and based on the patient's medical history, physical examination, social circumstances, seizure severity and the results of diagnostic testing. The aim of pre-surgical testing is to identify the site of the epileptogenic focus, map-associated brain function and establish whether the focus can be safely removed. EEG, 24 h EEG telemetry and brain imaging using MRI, PET scans and single-photon emission CT (SPECT) are used to localize the epileptogenic focus. Neurocognitive testing allows psychological and memory assessments. A Wada test may be performed to assess language lateralization and the ability of the contralateral mesial temporal structures to support memory. This is an invasive technique that involves the injection of 100–200 mg of sodium amytal into the internal carotid artery and is being replaced in some cases by functional MRI. If the results of these investigations are inconclusive, intracranial EEG recordings can be obtained by placing electrodes directly on or into the brain (strip, grid or depth electrodes) to improve precision in localizing epileptogenic foci.

Although the work-up for epilepsy surgery can take several years, the anaesthetist may not have the opportunity to meet the patient until shortly before surgery. It is important that a detailed pre-operative assessment and clinical evaluation is made and, because this is elective surgery, coexisting medical conditions should be optimized. Several genetic syndromes, e.g. tuberose sclerosis, are associated with epilepsy and many have anaesthetic implications. Assessment should also include a review of the patient's drug history as most will have been taking anticonvulsant medication for many years and may have significant side effects. Phenytoin and carbamazepine are potent hepatic enzyme inducers and can result in enhanced requirement for certain anaesthetic drugs such as some non-depolarizing muscle relaxants, narcotics and benzodiazepines. Sodium valproate may cause thrombocytopaenia and bleeding problems and is often stopped pre-operatively. Liver function tests and a clotting screen should be performed in patients who have been taking valproate. Other anticonvulsant drugs are sometimes stopped perioperatively for diagnostic purposes and familiarity with seizure presentation is important in order to recognize habitual seizures in the perioperative period.

Anaesthesia

Anaesthesia may be required for diagnostic procedures or definitive surgery and children often require sedation for neuroimaging procedures. General anaesthesia is used for placement of epidural strip electrodes via burr holes or implantation of subdural grids via a craniotomy. The patient should be sufficiently awake at the end of surgery so that a neurological examination can be conducted reliably.

General anaesthesia is often used for resection of well-delineated epileptogenic foci in non-eloquent areas of brain and the anaesthetic technique will depend on the need for intraoperative electrocorticography (ECoG). If neither ECoG nor cortical mapping is necessary, the patient's usual anticonvulsant medication should be continued prior to surgery. Pro-convulsant drugs and any physiological factors that might decrease seizure threshold (e.g. hypoxia, hypotension and hypocapnia) should be avoided during epilepsy surgery. All volatile agents reduce cerebral electrical activity in a dose-dependent manner, so, if ECoG is required during general anaesthesia, a total intravenous technique should be chosen. Neuromuscular blockade should not be used if cortical stimulation is used during general anaesthesia. Intraoperative cortical stimulation and mapping are necessary if the epileptogenic focus is located in or adjacent to eloquent areas of brain and an 'awake' technique may be indicated.

Post-operative management

Pre-operative alterations to anticonvulsant therapy may increase the risk of post-operative seizures. Patients should therefore be managed in a high-dependency area overnight for monitoring. They are usually able to be discharged home within 3 or 4 days.

Further reading

Apfel, C. C., Korttila, K., Abdalla, M. et al. (2004). A factorial trial of six interventions for the prevention of nausea and vomiting. New Engl J Med 350, 2441–51.

Basali, A., Mascha, E. J., Kalfas, I. and Schubert, A. (2000). Relation between perioperative hypertension and intracranial haemorrhage after craniotomy. Anesthesiology 93, 48–54.

Brat, D. J., Parisi, J. E., Kleinschmidt-DeMasters, B. K. et al. (2008). Surgical neuropathology update: a review of the changes introduced by WHO classification of tumours of the central nervous system, 4th edition. Arch Pathol Lab Med 132, 993–1007.

De Gray, L. C. and Matta, B. F. (2005). Acute and chronic pain following craniotomy: a review. Anaesthesia 60, 693–704.

Dinsmore, J. (2007). Anaesthesia for elective neurosurgery. Br J Anaesth 99, 68–74.

Frost, E. A. and Booij, L. H. (2007). Anesthesia in the patient for awake craniotomy. Curr Opin Anaesthesiol 20, 331–5.

Gelb, A. W., Craen, R. A., Rao, G. S. et al. (2008). Does hyperventilation improve operating condition during supratentorial surgery? A multicenter randomized crossover trial. Anesth Analg 106, 585–94.

Gottschalk, A. and Yaster, M. (2007). Pain management after craniotomy. Neurosurg Q 17, 64–73.

Hall, W. A. and Truwit, C. L. (2008) The surgical management of infections involving the cerebrum. Neurosurgery, 62 (Suppl. 2), 519–31.

Herrick, I. A. and Gelb, A. W. (2000). Anesthesia for temporal lobe epilepsy surgery. Can J Neurol Sci 27 (Suppl. 1), S64–67.

Kawano, Y., Kawaguchi, M., Inoue, S. et al. (2004). Jugular bulb oxygen saturation under propofol or sevoflurane/nitrous oxide anaesthesia during deliberate mild hypothermia in neurosurgical patients. J Neurosurg Anesthesiol 16, 6–10.

Leslie, K. and Williams, D. L. (2005). Postoperative pain, nausea and vomiting in neurosurgical patients. Curr Opin Anaesthesiol 18, 461–5.

McKinney, P.A. (2004). Brain tumours: incidence, survival, and aetiology. J Neurol Neurosurg Psychiatry 75, 12–17.

Pasternak, J., McGregor DG and Lanier, W. L. (2005). Effect of single dose dexamethasone on blood glucose concentrations in patients undergoing craniotomy. J Neurosurg Anesthesiol 16, 122–5.

Rasmussen, M., Bundgaard, H. and Cold, G. E. (2004). Craniotomy for supratentorial brain tumors: risk factors for brain swelling after opening the dura mater. J Neurosurg 101, 621–6.

Rozet, I., Tontisirin, N., Muangman, S. et al. (2007). Effect of equiosmolar solutions of mannitol versus hypertonic saline on intraoperative brain relaxation and electrolyte balance. Anesthesiology 107, 697–704.

Sagher, O. and Leveque, J.-C. (2004). Surgical management of central nervous system infections. In Scheld, W. M., Whitley, R. J. and Marr, C. M., eds., Infections of the Central Nervous System, 3rd edn. Lippincott Williams & Wilkins, pp. 843–58.

Serletis, D. and Bernstein, M. (2007). Prospective study of awake craniotomy used routinely and nonselectively for supratentorial tumors. *J Neurosurg* **107**, 1–6.

Skucas, A. P. and Artru, A. A. (2006). Anesthetic complications of awake craniotomies for epilepsy surgery. *Anesth Analg* **102**, 882–7.

Yang, J. J., Cheng, H. L., Shang, R. J. *et al.* (2007). Haemodynamic changes due to infiltration of the scalp with epinephrine-containing lidocaine solution, a hypotensive episode before craniotomy. *J Neurosurg Anesthesiol* **19**, 31–7.

Chapter

13

Anaesthesia for intracranial vascular surgery and carotid disease

Jane Sturgess and Basil F. Matta

Introduction

Recent improvements in neurosurgical and neuroanaesthetic techniques have reduced the morbidity and mortality traditionally associated with intracranial vascular abnormalities. Even patients presenting with significant neurological deficit may achieve good outcome provided appropriate therapy is instituted early in their illness. The success of the combined aggressive anaesthetic and surgical management is most notable in those patients with subarachnoid haemorrhage (SAH) or traumatic intracranial haematomas. Neuroanaesthetists play an important role in the pre-operative resuscitation and optimization, intraoperative management and post-operative neurointensive care of patients with intracranial vascular lesions.

This chapter discusses the anaesthetic management of intracranial vascular abnormalities with particular emphasis on SAH, arteriovenous malformations (AVMs) and carotid artery stenosis.

Intracranial vascular abnormalities

Aetiology

The pathological classification of intracranial haematomas is provided in Table 13.1.

Traumatic haematoma

Traumatic intracranial haematomas secondary to head injury usually occur in young males early in their working lives, with significant social and economic implications. Extradural, subdural and intracerebral haematomas often occur in association with other significant injuries such as cervical spine or intra-abdominal trauma, which may take priority in treatment. However, as 40% of comatose head-injured patients have an intracranial mass, an early CT scan once the patient is stabilized will differentiate operative from non-operative lesions.

Extradural haematoma

The majority of extradural haematomas (EDHs) are traumatic. Extradural haematomas are often found in the temporal region in association with a skull fracture involving the middle meningeal artery. Less frequently, they originate from the venous sinuses following disruption of the dural membranes. Although most EDHs are acute, they can present up to 48 h after the initial trauma and are an important cause for a late clinical deterioration.

The clinical presentation depends on the size, position and rate at which the haematoma forms. Only one-third of patients with EDH present with the classic initial loss of consciousness followed by a lucid interval and then a rapid decline in consciousness. Not all patients develop ipsilateral pupillary dilation and focal neurological deficits. Although poor outcome is associated with coma on admission, bilateral dilated pupils, a subdural component and delays in surgical intervention, the overall mortality following an extradural haematoma is <5%.

Subdural haematoma

A SDH is often associated with an underlying cerebral injury and is therefore associated with poorer prognosis. Bleeding occurs from torn cerebral tissues and bridging cortical veins. Over 50% of patients will be unconscious from the start, with a mortality of 40–80%. Poor outcomes are associated with a low Glasgow Coma Scale score (GCS 3–5) on presentation, age > 60 years, unreactive dilated pupils, high intracranial pressure (ICP), hypotension and hypoxaemia.

Core Topics in Neuroanaesthesia and Neurointensive Care, eds. Basil F. Matta, David K. Menon and Martin Smith. Published by Cambridge University Press. © Cambridge University Press 2011.

Table 13.1 Classification of intracranial haematomas

Traumatic

Non-traumatic

- Hypertensive
- Amyloid angiopathy
- Drug-induced
- Coagulopathy
- Neoplasia
- Vascular:
  - ° Aneurysm
  - ° Arteriovenous malformations
  - ° Cavernous malformations

Intracerebral haematoma

A traumatic intracerebral haematoma can follow all types of blunt cranial trauma. Penetrating skull injuries (stab or gunshot wound) and depressed skull fractures are also commonly associated with intracerebral bleeds. In the elderly, and in alcoholics with cerebral atrophy, the associated trauma may be modest, and the haematoma may only produce symptoms 48 h after the initial trauma.

Posterior fossa haematoma

Although uncommon, a posterior fossa haematoma (PFH) can lead to rapid deterioration as a result of brainstem compression. Occipital abrasions, an occipital fracture, respiratory irregularities and/or hypertension should alert the clinician to the possibility of a PFH. Without rapid decompression, the mortality rate is very high.

Non-traumatic haematoma

The causes of non-traumatic intracerebral haemorrhage (ICH) vary with age. Hypertension and tumours predominate in the elderly, while vascular abnormalities predominate in younger patients.

Hypertensive haematoma

Hypertension is probably the most significant risk factor for ICH in the elderly. Evidence of pre-existing high blood pressure, such as left ventricular hypertrophy, is common. The mechanisms believed to be responsible for hypertensive bleeds include the formation and rupture of microaneurysms affecting the lenticulo-striate vessels, and the degeneration of the media affecting small penetrating arteries (hyalinosis).

Amyloid angiopathy

This is associated with the deposition of amyloid in the media and adventitia of cerebral vessels causing calcific degeneration and rupture of the vessel wall in the elderly. The arteries and arterioles of the leptomeninges and the superficial layers of the cortex are involved causing lobar haemorrhages (most commonly the parietal and occipital lobes). Subarachnoid and subdural haemorrhages can also occur.

Drug and alcohol abuse

Cocaine and amphetamines cause intense sympathetic activity that can lead to extreme rises in blood pressure. In such circumstances, especially with amphetamine abuse, an ICH can occur without an underlying vascular lesion. Intravenous drug abusers are at increased risk of bacterial endocarditis with the subsequent development and rupture of cerebral mycotic aneurysms. Alcoholics can develop systemic hypertension and liver abnormalities, which predispose them to spontaneous ICHs.

Coagulopathies

All types of coagulopathies predispose to spontaneous intracerebral bleeds. These can be intrinsic (idiopathic thrombocytopaenia, disseminated intravascular coagulation, haemophilia) or drug related (aspirin, anticoagulants, fibrinolytics). Intracranial haematomas secondary to anticoagulant therapy are common.

Neoplasia

Patients with primary or secondary cerebral tumours may deteriorate suddenly because of haemorrhage into the lesion. This is more likely to occur in the more vascular tumours, which include malignant gliomas, malignant melanomas, bronchogenic carcinomas, choriocarcinomas and renal cell carcinomas.

Vascular anomalies

These include cerebral aneurysms, AVM and cavernous malformations. The majority of patients present with either an intracerebral haematoma or a SAH. Rarely, they may present with cerebral irritation, seizures or neurological deficits from an intracranial mass effect.

Pathophysiology

Autoregulation, arterial carbon dioxide and oxygen tension ($PaCO_2$ and PaO_2, respectively) and cerebral metabolism influence cerebral blood flow (CBF). In normal individuals, autoregulation ensures that CBF remains at an average of $50\,\text{ml}\,(100\,\text{g})^{-1}\,\text{min}^{-1}$ despite changes in cerebral perfusion pressure (CPP) between 60 and 160 mmHg. Hypocapnia can increase or restore impaired autoregulation, whereas hypercapnia impairs autoregulation. At CPP outside this range, CBF becomes pressure dependent.

In normal individuals, changes in cerebral blood volume (CBV) mirror changes in CBF. Therefore, following intracranial haemorrhage when autoregulation is often impaired either focally or globally, rapid changes in blood pressure have profound effects on CBF. While hypotension will lead to cerebral ischaemia, hypertension will result in increased CBV, raised ICP and secondary brain ischaemia.

Carbon dioxide is one of the major determinants of CBF. Cerebral blood flow changes almost linearly with changes in $PaCO_2$ between 3 and 10 kPa. While hyperventilation reduces CBF, CBV and ICP, hypoventilation has opposite effects. Intracranial haemorrhage may reduce cerebral vasoreactivity to carbon dioxide. Therefore, hyperventilation may be ineffectual in reducing ICP. Furthermore, as the relationship between CBF, CBV and ICP may no longer exist, hyperventilation may reduce CBF without changing CBV or ICP, thus exacerbating brain ischaemia.

There is little effect of PaO_2 on CBF within the physiological range. However, if PaO_2 decreases below 6 kPa, tissue oxygen delivery is maintained by cerebral vasodilation, which overrides any vasoconstriction induced by hyperventilation. Although a PaO_2 >100 kPa may cause cerebral vasoconstriction, a combination of moderate hyperventilation and hyperoxia may be used as a temporary measure to reduce brain bulk while maintaining cerebral oxygen delivery.

Cerebral blood flow and cerebral metabolism are tightly coupled. Any increase in regional or global cerebral activity will lead to an increase in cerebral metabolism and therefore CBF. This relationship may be uncoupled by an intracerebral bleed or head injury, a finding that is central to the management of intracranial haemorrhage.

Principles of management

Regardless of the causes of intracranial haemorrhage, the above pathology that affects the above physiological mechanisms may precipitate cerebral ischaemia. Therefore, the management of all patients with intracerebral haematomas irrespective of cause is aimed at maintaining adequate CBF and preventing and treating secondary cerebral ischaemia. The anaesthetic management of traumatic intracranial haematomas is described in detail in Chapter 21.

Subarachnoid haemorrhage

Cerebral aneurysms account for 75–80% of spontaneous SAH, cerebral AVMs for 4–5%, and in 15–20% of patients no source of haemorrhage can be found. Other causes of SAH include trauma, dural and spinal AVMs, mycotic aneurysms, sickle-cell disease, cocaine abuse and coagulation disorders.

Cerebral aneurysms occur mainly at vascular bifurcations within the circle of Willis or proximal cerebral artery. Most are supratentorial, and approximately 20% of patients will have multiple aneurysms. The incidence of aneurysmal SAH is 12–15 per 100,000 of the population per year with a peak incidence between 55 and 60 years of age. Females are affected more than males, and genetic factors may contribute.

Despite improvements in anaesthetic and surgical care, SAH is associated with high morbidity and mortality. One-third of patients will die before reaching hospital and the remaining patients will have a 30–50% mortality. The major risks facing patients who reach hospital are recurrent haemorrhage, the development of delayed ischaemic neurological deficits (vasospasm) and hydrocephalus. Conservative non-surgical management of SAH is associated with much higher mortality than surgical management (40 vs. <10%, respectively, within 6 months of the bleed). However, conservative medical management has recently been advocated in elderly patients (>64 years) with unruptured aneurysms <1 cm in diameter as the risks of surgery outweigh the benefits.

Clinical presentation

Subarachnoid haemorrhage classically presents with sudden-onset severe headache radiating to the occipital or cervical region with or without loss of consciousness. Photophobia, nausea, vomiting, lethargy and signs of meningism are all common. Hypertension, hyperpyrexia, seizures, motor or sensory deficits, cranial nerve palsies (IIIrd and VIth) and visual field defects may also occur. Elevated ICP and meningeal irritation cause loss of consciousness, headaches and neurological deficits. A sudden rise in ICP, in conjunction with normal coagulation, is thought to prevent continuing bleeding from the aneurysm site.

Early management

The immediate management of patients with SAH follows the principles of airway, breathing and circulation. Patients unable to protect their airway or obey commands, and those with a GCS <9 should have their airway secured by intubation and ventilation. Hypoxaemia and hypercarbia may result in a rapid increase in ICP that could precipitate a rebleed and aggravate cerebral ischaemia from the initial insult. Heart rate, blood pressure and tissue perfusion are assessed and treated when abnormal. Neurological examination includes level of consciousness, spontaneous movement, orientation, ability to follow commands, pupillary size, shape, reactivity, ocular movement, muscle tone and reflexes.

Information regarding previous trauma, ICHs, hypertension and hypertensive treatments, known vascular malformations or tumours, anticoagulant use, coagulopathies, prosthetic heart valves, ischaemic cerebrovascular disease and drug abuse should be obtained at the same time.

The clinical condition of the patient is graded using the World Federation of Neurological Surgeons (WFNS) system as shown in Table 13.2. Although morbidity and mortality varies widely between centres, it is commonly accepted that a higher WFNS grade generally results in worse outcome. This may be due to a combination of initial damage and the increased risk of developing intracranial hypertension, vasospasm, reduced CBF and impaired autoregulation.

A CT scan will identify the site and extent of the haemorrhage and assess ventricular size. It may also indicate the most likely site of the aneurysm. Once an intracranial bleed is identified, immediate referral to a neurosurgical centre is advisable. Although we will consider patients with SAH of all grades at our centre including those with unreactive pupils, in reality those elderly patients with a poor quality of life, extensive SAH on CT scan and with bilateral fixed dilated pupils are not usually suitable for neurosurgical intervention. Decisions on further management should not be based on pupillary size in isolation, as dilated pupils can accompany subclinical seizures and hydrocephalus and therefore are not an absolute contraindication for transfer.

When no SAH is detected on CT scan but the history is strongly suggestive of it, a lumbar puncture is performed. If xanthochromia is present, the patient should be transferred to a neurosurgical centre for cerebral angiography. Lumbar puncture should only

Table 13.2 World Federation of Neurological Surgeons (WFNS) grading of subarachnoid haemorrhage

Grade	Glasgow Coma Scale	Motor deficit (aphasia and/or hemiparesis or hemiplegia)
0	15	Absent
I	15	Absent
II	13–14	Absent
III	13–14	Present
IV	7–12	Present or absent
V	3–6	Present or absent

be performed after a negative CT scan and in the absence of signs of raised ICP, as the procedure may cause a rebleed or brain herniation with disastrous consequences.

Once a diagnosis of SAH has been made, the WFNS grade and the pre-morbid state of the patient influence further treatment. Patients with grades I or II are monitored on the neurosurgical high-dependency unit. Neurological assessments, vital signs and fluid balance are recorded hourly. A daily fluid intake of at least 3 litres is recommended. Intravenous fluids can supplement oral intake, but 5% dextrose solutions are best avoided because of hypotonicity and the possible risk of hyperglycaemia with its associated adverse effects in brain injury. Oral nimodipine (60 mg every 4 h) is started in an attempt to prevent delayed cerebral ischaemia. However, nimodipine can cause hypotension and the dose may need to be reduced or divided into more frequent doses (30 mg every 6 h). Ideally, systolic blood pressure should be maintained at 140–150 mmHg (slightly higher in previously hypertensive individuals). Paracetamol or codeine phosphate are prescribed for pain. Any electrolyte abnormalities are corrected and a haematocrit of 30% is aimed for. A central venous line or a pulmonary artery floatation catheter may be required to guide therapy in those with cardiac disease and the elderly, aiming for a filling pressure of 10–14 mmHg.

Patients with WFNS grades III and IV are cared for on the neurocritical care unit. The CT scan is studied for factors contributing to the poor grade of the patient. If hydrocephalus is present, an extraventricular drain is inserted. If a large intracerebral haematoma is present and the patient's condition is stable, urgent vascular studies are performed before clot evacuation and aneurysm clipping. However, in the event of deterioration with mass effect (such as a fixed pupil), surgical decompression is performed immediately.

Patients with evidence of raised ICP on CT scan should have their ICP monitored to help guide management (see Chapter 4). After resuscitation, these patients are assessed neurologically. Neuromuscular relaxants and sedation are withdrawn and at an appropriate time the response to a painful stimulus is observed. If the patient exhibits purposeful movement, they are resedated and cerebral angiography is performed with a view to definite aneurysm clipping. In the case of multiple aneurysms, only the culprit aneurysm is treated. Residual aneurysms may be treated electively a minimum of 3 months later depending on the outcome of the current episode.

If the patient displays no purposeful movement to painful stimuli, CBF studies are performed together with cerebral perfusion supported with ICP management and blood pressure control. Patients are assessed periodically for improvements in their neurological status. If no improvement occurs, outcome is likely to be poor and a decision regarding further treatment should be discussed with the relatives at an early stage.

Although CT scanning and magnetic resonance angiography can diagnose vascular lesions, cerebral angiography remains the gold standard. An acceptable angiogram must show all the intracranial vessels in at least two planes to identify the neck of the aneurysm and its surrounding vessels. Any radiographic evidence of vasospasm is noted. If multiple aneurysms are detected, the patient's symptoms, and the location, appearance and presence of regional vasospasm help identify the culprit aneurysm. For angiogram-negative patients in whom other causes have been excluded (such as dural fistulae, cerebral vasculitis and venous thrombosis), repeat angiography is performed 14 days later.

Timing of surgery

Definitive surgery can be early (1–3 days after SAH) or late (10–14 days after SAH). Historically, 'late' surgery was preferred as surgical exposure and aneurysm clipping was considered easier when less cerebral oedema and inflammation were present. However, although technically more difficult, 'early' surgery decreases the probability of rebleeding with its associated high morbidity and mortality. Furthermore, by removing the blood clot early, the risk of developing a delayed ischaemic deficit may be reduced. If a deficit should develop as a result of vasospasm, then induced hypertension can be used safely if the aneurysm is secured. Recent experience shows that early surgery does not increase the risk of intraoperative complications compared with later surgery.

Our policy is to perform definitive surgery within 4 days of the primary event especially in patients with good-grade SAH. This is based on published evidence suggesting that rebleeding is commonest in the first 24 h after SAH, and 70% of patients who rebleed will die. This has been confirmed recently in a prospective audit at our hospital, which identified a 4% risk of rebleeding within the first day rising to 20% in the first 2 weeks, with 85% mortality as a result of the second bleed. Surgery is performed during the day on elective lists except when a space-occupying mass needs urgent evacuation.

Pre-operative evaluation

A routine general anaesthetic assessment will include the patient's past medical history, medications, allergies and previous general anaesthetics. The extent of the neurological and myocardial injury is of particular interest. In addition, blood results, ECG and echocardiography when indicated, chest X-ray, CT scans, angiography and transcranial Doppler ultrasonography findings should be available. Proper communication between the anaesthetist and the operating surgeon is likely to lead to the best perioperative care.

Cardiovascular assessment

Although seen in the majority (50–100%) of patients with a SAH, ECG changes are more frequent in those with severe neurological impairment. They include T-wave abnormalities, ST segment depression, prominent U waves, prolonged QT intervals, and both atrial and ventricular dysrhythmias. The ECG abnormalities occur within 48 h of the SAH and may last up to 6 weeks. While the degree of myocardial dysfunction does not correlate with the SAH-induced ECG changes, the greatest degree of myocardial dysfunction occurs in those patients with worse WFNS grades. Post-mortem and creatine phosphokinase isoenzyme studies have shown that the majority of SAH-induced ECG changes are related to subendocardial ischaemia or localized areas of myocardial necrosis. It is postulated that these changes are caused by posterior hypothalamic stimulation leading to an acute increase in sympathetic activity. The resulting increase in myocardial and systemic norepinephrine levels may (by a direct toxic effect or by increasing myocardial afterload) cause this subendocardial ischaemia. The coronary arteries are usually normal. Some patients will develop pathological Q waves following a SAH. This is often misinterpreted as evidence of a recent myocardial infarction (MI). However, the differentiation between SAH-associated and myocardial ischaemia-related ECG changes is difficult, especially in patients with coexisting cardiac disease. An echocardiogram and/or a pulmonary artery catheter may be valuable in these patients.

Although non-specific ECG changes not accompanied by symptoms or signs of myocardial dysfunction are probably insignificant and should not delay surgery, it is probably prudent to wait as long as possible before proceeding with the surgery in those patients with changes suggestive of MI, as the risk of malignant dysrhythmias is high. The benefits of early surgery have to be weighed against possible perioperative myocardial ischaemia. Our policy is to wait at least 72 h unless there is mass effect or the patient's condition allows a 10–14-day wait.

Blood pressure abnormalities are frequent after SAH. When hypertension is a compensatory response to maintain CPP in the presence of an elevated ICP, it should not be treated unless it is severe. Systolic blood pressure >160 mmHg increases the risk of rupture and rebleeding in an unsecured aneurysm and therefore a compromise needs to be achieved. Patients with systolic blood pressures >160 mmHg may be treated judiciously with labetalol, which appears to have little if any effect on CBF or ICP. Sodium nitroprusside and hydralazine are vasodilators that increase CBF and therefore should not be used while the dura is closed, especially in the presence of raised ICP. In patients with symptomatic vasospasm, higher blood pressures may be tolerated.

Hypotension should be avoided at all costs and the blood pressure below which neurological deterioration occurs recorded. This can be used to guide blood pressure management intraoperatively.

Respiratory assessment

Respiratory dysfunction, common after SAH, can be the result of poor ventilatory drive, decreased level of consciousness and aspiration of stomach contents, and neurogenic pulmonary oedema. Therefore, a thorough evaluation of the respiratory system must include examination for evidence of pulmonary oedema, basal atelectasis and aspiration pneumonia. The oxygen and ventilatory requirements, arterial blood gases and chest X-ray are assessed. Patients requiring high levels of inspired oxygen and positive end-expiratory pressure to maintain borderline arterial blood gases should have their operation postponed until their respiratory function improves. Avoiding secondary hypoxaemic insults is paramount.

Volume status and blood chemistry

Autonomic hyperactivity is thought to be responsible for the reduction in plasma and red blood cell volume. Other factors include bedrest, negative nitrogen balance and diuretics. A haematocrit of 30% is considered optimum. A central venous pressure line or a pulmonary artery floatation catheter may be required to guide fluid management.

Hyponatraemia is common (10–34%) and can be associated with an impaired level of consciousness, cerebral oedema, seizures and vasospasm. Hyponatraemia may be iatrogenic because of the administration of hyponotic maintenance fluids instead of 0.9% sodium chloride. It may also result from either cerebral salt-wasting syndrome or from the syndrome of inappropriate secretion of antidiuretic hormone (SIADH). In both groups, the plasma sodium concentration is low (<134 mmol l^{-1}). Patients with salt-wasting syndrome are hypovolaemic and require fluid to prevent intravascular volume contraction. Atrial natriuretic factor may also be involved. In contrast, patients with SIADH require fluid restriction. Central venous pressure monitoring is required in these circumstances.

Normoglycaemia should be maintained, as hyperglycaemia is associated with worse neurological outcome after brain injury. Dextrose-containing solutions are best avoided and an insulin infusion may be required to control stress-induced hyperglycaemia when present.

Neurological assessment

A detailed examination to assess the level of consciousness and the presence of focal neurological deficits should be performed. Evidence of raised ICP, cerebral vasospasm, hydrocephalus and an intracranial mass effect should be sought.

Blood in the subarachnoid space may occlude the arachnoid villae and lead to the development of hydrocephalus. Mortality is higher in patients who develop hydrocephalus. Symptoms include headache, drowsiness, confusion and agitation. If hydrocephalus develops before the aneurysm has been secured, a ventricular drain may improve the neurological state of the patient. The cerebrospinal fluid (CSF) should be drained to 15–20 cmH$_2$O to avoid excess ventricular decompression, which may cause the aneurysm to re-rupture.

Seizures can occur following a SAH and lead to acute increases in blood pressure and rebleeding. When present, seizures should be controlled with anticonvulsants; however, there is currently no evidence to support the prophylactic use of anticonvulsants in patients following SAH and hence they are not routinely administered at our institution.

Medications

Pre-operative drugs are usually continued unless contraindicated; for example, diuretics are discontinued if the patient is dehydrated. Patients presenting for aneurysm surgery after SAH are usually receiving calcium-channel blockers (nimodipine) to reduce the risk of developing delayed ischaemic deficits. Therefore, relative hypotension secondary to systemic vasodilation with an increased cardiac output is not an uncommon finding in these patients. Patients must be well hydrated before general anaesthesia to prevent hypotension on induction of anaesthesia.

Pre-medication

The use of sedative pre-medications is controversial as pre- and post-operative neurological assessment may be difficult. Pre-medicants may also cause respiratory depression leading to hypercarbia, hypertension and increased CBF, CBV and ICP. Generally, grade III and V patients rarely require sedative pre-medication. Grade I and II patients may require an anxiolytic to prevent the haemodynamic fluctuations associated with anxiety. Intravenous midazolam can be administered in the anaesthetic room. Midazolam reduces the cerebral metabolic rate, and hence CBF and CBV, without significantly affecting cerebral carbon dioxide reactivity or autoregulation. However, the agent should be titrated carefully, as hypotension must be avoided. Patients at risk of aspiration will need standard antacid prophylaxis.

Monitoring

Routine monitoring will include ECG, pulse oximetry, end-tidal capnography, urinary output, and temperature. Direct blood pressure measurement is established before induction of anaesthesia, as this will allow accurate, beat-to-beat observation of blood pressure.

It will also be useful for intraoperative blood gas and haemoglobin measurements. Central venous pressure is measured in all patients presenting for aneurysm surgery to guide fluid management as these patients often receive repeated doses of diuretics and/or mannitol. A pulmonary artery catheter is used in elderly patients, those with cardiac disease and in poor-grade SAH patients, especially if hypertensive–hypervolaemic–haemodilution (triple H) therapy is contemplated.

A jugular bulb catheter measures jugular venous oxygen saturation and lactate, and is used to monitor alterations in ventilation and blood pressure. A cerebral function analysing monitor is used when burst suppression is planned (e.g. prolonged temporary clipping). An intraparenchymal probe, which measures cerebral oxygenation, carbon dioxide, pH and temperature, can be sited in the territory of the operative site by the surgeon.

Induction of anaesthesia

The aims are to titrate the depth of anaesthesia and the blood pressure to match surgical need, control ICP, minimize cerebral metabolic demands, prevent cerebral ischaemia, ensure good operating conditions and allow rapid awakening. As transmural pressure determines the likelihood of aneurysmal rupture, abrupt increases in arterial blood pressure or sudden decreases in ICP may cause a rebleed. Although rebleeding is rare during induction of anaesthesia and tracheal intubation (<0.5% at our institution), it is associated with high mortality and post-operative morbidity. Aneurysmal rupture is suspected when a sustained rise in blood pressure with or without bradycardia is observed on or shortly after induction or tracheal intubation. The surgery is best deferred for 24–48 h during which detailed assessment of the patient is made.

With the exception of ketamine, any intravenous induction agent can be used. Thiopentone, etomidate and propofol are the main agents used for induction of anaesthesia, with muscle relaxation usually achieved with vecuronium, atracurium or pancuronium. When rapid control of the airway is required, suxamethonium can be used, but it may result in a transient increase in ICP. This potential increase in ICP and its possible effect on aneurysmal rupture is balanced against the risk of aspiration, hypoxaemia and hypercapnia.

If a rapid sequence is not required, the patient's lungs are denitrogenated and anaesthesia is induced with the intravenous agent of choice in combination with a short-acting opioid (e.g. fentanyl 1 μg kg^{-1} or remifentanil 1 μg kg^{-1} followed by an infusion). The agent is titrated to blood pressure and heart rate. There is no place for high-dose opioid anaesthesia as this will result in catastrophic hypotension, cerebral vasodilation, reduced CPP and cerebral ischaemia. Once the patient is judged ready for tracheal intubation (by the use of peripheral nerve stimulator), further aliquots of induction agent, fentanyl, labetalol, esmolol or lidocaine can be used to attenuate the response to laryngoscopy and intubation. The lungs are then ventilated to mild hypocapnia at PaCO$_2$ ~4 kPa. Marked hyperventilation reduces ICP and may increase transmural pressure leading to aneurysmal rupture. The endotracheal tube is then secured, wide-bore intravenous access is established and the eyes are protected. Local anaesthesia or further doses of induction agent or opioid can be used to attenuate the response to head pin insertion. Lumbar drains, although not used routinely, may be employed for posterior circulation and giant aneurysms where a greater degree of brain retraction is anticipated. Rapid decompression should be prevented when a lumbar drain is inserted as this will lead to a sudden reduction in ICP and rebleeding. Patients are then transferred into theatre and positioned at 15–30° head up to aid venous drainage.

Maintenance

There is currently no evidence from prospective randomized trial to suggest that a particular anaesthetic technique is superior in patients undergoing aneurysm surgery. However, the 'best' anaesthetic technique produces a 'slack' brain so that retraction pressure is low while ensuring maximal cerebral protection by keeping cerebral metabolic requirements to a minimum. Those agents that maintain cerebral vasoreactivity to carbon dioxide and autoregulation may reduce fluctuations in CBF, ICP and CPP when blood pressure changes with varying surgical stimuli.

A combination of a propofol infusion and an opioid are increasingly used to maintain anaesthesia during aneurysm surgery. Propofol allows rapid adjustment of anaesthetic depth with more rapid recovery than either thiopentone or isoflurane. Propofol has no intrinsic vasodilatory effect and therefore does not result in increases in CBF, CBV or ICP. It also reduces the cerebral metabolic rate, with cortical structures being depressed to a greater extent than subcortical structures, and may be neuroprotective.

Inhalational anaesthetic agents have a dual effect on CBF: a reduction consequential to the decrease in cerebral metabolism and an increase secondary to their direct cerebral vasodilatory effect. The 'net' effect of an inhalational agent on CBF is therefore dependent on the level of cerebral metabolism at the time the agent is introduced. When cerebral metabolism is low, as in patients with SAH grades III or IV, the net effect may be vasodilatory, with increases in CBF and ICP accompanying the introduction of the agent. However, in patients with good-grade SAH I or II in whom cerebral metabolism is high, inhalational agents primarily reduce CBF secondary to the reduction in cerebral metabolism. Therefore, inhalational agents can be used safely in patients with good-grade SAH. When there is uncertainty about the level of cerebral metabolism, or when sign of significant cerebral oedema is present, total intravenous anaesthesia is the preferred option.

Inhalational agents with the exception of sevoflurane impair autoregulation in a dose-dependent manner. Therefore, isoflurane in concentrations <1.0% can be used to supplement intravenous anaesthesia. The epileptic activity of enflurane prevents its use in neurosurgery. Desflurane increases ICP and this may be related to its sympathoadrenal effects. Sevoflurane has been shown not to alter cerebral autoregulation in concentrations up to 1.5 MAC (minimum alveolar concentration).

Nitrous oxide (N$_2$O) has a number of advantages. It has a rapid onset and offset, easy to use and relatively inexpensive. However, its routine use in neuroanaesthesia is discouraged at our institution, as there is evidence to suggest that N$_2$O increases ICP and CBF by stimulating cerebral metabolism. Although N$_2$O increased CBF velocity when used in combination with isoflurane, this effect can be attenuated by hyperventilation and propofol.

Opioids generally have negligible effects on CBF and metabolism. However, the newer synthetic opioids fentanyl, sufentanil, alfentanil and remifentanil can increase ICP in patients with tumours and head trauma. This increase, originally assumed to be secondary to an increase in CBF, is more likely to be the result of changes in PaCO$_2$ and systemic hypotension. Irrespective of the actual mechanism causing the increase in ICP, these observations underscore the importance of administering these agents judiciously and carefully to avoid systemic hypotension. Fentanyl, with its medium duration of action and its negligible cerebral vascular effects, is the agent of choice in many neurosurgical intensive care units. Remifentanil, a new opioid with a rapid onset and short half-life, is being investigated for neurosurgery. Remifentanil appears to compare favourably with fentanyl in patients undergoing elective supratentorial surgery. We have shown that remifentanil, when combined with 0.5 MAC sevoflurane, does not alter cerebral autoregulation in individuals undergoing non-intracranial neurosurgical procedures.

Brain relaxation

The aim is to produce a 'slack' brain so that retraction pressure can be kept to a minimum. There are several methods employed to reduce the brain bulk, CSF volume and CBV. These include a 15–30° head-up position, mild hypocarbia (~4 kPa), mannitol and furosemide.

Mannitol is an osmotic diuretic used to reduce cerebral tissue water. It is usually administered (0.5–1.0 g kg^{-1}) as a 20% solution. Mannitol probably acts on all three intracranial compartments via different mechanisms. It may reduce brain bulk by osmotic dehydration, CBV by improving rheology of red blood cells and thus decreasing blood viscosity, and CSF production. Mannitol is also a free-radical scavenger. Mannitol's high osmolarity causes an immediate but transient increase in intravascular volume, CBF, CBV and ICP. This is followed by a reduction in ICP and CBV, which is maximum at 45–60 min. Therefore, care must be taken when administering mannitol to patients with poor cardiac function as they may develop congestive cardiac failure and pulmonary oedema. Furosemide can be used in conjunction with mannitol or it can be used alone in those patients with poor myocardial function who may be sent into cardiac failure with mannitol. Hypertonic saline has been advocated as an alternative to mannitol, although its action is transient and its overall effects remain untested in SAH.

The potential ischaemic effects of marked hyperventilation must be balanced against the benefits of reducing CBV. When used properly, hyperventilation is a quick and effective tool for reducing CBV, provided a measure of cerebral oxygenation is employed. Although it cannot detect regional ischaemia, jugular bulb oximetry (measuring bulb venous oxygen saturation, SjO$_2$) will reflect the balance between cerebral oxygen supply and demand. It is probably unwise to induce hypocapnia if SjO$_2$ is <50%.

Cerebral blood volume can also be reduced pharmacologically by reducing cerebral metabolism and hence CBF. This is achieved by bolus intravenous administration of thiopentone (3–5 mg kg^{-1}), propofol (1–2 mg kg^{-1}) or lidocaine (1.5 mg kg^{-1}). If brain condition improves after the bolus, a continuous infusion is started.

The amount of fluid given intraoperatively depends on the maintenance requirements, blood loss and filling pressures. Urine output is a poor marker of circulatory volume in the presence of mannitol and furosemide. We maintain hypervolaemia prior to clipping to optimize CBF and reduce the effects of perioperative vasospasm.

Hyponatraemia is associated with an increased incidence of delayed ischaemic neurological deficits, and glucose solutions are avoided as they may worsen cerebral acidaemia and ischaemia. With difficult aneurysms, measures are taken to reduce the transmural pressure across the wall of the aneurysm before a permanent clip is placed. This reduces the risk of rupture and the rate of bleeding should the aneurysm rupture during dissection. There are two methods by which this can be achieved: deliberate hypotension and temporary clipping.

- *Deliberate hypotension*. Although the use of induced hypotension during surgical clipping of cerebral aneurysms is in decline, many North American neurosurgical centres continue to use it regularly. Hypotension increases 'slack' in the structures around the aneurysm and aneurysmal sac and decreases the risk of rupture during surgical dissection and clipping of the aneurysm. Hypotension also decreases bleeding from surrounding small vessels, which allows better visualization of the anatomy of the aneurysm and the perforating vessels. Some of the drugs used include isoflurane, thiopentone (3–5 mg kg^{-1}), propofol (1–4 mg kg^{-1}), labetalol in 5–10 mg increments, esmolol and sodium nitroprusside. The mean arterial pressure (MAP) is not usually reduced below 50 mmHg in normotensive individuals, and chronically hypertensive patients may require a higher mean pressure (systolic is best kept greater than the pre-operative diastolic value). However, there are numerous problems associated with deliberate hypotension. Many SAH patients will have impaired autoregulation or cerebral vasospasm, and hypotension may therefore lead to focal or global cerebral ischaemia. Furthermore, the ischaemic threshold cannot be predicted accurately. Hypotension is rarely employed at our institution.

- *Temporary clipping.* This is the preferred technique in our unit. When exposure of the aneurysm is difficult and temporary clip placement is anticipated, maximal cerebral protection is aimed for: moderate hypothermia (33°C), induced hypertension (20% above baseline) and propofol- or thiopentone-induced burst suppression. A temporary clip occludes the vessels feeding the aneurysm and reduces transmural pressure, thus decreasing the risk of rupture. Although the safe length of time temporary clipping can be used before cerebral infarction occurs is unknown, the risk of infarction increases with the duration of clip application and varies from 15–120 min. Factors thought to contribute to new neurological deficit include age >61 years and poor pre-operative neurological condition.

Cerebral protection

Various cerebroprotective methods have been used including hypothermia, additional doses of intravenous or inhalational anaesthetics, deliberate hypertension, and drugs such as mannitol, phenytoin and calcium-channel blockers. These methods may be used routinely or their use may be guided by changes to the EEG or evoked potentials. Although the exact mechanism for neuroprotective action of anaesthetic agents is not fully understood, barbiturates and propofol may produce their effect by reducing the cerebral metabolic rate. However, doses of intravenous anaesthetic high enough to suppress EEG activity cause marked cardiovascular depression. The cerebral protective effects of barbiturates may be secondary to their ability to reduce calcium influx, inhibit free radical formation, potentiate γ-aminobutyric acid (GABA)-ergic activity, reduce cerebral oedema and inhibit glucose transfer across the blood–brain barrier.

In contrast to pharmacological agents that only reduce the active component of cerebral metabolism, hypothermia reduces both the active and basal components, thereby increasing the period of ischaemia tolerated. Cerebral metabolism is approximately 15% of normal at 20°C. Despite the long-held view that hypothermia may be protective, the routine use of moderate hypothermia during surgical clipping of cerebral aneurysms failed to demonstrate a benefit. Problems associated with hypothermia include reliability of temperature measurement, the optimal temperature needed to offer the best benefit:risk ratio and the best method of rewarming the patient safely so that normothermic temperatures are reached before emergence. Other problems include delayed awakening, post-operative shivering, coagulation disorders and aggravation of myocardial disease.

Ketamine, an *N*-methyl-D-aspartate (NMDA) receptor antagonist, has been traditionally avoided in neurosurgery because it increases CBF and ICP. However, NMDA receptor antagonists can prevent neuronal injury by decreasing cellular influx of calcium. There is renewed interest in the use of ketamine for neuroanaesthesia as it has been shown to be neuroprotective in an experimental head-injured rat model. Furthermore, when ketamine is administered ($1\,mg\,kg^{-1}$) during isoflurane and N_2O anaesthesia in mechanically ventilated patients it reduced ICP, CBF velocity and total EEG power. The role of ketamine in neuroprotection requires further evaluation.

Induced hypertension

This is often employed to improve collateral blood flow during temporary clipping and in patients with areas of critical perfusion. Adequate volume loading and inotropes such as dopamine are often sufficient for producing the desired hypertension. However, in patients with abnormal autoregulation, CBF is pressure dependent and increases in MAP will increase CBF and may result in blood–brain barrier damage and vasogenic oedema. Patients with myocardial disease or unsecured aneurysms are at risk for myocardial ischaemia and aneurysm rupture, respectively.

Intraoperative rupture

If the aneurysm ruptures intraoperatively, intravenous fluids are increased to maintain the CPP. Cerebral protection is provided by propofol- or thiopentone-induced EEG burst suppression. Normovolaemia must be maintained. The afferent and efferent blood vessels supplying the aneurysm may be temporarily occluded by the surgeon. However, if bleeding persists, a short period of induced hypotension may be used to facilitate control.

Giant aneurysms and circulatory arrest

Approximately 2% of cerebral aneurysms are >2.5 cm in diameter. These giant aneurysms are a challenge because of their size, the lack of an anatomic neck and the perforating vessels that often originate from their walls. They often present with symptoms of mass lesion such as headaches and nerve palsies. Although improvements in microsurgical techniques and neuroanaesthesia have improved outcome considerably after giant aneurysm surgery, the morbidity and mortality remains higher than that after surgery for smaller aneurysms. Three main techniques are used: temporary clipping, hypothermic circulatory arrest and arterial bypass surgery (e.g. extracranial to intracranial (EC-IC) bypass).

Circulatory arrest ensures haemorrhage during dissection and exposure of the aneurysm is minimized. After induction of anaesthesia, and with all routine monitors in place, surface cooling is started. Barbiturates are administered to induce and maintain burst suppression (5 mg kg^{-1} bolus followed by 5–10 mg kg^{-1} h^{-1} infusion). Haemodilution to a haematocrit of 30% is achieved by collecting blood and administering cold intravenous saline containing potassium. After the aneurysm is dissected, femoral-artery-to-vein bypass is established following the administration of heparin 300 IU kg^{-1} aiming for an activated clotting time (ACT) between 450 and 500 s. The patient is cooled to 18°C. Cardiac fibrillation, which commonly begins at temperatures <28°C, is stopped by potassium chloride. Once the desired temperature is reached and the EEG is isoelectric, circulatory arrest is performed. This should only be for the duration of clip application and should not exceed 60 min. Once the aneurysm is secured, bypass is re-established and warming at a rate not exceeding 0.5°C min^{-1} proceeds with the help of a vasodilator (sodium nitroprusside). Normal sinus rhythm is established by cardioversion when the heart fibrillates and by the administration of anti-arrhythmic drugs. Bypass is discontinued when the patient's temperature reaches 36°C. Heparin is reversed with protamine and coagulation factors, and blood is administered as necessary. The bypass is best coordinated with a cardiac anaesthetist.

Arteriovenous malformations

Arteriovenous malformations are congenital abnormalities that shunt blood from the arterial to the venous side with flow rates out of proportion to the low metabolism within this abnormal vascular network. The majority of AVMs are supratentorial and superficial. In approximately 5% of cases, they are found in association with cerebral aneurysms. While the risk of bleeding averages 2% per year, the risk of rebleeding is closer to 5% per year.

Patients with AVMs commonly present with intracranial haemorrhage and less frequently with seizures, headaches and/or signs of intracranial hypertension. In our institution, the majority of AVMs are embolized and only small superficial ones are resected surgically. The embolization is carried out as staged procedures over a period of several weeks. The AVM 'feeder' vessels are characterized by high blood flow, low resistance, low perfusion pressure and decreased carbon dioxide reactivity. Embolization or resection of the AVM results in normalization of flow velocity and carbon dioxide reactivity.

The principles of intraoperative management are similar to those already described for aneurysm surgery. A notable exception is the meticulous control of blood pressure control both intra- and post-operatively. It is well recognized that some patients are at risk of brain swelling and haemorrhage after AVM resection. Risk factors include the volume of the AVM (>20 cm^3), the presence of deep feeders, the location of the AVM (rolandic, inferior limbic and insular region) and the pre-excision mean feeder transcranial Doppler flow velocity (>120 cm s^{-1}). According to the normal perfusion pressure breakthrough theory initially proposed by Spetzler and colleagues, the hyperaemia occurs as a result of the loss of autoregulatory capacity in normal brain tissue adjacent to the AVM. However, Young and colleagues were not able to demonstrate this loss of autoregulation with xenon wash-out studies, and occlusive hyperaemia has been proposed as the cause of this hyperperfusion. Regardless of the underlying mechanism, there is little doubt that brain swelling/haemorrhage that occurs after AVM resection is related to an increase in hemispheric perfusion, and the only effective treatment is adequate control of blood pressure and optimal cerebral vasoconstriction. High-dose propofol infusion and labetalol are effective in controlling blood pressure.

Recovery

In patients with initial good-grade SAH, a rapid return of consciousness is aimed for to allow early neurological assessment. Provided no untoward events occurred intraoperatively, grade I and II patients are extubated. In patients with WFNS grade III, recovery depends on their pre-operative conscious level and ventilatory state. Grade IV and V patients are usually transferred to the neurocritical care unit for a 24–48 h period of elective post-operative ventilation.

When surgery is complete, the anaesthetic agents are discontinued and 100% oxygen is given. Residual neuromuscular blockade is reversed, the airway suctioned and the patient extubated on regaining consciousness. Boluses of short-acting opioids, propofol or lidocaine can be used to facilitate extubation and control the blood pressure. Uncontrolled hypertension in the immediate post-operative phase can precipitate ICH. In patients with unsecured aneurysms, the blood pressure is kept to within 20% of normal. If the patient remains hypertensive (systolic pressure >200 mmHg) in recovery despite adequate pain relief, esmolol, labetalol or nifedipine are used.

If the patient fails to regain their pre-operative neurological state, the following need to be excluded:

- Anaesthetic causes (partial neuromuscular blockade)
- Residual narcotic and sedative drugs
- Hypoxia and hypercarbia
- Metabolic factors (hyponatraemia)
- Post-ictal state.

It is important that the airway is not compromised post-operatively so that hypercapnia and hypoxaemia are avoided. Reintubation will be required in those patients unable to protect their airway or maintain adequate gas exchange. Once the above possible causes have been excluded, a CT scan is performed to exclude hydrocephalus, cerebral oedema, intracranial haemorrhage, haematoma or a rebleed (multiple aneurysms). If the scan is negative, a cerebral angiogram is required to exclude vascular occlusion (e.g. misplaced clip). Vasospasm can be detected using transcranial Doppler.

All patients are transferred to the neurocritical care unit or high-dependency unit for their post-operative management. Cerebral vasospasm and delayed ischaemic neurological deficits remain the major post-operative complication once the aneurysm has been clipped. The management of this condition is described in Chapter 22.

Interventional neuroradiological treatment of vascular abnormalities

Interventional neuroradiology is being used increasingly to treat central nervous system (CNS) disease by either delivering therapeutic devices (coils, stents or glue) or by administering drugs at the point of need (e.g. thrombolytics in acute ischaemic stroke). As a result of this, the demand for administering neuro-anaesthetics in the radiology suite is on the increase. Recent evidence (from the International Subarachnoid Aneurysm Trial (ISAT)) supports the use of the international normalized ratio (INR) for the treatment of SAH due to aneurysm rupture, with improvements in mortality and morbidity in the short and long term.

The neuroangiography suite presents a unique environment for the anaesthetist. It is often isolated from other hospital areas, the patient is distant from the anaesthetist and the fluoroscopy tube presents both a radiation hazard and a physical obstacle when accessing the patient's airway. Nonetheless, it should be equipped for the anaesthetized patient similar to the operating theatre. Piped gases, suction, an anaesthetic machine and an anaesthetic assistant must be available. Anaesthetic, radiological equipment and monitors should be organized to allow both procedures to take place with minimum disruption to team members. All staff are potentially exposed to radiation either from the tube or from scatter. Team members need to understand the principles of radiation safety and must wear personal protective devices. This is best achieved by the use of 0.5 mm thick lead aprons, and only entering the screening area when necessary. At all other times, the patient should be monitored from behind a glass leaded screen. Dosimeter badges should be worn and checked on a regular basis.

Pre-operative assessment

Patients may present as an emergency (as an intensive care patient) or for an elective procedure in good health. A detailed anaesthetic assessment, similar to the process already described earlier on in this chapter, is mandatory. This should include previous anaesthetic history, past medical history and medications. A detailed airway assessment is mandatory to prepare for anticipated difficult intubation in the isolated environment. Routine investigations must include a full blood count, coagulation studies, urea and electrolytes, and ECG. Further investigations may include chest X-ray, CT head, echocardiography and transcranial Doppler, and others as appropriate. Particular attention should be paid to any previous exposure or allergy to contrast media, protamine and shellfish. Anticoagulation history is of particular importance as these patients are often on dual antiplatelet therapy. All female patients of childbearing age must have their pregnancy status established with a pregnancy test if necessary. If there is a significant chance of the patient being pregnant, extra radiation protection must be available. For those patients with SAH secondary to ruptured aneurysm, the pre-operative assessment is otherwise exactly the same as those presenting for craniotomy and clipping. This has been described in detail earlier in this chapter.

Anaesthetic management

As interventional neuroradiology is a relatively painless procedure some centres choose to use conscious sedation instead of general anaesthesia, although the overall trend is towards general anaesthesia. No single technique has been shown to be superior. As with other neuroanaesthetic procedures, rapid recovery is necessary to accurately assess the patient's neurological status post-operatively. The same principles apply to pre-medication for interventional neuroradiology as for craniotomy in patients with cerebrovascular abnormalities. Importantly, patients should not omit nimodipine prior to intervention.

Monitoring

Routine monitoring (pulse oximetry, non-invasive blood pressure, ECG, end-tidal carbon dioxide and gas analysis) as for any general anaesthetic is mandatory. A peripheral nerve stimulator should be used to assess muscle relaxation during the procedure and suitability of reversal at the end of the procedure. In addition, temperature monitoring is used, as the procedure may be long and the ambient temperature in the neuroradiology suite is often cold. Methods to warm the patient should be available and normothermia should be maintained. A urinary catheter is useful, as a diuretic reaction to the contrast media used and from fluid loading is common. Invasive blood pressure monitoring may often be required prior to induction of anaesthesia, and provides beat-to-beat blood pressure monitoring at times of anticipated haemodynamic instability. It is also a convenient way for the interventional team to take blood to assess anticoagulation. If it is difficult to site a radial arterial catheter, it is possible to transduce the femoral artery introducer sheath, although this can result in underestimation of systolic and overestimation of diastolic blood pressures. The mean arterial pressure is more reliable. Central venous pressure measurement is often not required, as fluid shifts and major blood loss are not anticipated during interventional procedures. However, should the cardiac status

of the patient require central venous access, it should be sited prior to the procedure and its position can be checked using fluoroscopy in suite. Neurophysiological monitoring may be considered, but its sensitivity in all vascular territories is poor, results can be altered by general anaesthesia and it requires the constant presence of a neurophysiologist or technician. Hence, it is not widely used. Transcranial Doppler may provide more information about cerebral vasospasm but again is not widely used.

The intravenous and intra-arterial access should be easily accessible at all times during the procedure. This often means siting all lines in the same arm, usually on the side opposite to the radiologist. It is advisable to have two secure lines. Extension tubing for all lines will be required. The drug effect may be delayed after administration due to passage through the extension tubing before reaching the patient.

Interventional neuroradiological procedures are long and require the patient to lie supine and motionless. Lying still for long periods of time can be uncomfortable and the procedure can be psychologically stressful. Some units use intravenous sedation. A number of techniques have been used. The technique chosen depends on the experience of the anaesthetist and the goals of the sedation/procedure. Regimens include intermittent midazolam and fentanyl boluses, low-dose propofol infusion ($25–75\,\mu g\;kg^{-1}\;min^{-1}$), remifentanil ($0.03–0.1\,\mu g\;kg^{-1}\;min^{-1}$), or dexmedetomidine ($0.3–0.7\,\mu g\;kg^{-1}\;h^{-1}$). There is a risk of upper airway obstruction with this technique, with subsequent hypoxia and hypercapnia. A nasopharyngeal airway in an anticoagulated patient should be avoided. Another potential problem is behavioural disturbance and disinhibition leading to movement and loss of imaging quality, and of course the risk of aneurysm rupture if the microcatheter tip is at or in the aneurysm. Patients with movement disorders and poorly controlled epilepsy are not suitable candidates for sedation techniques.

General anaesthesia

General anaesthesia with endotracheal intubation is being increasingly employed. Again, the aim during induction of general anaesthesia is maintenance of adequate CPP while avoiding sudden and profound changes to the transmembrane pressure gradient of cerebral aneurysms. One should also avoid changes to perfusion across AVMs and their surrounding tissue. Dysfunctional autoregulation can cause cerebral ischaemia or hyperperfusion with small changes in systolic pressure. A combination of 'sleep'-dose propofol and an opiate is a reliable induction technique. Alfentanil up to $10\,\mu g\ kg^{-1}$, fentanyl 0.1–$0.2\,\mu g\ kg^{-1}$ or remifentanil 0.05–$0.5\,\mu g\ kg^{-1}\ min^{-1}$ have all been used at induction. Muscle relaxation and endotracheal intubation are achieved with atracurium ($0.5\,mg\ kg^{-1}$), vecuronium ($0.1\,mg\ kg^{-1}$) or rocuronium ($0.5\,mg\ kg^{-1}$).

The goals of anaesthesia during interventional neuroradiological procedures are the same as for aneurysm clipping: haemodynamic stability, avoidance of rises in ICP and complete immobility. The choice of anaesthetic agents and techniques are similar to those described earlier for aneurysm surgery. On the whole, the procedure is unstimulating and anaesthetic requirements are low. There are predictable points of stimulation, namely femoral cannulation, manipulation of the microcatheter in the cerebral vessels and injection of contrast material. Deep anaesthesia can result in hypotension, which must be avoided, especially during aneurysm intervention, and slow 'awakening'. While every attempt is made to avoid hypotension, essential or reactive hypertension may require treatment to prevent cerebral oedema or rebleeding. In these cases, a short-acting agent that can readily be titrated to effect should be chosen. Labetalol and esmolol have both been used successfully with little direct effect on the cerebral vasculature.

Anticoagulation

During the procedure, the patient is anticoagulated to prevent thromboembolic complications. A baseline ACT is taken shortly after femoral cannulation. Heparin is administered before insertion of the first coil/intervention, commonly as a bolus of 70–$100\,U\ kg^{-1}$, with the intention of producing a prolonged ACT of two to three times baseline. This is maintained with further boluses or a continuous infusion of heparin throughout the procedure. If there is no response to heparin, porcine heparin instead of bovine can be used. Fresh frozen plasma may be required if the patient has or is suspected to have antithrombin III deficiency. Heparinization may need to be reversed either at the end of the procedure or in the emergency setting, and protamine should be available. In addition to heparin, many patients listed for carotid stenting will also be receiving antiplatelet agents – aspirin and/or clopidogrel. In the event of haemorrhagic complications (cerebrovascular accident or those requiring surgery),

platelets should be ordered and the case discussed urgently with the haematology consultant. Other antiplatelet agents that have been used in coronary stenting (glycoprotein IIb/IIIa receptor antagonists, ticlopidine) have not found favour in interventional neuroradiology.

Deliberate alterations of blood pressure

Deliberate hypotension can sometimes be required to slow down forward flow in the feeding artery, or back flow in the draining vein of an AVM as glue is injected. High blood flow risks pulmonary embolization of glue. It is also used to assess cerebrovascular reserve prior to proximal vessel occlusion procedures. The drug of choice should be short acting, have predictable actions and be rapidly reversible. Increasing anaesthetic depth has been used, as have specific antihypertensives such as β-blockade, sodium nitroprusside, hydralazine and nitroglycerine.

During periods of acute vascular occlusion or vasospasm, induced hypertension can maintain cerebral perfusion by increasing flow across the circle of Willis, as discussed earlier in the chapter.

Intraprocedural complications

The ISAT trial has resulted in the majority of intracranial aneurysms being treated in the neuroradiology suite. Aneurysm rupture can occur spontaneously, during induction of anaesthesia and intubation, or during the procedure. Small leaks may be tolerated with little change in either the haemodynamics or ICP. Larger leaks need prompt treatment to improve outcome. Clear communication between the radiologist and anaesthetist is essential. Rupture may be diagnosed by identification of extravascular contrast material, or by hypertension (with or without bradycardia) as ICP rises. Procedural rupture may occur on insertion of the microcatheter or the coils. Anticoagulation should be reversed and arterial blood pressure supported. Control of haemorrhage may be achieved by rapid deployment of coils. If this is not possible, the anaesthetist must prepare the patient, surgeon and the theatre for urgent transfer and surgical intervention.

Patients with SAH undergoing interventional radiological procedures are at risk for developing cerebral vasospasm. Patients will already be receiving oral nimodipine and this should be continued throughout the perioperative period. In those with established vasospasms, 'chemical angioplasty' can be achieved by the intra-arterial administration of repeated doses of papaverine. Papaverine has a number of adverse CNS side effects including seizures, cerebral haemorrhage and new neurological deficits. Other intraluminal agents have been assessed with varying degrees of success in the short and longer term, including magnesium sulfate, 3-hydroxy-3-methylglutaryl-CoA reductase inhibitors and nitric oxide donors. Clinical trials have shown marked prevention of vasospasm with clazosentan, an endothelin receptor antagonist, yet patient outcome was not improved.

Triple H therapy – namely hypertension, hypervolaemia and haemodilution – can be used to attempt to improve CBF. However, while potentially improving CBF, the effects of high-dose vasopressors on other organ systems must be considered, and a balance between brain and other vital organ perfusion met.

Angioplasty of the affected vasospastic vessels may be performed when medical management is unsuccessful. A compliant balloon that will conform to the vessel wall and exert a low dilation pressure to resolve the spasm is inserted via the femoral vessels and positioned at the level of the vessel with vasospasms. Although often successful initially, this benefit seems to be short lived and has not been shown to affect patient outcome.

Anaesthesia for carotid endarterectomy

Carotid endarterectomy (CEA) prevents strokes in patients with symptomatic severe (>70%) internal carotid artery (ICA) stenosis. Its effectiveness remains debatable in asymptomatic patients or in those with mild or moderate stenosis. As the aim of CEA is to prevent stroke, the major indications for CEA are recurrent strokes, transient ischaemic attacks (TIA) and reversible ischaemic neurological deficit (RIND). Patients with carotid stenosis often have concurrent coronary artery disease and are at 6% risk of stroke or death 30 days after the procedure. The prevalence of moderate ICA stenosis (>50% reduction in lumen diameter) rises from about 0.5% in people in their 50s to around 10% in those over the age of 80 years. As the incidence of coronary artery disease also increases with age, it is not surprising that the major cause of mortality and morbidity from CEA is MI, accounting for almost 50% of post-operative deaths. Irrespective of the surgical and anaesthetic technique used, the procedure-related risk of stroke or death should be <3% in asymptomatic

Table 13.3 Perioperative risk factors

Medical risk factors
• Angina
• Myocardial infarction within 6 months of surgery
• Congestive cardiac failure
• Uncontrolled hypertension
• Advanced peripheral vascular disease
• Chronic obstructive pulmonary disease
• Obesity
Neurological risk factors
• Progressive neurological deficit
• Recent deficit (within 24 h)
• Active transient ischaemic attacks
• Recent cerebral infarction (<7 days)
• Generalized cerebral ischaemia
Angiographic risk factors
• Contralateral occlusion of internal carotid artery (ICA)
• Coexisting ipsilateral carotid siphon disease
• Extensive plaque extension >3 cm distally or >5 cm proximally
• Thrombus extending from an ulcerative lesion
• Carotid bifurcation at cervical vertebral level C2 with short thick ICA

patients and <6% in symptomatic patients. A complication rate exceeding these figures should prompt a review of the surgical and/or anaesthetic technique. Angioplasty and stenting of carotid stenosis, increasing in popularity, may be as effective and safe as CEA in selected patients, particularly in those who have undergone previous carotid artery surgery.

Pre-operative assessment

Patients with carotid artery atheroma and embolic phenomena should be considered for urgent surgery. These patients are at high risk of developing neurological and cardiac post-operative complications. Many models have been proposed to assess this risk and some are summarized in Tables 13.3 and 13.4. Although the risk factors in individuals vary, patients with the greatest risk are also those most likely to suffer a severe stroke and they therefore have the most to gain from prophylactic surgery.

Patients presenting for carotid surgery are elderly and often have coexisting medical problems common

Table 13.4 Grading of patients undergoing carotid endarterectomy

Grade	Neurological findings	Medical findings	Angiographic risk	Risk of MI/RND
1	Stable	No defined risk	No major risk	1%
2	Stable	No defined risk	No major risk	2%
3	Stable	Major risk	With or without risk	7%
4	Unstable	With or without risk	With or without risk	10%

Patients are at increased risk if they have suffered an acute internal carotid artery occlusion or recurrent carotid stenosis having previously undergone carotid endarterectomy.
MI, myocardial infarction; RND, residual neurological deficit.

to patients with vascular disease. These include coronary artery disease, chronic pulmonary airway disease and diabetes mellitus. As part of the routine pre-operative assessment, special emphasis should be laid on a thorough evaluation of the cardiovascular system, neurological system, respiratory system and endocrine system.

Cardiovascular system

Stroke and TIA are markers of general atherosclerosis. Many patients presenting for CEA will have concomitant coronary artery disease and up to 20% have a history of MI. In one reported series following over 9000 patients, cardiac complications (either myocardial, unstable angina, pulmonary oedema or ventricular tachycardia) occurred in 3.9% and was associated with a greater risk of post-operative stroke or death. The cardiac risk is further increased by other associated medical conditions such as hypertension and obesity. The high prevalence of coronary artery disease, as determined by history, ECG or cardiac catheterization present in over 55% of these patients, is responsible for the increased risk of post-operative MI (5%) when compared with those patients without coronary artery disease (0.5%). Evidence of cardiac disease should be sought by careful history and thorough examination, noting the presence of angina and its severity, previous MI, and symptoms and signs of cardiac failure. The ECG should be examined for abnormalities of rhythm and evidence of previous infarction and ischaemia. When indicated, a chest radiograph is examined for evidence of cardiac failure. Further cardiac work-up, including an exercise ECG, radionuclide studies or coronary angiography, may be necessary and is best coordinated with a cardiologist. In order to assess the risk to patients with coronary artery disease having non-cardiac surgery, a number of risk indexes have been proposed, the most common of which are the American Society of Anesthesiologists

(ASA) index, the Goldman index, the Detsky index and the Revised Cardiac Risk (RCR) index. However, there are two scores specific to CEA – the Tu score and the Halm score. These scores have been compared for their ability to predict complications specifically following CEA. The Halm score CEA-specific risk model and the RCR index were found to be most favourable. In addition the Vascular Anaesthesia Society of Great Britain and Ireland has produced an on-line risk calculator to help in the assessment of risk to your patient.

Hypertension must be well controlled in the pre- and post-operative period. Poorly controlled hypertension (blood pressure >170/95) is associated with post-operative hypertension and transient neurological deficits. Therefore, unless urgent, surgery should not be performed in poorly controlled hypertensive patients, and sudden normalization of blood pressure should be avoided to reduce the risk of hypoperfusion and stroke. In some unstable patients, combined coronary artery bypass and CEA may be necessary and are discussed later in this chapter.

Neurological system

Evaluation of the cerebrovascular system should document carefully the presence of transient or permanent neurological deficit. This is essential for assessing post-operative progress as well as quantifying perioperative risk of stroke. Frequent daily TIAs, multiple neurological deficits secondary to cerebral infarctions or a progressive neurological deficit increase the risk of a new post-operative neurological deficit. The results of tests assessing the cerebral vascular system such as a Duplex ultrasound scan, cerebral angiography and carbon dioxide reactivity should be available.

Respiratory system

Chronic obstructive pulmonary disease is often present in these patients and needs optimal medical treatment pre-operatively, which may include bronchodilators, corticosteroids, physiotherapy and incentive spirometry. Cigarette smoking should be stopped 6–8 weeks pre-operatively. If necessary, pre-operative pulmonary function tests such as peak expiratory flow rate, FVC/FEV1 (forced vital capacity/forced expiratory volume in 1 s) ratio and a baseline arterial blood gas analysis with the patient breathing air should be carried out to guide perioperative care of the patient.

Endocrine system

Diabetes mellitus has been shown to exist in about 20% of patients presenting for CEA and most of these patients are insulin dependent. Adequate blood glucose control with absence of ketoacidosis pre-operatively must be established. In experimental studies, even modest elevations in blood glucose have been shown to augment post-ischaemic cerebral injury. Manifestations of diabetes mellitus such as renal failure, silent MI, autonomic and sensory neuropathy, and ophthalmic complications must be looked for.

Medications

It is very important that the patient's pre-operative medications are reviewed. These patients are often receiving cardiac and antihypertensive drugs, antiplatelet agents, antacids, steroids, insulin and anticoagulants. Antihypertensives should be given, but the anaesthetist needs to be aware of and anticipate the hypotension that may occur on induction of anaesthesia. A sliding scale may be required to ensure tight control of blood glucose levels. Antiplatelet and anticoagulant agents are common in this population; usually aspirin is continued, but warfarin is discontinued. The need for clopidogrel should be discussed with the surgeon, but it should be continued for carotid stenting.

Anaesthetic management

The aim of the perioperative anaesthetic management is to minimize the risk of occurrence of the two major complications, namely cerebrovascular accident and MI. Strokes can be either haemodynamic or embolic in origin. GALA, a multicentre randomized controlled trial set up to determine whether perioperative stroke could be both predicted and avoided more easily in an awake patient than in one receiving a general anaesthetic, failed to establish a difference between the two groups. No randomized clinical trial has identified a superior anaesthetic technique. Therefore, many of the

anaesthetic techniques advocated, including the one provided here, are the result of indirect evidence based on animal data or surrogate end points, and are biased by personal experience.

Pre-medication

A good rapport should be established with the patient in the pre-operative period. This will help to reduce anxiety, which may exacerbate perioperative blood pressure abnormalities with increased risk of myocardial ischaemia and cardiac arrhythmias. An anxiolytic pre-medicant is especially important in those patients undergoing the procedure under regional or local blockade. Regional anaesthesia allows neurological assessment during and immediately following the procedure but necessitates judicious use of pre-operative sedation. A balance must be struck between adequate sedation and 'oversedation' as the latter depresses neurological function. Oversedation often leads to hypoventilation with carbon dioxide retention and blood pressure abnormalities, often with detrimental effects on the cerebral circulation. Benzodiazepine is used routinely in our institution for pre-medication.

Regional or local versus general anaesthesia

The type of anaesthetic used seems to depend on individual practice rather than hard evidence. Local anaesthesia or a cervical plexus block allows evaluation of neurological status during carotid cross-clamping to assess the need for shunting and therefore prevention of stroke from hypoperfusion. However, perioperative strokes are more likely to be embolic than low flow in origin. Other potential advantages include a lower incidence of post-operative hypertension and a reduced need for vasoactive drugs with a shorter stay in the ICU. Unfortunately, this technique has numerous disadvantages. It requires patient cooperation and the ability to remain supine for the duration of the procedure. Many of the patients presenting for CEA are unable to lie flat and not cough for the duration of surgery. The procedure may be uncomfortable for the patient, many of whom would prefer to be unaware during surgery. Anxiety, especially with the proximity of the surgical drapes, may lead to hyperventilation with a concomitant reduction in CBF and increased risk of cerebral ischaemia. Autonomic responses to surgical manipulation of the carotid bulb may be excessive, resulting in hypotension, hypertension or bradycardia. There is also an ever-present risk of airway obstruction, as well as the occurrence of nausea and vomiting. Uncontrolled haemorrhage or sudden neurological deterioration may require general anaesthesia with rapid tracheal intubation. Nevertheless, when used properly in carefully selected patients by experienced surgeons, regional anaesthesia has a good safety record and is not associated with any increase in the rate of perioperative MI.

Regional or local anaesthesia

The patient is attached to all the standard monitors as for general anaesthesia. An appropriate dose of sedation is given. Regional anaesthesia is achieved with a deep cervical plexus block. This may be performed by a single injection or a multiple injection technique (performed by the surgeon). For the single injection technique, the patient is placed supine with the head turned to the opposite side. The area is prepped and draped. The lateral margin of the clavicular head of the sternocleidomastoid muscle is identified at the level of C4 (level with the superior margin of thyroid cartilage). The middle and index fingers are rolled laterally over the anterior scalene muscle until the interscalene groove, between the anterior and middle scalene muscle, is palpated. Asking the patient to lift the head off the table slowly may further enhance the groove. After raising a skin wheal with 1% lidocaine, a short-bevel needle is inserted between the palpating fingers, perpendicular to all levels and slightly caudad in direction until paresthesia is elicited. Ultrasound can be used to confirm position and identify the nerves. After careful aspiration, 5–6 ml of local anaesthetic suitable for the duration of surgery is injected (1% lidocaine or 0.5% bupivacaine with 1:200,000 epinephrine). The local anaesthetic should spread in the fascial sheath extending from the cervical transverse processes to beyond the axilla, investing the cervical plexus in between the middle and anterior scalene muscles. The slight caudad direction is important, because, should the nerve not be encountered, advancing the needle in this direction is less likely to result in epidural or subarachnoid puncture, as this complication is prevented by the transverse process of the cervical vertebra. There is no need to perform a superficial cervical plexus block with this technique, as the nerve roots are already anaesthetized. It may be more comfortable for the patient, who is going to have his or her head turned laterally intraoperatively, if 5 ml of local anaesthetic is deposited below

the attachment of the sternocleidomastoid muscle, thus anaesthetizing the accessory nerve. Local infiltration by the surgeon may be required if the upper end of the incision is in the trigeminal nerve area or if the midline is crossed. Judicious administration of intravenous midazolam or propofol can provide sedation without compromising the ability to evaluate the patient's neurological function.

Possible complications of interscalene cervical plexus block include epidural, subarachnoid and intervertebral artery injection, which can be minimized by the caudad direction of the needle and by repeated aspiration before injecting the local anaesthetic. Hoarseness may occur if the recurrent laryngeal nerve is blocked, and Horner's syndrome if the cervical sympathetic chain is blocked. The lower roots of the brachial plexus may also be blocked by spread of local anaesthetic. Local infiltration with or without superficial cervical plexus block has been used. A large volume of local anaesthetic is required and the results are not as satisfactory as deep cervical plexus block.

General anaesthesia

These patients in general have a tendency for extreme blood pressure lability under general anaesthesia. However, general anaesthesia reduces cerebral metabolic demand and may offer some degree of cerebral protection. It also allows for the precise control and manipulation of systemic blood pressure and arterial carbon dioxide tension to optimize CBF. Several techniques are available and the precise one used depends on the experience and preference of the anaesthetist. A balanced general anaesthesia that maintains the blood pressure at the pre-operative level is preferred to 'deep' general anaesthesia that may necessitate the use of vasopressors to maintain blood pressure, as the risk of myocardial ischaemia may be increased in the latter.

Induction

The aim is to maintain cerebral and myocardial perfusion as close to baseline values as possible. A pre-induction intra-arterial line is useful to monitor blood pressure during and after induction. Anaesthesia can be induced in several ways. After pre-oxygenation, fentanyl or remifentanil, and thiopentone or propofol are given in incremental doses, titrated against the patient's haemodynamic responses. Muscle relaxation is achieved using a cardiostable non-depolarizing agent such as vecuronium, and a peripheral nerve stimulator is used to monitor the neuromuscular junction. To obtund the intubation response, lidocaine 1–1.5 mg kg^{-1} may be given 2–3 min before laryngoscopy and intubation. When muscle relaxation is complete, laryngoscopy and intubation are performed. After confirmation of tracheal tube placement by breath sounds and end-tidal capnometry, the tube is secured away from the operative side. Some surgeons may prefer nasotracheal placement of the tube to allow maximum extension of the neck and therefore better exposure. The lungs are ventilated to maintain adequate arterial oxygen saturation and normocarbia.

Maintenance

Once again, the aim is to provide stable cerebral perfusion while minimizing stress to the myocardium. This may be provided with either total intravenous anaesthesia or inhalational anaesthesia, and muscle relaxation. The use of isoflurane is associated with a lower critical CBF needed to maintain a normal EEG, as well as a lower incidence of ischaemic EEG changes compared with halothane and enflurane. It may also serve to offer myocardial protection from ischaemic damage. Sevoflurane is another inhalational agent that can be used successfully in this patient population. In addition to its low blood gas solubility coefficient allowing early awakening, sevoflurane maintains cerebral autoregulation, and has minimal direct cerebral vascular effects. Total intravenous anaesthesia with propofol and a fentanyl or remifentanil infusion can also be used. Remifentanil is an ultra-short-acting synthetic opioid that can cause hypotension and bradycardia in overdose. It has been used successfully in combination with propofol to provide anaesthesia and allows a rapid change of anaesthetic depth as needed. Even though it is a powerful analgesic while administered, there is a concern about hyperalgesia and subsequent hypertension following its use. Adequate longer-acting analgesics must be given early in the anaesthetic to avoid this problem. Alternatively, fentanyl can be used. Whichever technique is chosen, the regimen should allow early awakening so that neurological function can be assessed.

Before carotid cross-clamping, heparin (75–100 units kg^{-1}) is administered intravenously. Application of the carotid cross-clamp is often associated with an increase in blood pressure. Mild increases in blood pressure up to about 20% above pre-operative levels are acceptable, but excessive increases should be controlled. Heparin is generally not reversed after closure of the artery, but if the surgeon is not satisfied with haemostasis at the time of wound closure, a small dose of protamine (0.5 mg kg^{-1}) may be given.

Blood pressure and arterial carbon dioxide management

Arterial blood gases are checked after tracheal intubation and when necessary during the surgical procedure to ensure adequate oxygenation and normocapnia. Hypercapnia should be avoided, as it will only vasodilate blood vessels supplying the normal brain without affecting those supplying the ischaemic regions, which are presumably already maximally dilated. This diverts blood from the ischaemic areas to the normal areas (intracranial steal), thus further aggravating cerebral ischaemia. Hypocapnia, on the other hand, may increase flow to the ischaemic area by constricting the blood vessels in the normal areas (Robin Hood effect) and could be beneficial. However, hypocapnia causes a global reduction in CBF, and it is generally accepted that the changes in CBF associated with changes in carbon dioxide in these individuals are unpredictable. Normocapnia is therefore preferred.

The pre-operative blood pressure of individual patients should give guidance to a 'target' mean arterial blood pressure in the perioperative period. Cerebral autoregulation in these patients may be impaired, and the autoregulation curve is shifted to the right in uncontrolled or poorly controlled hypertensive patients. As autoregulation may be lost completely in ischaemic areas, maintaining an adequate blood pressure is a critical factor in the maintenance of CBF. If the blood pressure decreases below the individual patient's normal level, 'lightening' anaesthesia by reducing isoflurane concentration or decreasing the propofol infusion rate within acceptable limits should be done before using a vasopressor. Use of a vasopressor to elevate blood pressure during the cross-clamp may be necessary, but it has been shown to induce ventricular dysfunction and may increase the incidence of MI. If necessary, a phenylephrine (0.1–0.5 µg kg^{-1} min^{-1}) infusion can be administered judiciously. On the other hand, patients who remain hypertensive during anaesthesia may require intravenous hypotensive agents (nitroglycerine infusion 1–5 µg kg^{-1} min^{-1}) for control. Surgical manipulation of the carotid sinus may cause a marked alteration in heart rate and blood pressure. These reflexes can be minimized by prior local infiltration with lidocaine. Should EEG changes occur shortly after infiltration, one must be aware that the injection may have been into the carotid artery, resulting in transient CNS lidocaine toxicity.

Monitoring

Cardiovascular and respiratory monitoring

In addition to routine monitoring, an intra-arterial cannula is placed under local anaesthesia, before induction, to continuously monitor blood pressure throughout the perioperative period and facilitate the sampling of arterial blood gases. In low-risk patients, a rapidly cycling non-invasive blood pressure device can be used during induction, and invasive monitoring sited once the patient is anaesthetized but before the start of surgery. Central venous pressure, pulmonary capillary wedge pressure, cardiac output and urine output may be indicated in high-risk cardiac patients. End-tidal carbon dioxide, checked against an arterial sample obtained after induction, helps to maintain normocapnia in ventilated patients.

Central nervous system monitoring

No special monitoring is required in awake patients operated on under regional anaesthesia. Under general anaesthesia, brain function has been monitored in a number of ways, summarized in Table 13.5 below.

Electrophysiological monitoring

The 16-channel conventional EEG remains the gold standard as a sensitive indicator of inadequate cerebral perfusion in the anaesthetized patient. The unprocessed EEG displays voltage as a function of time. Proper use of this technique is tedious and time-consuming, and interpretation of the raw EEG is not easy – certainly in the setting of an operating theatre. Furthermore, at the usual rate of $25\,\mathrm{mm\ s^{-1}}$, a 270 m strip of paper is produced for a 3 h case. Nevertheless, intraoperative neurological complications have been shown to correlate well with EEG changes indicative of ischaemia. Ipsilateral or bilateral attenuation of high-frequency amplitude or development of low-frequency activity seen during carotid cross-clamping is indicative of cerebral hypoperfusion. The computer-processed EEG and somatosensory evoked potential have also been found to be useful.

The processed EEG generally simplifies the raw data and displays them as either average power or voltage. This allows less experienced observers to concentrate on how the parameters are changing with respect to time instead of trying to mentally analyse them. Although computer-processed EEGs are easier to interpret, they have been shown to be less accurate than the 16-channel EEG. Nonetheless, the use of EEG monitoring has still not decreased the incidence of perioperative stroke.

Somatosensory evoked potentials

Somatosensory evoked potentials (SSEPs) have been shown to be useful during CEA, yet the need for computer averaging means that this technique does not provide a continuous real-time monitor. Stable anaesthesia must be maintained to minimize the influence of anaesthetic agents on the amplitude. In general, >50% reduction or complete loss of amplitude of the cortical component is considered to be a significant indicator of inadequate cerebral perfusion. In contrast to conventional EEG, SSEPs monitor the cortex as well as the subcortical pathways in the internal capsule, an area not reflected in the cortical EEG. Not all studies agree that the use of SSEPs is either sensitive or specific for cerebral ischaemia and they are not therefore universally used.

Measurement of stump pressure (internal carotid artery back pressure)

As one important determinant of CBF is perfusion pressure, it seems reasonable to assume that the distal arterial pressure in the ipsilateral hemisphere during carotid occlusion would provide some indication of collateral CBF. Stump pressure represents the mean arterial pressure measured in the carotid stump (the ICA cephalad to the common carotid cross-clamp) after cross-clamping of the common and external carotid arteries, and the retrograde pressure transmitted along the ipsilateral carotid artery from the vertebral and contralateral carotid arteries. Stump pressure has been found useful to indicate intraoperative cerebral ischaemia and direct the use of shunt placement in a large case series and also when compared with near-infrared spectroscopy (NIRS) and transcranial Doppler ultrasonography (TCD).

Intraoperative measurement of cerebral blood flow

Intraoperative CBF measurement has also been used to determine the need for placement of shunts, but the associated cost makes it prohibitive for general use. This involves the intra-arterial injection of $20\,\mathrm{mCi}$ of the inert radioactive gas ^{133}Xe and measuring the wash-out of β emissions by an extracranial collimated sodium iodide scintillation counter focused on the

Table 13.5 Summary of available central nervous system monitoring

Monitor	Advantages	Disadvantages
Awake patient	Continuous neurological assessment Avoids the risks of general anaesthesia Lower incidence of post-operative hypertension Shorter ICU stay	Requires patient cooperation, ability to lie flat, anxiety, hyperventilation with potential risk of cerebral ischaemia Risk of autonomic disturbances, nausea, vomiting and airway obstruction
EEG (16-channel)	Gold standard	Cumbersome, difficult to interpret Not suitable for theatre environment
EEG (computer processed), cerebral function monitor, digital subtraction angiography, etc.	Easier to use than 16-channel Less cumbersome set-up	More than one channel needed for reasonable detection of ischaemia Embolic events not easily detectable
Somatosensory evoked potentials	Can detect subcortical ischaemia	Cumbersome Intermittent monitor with 'time lag' Affected by anaesthetic agents
Stump pressure	Measures retrograde perfusion pressure Easy to perform Cheap	Unreliable Does not reflect regional blood flow
Regional cerebral blood flow	Measures cerebral blood flow	Expensive Invasive Requires steady state Intermittent
Transcranial Doppler ultrasound	Continuous Non-invasive Relatively easy to use Can be used pre-, intra- and post-operatively Detects emboli Detects shunt malfunction	Not as sensitive as EEG Measures flow velocity and not cerebral blood flow Failure rate of 5–10% due to lack of ultrasonic window
Near-infrared spectroscopy	Continuous Non-invasive Easy to use	Extracranial contamination a problem No defined ischaemic thresholds yet

parietal cortex. The initial slope or fast component of the wash-out curve relates directly to regional blood flow. Newer measurement techniques involve single-photon emission CT (SPECT) of inhaled xenon. Both techniques are useful as research tools, but very few centres have the equipment and expertise required to produce accurate results.

Transcranial Doppler ultrasonography

Transcranial Doppler ultrasonography is an attractive technique for the detection of embolic events and cerebral ischaemia during cross-clamping of the carotid artery because it is continuous and non-invasive, and the transducer probes can be used successfully without impinging on the surgical field. It is also an important tool in the pre-operative assessment and post-operative care of patients with carotid disease.

Cerebral ischaemia is considered severe if the mean flow velocity in the middle cerebral artery (FV) after clamping is 0–15% of the pre-clamping value, mild if FV is 16–40% and absent if FV >40%. This criterion correlates well with subsequent ischaemic EEG changes and hence can be used as an indication for shunt placement (Fig. 13.1). Transcranial Doppler ultrasonography has been used successfully to detect intraoperative cerebral ischaemia, malfunctioning of shunts due to kinking

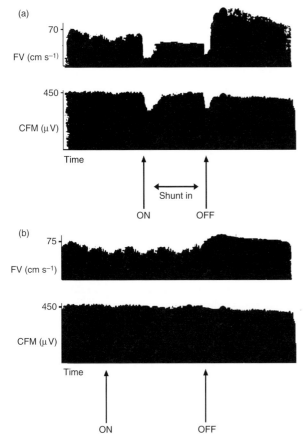

Fig. 13.1. Graphic display of right middle cerebral artery flow velocity (FV) and cerebral function analysing monitor (CFM) in two patients undergoing carotid endarterectomy. (a) On cross-clamping the carotid artery (ON), FV and CFM decrease, indicating cerebral ischaemia. Insertion of a shunt restores the signals to near pre-clamping value. Hyperaemia is observed upon release of the carotid artery cross-clamp at the end of the procedure (OFF). (b) Cross-clamping of the carotid artery results in no significant change in either FV or CFM and hence no shunt was used. Hyperaemia is also observed upon release of the clamp, but to a lesser degree than in (a).

and high-velocity states associated with hyperperfusion syndromes, as well as intra- and post-operative emboli. It appears to be a useful adjunct to other monitoring modalities such as EEG.

Emboli, or high-intensity 'chirps', are easily detectable using TCD. They can occur throughout the operation but are more frequent during dissection of the carotid arteries, upon release of the ICA cross-clamp and during wound closure. The rate of microembolus generation can indicate incipient carotid artery thrombosis, has been related to intraoperative infarcts and can predict post-operative neuropsychological morbidity. Many units use TCD monitoring routinely.

Following closure of the arteriotomy and release of the carotid clamps, the FV will typically increase immediately to levels above baseline and gradually correct back to the pre-clamping baseline over the course of a few minutes. This hyperaemic response is to be expected, as the vascular bed vasoconstricts in an autoregulatory response to increased perfusion pressure. However, approximately 10% of patients are at risk of cerebral oedema or haemorrhage because of gross hyperaemia with velocities of 230% of the baseline value lasting for several hours to days. This persistent post-operative hyperaemia or reperfusion, more likely to occur in patients with high-grade stenosis, is probably the result of defective autoregulation in the ipsilateral hemisphere. A reduction in blood pressure is effective in normalizing the FV and alleviating the symptoms. Transcranial Doppler ultrasonography provides the means of early detection and effective treatment of this potentially fatal complication.

Finally, a progressive fall in FV post-operatively to below pre-clamping baseline levels can be indicative of post-operative occlusion of the ipsilateral carotid artery and can be an indication for re-exploration of the endarterectomy. The development of sudden symptoms post-operatively should prompt an immediate TCD examination and early re-exploration.

Near-infrared spectroscopy

Near-infrared spectroscopy, first described by Jöbsis in 1977, continues to receive attention as a monitor of cerebral oxygenation. By using near-infrared light, cerebral oximetry can theoretically be used to monitor haemoglobin oxygen saturation (HbO_2) in the total tissue bed including capillaries, arterioles and venules. One of the limitations of this technology is its inability to differentiate reliably between intra- and extra-cranial blood. However, during CEA, as the external carotid artery is clamped, most of the contamination due to extracranial blood flow is removed. There is now evidence to suggest that it is possible to obtain useful intraoperative information about cerebral oxygenation in patients undergoing CEA using NIRS. In patients undergoing CEA under general anaesthesia, changes in jugular venous oxyhaemoglobin saturation and middle cerebral artery blood velocity correlate well with changes in cerebrovascular haemoglobin oxygen saturation (ScO_2). Similarly, Samara and colleagues demonstrated that NIRS can be used to track changes in carotid blood flow in the majority of patients undergoing CEA under regional anaesthesia. Kirkpatrick and co-workers observed that NIRS-based measurements can provide a warning of severe cerebral ischaemia (SCI) with high specificity and sensitivity provided the extracranial vascular contamination is accounted for. Despite numerous publications on the use of NIRS in CEA, its use as a monitoring tool for detecting cerebral ischaemia remains undefined. A recent study has suggested that it may be of use in predicting hyperperfusion syndrome after carotid stenting (see Chapter 9).

Intraoperative cerebral protection

A detailed account of this appears in Chapter 3, but a pragmatic approach to cerebral protection during anaesthesia is briefly discussed here. Ischaemia from hypoperfusion is most likely to occur during carotid cross-clamping. Therefore, cerebral protection is 'most' effective when a carotid shunt is never used, at which time it is reasonable to administer a bolus of either thiopentone 5 mg kg^{-1} or propofol 2 mg kg^{-1} prior to cross-clamping of the carotid artery. With selective shunting based on monitoring cerebral ischaemia EEG, evoked potentials or a reduction in CBF detected by TCD, thiopentone should not be given as it will interfere with monitoring, and a shunt is inserted.

The decision on whether to shunt or not is generally made by the surgeon. There are those who shunt routinely, some who never use shunts and others that shunt selectively according to signs of cerebral ischaemia detected by monitoring of the CNS during carotid artery cross-clamping. There does not appear to be any difference in stroke or mortality rates among the groups.

The anaesthetic itself may provide neuroprotection. Isoflurane may pre-condition the brain so that it is better able to tolerate an ischaemic insult, and can be used to provide anaesthesia or in low doses to supplement an intravenous technique. Propofol (and benzodiazepines) produces a dose-related decrease in cerebral metabolic rate and CBF, and can be used in combination with a short-acting opioid to provide balanced intravenous anaesthesia. In addition to anaesthetic drugs, several other drugs have been evaluated, with varying degrees of success, to provide neuroprotection. Sadly, drugs that have shown promise in animal studies have failed to translate into effective drugs in humans. To date, there is no 'silver bullet', which probably reflects the complex timing of events and series of pro- and anti-inflammatory cascades initiated by an ischaemic insult to the brain.

Non-pharmacological methods of cerebral protection include mild hypothermia (temperature of about 35°C), which may easily be achieved and may decrease cerebral metabolism sufficiently with no obvious disadvantages. Should stroke occur on the table, hypothermia should be continued, the patient transferred to intensive care and gradually rewarmed after 24 h of continuous cooling.

Carotid stenting

During work-up of patients with carotid disease, some are considered too high risk for surgical intervention or general anaesthesia. These patients are increasingly being offered carotid stenting. Carotid stenting is not without risk, and despite its initial popularity as an alternative to surgery (and the thought that it may even supersede surgical intervention), comparisons of patient groups have shown poorer outcome in the stenting group. The worst outcome in this group of patients may be due to their worse pre-morbid state preventing general anaesthesia and surgery. Patients undergoing carotid stenting have a greater risk of stroke (even when filters are used to catch emboli) and adverse cardiovascular events. Nonetheless, there are patients in whom endovascular therapy remains their only treatment option.

Deployment of the stent can cause parasympathetic stimulation with subsequent bradycardia and nausea. It is our practice to site a peripheral intravenous cannula prior to intervention and to administer an anticholinergic. In our institute, we choose to use 200 µg of glycopyrrolate, as it is less likely to cause sedation than atropine. An intra-arterial catheter is also placed to monitor blood pressure and facilitate blood sampling. Standard monitoring is used including a five-lead ECG. Supplemental oxygen is provided throughout the procedure by a face mask or nasal cannulae, as tolerated by the patient. No sedation is given unless the patient is especially anxious.

For those considered at high risk of hyperperfusion syndrome, tight blood pressure control is maintained after the stent has been deployed. An intravenous infusion of β-blocker, either labetalol or esmolol, may be necessary. At times, a second agent may be required; hydralazine, nitrate and sodium nitroprusside have been used with success. Blood pressure control is titrated against the patient's symptoms, predominantly headache relief. Oral antihypertensives are commenced and the patient transferred to a high-dependency environment to continue blood pressure control and wean the antihypertensive infusion.

Combined or staged carotid endartarectomy and coronary artery bypass grafts

More than 50% of patients undergoing CEA have overt coronary artery disease: previous infarct, angina or ischaemic ECG abnormalities. Similarly, up to one-fifth of patients undergoing coronary artery bypass grafting have duplex ultrasound-detected moderate (>50%) carotid stenosis, with 5.9–12% of those having severe (>80%) stenosis. Therefore, it is not surprising that stroke complicates up to 4% of all coronary artery bypass operations. There are many potential causes for coronary bypass-related stroke, namely embolization from the carotid arch, endocardium or pump oxygenator, hypoperfusion related to occlusive arterial lesion or ICH. Coronary angiography has been used to select high-risk patients for staged CEA or combined with coronary artery bypass grafting.

If the procedures are combined, the risk of stroke and mortality is increased. When staged procedures are planned, it is preferable to operate on the presenting lesion first. One centre has reported success when performing combined coronary artery bypass and carotid stenting for those patients with severe disease.

Extracranial–intracranial bypass grafting

Anastomosing the extracranial to the intracranial arterial circulation (an EC/IC bypass) should in theory increase CBF to ischaemic areas, thus reducing the risk of stroke. The only large prospective randomized trial on EC/IC failed to demonstrate a benefit when compared with medical therapy alone. Hence, the popularity of this procedure for preventing strokes in patients with carotid stenosis has declined markedly.

Prophylactic EC/IC bypass procedures are increasingly performed for patients in whom therapeutic occlusions are required for controlling aneurysmal or vascular lesions not amenable to surgical clipping, such as giant internal carotid artery aneurysms with wide necks. The procedures carry a significantly higher mortality than CEA, which may in part be due to patient selection. The perioperative management of patients presenting for EC/IC bypass surgery is similar to those presenting for CEA, and particular attention is focused on preventing coughing and control of blood pressure to ensure patency of the graft.

Post-operative care and complications

In order to continue the benefits of a carefully conducted anaesthetic, recovery should be smooth and prompt to allow immediate post-operative neurological assessment. We find that careful reduction in anaesthetic concentration with discontinuation upon wound closure results in satisfactory haemodynamics. Lidocaine $1–1.5\,mg\,kg^{-1}$ may be given intravenously to minimize cough during emergence. When the patient is responsive and awake, the trachea is extubated. It is advisable to leave the intra-arterial cannula in the immediate post-operative period to permit continuous blood pressure monitoring and blood gas analyses. All our patients receive supplemental oxygen and are monitored in recovery for a prolonged period (2 h or more if necessary). This allows rapid intervention should wound haematoma or intimal flap thrombosis develops.

Although the need for intensive care depends on the pre-morbid state and the intraoperative course, a neurovascular unit staffed with nurses familiar with the post-operative course and potential complications allows the majority of patients to be monitored closely for cardiac, respiratory and neurological complications without the need for intensive care.

Carotid chemoreceptor and baroreceptor dysfunction

Post-operative haemodynamic instability is common (incidence >40%) after CEA and is thought to be due to carotid baroreceptor dysfunction. It is postulated that the atheromatous plaques dampen the pressure wave reaching the carotid sinus baroreceptors and with the removal of these plaques increased stimulation of baroreceptors may result in bradycardia and hypotension. The hypotension can be prevented or treated by blocking the carotid sinus nerve with a local anaesthetic, intravenous fluid administration or, if necessary, the administration of vasopressor drugs such as phenylephrine.

Hypertension after CEA is less well understood and has been reported to be more common in patients with pre-operative hypertension, particularly if poorly controlled, and in patients undergoing CEA if the carotid sinus is denervated. Hypertension after CEA in which the sinus nerve is preserved has been postulated to be due to temporary dysfunction of the baroreceptors or nerve, caused by intraoperative trauma. Mild increases in blood pressure are acceptable (up to about 20% above pre-operative levels), but marked increases are treated with an infusion of antihypertnsive drugs such as nitroglycerine or β-blockers, depending on the patient's condition in the immediate post-operative period.

Other causes of haemodynamic instability after CEA include myocardial ischaemia/infarction, dysrhythmias, hypoxia, hypercarbia, pneumothorax, pain, confusion and bladder distension, which should be treated appropriately.

Hypotension may lead to hypoperfusion and ischaemic infarction of the brain. Hypertension may increase the incidence of wound haematoma formation with possible airway obstruction. Similarly, myocardial ischaemia/infarction may occur as a result of either complication. Therefore, the blood pressure must be closely monitored and controlled in the immediate post-operative period. Regional anaesthesia appears to be associated with a higher incidence of post-operative hypotension while general anaesthesia is more often associated with post-operative hypertension.

Carotid endarterectomy may result in loss of carotid body function with reduced ventilatory response to hypoxaemia and hypercarbia. This effect is further exaggerated in patients with coexisting pulmonary disease, especially in the presence of respiratory depressant drugs. Provision of supplemental oxygen and close monitoring of ventilatory status is particularly important in these patients and, if necessary, they should be admitted to the high-dependency unit/ICU for observation.

Hyperperfusion syndrome

Patients who become hypertensive in the post-operative period (defined as systolic blood pressure >200 mmHg) are at much greater risk of developing neurological deficit (10.2%) than patients who remain normotensive (3.4%). Hypertension may cause excessive cerebral perfusion in a circulation unable to autoregulate, resulting in hyperperfusion syndrome and ICH. Patients at greater risk include those with reduced pre-operative hemispheric CBF caused by bilateral high-grade stenosis, unilateral high-grade carotid stenosis with poor collateral cross-flow or unilateral carotid occlusion with contralateral high-grade stenosis. The syndrome is thought to develop after restoration of perfusion to an area of the brain that has lost its ability to autoregulate because of chronic maximal vasodilation.

Restoration of blood flow after CEA thus leads to a state of hyperperfusion until autoregulation is re-established, which occurs over a period of days. Clinical features of this syndrome include headache (usually unilateral), face and eye pain, cerebral oedema, seizures and ICH. Patients at risk for this syndrome should be closely monitored in the perioperative period, and their blood pressure should be meticulously controlled.

Rapid management of haemodynamic instability in the post-operative period can alter patient outcome. A guideline in each unit to direct therapy and offer targets may help.

Myocardial ischaemia and infarction

Perioperative MI is the most frequent cause of mortality following CEA. In general, the reported incidence of fatal post-operative MI is 0.5–4% and the proportion of total perioperative mortality (within 30 days of operation) attributed to cardiac causes is high. All causes of increased cardiac work must be minimized in order to avoid myocardial ischaemia. The patient should be warm, pain free, well oxygenated and normotensive with no tachycardia. Any signs of myocardial ischaemia should be treated immediately. β-Blockade should not be started in the perioperative period, but should be continued if the patient is already taking this medication.

Haemorrhage and airway obstruction

Persistent oozing from deep tissues, insecure ligation of vessels and the disruption of suture lines may all lead to bleeding from the wound site. This can be further aggravated by compromised coagulation due to the use of anticoagulants or antiplatelet agents. An expanding haematoma in the neck may cause airway obstruction and may necessitate re-exploration of the wound site. Difficult intubation may result from this complication and the unwary may mismanage these patients with catastrophic results. Clinical assessment of the airway can underestimate the potential hazard of a rapid sequence induction technique. Opening the sutures and letting the haematoma out or surgical evacuation of the haematoma under local anaesthesia are possible options. If general anaesthesia is necessary, an inhalational induction with halothane or sevoflurane, or a fibre-optic awake intubation, are the methods of choice.

Neurological complications

Post-operative neurological deficit occurs in 1–7% of patients after CEA, regardless of the anaesthetic technique. Neurological deficits following CEA are multifactorial in origin: they may result from embolization at the site of surgery, cerebral ischaemia due to hypoperfusion or thrombosis at the endarterectomy site and intimal flap, or ICH. The manifestations include transient deficits and ischaemic strokes. All potentially treatable causes including thrombosis must be sought and re-exploration may be necessary. Re-exploration for evacuation of a haematoma requires meticulous airway management as discussed above. Cranial nerve injuries have also been reported, the most commonly injured nerves being the hypoglossal and recurrent laryngeal nerves, leading to possible problems with upper-airway control. Damage to the recurrent laryngeal nerves may reduce the upper-airway protective reflexes and place the patient at risk of aspiration, as well as cause airway obstruction (if the abductor fibres are not the only ones affected).

Conclusions

The maintenance of adequate cerebral perfusion, the avoidance of hypotension and the prevention and treatment of raised ICP are essential for good recovery in patients with intracranial haemorrhage, cerebral trauma or encephalopathies. Therefore, clinicians caring for these patients must have a thorough understanding of cerebral physiology and the factors that affect cerebral haemodynamics. The principles of anaesthetic management of patients with SAH described above are applicable to any patient with an intracranial vascular lesion.

Further reading

Bart, R. D., Takaoda, S., Pearlstein, R. D., Dexter, F. and Warner, D. S. (1998). Interactions between hypothermia and the latency to ischemic depolarisation – implications for neuroprotection. *Anesthesiology* **88**, 1266–73.

Bricolo, A. P. and Paust, L. M. (1984). Extradural haematoma: toward zero mortality. A prospective study. *Neurosurgery* **14**, 8–12.

Bromberg, J. E. C., Rinkel, G. J. E., Algra, A. *et al.* (1995). Subarachnoid haemorrhage in first and second degree relatives of patients with subarachnoid haemorrhage. *BMJ* **311**, 288–9.

Drake, C. G., Hunt, W. E., Sano, K. *et al.* (1988). Report of World Federation of Neurological Surgeons Committee on a Universal Subarachnoid Hemorrhage Grading Scale. *J Neurosurg* **68**, 985–6.

Fiorella, D., Albuquerque, F. C., Han, P. and McDougall, C. G. (2004). Strategies for the management of intraprocedural thromboembolic complications with abciximab (ReoPro). *Neurosurgery* **54**, 1089–98.

Franke, C. L., de Jonge, J., van Swieten, J. C., Op de Coul, A. A. and van Gijn, J. (1990). Intracerebral hematomas during anticoagulant treatment. *Stroke* **21**, 726–30.

GALA Trial Collaborative Group, Lewis, S. C., Warlow, C. R. *et al.* (2008). General anaesthesia versus local anaesthesia for carotid surgery (GALA): a multicentre, randomised controlled trial. *Lancet* **372**, 2132–42.

Giannotta, S. L., Oppenheimer, J. H., Levy, M. L. and Zelman, V. (1991). Management of intraoperative rupture of aneurysms without hypotension. *Neurosurgery* **28**, 531–5.

Green, R. M., Kelly, K. M., Gabrielson, T., Levine, S. R. and Vanderzant, C. (1990). Multiple intracerebral hemorrhages after smoking "crack" cocaine. *Stroke* **21**, 957–62.

Greenstein, A. J., Chassin, M. R., Wang, J. *et al.* (2007). Association between minor and major surgical complications after carotid endarterectomy: results of the New York Carotid Artery Surgery study. *J Vasc Surg* **46**, 1138–44; discussion 1145–6.

Gupta, S., Heath, K. and Matta, B. F. (1997). Effect of incremental doses of sevoflurane on cerebral pressure autoregulation in humans. *Br J Anaesth* **79**, 469–72.

Howell, S. J. (2007). Carotid endarterectomy. *Br J Anaesth* **99**, 119–31.

International Study of Unruptured Intracranial Aneurysms Investigators (1998). Unruptured intracranial aneurysms – risk of rupture and risks of surgical intervention. *N Engl J Med* **339**, 1725–33.

Kelly, D. F. (1997). Timing of surgery for ruptured aneurysms and initial critical care. *J Stroke Neurovasc Dis* **6**, 235–6.

Lakhani, S., Guha, A. and Nahser, H. C. (2006). Anaesthesia for endovascular management of cerebral aneurysms. *Eur J Anaesthesiol* **23**, 902–13.

Lam, A. M., Winn, H. R., Cullen, B. F. and Sundling, N. (1991). Hyperglycemia and neurological outcome in patients with head injury. *J Neurosurgery* **75**, 545–51.

Lanzino, G., Rabinstein, A. A. and Brown, R. D. Jr (2009). Treatment of carotid artery stenosis: medical therapy, surgery or stenting? *Mayo Clin Proc* **84**, 362–87.

Lawton, M. T. and Spetzler, R. F. (1995). Surgical management of giant intracranial aneurysms, experience with 171 patients. *Clin Neurosurg* **42**, 245–66.

Marion, D. W., Penrod, L. E., Kelsey, S. F. *et al.* (1997). Treatment of traumatic brain injury with moderate hypothermia. *N Engl J Med* **336**, 540–6.

Mas, J. L., Trinquart, L., Leys, D. *et al.* (2008). Endarterectomy versus angioplasty in patients with symptomatic severe carotid stenosis (EVA-3S) trial: results up to 4 years from a randomised, multicentre trial. *Lancet Neurol* 7, 885–92.

Matsumoto, S., Nakahar, I., Higashi, T. *et al.* (2009). Near-infrared spectroscopy in carotid artery stenting predicts cerebral hyperperfusion syndrome. *Neurology* 72, 1512–8.

Matta, B. and Czosnyka, M. (2010) Transcranial Doppler Ultrasonography in anaesthesia and neurosurgery. In Cottrell, J. E. and Young, W. L., eds., *Cottrell and Young's Neuroanesthesia*, 5th edn. Philadelphia: Mosby.

Matta, B. F. and Lam, A. M. (1995). Nitrous oxide increases cerebral blood flow velocity during pharmacologically induced EEG silence in humans. *J Neurosurg Anesthesiol* 7, 89–93.

Matta, B. F., Lam, A. M. and Mayberg, T. S. (1994). The influence of arterial hyperoxygenation on cerebral venous oxygen content during hyperventilation. *Can J Anaesth* 41, 1041–6.

Matta, B. F., Lam, A. M., Mayberg, T. S., Shapira, Y. and Winn, H. R. (1994). A critique of the intraoperative use of jugular venous bulb catheters during neurosurgical procedures. *Anesth Analg* 79, 745–50.

Matta, B. F., Mayberg, T. S. and Lam, A. M. (1995). Direct cerebrovasodilatory effects of halothane, isoflurane, and desflurane during propofol induced isoelectric electroencephalogram in humans. *Anesthesiology* 83, 980–85.

Mayer, S. A. and Swarup, R. (1996). Neurogenic cardiac injury after subarachnoid hemorrhage. *Curr Opin Anaesthesiol* 9, 356–61.

Molyneux, A. J., Kerr, R. S., Birks, J. *et al.* (2009). Risk of recurrent subarachnoid haemorrhage, death, or dependence and standardised mortality ratios after clipping or coiling of an intracracnial aneurysm in the International Subarachnoid Aneurysm Trial (ISAT): long-term follow-up. *Lancet Neurol* 8, 427–33.

Moritz, S., Kasprzak, P, Arit, M., Taeger, K. and Metz, C. (2007). Accuracy of cerebral monitoring in detecting cerebral ischaemia during carotid endarterectomy: a comparison of transcranial Doppler sonography, near-infrared spectroscopy, stump pressure, and somatosensory evoked potentials. *Anesthesiology* 107, 563–9.

Poon, W. S., Rehman, S. U., Poon, C. Y. and Li, A. K. (1992). Traumatic extradural haematoma of delayed onset is not a rarity. *Neurosurgery* 30, 681–6.

Press, M. J., Chassin, M. R., Wang, J., Tuhrim, S. and Halm, E. A. (2006). Predicting medical and surgical complications of carotid endarterectomy. *Arch Int Med* 166, 914–20.

Schievink, W. I., Wijdicks, E. F. M., Parisi, J. E., Piepgras, D. G. and Whisnant, J. P. (1995). Sudden death from aneurysmal subarachnoid hemorrhage. *Neurology* 45, 871–4.

Strebel, S., Lam, A. M., Matta, B. F. *et al.* (1995). Dynamic and static cerebral autoregulation during isoflurane, desflurane and propofol anesthesia. *Anesthesiology* 83, 66–76.

Todd, M. M., Hindman, B. J., Clarke, W. R. and Torner, J. C. (2005). Intraoperative Hypothermia for Aneurysm Surgery Trial (IHAST) Investigators. Mild intraoperative hypothermia during surgery for intracranial aneurysm. *N Engl J Med* 352, 135–45.

Warner, D. S. (1994). Perioperative neuroprotection. *Curr Opin Anaesthesiol* 7, 416–20.

Warner, D. S. and Laskowitz, D. T. (2006). Changing outcome from aneurysmal subarachnoid haemorrhage. *Anesthesiology* 104, 629–30.

Werner, C., Kochs, E., Bause, H. *et al.* (1995). Effects of sufentanil on cerebral hemodynamics and intracranial pressure in patients with brain injury. *Anesthesiology* 83, 721–6.

Wilberger, J. E., Harris, M. and Diamond, D. L. (1990). Acute subdural hematoma. *J Trauma* 30, 733–6.

Young, W. L., Prohovnick, I., Ornstein, E. *et al.* (1994). Monitoring of intraoperative cerebral haemodynamics before and after arteriovenous malfomations. *Stroke* 25, 611–14.

Chapter 1

Principles of paediatric neurosurgery

Craig D. McClain and Sulpicio G. Soriano

Introduction

The perioperative management of paediatric patients undergoing neurosurgical procedures should be based on the developmental stage of the patient. Age-dependent differences in cranial bone development, cerebral vascular physiology and neurological lesions distinguish neonates, infants and children from their adult counterparts. In particular, the central nervous system (CNS) undergoes a tremendous amount of structural and physiological change during the first 2 years of life. The goal of this chapter is to highlight these age-dependent differences and their effect on the perioperative management of the paediatric neurosurgical patient.

The neonate

Neurological pathologies that require surgery during the neonatal period are mainly due to life-threatening congenital anomalies or intracranial haemorrhage. There are a variety of reasons why neonates undergoing neurosurgical procedures present special challenges to anaesthesiologists. For one, neonatal physiology is different from adult physiology. For example, the anaesthesiologist must be mindful of the additional perioperative concerns that newborn cardiac physiology presents during perioperative care. The possibility of intracardiac shunts, elevated pulmonary pressures and a stiff ventricle result in fundamentally different perioperative management strategies. In addition to physiological differences, neonates may also have different drug metabolism from adults, especially with hepatically metabolized drugs. Closed claim analysis studies have revealed that neonates are at higher risk for morbidity and mortality than any other age group. Respiratory- and cardiac-related events account for the majority of these complications. Given the urgent nature of many neonatal neurosurgical procedures, a thorough pre-operative evaluation may be difficult, and other coexisting congenital anomalies may not be detected. Thus, thorough understanding of the fundamental differences inherent in neonates is essential.

Anatomy

The diminutive size of the premature and term neonate has a significant impact on the perioperative course. As noted above, neonates and infants are at higher risk for morbidity and mortality than any other age group, with respiratory- and cardiac-related events accounting for the majority of these complications. Anatomic differences between the paediatric and adult airway are primarily due to the size and orientation of the components of the upper airway, larynx and trachea. In addition, neonates and infants have the greatest differences from adults in this respect. However, the configuration of the larynx becomes similar to the adult after the second year of life. The infant's larynx is also funnel-shaped and narrowest at the level of the cricoid, making this the smallest cross-sectional area in the infant airway. This feature places the infant at particular risk for life-threatening subglottic obstruction secondary to mucosal swelling after prolonged intubation with a tight-fitting endotracheal tube. The use of a cuffed endotracheal tube should be undertaken with great caution in this age group, and cuff pressures should be monitored carefully, especially when using nitrous oxide (N_2O). The distance between the vocal cords and the carina can be quite short in small babies, and thus the difference between extubation and mainstem intubation can be only a few centimetres. If the infant's head is flexed for a suboccipital approach to the posterior fossa or the cervical spine, an endotracheal tube can migrate into a mainstem bronchus. Given these conditions, the anaesthesiologist should auscultate both

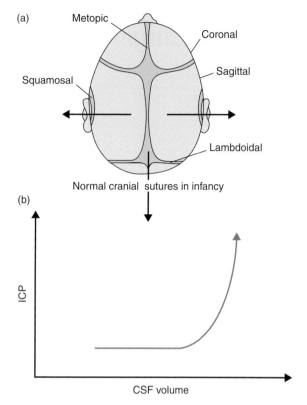

(a)

Metopic

Coronal

Squamosal

Sagittal

Lambdoidal

Normal cranial sutures in infancy

(b)

ICP

CSF volume

Fig. 14.1. Functional anatomy of cranial sutures and fontanelles in neonates and infants. Initially the compliant skull of the neonate will minimize insidious increases in intracranial volume. However, acute increases in intracranial volume (haemorrhage and obstructed ventriculoperitoneal shunt) will lead to rapid rises in intracranial pressure.

lung fields after the patient is positioned for the surgical procedure to rule out inadvertent intubation of a mainstem bronchus.

The neonatal cranial vault is in a state of flux. Open fontanels and cranial sutures lead to a compliant intracranial space (Fig. 14.1). Unlike an adult cranium, the neonatal cranium has a 'pop-off' valve when the fontanels are open. Frequent measurement of head circumference is often utilized to assess concerns for expanding intracranial lesions. The mass effect of an insidious haemorrhage is often masked by a compensatory increase in intracranial volume due to widening of the fontanels and cranial sutures. However, like adults, acute increases in cranial volume due to massive haemorrhage or an obstructed ventricular system cannot be attenuated by expansion of the immature cranial vault, which frequently results in life-threatening intracranial hypertension.

Congenital anomalies of the CNS generally occur as midline defects. This dysraphism may occur anywhere along the neural axis (from cranium to sacrum), involving the head (encephalocele) or spine (meningomyelocele). The extent of such defects is incredibly varied, and can range from relatively minor defects that affect only superficial bony and membranous structures to more serious defects that include a large segment of malformed neural tissue (Fig. 14.2).

Physiology

Developmental cerebral blood flow (CBF) is coupled tightly to metabolic demand, and both increase proportionately immediately after birth. Cerebral blood flow peaks between 2 and 4 years and stabilizes at 7–8 years. These alterations in CBF mirror changes in neuroanatomical development. Even in the neonate, autoregulatory mechanisms are present. The autoregulatory range of blood pressure in a normal newborn is between 20 and 60 mmHg, which reflects the relatively low cerebral metabolic requirements and blood pressure during the perinatal period. More importantly, the slope of the autoregulatory curve is quite steep at the upper and lower limits of the curve, while the flatter portion occurs over a relatively narrow range (Fig. 14.3). Neonates are especially vulnerable to cerebral ischaemia and intraventricular haemorrhage due to this narrow autoregulatory range.

Certain neonates are at an even higher risk of morbidity and/or mortality. Tsuji and colleagues demonstrated that sick premature neonates have a linear correlation between CBF and systemic blood pressure, placing these patients at particular risk for cerebral ischaemia as well as intraventricular haemorrhage due to this direct relationship and a lack of autoregulatory protection. Also, CBF pressure passivity occurs in premature neonates with low gestational age, birthweight and systemic hypotension. Furthermore, Boylan and colleagues reported that high-risk term as well as premature neonates did not demonstrate autoregulation of CBF.

Extreme vigilance and care must be taken when anaesthetizing neonates but particularly with sick premature infants. The balance between adequate cerebral perfusion and maintenance of adequate anaesthetic depth can be difficult. It is crucial to take into account the physiological differences in this patient population, and thus tight blood pressure control is essential in the management of neonates to minimize both cerebral ischaemia and intraventricular haemorrhage.

Premature and term neonates have functionally immature organ systems. The immaturity of the renal

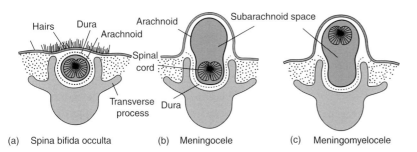

Fig. 14.2. Spinal dysraphism. (a) Spina bifida occulta – skin or skin with hair covers a bony defect only. (b) Meningocele – protrusion of a fluid-filled sac only (no neural tissue present). (c) Meningomyelocele – protrusion of a fluid-filled sac plus neural tissue.

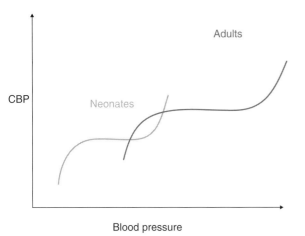

Fig. 14.3. Autoregulation of cerebral blood flow in neonates and adults. The slope of the autoregulatory curve drops and rises significantly at the lower and upper limits of the curve and is shifted to the left in neonates and infants (left curve) when compared with adults (right curve).

system is of particular concern during many neurosurgical procedures where significant fluid shifts may occur. The neonatal renal system is characterized by a decreased glomerular filtration rate and ability to concentrate urine in response to dehydration states. These differences result in diminished excretion of sodium and water, thus limiting the neonate's ability to compensate for fluctuations in fluid and solute loads. Drugs that are renally excreted may have a prolonged half-life. Furthermore, hepatic function is also diminished in neonates, and metabolism of drugs may be delayed due to decreased activity of hepatic enzymes. Neonates demonstrate a decreased ability to glucuronidate drugs, and thus drugs like morphine may have quite extended half-lives in the neonate. Total body water decreases from 85% in premature infants to 65% in adults, while body fat content increases from < 1% in premature infants to 15% in term infants and 35% in adults. Total body protein also follows a similar trend, and therefore hydrophilic drugs have more binding

sites and hydrophobic drugs have fewer in infancy. The constellation of these factors should prompt the clinician generally to decrease the weight-adjusted dose and frequency of administration of drugs given to the newborn. Judicious titration of potent drugs is critical in these patients.

Most neonatal surgery is performed on an emergent basis, which increases risk in the perioperative period due to undiagnosed congenital anomalies. Premature neonates may have persistence of the transitional circulation, which is the period of transition from fetal circulation to adult circulation. Of particular concern during this period are the presence of physiological intracardiac shunts (patent foramen ovale and patent ductus arteriosus), relatively elevated pulmonary vascular resistance and a stiff ventricle. The neonatal heart is characterized by fewer contractile elements and fewer elastic elements. This means that the neonatal heart cannot increase cardiac output with volume via the Frank–Starling method and that there is decreased ventricular compliance. Congestive heart failure can occur in neonates with large cerebral arteriovenous malformations and this condition requires aggressive haemodynamic support. More commonly, intracardiac right-to-left shunting occurs through patent ductus arterious or foramen ovalae that have not yet closed.

Finally, the respiratory system in neonates also presents a number of challenges. As with both neurological and cardiac physiology, respiratory physiology in neonates is different from adult patients. Neonates have a lower functional residual capacity, as well as a higher rate of oxygen consumption. This can make airway management and particularly rapid sequence inductions challenging. Premature infants may have some degree of lung disease, which can predispose these patients to bronchospasm and significant oxygen desaturations. Management of the neonatal respiratory system may be difficult for a variety of reasons, including the diminutive size of the airway, craniofacial anomalies, laryngotracheal lesions, and acute (hyaline membrane disease, retained amniotic fluid) or chronic (bronchopulmonary dysplasia) disease. As these conditions are dynamic, they should be addressed pre-operatively in order to anticipate problems and minimize perioperative morbidity.

The infant

Neurosurgery in infants encompasses a myriad of acute and chronic conditions. Children in this age group can present with a wide variety of pathologies requiring surgical intervention including trauma, congenital abnormalities such as craniosynostosis, hydrocephalus, intracranial tumours, intracranial vascular lesions and seizure disorders. Infants are prone to accidental as well as inflicted traumatic head injury and often require emergent craniotomies. Craniosynostosis surgery is frequently performed in this period in order to minimize restriction on brain growth. Given the compliance of the infant cranial vault, occulted slow-growing tumours will manifest as abnormal cranial enlargement.

Anatomy

The infant cranial vault consists of six separate bones (frontal, occipital, two parietal and two temporal) that are coupled by cranial sutures. The cranial bones fuse at approximately 12–18 months. These sutures come together at the anterior and posterior fontanelles. The posterior fontanelle closes first, usually by 1 or 2 months, or may already be closed at birth. The anterior fontanelle usually closes later, usually between 9 months and 18 months.

The Monro–Kellie hypothesis states that the sum of all intracranial volumes is constant, which is certainly true for adult patients and informs neuroanaesthetic management. However, neonates and infants are an exception to this rule due to their open fontanelles and unfused cranial sutures. Given the nature of the infant's fontanelles and unfused cranial sutures, the mass effect of a slow-growing tumour or insidious haemorrhage is often masked by a compensatory increase in intracranial volume accompanied by head growth. Thus, in infants where such processes are suspected, a component of the ongoing clinical assessment is usually serial measurements of cranial circumference. When intracranial pressure (ICP) increases occur slowly, open fontanelles and cranial sutures separate allowing the intracranial volume to increase. Therefore, the symptomatic manifestations of an expanding intracranial mass may be delayed. As a result, infants presenting with signs and symptoms of intracranial hypertension frequently have fairly advanced pathology. In this situation, the most obvious finding on physical examination may be an abnormally large head. However, rapid increases in cranial volume due to acute massive haemorrhage or acutely obstructed cerebrospinal fluid (CSF) flow cannot be attenuated by expansion of the immature cranial vault and frequently result in life-threatening intracranial hypertension. Once the fontanelles and sutures have fused, children have a lower intracranial compliance than adults. Contributory factors include a higher ratio of brain water content, less CSF volume and a higher ratio of brain content to intracranial capacity. Consequently, when similar relative increases in ICP occur, children may be at increased risk of herniation compared with adults. Thus, in children with fused sutures and closed fontanelles, signs and symptoms of intracranial hypertension must be assessed rapidly and addressed in order to avoid undesired outcomes.

Children over 2 years of age

Physiology

Age-dependent differences in cerebrovascular physiology have a significant impact on the perioperative management of neurosurgical patients. An understanding of these differences is the foundation of good paediatric neuroanaesthetic care. Cerebral blood flow is coupled tightly to cerebral metabolic rate for oxygen, and both increase proportionally immediately following birth. Wintermark and colleagues determined the effect of age on CBF. Using CT perfusion techniques, they reported that CBF peaked between 2 and 4 years and settled at 7–8 years. These changes mirror changes in neuroanatomical development. In healthy awake children, CBF is approximately 100 ml (100 g brain tissue)$^{-1}$. Neonates and infants have a lower CBF than older children at approximately 40 ml (100 g)$^{-1}$. In children, CBF can represent up to 25% of cardiac output. The proportion of cardiac output devoted to the brain varies with age, with infants and children having a larger distribution. The autoregulatory range of blood pressure in a normal term newborn lies between 20 and 60 mmHg, reflecting the relatively low cerebral metabolic requirements and vascular resistance of the perinatal period. Although children younger than 2 years of age have lower baseline mean arterial pressures, they have a lower autoregulatory reserve and can

Table 14.1 Common perioperative concerns for infants and children with neurological problems

Condition	Anaesthetic implications
Denervation injuries	Hyperkalaemia after succinylcholine Resistance to non-depolarizing muscle relaxants Abnormal response to nerve stimulation
Chronic anticonvulsant therapy	Hepatic and haematological abnormalities Increased metabolism of anaesthetic agents
Arteriovenous malformation	Congestive heart failure
Neuromuscular disease	Malignant hyperthermia Respiratory failure Sudden cardiac death
Chiari malformation	Apnoea Aspiration pneumonia
Hypothalamic/pituitary lesions	Diabetes insipidus Hypothyroidism Adrenal insufficiency

theoretically be at greater risk of cerebral ischaemia. These factors place the infant at risk for significant neurological insults during neurosurgical procedures compared with adults.

General considerations

Pre-operative evaluation

History and physical examination

The importance of proper and thorough preparation of the paediatric patient for anaesthesia and surgery is frequently overlooked in the perioperative period. Given the systemic effects of general anaesthesia and the physiological stress of surgery, an organ system-based approach is optimal for anticipating potential physiological derangements and coexisting disease states that may increase the risk of perioperative complications. Many potential perioperative problems can be pre-emptively addressed with such an approach. As some children are either pre-verbal or do not fully understand their medical condition, their parents or primary carers should be interviewed carefully to obtain information regarding coexisting medical problems. A thorough review of the patient's history can reveal conditions that may increase the risk of adverse reactions to anaesthesia and perioperative morbidity, and identify patients who need more extensive evaluation or whose medical condition needs to be optimized before surgery. There are also special perioperative concerns regarding children with neurological abnormalities

(Table 14.1). A thorough neurological examination should be a routine component of the pre-operative evaluation of children undergoing any neurosurgical procedure. It is critical to be able to document accurately any change in neurological status from baseline. Pre-operative fasting is necessary to minimize aspiration of gastric contents during the operative procedure, and guidelines vary according to local practices. Certain patients presenting for neurosurgical procedures may be at particular risk for aspiration of gastric contents, and caution should be exercised during induction of anaesthesia in these children.

Laboratory evaluation

Pre-operative evaluation and laboratory tests should be tailored to the proposed neurosurgical procedure. Given the risk of significant blood loss associated with surgery, a haematocrit, prothrombin time (PT) and partial thromboplastin time (PTT) should be obtained in order to uncover any insidious haematological disorder. Patients with suprasellar pathology should get serum thyroid hormone levels, as hypothyroidism may delay emergence from anaesthesia and complicate the post-operative neurological evaluation of infants or children. Type and cross-matched blood should be ordered prior to all craniotomies. Electrolyte disturbances may exist in some children with particular intracranial pathologies. Tumours such as craniopharyngiomas and other lesions affecting the hypothalamic–pituitary axis may cause significant perturbations in serum sodium. Some patients with such lesions will present for surgical procedures already on therapeutic agents such as 1-deamino-8-D-arginine vasopressin (DDAVP). Evaluation of serum electrolytes and serum osmolality is necessary for optimal perioperative management of these patients.

Induction of anaesthesia

The perioperative approach to the paediatric patient should take into account the patient's developmental age and neurological status. Paediatric neurosurgical patients may not fully comprehend the gravity of the proposed surgery and are non-cooperative. Sedatives given before the induction of anaesthesia can ease separation of the child from the parents and the transition from the pre-operative holding area to the operating room. Midazolam given orally is particularly effective in relieving anxiety and producing amnesia. Pre-operative sedation should be withheld or administered only with close observation in patients with deteriorating findings on neurological examination or lethargy, because it can induce respiratory depression and interfere with serial neurological examinations. A common problem is an uncooperative toddler who has an intracranial tumour and moderately decreased intracranial compliance, yet is agitated and resistant to separation from parents. Behaviours such as crying can elevate ICP and can present the anaesthesiologist with a dilemma regarding the approach to induction. Patients with elevated ICP may be at increased risk for delayed gastric emptying and thus aspiration. However, a crying, agitated child has demonstrated a tolerance to increased ICP, and the stress of inserting an intravenous catheter for induction of anaesthesia should be inconsequential.

The patient's neurological status and coexisting medical conditions will dictate the appropriate technique and drugs for induction of anaesthesia. In infants and young children, general anaesthesia can be induced with inhalation of sevoflurane in oxygen. Many practitioners will also use N_2O as a component of an inhalational induction. However, there is much debate regarding the use of N_2O during neurosurgical procedures. The use of N_2O should probably be considered on an individual case basis. Sevoflurane is not without neurological consequences, as it has been shown to have epileptogenic potential. However, the mechanism of this phenomenon is unclear. Alternatively, if the patient already has an intravenous catheter, anaesthesia can be induced with sedative/hypnotic drugs such

thiopental (5–8 mg kg^{-1}) or propofol (3–4 mg kg^{-1}). These drugs rapidly induce unconsciousness and can blunt the haemodynamic effects of tracheal intubation. A non-depolarizing muscle relaxant is then administered after induction of general anaesthesia in order to facilitate intubation of the trachea. Patients with nausea or gastro-oesophageal reflux disorder are at risk for aspiration pneumonitis and should have a rapid-sequence induction of anaesthesia performed with thiopental or propofol immediately followed by a rapid-acting muscle relaxant and cricoid pressure. Rocuronium can be used when succinylcholine is contraindicated, such as for patients with spinal cord injuries or paretic extremities. In these instances, succinylcholine can result in sudden, catastrophic hyperkalaemia. In children, the routine use of succinylcholine is uncommon. Concerns over occult myopathies, particularly in young males, are the reason. Once again, the use of succinylcholine should be an individualized decision based on the particular risks identified during the pre-operative evaluation.

Maintenance of anaesthesia

There are several classes of drugs used to maintain general anaesthesia. Potent, volatile anaesthetic agents (i.e. sevoflurane, isoflurane and desflurane) are administered by inhalation. These drugs are potent cerebral vascular dilators and cerebral metabolic depressants, which can mediate dose-dependent uncoupling of cerebral metabolic supply and demand while increasing cerebral blood volume and ICP. Moreover, the use of these agents can be associated with a significant decrease in cerebral perfusion pressure (CPP), primarily due to a dose-dependent reduction in arterial blood pressure. They depress the EEG and may interfere with intraoperative electrocorticography (ECoG). Given these issues, volatile anaesthetics are rarely used as the sole anaesthetic for neurosurgery. Nitrous oxide also acts as a cerebral vascular dilator.

Intravenous anaesthetics include sedative-hypnotics and opioids. These agents are also potent cerebral metabolic depressants but do not cause cerebral vasodilation. The sedative-hypnotics propofol, midazolam and thiopental rapidly induce general anaesthesia and attenuate the EEG. Opioid drugs can depress the EEG but not to the same degree as the sedative hypnotics. Fentanyl and other related synthetic opioids including sufentanil have their context-sensitive half-times increase with repeated dosing or prolonged infusions and require hepatic metabolism. As a result, the narcotic effects of these drugs, such as respiratory depression and sedation, may be prolonged. Remifentanil is a unique opioid that is rapidly cleared by plasma esterases whose context-sensitive half-life remains constant unrelated to the length of infusion. This makes it, when administered at a rate of $0.2–1.0 \,\mu\mathrm{g}\,\mathrm{kg}^{-1}\,\mathrm{min}^{-1}$, an ideal opioid for rapid emergence from anaesthesia. However, this rapid recovery is frequently accompanied by delirium and inadequate analgesia. Although craniotomies generally do not require aggressive post-operative pain management, the immediate post-operative period generally requires the use of intravenous opioids. Thus, when remifentanil is utilized for maintenance of general anaesthesia, a longer-acting opioid such as morphine or hydromorphone should be part of the plan for the immediate post-operative period. Deep neuromuscular blockade with a non-depolarizing muscle relaxant is maintained to avoid patient movement and minimize the amount of anaesthetic agents needed. Muscle relaxants should be withheld or permitted to wear off when assessment of motor function during neurosurgery is planned. During many neurosurgical procedures, head fixation devices such as the Mayfield head clamp are employed. The use of muscle relaxation when these devices are employed is extremely important to prevent inadvertent patient movement while fixed in these clamps and pins. Sudden uncontrolled patient movement while in a head fixation device can result in scalp lacerations and even cervical spine injuries.

Positioning

Children with elevated ICP should be transported to the pre-operative holding area and operating room with the head elevated in the midline position to maximize cerebral venous drainage. Once a patient is in the operating room, the neurosurgeons and anaesthesiologists must all have adequate access to the patient. This can be particularly challenging in infants and small children, for whom slight displacement of the head or small movements of the endotracheal tube can result in tracheal extubation or endobronchial intubation, so extra care must be taken to ensure the airway is secured after final positioning. Given the fact that many neurosurgical procedures can be quite lengthy, it is important to carefully establish and evaluate adequate positioning prior to prepping and draping of the patient. Additionally, major positional adjustment of the patient during

the procedure may be contraindicated if the patient is placed in a head fixation device due to potential for cervical spine injury under anaesthesia.

The prone position is commonly used for posterior fossa and spinal cord surgery in paediatric patients. In addition to the physiological sequelae of this position, a whole spectrum of compression and stretch injuries has been reported. Padding under the chest and pelvis can support the torso. It is important to ensure free abdominal wall motion, because increased intra-abdominal pressure can impair ventilation, cause venocaval compression and increase epidural venous pressure and bleeding. In males, the penis and testicles should be checked to ensure there is no compression. Soft rolls are used to elevate and support the lateral chest wall and hips in order to minimize any increase in abdominal and thoracic pressure. In addition, this allows a Doppler probe to be placed on the chest without pressure. The head must be carefully flexed to avoid kinking of the endotracheal tube, inadvertently advancing the tube into an endobronchial position or compressing the chin on the chest. Too much flexion for an extended time can cause lower brainstem and upper spinal cord ischaemia, as well as head and tongue swelling from blockage of venous or lymphatic drainage. This can lead to post-extubation airway obstruction or croup.

Most neurosurgical procedures are performed with the head slightly elevated to facilitate venous and CSF drainage from the surgical site. However, superior sagittal sinus pressure decreases with greater head elevation, and this increases the likelihood of venous air embolism (VAE). Extreme head flexion can cause brainstem compression in patients with pathological conditions of the posterior fossa, such as mass lesions or Arnold–Chiari malformations. It can also cause endotracheal tube problems, including obstruction from kinking or displacement to the carina or the right mainstem bronchus. Extreme rotation of the head can impede venous return through the jugular veins and lead to impaired cerebral perfusion, increased ICP and cerebral venous bleeding.

Monitoring

Standard monitoring equipment used for all patients undergoing anaesthesia include an ECG, pulse oximeter, blood pressure gauge, end-tidal carbon dioxide analyser and thermometer. A precordial or oesophageal stethoscope is commonly used in North American practice, but less so in Europe. Given the potential for sudden haemodynamic instability due to VAE, haemorrhage, herniation syndromes, or manipulation of cranial nerves, placement of an intra-arterial cannula for continuous blood pressure monitoring is appropriate for most neurosurgical procedures. An arterial catheter also provides access for sampling serial blood gases, electrolytes, haematocrit and serum osmolality. Central venous pressures may not accurately reflect vascular volume, especially in a child in the prone position. Therefore, the risks of a central venous catheter may outweigh the benefits. Certain patients may arrive in the operating room with ICP monitoring devices. The intraoperative use of these devices may be useful in particular cases but should not be considered a necessary routine monitor for children undergoing neurosurgical procedures.

Vascular access

Owing to limited access by the anaesthesiologist to the child during many neurosurgical procedures, optimal intravenous access is mandatory prior to the start of surgery. Central venous catheters are often inserted for intravenous access, central pressure monitoring and infusion of vasoactive drugs in adult neurosurgical procedures. However, paediatric central vein catheters have a small internal diameter (gauge) and are resistant to high flow rates. Two large peripheral venous cannulae are sufficient for most paediatric craniotomies. In the child that has difficult peripheral venous access, central venous cannulation may be necessary. Utilization of the femoral vein avoids the risk of pneumothorax associated with subclavian catheters, and does not interfere with cerebral venous drainage, as may be the case with jugular venous catheters. Furthermore, femoral catheters are more easily accessible to the anaesthesiologist during intracranial operations. As significant blood loss and haemodynamic instability can occur during craniotomies, an intra-arterial cannula provides direct blood pressure monitoring and sampling for blood gas analysis.

Venous air embolism occurs when ambient air enters the vascular system through open venous sinuses in the surgical field during surgical procedures. The incidence of VAE in children undergoing suboccipital craniotomy in the sitting position is not significantly different from that in adults. However, children appear to have a higher incidence of hypotension and a lower likelihood of successful aspiration of intravascular air via central venous catheters.

Post-operative issues

Close observation in an intensive care unit (ICU) with serial neurological examinations and invasive haemodynamic monitoring is helpful for the prevention and early detection of post-operative problems. In certain patients, seizures can occur during the post-operative period and may lead to significantly increased morbidity. When seizures do occur, the response must be prompt: first with basic life support algorithms addressing airway, breathing and circulation, and then with administration of sufficient anticonvulsant drug to stop the seizure. A common approach involves lorazepam 0.1 mg kg^{-1} IV (repeated after 10 min if necessary) for immediate control, followed by fosphenytoin 20 mg kg^{-1}, phenobarbitol 20 mg kg^{-1} or levetiracetam 10 mg kg^{-1} on a regular schedule for more lasting coverage. Levetiracetam is becoming an increasingly common agent used for seizure prophylaxis in the perioperative period. The reasons for this change from fosphenytoin and phenobarbitol include the generally more favourable side effect profile of levetiracetam as well as the lack of the need for following drug levels. Phenytoin levels may be altered in sick children in the hospital and free drug levels should be followed rather than total drug levels.

Pain control and sedation present unique challenges in the paediatric ICU. Ideally, post-operative neurosurgical patients are comfortable, awake and cooperative in order to obtain serial neurological examinations. In paediatrics, these goals can be difficult to achieve due to the cognitive level of the patient. The mainstay of sedation in the paediatric ICU remains a combination of opioid and benzodiazepine administered via continuous infusion. Infants and children receiving sedative infusion for >3–5 days are subject to tolerance and experience symptoms of withdrawal when infusions are discontinued. Propofol is a potent, ultra-short-acting sedative-hypnotic that is extremely useful in adult neurocritical care but has only limited utility in paediatrics because of its association with a fatal syndrome of bradycardia, rhabdomyolysis, metabolic acidosis and multiple organ failure when used over extended periods in small children. While some centres have advocated its use in children under strict controls, propofol is generally limited to operative anaesthesia, procedural sedation and continuous infusions of limited duration (<24 h).

A newer agent, dexmedetomidine, an intravenous α$_2$-agonist, is an ultra-short-acting, single-agent sedative that is often used in the post-operative period. The purported advantage of this agent is its ability to provide sedation while allowing easy and frequent neurological assessment. Studies involving children are preliminary, but the drug appears to be safe and effective when used for periods of 24 h or less. Opioid cross-tolerance makes it a useful agent for treatment of fentanyl or morphine withdrawal. Transient increases in blood pressure can be seen with boluses followed by hypotension and bradycardia as sedation deepens. Further experience and vetting will be necessary to determine the proper place for this agent in the routine perioperative care of neurosurgical patients.

Anaesthesia for specific neurosurgical procedures

Neonatal emergencies

Myelomeningocele

Myelomeningocele is due to failure of closure of the posterior neural tube, resulting in malformation of the vertebral column and spinal cord and other CNS anomalies. This defect occurs during the fourth week of gestation. Thus, there is a problem that arises very early in gestation that results in a wide spectrum of CNS abnormalities. McLone and Knepper hypothesized that the aetiology of this spectrum of abnormalities results from failure of fusion of the neural tube leading to leakage of CSF through this defect during critical CNS development. This leakage does not create the conditions necessary for distension of the cranial end of the neural tube, which leads to abnormal development of the CNS and, in particular, the posterior fossa and its contents. Thus, the myelomeningocele itself is essentially the most identifiable external manifestation of a spectrum of potential CNS pathologies whose common aetiology can be traced to very early embryologic development.

The spinal defect can occur anywhere along the vertebral column, although lumbar and low thoracic defects are most common. In the most severe forms (rachischisis), the neural plate appears as a raw, fleshy plaque through a vertebral column defect (spina bifida) and the skin. A protruding membranous sac containing meninges, CSF, nerve roots and a dysplastic spinal cord often protrudes through the defect in meningocele or myelomeningocele. Tracheal intubation of a neonate with a myelomeningocele can be challenging

depending on the size and location of the defect. The supine patient may be elevated on towel rolls taking care to create a port through which the myelomeningocele may protrude. Likewise, the neonate can be positioned in the right lateral decubitus position to allow an unimpeded arc from right to left for laryngoscopy and intubation. Blood and insensible fluid loss is dependent on the size of the myelomeningocele and the amount of tissue dissection required to repair the defect. Hydrocephalus occurs in 80% of neonates with myelomeningocele or encephalocele, and a ventriculoperitoneal shunt will often need to be inserted immediately after the myelomeningocele is initially repaired or within several days after primary closure.

Intraventricular haemorrhages

Given the fragile nature of their cerebral vascular system, low-birthweight premature neonates frequently develop intraventricular haemorrhage, which can lead to post-haemorrhagic hydrocephalus. Exaggerated fluctuations in blood pressure have been implicated in the development of intraventricular haemorrhage. Evaluation for intraventricular haemorrhage involves a head ultrasound, made easier in infants because of their open fontanelles. Evaluation of the presence and extent of intraventricular haemorrhage should take place prior to administration of any systemic anticoagulants such as heparin or enoxaparin.

Signs and symptoms of post-haemorrhagic hydrocephalus include enlarging occipital-to-frontal circumference, a tense anterior fontanelle and periods of bradycardia. Serial lumbar punctures will temporize the symptoms. However, the definitive surgical approach to this problem is to insert a shunt attached to a subgaleal reservoir. The major anaesthetic issues in managing these premature neonates are the transport from and to the neonatal ICU and continuation of ventilator and haemodynamic support.

Hydrocephalus

Hydrocephalus is a vexing paediatric neurosurgical condition that has a laundry list of aetiologies including haemorrhage (neonatal intraventricular or subarachnoid), congenital problems (aqueductal stenosis), trauma, infection and tumours (especially in the posterior fossa). Unless the aetiology of the hydrocephalus can be definitively treated, treatment entails surgical placement of a ventricular drain or ventriculoperitoneal shunt. Alternatively, the shunt can drain into the right atrium or pleural cavity. Acute obstruction of these shunts should be treated urgently because acute rises in ICP in the relatively small cranial vault of the infant or child can be lethal. Anaesthesia should be established in the obtunded patient with a rapid sequence induction technique followed by tracheal intubation. If intravenous access cannot be established, an inhalation induction with sevoflurane and gentle cricoid pressure may be an alternative in the conscious patient. The possibility of VAE during placement of the distal end of a ventriculoatrial shunt should always be kept in mind. Post-operatively, patients should be observed carefully because an altered mental status and recent peritoneal incision place them at high risk for pulmonary aspiration once feedings are begun.

Chiari malformations

There are four types of Chiari malformations (Table 14.2). The Arnold–Chiari malformation (type II) almost always coexists in children with myelodysplasia. This defect consists of a bony abnormality in the posterior fossa and upper cervical spine with caudal displacement of the cerebellar vermis, fourth ventricle and lower brainstem below the plane of the foramen magnum. Medullary cervical cord compression can occur. Vocal cord paralysis with stridor and respiratory distress, apnoea, abnormal swallowing and pulmonary aspiration, opisthotonos and cranial nerve deficits may be associated with the Arnold–Chiari malformation and usually present during infancy. Patients with vocal cord paralysis or a diminished gag reflex may require tracheostomy and gastrostomy to secure the airway and minimize chronic aspiration. Patients of any age may have abnormal responses to hypoxia and hypercarbia because of cranial nerve and brainstem dysfunction. Extreme head flexion may cause brainstem compression in otherwise asymptomatic patients.

Type I Chiari malformations can occur in healthy children without myelodysplasia. These defects involve caudal displacement of the cerebellar tonsils below the foramen magnum, but patients generally have much milder symptoms, sometimes presenting only with headache or neck pain.

Surgical treatment usually involves a decompressive suboccipital craniectomy with cervical laminectomies in the prone position. Given the proximity of the straight and transverse sinus under the occipital bone, massive blood loss and VAE can occur as the bone flap is lifted.

Table 14.2 Chiari malformations

Type	Malformation
Type I	Caudal displacement of cerebellar tonsils below the plane of the foramen magnum
Type II	Arnold–Chiari, associated with myelomeningocele: caudal displacement of the cerebellar vermis, fourth ventricle and lower brainstem below the plane of the foramen magnum. Dysplastic brainstem with characteristic 'kink', elongation of the fourth ventricle, 'beaking' of the quadrigeminal plate, hypoplastic tentorium with small posterior fossa, polymicrogyria and enlargement of the massa intermedia
Type III	Caudal displacement of the cerebellum and brainstem into a high cervical meningocele
Type IV	Cerebellar hypoplasia

Tumours

Posterior fossa tumours

As the majority of intracranial tumours in children occur in the posterior fossa, CSF flow is often obstructed and intracranial hypertension and hydrocephalus are often present. Most neurosurgeons approach this region with children in the prone position. The patient's head is generally secured with a Mayfield head frame, although pins used in small children can cause skull fractures, dural tears and intracranial haematomas. Elevation of the bone flap can result in sinus tears, massive blood loss and/or VAE. Surgical resection of tumours in the posterior fossa can also lead to brainstem and/or cranial nerve damage. Table 14.3 lists some of the signs of encroachment on these structures. Damage to the respiratory centres and cranial nerves can lead to apnoea and airway obstruction after extubation of the patient's trachea.

Suprasellar tumours

Craniopharyngiomas are the most common periosellar tumours in children and adolescents and may be associated with hypothalamic and pituitary dysfunction. Steroid replacement (dexamethasone or hydrocortisone) is generally administered, as the integrity of the hypothalamic–pituitary–adrenal axis may be uncertain. In addition, diabetes insipidus occurs preoperatively in some patients and is a common postoperative problem. Nocturnal enuresis may result in

Table 14.3 Effects of surgical brainstem manipulation

Brainstem area	Signs	Changes in monitor
Cranial nerve V	Hypertension, bradycardia	Arterial pressure, ECG
Cranial nerve VII	Facial muscle movement	EMG
Cranial nerve X	Hypotension, bradycardia	Arterial pressure, ECG
Pons, medulla	Arrhythmias, hypotension, hypertension, tachy- or bradycardia, irregular breathing pattern	ECG, arterial pressure, end-tidal carbon dioxide

Table 14.4 Diagnostic criteria for diabetes insipidus

Criterion	Measurement
Urine output	$4\,ml\,kg^{-1}\,h^{-1}$
Serum sodium	$>145\,mEq\,l^{-1}$
Serum osmolality	$>300\,mOsm\,kg^{-1}$
Urine osmolality	$<300\,mOsm\,kg^{-1}$
Polyuria persisting	$>30\,min$

pre-operative hypovolaemia. If diabetes insipidus does not exist pre-operatively, it usually does not develop until the post-operative period. This is because there appears to be an adequate reserve of antidiuretic hormone in the posterior pituitary gland capable of functioning for many hours, even when the hypothalamic–pituitary stalk is damaged intraoperatively. The surgical approach to the sella is between the frontal lobes in infants and young children and transnasal in adolescences. The frontal approach tends to provoke more surgical bleeding and places the infant or child at risk for venous air embolism due the elevated position of the head during the surgery. Therefore, patients undergoing a frontal craniotomy should have adequate intravenous access and monitors such as an arterial catheter and pre-cordial Doppler. Although it occurs primarily after surgery, diabetes insipidus is associated with suprasellar surgery. The diagnosis of intraoperative diabetes insipidus is straightforward and is characterized by the criteria described in Table 14.4. Other causes of polyuria must be ruled out (e.g. administration of mannitol, furosemide or osmotic contrast agents, and the presence of hyperglycaemia). Once the diagnosis of diabetes insipidus is established, a vasopressin infusion is commenced at $1\,mU\,kg^{-1}\,h^{-1}$ and is increased every 5–10 min to a maximum of $10\,mU\,kg^{-1}\,h^{-1}$ to decrease the urine output to $<2\,ml\,kg^{-1}\,h^{-1}$. Total maintenance fluids (intravenous and oral fluids) should not exceed the insensible losses plus the obligate urinary losses. It is convenient to calculate the total intravenous fluids as two-thirds of maintenance. The appropriate intravenous fluid is 5% dextrose/0.9% saline with 0–$40\,mEq$ $KCl\,l^{-1}$. The antidiuretic effect of vasopressin is an 'all or none' phenomenon. Once the patient's urine output is $<2\,ml\,kg^{-1}\,h^{-1}$, the vasopressin and crystalloid infusion rate should be maintained until the patient is alert enough to take oral fluids and vasopressin derivatives such as DDAVP.

Epilepsy

Surgical treatment has become a viable option for many patients with medically intractable epilepsy. Two major considerations should be kept in mind. Chronic administration of anticonvulsant drugs, such as phenytoin and carbamazepine induces rapid metabolism and clearance of several classes of anaesthetic agents including neuromuscular blockers and opioids. Therefore, the anaesthetic requirements for these drugs are increased and require close monitoring of their effect and frequent redosing. Intraoperative neurophysiological monitors can be used to guide the actual resection of the epileptogenic focus and general anaesthetics can compromise the sensitivity of these devices. Furthermore, if cortical stimulation is utilized to mimic the seizure pattern or identify areas on the motor strip, neuromuscular blockade should be antagonized.

Occasionally, a repeat craniotomy must be performed in a child shortly after the primary procedure. An elective repeat craniotomy may be necessary for removal of grids and strips used for invasive EEG monitoring and subsequent resection of the seizure focus. It is important to avoid administration of N_2O until the dura is opened, as intracranial air can persist up to 3 weeks following a craniotomy, and N_2O in these situation can cause rapid expansion of air cavities and result in tension pneumocephalus.

Post-operative seizures are an uncommon but devastating complication. Prophylaxis in the peri-operative period and aggressive treatment of new convulsions are well-recognized mainstays of care. While phenytoin is the agent used most commonly for prophylaxis, maintaining therapeutic serum levels can be challenging. Levetiracetam is becoming increasingly common and in many instances supplanting phenytoin as the choice for prophylaxis. Both drugs can be administered intravenously, but, unlike phenytoin, administration of levetiracetam does not require following serum drug levels to monitor for toxicity. Alternative agents frequently used in paediatrics include pheno-barbital, carbamazepine and valproic acid. Status epilepticus can be treated with lorezepam 0.1 mg kg^{-1} IV push over 2 min or diazepam 0.5 mg kg^{-1} PR as effective agents. Lorezapam may be repeated after 10 min and accompanied by fosphenytoin 20 mg kg^{-1} IV or IM if initial doses are ineffective. Although potentially compounding respiratory depression, phenobarbital 20 mg kg^{-1} is also an effective first-line anti-epileptic drug.

The vagal nerve stimulator is another advance in the surgical treatment of epilepsy. Although its exact mechanism of action is not understood, it appears to inhibit seizure activity at brainstem or cortical levels. Its placement has shown benefit with minimal side effects in many patients who are disabled by intractable seizures. At this time, there are few published series of vagal nerve stimulation studies in children, but it is estimated that there is a 60–70% improvement in seizure control in children receiving vagal nerve stimulation, with the best results in those with drop attacks. The anaesthetic management of patients for implantation of vagal nerve stimulators should focus on the coexisting diseases. The procedure itself involves creation of a left subpectoral muscle pocket for the impulse generator and isolation of the left vagal nerve for positioning of the electrode.

Neurovascular disease

The perioperative management of paediatric patients with vascular anomalies should focus on optimizing cerebral perfusion. Operative management is commonly associated with massive blood loss and these patients require several IV access sites and invasive haemodynamic monitoring. Haemodynamic stability during intracranial surgery requires careful maintenance of intravascular volume. Massive blood loss should be anticipated and treated with blood replacement therapy. Hypotension can transiently be treated with vasopressor infusion (dopamine) during fluid resuscitation.

Moyamoya syndrome

Moyamoya syndrome is a rare, chronic vaso-occlusive disorder of the internal carotid arteries that presents as transient ischaemic attacks or recurrent strokes in childhood. The cause is unknown, but the syndrome can be associated with previous intracranial radiation, neurofibromatosis, Down's syndrome and a variety of haematological disorders. The anaesthetic management of these patients is directed at optimizing cerebral perfusion. This includes ensuring generous pre-operative hydration and maintaining the blood pressure within the patient's pre-operative range. Moyamoya syndrome is a vasculopathy characterized by chronic progressive stenosis to occlusion at the apices of the intracranial internal carotid arteries including the proximal anterior cerebral arteries and middle cerebral arteries, and is associated with: prior radiotherapy to the head or neck for optic gliomas, craniopharyngiomas and pituitary tumours; genetic disorders such as Down's syndrome, neurofibromatosis type I (NF1) (with or without hypothalamic–optic pathway tumours), large facial haemangiomas, sickle-cell anaemia and other haemo-globinopathies; and autoimmune disorders such as Graves' disease, congenital cardiac disease, renal artery stenosis and others. Moyamoya disease is the idiopathic form of moyamoya, while moyamoya syndrome is defined as the vasculopathy found in association with another condition, such as neurofibromatosis, sickle-cell disease or Down's syndrome. Maintenance of normocapnia is essential in patients with Moyamoya syndrome because both hyper- and hypocapnia can lead to steal phenomenon from the ischaemic region and further aggravate cerebral ischaemia. An opioid-based anaesthetic provides a stable level of anaesthesia for these patients and is compatible with intraoperative EEG monitoring. Once the patient emerges from anaesthesia, the same manoeuvres that optimize cerebral perfusion should be extended into the post-operative period. These patients should receive intravenous fluids to maintain adequate cerebral perfusion and adequate narcotics to avoid hyperventilation induced by pain and crying.

Arteriovenous malformations

Arteriovenous malformations (AVMs) result from improper formation of the arteriolar-capillary network that provides a connection between arteries and veins in the brain. The embryonic origins of these malformations are unclear. Malformations not large enough to produce congestive heart failure usually remain clinically silent unless they cause seizures or a stroke or until the acute rupture of a communicating vessel results in subarachnoid or intracerebral haemorrhage. Overall, 80–85% of all paediatric AVMs present with haemorrhage. It may present with seizures, headache or focal neurological deficits. Haemorrhagic AVMs have been associated with a 25% mortality rate. Rebleeding rates are approximately 6% for the first 6 months, then 3% per year afterwards. This lesion produces neurological deficits through mass effect or from cerebral ischaemia that is due to diversion of blood to the AVM from the normal cerebral circulation ('steal').

Vein of Galen malformations

Vein of Galen malformations (VOGMs) are direct connections between cerebral arteries and existing veins. Unlike AVMs, they do not usually have a nidus and, in some cases of arteriovenous fistula, may exist as a single pathological connection between an artery and vein. In VOGMs, single or multiple small arterial vessels directly drain into the vein of Galen. The result of this type of direct connection is markedly increased cerebral venous pressure, leading to increased ICP and potential haemorrhage. In some VOGMs, the connections have such rapid flow rates that children develop high-output cardiac failure and hydrocephalus. The management of the neonate with VOGM is primarily supportive with vasopressors and mechanical ventilation for progressive congestive heart failure. Aggressive embolizations in the interventional radiology suite are first-line therapies for neonates with VOGM. Infants and children with residual lesions may require additional embolizations and surgery for the placement of ventriculoperitoneal shunts for hydrocephalus.

Ventriculoscopy

Technological advances in minimally invasive endoscopic surgery have entered the neurosurgical arena. The anaesthetic considerations for these evolving techniques are the same as for any other neurosurgical procedures, as discussed in this chapter. Endoscopic third ventriculoscopy has become an accepted procedure for the treatment of obstructive hydrocephalus in infants and children. Despite the relative safety of this procedure, bradycardia and other arrhythmias have been reported in conjunction with irrigation fluids and/or manipulation of the floor of the third ventricle.

Traumatic brain injury

Paediatric head trauma requires a multiorgan approach to minimizing morbidity and mortality. A small child's head is often the point of impact in injuries, but other organs can also be damaged. As secondary insults can progressively worsen outcome, basic life-support algorithms should be applied immediately to assure a patent airway, spontaneous respiration and adequate circulation. Immobilization of the cervical spine is essential to avoid secondary spinal cord injury with manipulation of the patient's airway until radiological clearance is confirmed. Blunt abdominal trauma and long-bone fractures frequently occur with head injury and can be major sources of blood loss. In order to assure tissue perfusion during the operative period, the patient's blood volume should be restored with crystalloid solutions and/or blood products. Ongoing blood loss can lead to coagulopathies and should be treated with specific blood components.

Infants with shaken baby syndrome often present with a myriad of chronic and acute subdural haematomas. As with all traumatic events, the presence of other coexisting injuries, fractures and abdominal trauma should be identified. Craniotomies for the evacuation of either epidural or subdural haematomas are at high risk for massive blood loss and VAE. Postoperative management of these victims is marked by the management of intracranial hypertension and, in the most severe cases, determination of brain death.

Resuscitation

Traumatic brain injury (TBI) is an evolving process that extends beyond the initial insult. Progression of the primary neuronal injury can be attenuated by preventing hypotension and hypoxia. Rapid implementation of advanced life-support algorithms is an essential first step in the management of head-injured patients.

Securing a patent airway and restoring oxygenation and ventilation are paramount in advanced life-support algorithms. Secondary injury results from the pathological sequelae of the primary injury: oedema and ischaemia due to cortical compression, hypotension, hypoxia and so on. Inappropriate manipulation of a patient with an unstable fracture can exacerbate both primary and secondary injuries. Anaesthesiologists caring for a child with a potential cervical spine injury should know that spinal cord injuries in children commonly occur without actual evidence of spinal bone fractures on plain cervical radiographs. These injuries are known as SCIWORA (spinal cord injuries without radiologic abnormality). Injuries to the cervical spine in particular are often difficult to recognize but may sometimes be identified by odontoid displacement or pre-vertebral swelling on a radiograph. As a result, CT is frequently indicated when a spinal injury is initially suspected in a child with trauma. Sometimes, as with brain injury, there can be a delay in the onset of neurological deficits with SCIWORA injuries. However, infants and young children are predisposed to C1–2 cervical disruptions, which may be difficult to diagnose in cervical spine X-rays. There should be minimal cervical spine manipulation during tracheal intubation of the head-injured infant.

Age-appropriate normograms of blood pressure in paediatric patients should dictate the end points of resuscitation. Hypotension is associated with greater mortality in children than in adults. Vavilala and colleagues confirmed this notion by correlating hypotension to increased morbidity and mortality. Therefore, hypotension secondary to trauma should be treated aggressively by securing large-bore intravenous catheters and restoration of fluid deficits. After normotension has been achieved, CPP management should be instituted according to the haemodynamic parameters listed below. The choice of resuscitation fluids remains controversial, whether it is crystalloid, colloid or hypertonic saline. However, the administration of hypertonic saline has been shown to improve various clinical parameters, although not survival rate.

Intracranial pressure monitoring

The use of ICP monitoring in infants and children with severe head injury with a Glasgow Coma Scale score <8 is strongly supported by several clinical studies. However, as noted above, age-specific differences in cerebral haemodynamics necessitate modifying these variables. All retrospective studies on the effects of ICP have demonstrated that pronounced morbidity and mortality occur after the ICP is persistently elevated above 20 mmHg. Although there is an age-related decrease in normal ICP in infants and young children, these retrospective studies demonstrate that the 'safe' upper limit for ICP is similar in adults. However, the value of '<20 mmHg' was artificially set, and lower increments were not fully tested in paediatric patients. Intracranial pressure measurements from ventricular

catheters and fibre-optic intraparenchymal transducers have a good correlation. However, ventricular catheters also provide a conduit to withdraw CSF.

Management of cerebral perfusion pressure

One of the most controversial topics in the management of TBI patients is the goal of cerebral perfusion. The goals of therapy should be based on the data obtained from cerebral vascular monitors. Several paediatric studies have demonstrated that lower CPP is associated with better outcome when compared with adult values. Downard and colleagues retrospectively reviewed the course of 188 children with TBI and concluded that there were no survivors with CPP <40 mmHg. Furthermore, 10 mmHg increases in CPP up to 70 mmHg did not improve the Glasgow Outcome Scale score. Chambers and colleagues determined the critical thresholds for CPP in relation to the patient's age. They reported that CPP in head-injured patients should be 48 mmHg at 2–6 years, 54 mmHg at 7–10 years and 58 mmHg at 11–15 years. Therefore, maintaining CPP above 40 mmHg appears to be associated with the best outcome in paediatric patients. However, studies in infants need to be performed in order to assess the efficacy of even lower CPP.

Drugs

Endotracheal intubation and mechanical ventilation mandates prolonged sedation and, in severe cases, neuromuscular blockade. Sedation is carried out with intermittent doses of midazolam, fentanyl or morphine as first-line drugs to minimize discomfort and agitation. Brain swelling can initially be managed by hyperventilation and elevating the head above the heart. Should these manoeuvres fail, mannitol can be given at a dose of 0.25–1.0 g kg^{-1} IV. This will transiently alter cerebral haemodynamics and raise serum osmolality by 10–20 mOsm kg^{-1}. Furosemide is a useful adjunct to mannitol in decreasing acute cerebral oedema and has been shown in vitro to prevent rebound swelling due to mannitol. All diuretics will interfere with the ability to utilize urine output as a guide to intravascular volume status. The use of hypertonic saline (3% NaCl) has been shown to decrease ICP and improve CPP in paediatric patients.

High-dose barbiturate therapy produces a burst suppression pattern on the EEG and results in a reduction in cerebral metabolic rate. Refractory intracranial hypertension can be treated by thiopental infusions. However, myocardial depression and hypotension are unacceptable side effects of this therapy and need to be countered by volume loading and ionotropic support.

Decompressive craniotomy

Reduction of severe intracranial hypertension that is refractory of less invasive manoeuvres may warrant surgical decompression of haemorrhagic and oedematous brain tissue. Polin and colleagues reported the effect of bifrontal decompressive craniectomy in a mixed population of head-injured patients. Favourable outcome correlated with pre-operative ICP <40 mmHg, treatment within 48 h of presentation and age <18 years. Taylor and colleagues prospectively evaluated the utility of early decompressive craniectomy within 24 h after the time of injury. They reported a significant decrease in ICP and improved 6-month outcome in the children undergoing the decompressive craniectomy. Cho and colleagues reported their experience with bifrontal or frontotemporal craniotomy for management of refractory intracranial hypertension due to shaken baby syndrome. They found a significant decrease in mortality in the craniotomy group when compared with the medically managed children. Jagannathan and colleagues reported the outcome of 23 craniotomies performed on children (mean age of 11.9 years). Sixteen patients survived and 81% of the survivors returned to school and had a reasonable quality of life. Despite the severity of this surgical approach, studies in children and adults demonstrate the utility in reducing refractory intracranial hypertension and an improvement in outcome. Therefore, decompressive craniotomy has a role as a last attempt at managing moribund head-injured infants and children.

Induced hypothermia

Induced hypothermia has been shown unequivocally to reduce neurological injury in pre-clinical studies. Its efficacy in the clinical setting has been controversial. Head cooling and mild hypothermia have been demonstrated to be protective in asphyxiated neonates. However, induced hypothermia in adult TBI has mixed results. Adelson and colleagues demonstrated in a Phase II trial that induced hypothermia can be a safe therapeutic option in children with TBI. A National Institutes of Health-sponsored Phase III trial is underway. Recently, an international multicentre trial of induced hypothermia in paediatric patients reported that hypothermia did not improve the neurological outcome and may increase mortality.

Conclusion

The management of paediatric patients for neurosurgery is currently based on a few randomized trials and draws heavily from data derived from adult series. Evidence-based management of paediatric patients is still evolving. Therefore, fundamental knowledge of age-related differences in cerebral vascular physiology and anatomy is essential for the perioperative management of paediatric neurosurgical patients.

Further reading

Adelson, P. D., Bratton, S. L., Carney, N. A. et al. (2003). Guidelines for the acute medical management of severe traumatic brain injury in infants, children, and adolescents. Chapter 5. Indications for intracranial pressure monitoring in pediatric patients with severe traumatic brain injury. *Pediatr Crit Care Med* **4** (Suppl.) S19–S24.

Adelson, P. D., Ragheb, J., Kanev, P. et al. (2005). Phase II clinical trial of moderate hypothermia after severe traumatic brain injury in children. *Neurosurgery* **56**, 740–54.

Arieff, A. I., Ayus, J. C. and Fraser, C. L. (1992). Hyponatraemia and death or permanent brain damage in healthy children. *BMJ* **304**, 1218–22.

Boylan, G. B., Young, K., Panerai, R. B., Rennie, J. M. and Evans, D. H. (2000). Dynamic cerebral autoregulation in sick newborn infants. *Pediatr Res* **48**, 12–17.

Chambers, I. R., Jones, P. A., Lo, T. Y. et al. (2006). Critical thresholds of intracranial pressure and cerebral perfusion pressure related to age in paediatric head injury. *J Neurol Neurosurg Psychiatry* **77**, 234–40.

Cho, D. Y., Wang, Y. C. and Chi, C. S. (1995). Decompressive craniotomy for acute shaken/impact baby syndrome. *Pediatr Neurosurg* **23**, 192–8.

Clifton, G. L., Miller, E. R., Choi, S. C. et al. (2001). Lack of effect of induction of hypothermia after acute brain injury. *N Engl J Med* **344**, 556–63.

Cohen, M. M., Cameron, C. B. and Duncan, P. G. (1990). Pediatric anesthesia morbidity and mortality in the perioperative period. *Anesth Analg* **70**, 160–7.

Constant, I., Seeman, R. and Murat, I. (2005). Sevoflurane and epileptiform EEG changes. *Paediatr Anaesth* **15**, 266–74.

Cray, S. H., Robinson, B. H. and Cox, P. N. (1998). Lactic acidemia and bradyarrhythmia in a child sedated with propofol [see comments]. *Crit Care Med* **26**, 2087–92.

Cucchiara, R. F. and Bowers, B. (1982). Air embolism in children undergoing suboccipital craniotomy. *Anesthesiology* **57**, 338–9.

Diaz, S. M., Rodarte, A., Foley, J. and Capparelli, E. V. (2007). Pharmacokinetics of dexmedetomidine in postsurgical pediatric intensive care unit patients: preliminary study. *Pediatr Crit Care Med* **8**, 419–24.

Downard, C., Hulka, F., Mullins, R. J. *et al.* (2000). Relationship of cerebral perfusion pressure and survival in pediatric brain-injured patients. *J Trauma* **49**, 654–8.

Duhaime, A. C., Christian, C. W., Rorke, L. B. and Zimmerman, R. A. (1998). Nonaccidental head injury in infants – the "shaken-baby syndrome". *N Engl J Med* **338**, 1822–9.

El-Dawlatly, A. A., Murshid, W., Alshimy, A. *et al.* (2001). Arrhythmias during neuroendoscopic procedures. *J Neurosurg Anesthesiol* **13**, 57–8.

Eldredge, E. A., Soriano, S. G. and Rockoff, M. A. (1995). Neuroanesthesia. In Adelson, P. D. and Black, P. M., eds., *Surgical Treatment of Epilepsy in Children*, vol. 6. Philadelphia: W. B. Saunders, pp. 505–20.

Ferrari, L. R. (1999). *Anesthesia and Pain Management for the Pediatrician*. Baltimore: Johns Hopkins University Press.

Ferrari, L. R., Rooney, F. M. and Rockoff, M. A. (1999). Preoperative fasting practices in pediatrics. *Anesthesiology* **90**, 978–80.

Gambardella, G., Zaccone, C., Cardia, E. and Tomasello, F. (1993). Intracranial pressure monitoring in children: comparison of external ventricular device with the fiberoptic system. *Childs Nerv Syst* **9**, 470–3.

German, J. W., Aneja, R., Heard, C. and Dias, M. (2000). Continuous remifentanil for pediatric neurosurgery patients. *Pediatr Neurosurg* **33**, 227–9.

Grady, M. S., Bedford, R. F. and Park, T. S. (1986). Changes in superior sagittal sinus pressure in children with head elevation, jugular venous compression, and PEEP. *J Neurosurg* **65**, 199–202.

Hertzog, J. H., Dalton, H. J., Anderson, B. D. *et al.* (2000). Prospective evaluation of propofol anesthesia in the pediatric intensive care unit for elective oncology procedures in ambulatory and hospitalized children. *Pediatrics* **106**, 742–7.

Hutchison, J. S., Ward, R. E., Lacroix, J. *et al.* (2008). Hypothermia therapy after traumatic brain injury in children. *N Engl J Med* **358**, 2447–56.

Jagannathan, J., Okonkwo, D. O., Dumont, A. S. *et al.* (2007). Outcome following decompressive craniectomy in children with severe traumatic brain injury: a 10-year single-center experience with long-term follow up. *J Neurosurg* **106** (Suppl.), 268–75.

Johnson, J. O., Jimenez, D. F. and Tobias, J. D. (2002). Anaesthetic care during minimally invasive neurosurgical procedures in infants and children. *Paediatr Anaesth* **12**, 478–88.

Khanna, S., Davis, D., Peterson, B. *et al.* (2000). Use of hypertonic saline in the treatment of severe refractory posttraumatic intracranial hypertension in pediatric traumatic brain injury. *Crit Care Med* **28**, 1144–51.

Kuwabara, Y., Ichiya, Y., Sasaki, M. *et al.* (1997). Response to hypercapnia in moyamoya disease. Cerebrovascular response to hypercapnia in pediatric and adult patients with moyamoya disease. *Stroke* **28**, 701–7.

Lam, W. H. and MacKersie, A. (1999). Paediatric head injury: incidence, aetiology and management. *Paediatr Anaesth* **9**, 377–85.

Luerssen, T. G., Klauber, M. R. and Marshall, L. F. (1988). Outcome from head injury related to patient's age. A longitudinal prospective study of adult and pediatric head injury. *J Neurosurg* **68**, 409–16.

McClain, C. D., Soriano, S. G., Goumnerova, L. C., Black, P. M. and Rockoff, M. A. (2007). Detection of unanticipated intracranial hemorrhage during intraoperative magnetic resonance image-guided neurosurgery. Report of two cases. *J Neurosurg* **106**, (Suppl.) 398–400.

McLone, D. G. and Knepper, P. A. (1989). The cause of Chiari II malformation: a unified theory. *Pediatr Neurosci* **15**, 1–12.

Modica, P. A., Tempelhoff, R. and White, P. F. (1990). Pro- and anticonvulsant effects of anesthesia (part I). *Anesth Analg* **70**, 303–15.

Morray, J. P., Geiduschek, J. M., Ramamoorthy, C. *et al.* (2000). Anesthesia-related cardiac arrest in children: initial findings of the Pediatric Perioperative Cardiac Arrest (POCA) Registry. *Anesthesiology*, **93**, 6–14.

Polin, R. S., Shaffrey, M. E., Bogaev, C. A. *et al.* (1997). Decompressive bifrontal craniectomy in the treatment of severe refractory posttraumatic cerebral edema. *Neurosurgery* **41**, 84–92.

Pryds, O. and Edwards, A. D. (1996). Cerebral blood flow in the newborn infant. *Arch Dis Child Fetal Neonatal Ed* **74**, F63–F69.

Reasoner, D. K., Todd, M. M., Scamman, F. L. and Warner, D. S. (1994). The incidence of pneumocephalus after supratentorial craniotomy. Observations on the disappearance of intracranial air. *Anesthesiology* **80**, 1008–12.

Rhoney, D. H. and Murry, K. R. (2002). National survey on the use of sedatives and neuromuscular blocking agents in the pediatric intensive care unit. *Pediatr Crit Care Med* **3**, 129–33.

Scott, R. M., Smith, J. L., Robertson, R. L. *et al.* (2004). Long-term outcome in children with moyamoya syndrome after cranial revascularization by pial synangiosis. *J Neurosurg* **100**, 142–9.

Shapiro, K., Marmarou, A. and Shulman, K. (1980). Characterization of clinical CSF dynamics and neural axis compliance using the pressure–volume index: I. The normal pressure–volume index. *Ann Neurol* **7**, 508–14.

Sharples, P. M., Stuart, A. G., Matthews, D. S., Aynsley-Green, A. and Eyre, J. A. (1995). Cerebral blood flow and metabolism in children with severe head injury. Part 1: Relation to age, Glasgow coma score, outcome, intracranial pressure, and time after injury. *J Neurol Neurosurg Psychiatry* **58**, 145–52.

Simma, B., Burger, R., Falk, M., Sacher, P. and Fanconi, S. (1998). A prospective, randomized, and controlled study of fluid management in children with severe head injury: lactated Ringer's solution versus hypertonic saline. *Crit Care Med* **26**, 1265–70.

Soriano, S. G. and Martyn, J. A. (2004). Antiepileptic-induced resistance to neuromuscular blockers: mechanisms and clinical significance. *Clin Pharmacokinet* **43**, 71–81.

Soriano, S. G., Sethna, N. F. and Scott, R. M. (1993). Anesthetic management of children with moyamoya syndrome. *Anesth Analg* **77**, 1066–70.

Sponheim, S., Skraastad, O., Helseth, E. *et al.* (2003). Effects of 0.5 and 1.0 MAC isoflurane, sevoflurane and desflurane on intracranial and cerebral perfusion pressures in children. *Acta Anaesthesiol Scand* **47**, 932–8.

Taylor, A., Butt, W., Rosenfeld, J. *et al.* (2001). A randomized trial of very early decompressive craniectomy in children with traumatic brain injury and sustained intracranial hypertension. *Childs Nerv Syst* **17**, 154–62.

Tobias, J. D. (2006). Dexmedetomidine to treat opioid withdrawal in infants following prolonged sedation in the pediatric ICU. *J Opioid Manag* **2**, 201–5.

Tobias, J. D. (2007). Dexmedetomidine: applications in pediatric critical care and pediatric anesthesiology. *Pediatr.Crit Care Med* **8**, 115–31.

Tsuji, M., Saul, J. P., du Plessis, A. *et al.* (2000). Cerebral intravascular oxygenation correlates with mean arterial pressure in critically ill premature infants. *Pediatrics* **106**, 625–32.

Valencia, I., Holder, D. L., Helmers, S. L., Madsen, J. R. and Riviello, J. J. Jr (2001). Vagus nerve stimulation in pediatric epilepsy: a review. *Pediatr Neurol* **25**, 368–6.

Vardi, A., Salem, Y., Padeh, S., Paret, G. and Barzilay, Z. (2002). Is propofol safe for procedural sedation in children? A prospective evaluation of propofol versus ketamine in pediatric critical care. *Crit Care Med* **30**, 1231–6.

Vavilala, M. S., Bowen, A., Lam, A. M. *et al.* (2003). Blood pressure and outcome after severe pediatric traumatic brain injury. *J Trauma* **55**, 1039–44.

Vavilala, M. S., Lee, L. A. and Lam, A. M. (2003). The lower limit of cerebral autoregulation in children during sevoflurane anesthesia. *J Neurosurg Anesthesiol* **15**, 307–12.

Wheeler, D. S., Vaux, K. K., Ponaman, M. L. and Poss, B. W. (2003). The safe and effective use of propofol sedation in children undergoing diagnostic and therapeutic procedures: experience in a pediatric ICU and a review of the literature. *Pediatr Emerg Care* **19**, 385–92.

Wintermark, M., Lepori, D., Cotting, J. *et al.* (2004). Brain perfusion in children: evolution with age assessed by quantitative perfusion computed tomography. *Pediatrics* **113**, 1642–52.

Wise-Faberowski, L., Soriano, S. G., Ferrari, L. *et al.* (2004). Perioperative management of diabetes insipidus in children. *J Neurosurg Anesthesiol* **16**, 220–5.

Wolf, G. K., McClain, C. D., Zurakowski, D., Dodson, B. and McManus, M. L. (2006). Total phenytoin concentrations do not accurately predict free phenytoin concentrations in critically ill children. *Pediatr Crit Care Med* **7**, 434–9.

Wyatt, J. S., Gluckman, P. D., Liu, P. Y. *et al.* (2007). Determinants of outcomes after head cooling for neonatal encephalopathy. *Pediatrics* **119**, 912–21.

Anaesthesia for spinal surgery

Ian Calder

The scope of spinal surgery

Surgical interventions may be required from the craniocervical junction to the sacrum. The approaches include maxillotomy, mandibular and tongue split, thoracotomy and anterior abdominal incision, as well as the more usual posterior route. Pathology includes disc protrusions, primary and secondary tumours, infections, trauma, arthritides and congenital disease. Most surgical endeavours are directed towards relieving stenosis of root canals or the spinal canal and/or stabilizing the spinal column. Correction of spinal curvatures (kyphosis and scoliosis) is one of the major endeavours of spine surgeons. There has been an explosion in technology in the last 20 years and there are now many different fixation systems and implants to facilitate stabilization of the spinal column (Fig. 15.1).

The language of spinal surgery

Anaesthetists unfamiliar with spinal surgery will find it helpful to be aware of some of the terms in common usage (Table 15.1). Some, such as the 'clivus' – the bone forming the base of the skull anterior to the foramen magnum – are common parlance in spinal units but are rarely used elsewhere.

Spinal instability

Symptomatic spinal instability has been defined as the 'loss of the ability under normal physiological loads to maintain relationships between vertebrae in such a way that there is neither initial nor subsequent damage to the spinal cord or nerve roots, and there is neither development of incapacitating deformity or severe pain.' However, instability can be asymptomatic.

For example, in rheumatoid arthritis, up to 50% of patients with anterior atlanto-axial subluxation (AAS) may be unaware of their abnormality. Symptoms of AAS include neck, occipital and facial pain, which is sometimes lancinating (L'Hermitte's phenomenon). Neurological impairment related to AAS is characteristically subtle, although sudden death has been described. The question is often asked whether symptomless rheumatoid patients should have flexion/extension radiographs before anaesthesia. Although there is no evidence of benefit in terms of outcome, it is sensible to get the radiographs because of 'outcome bias' and also because current opinion recommends early fixation of AAS.

The spine can be regarded as two columns – anterior and posterior. The anterior column comprises the ligaments and bones back to the posterior longitudinal ligament (PLL) and the posterior column the elements posterior to the PLL. Disruption of the anterior column tends to make the spine unstable in extension, and posterior column damage favours instability in flexion (Fig. 15.2).

Radiological measurements can also be used to assess spinal instability, although there is poor correlation between radiographic abnormality and neurological symptoms and signs. The most commonly used descriptors of instability are:

- Translation:
  - C1–2: anterior atlanto-dental interval (ADI) >5 mm, posterior ADI <13 mm
  - C2–T1: >3.5 mm between points on adjacent vertebrae

- Angulation:
  - >11° between vertebrae.

Core Topics in Neuroanaesthesia and Neurointensive Care, eds. Basil F. Matta, David K. Menon and Martin Smith. Published by Cambridge University Press. © Cambridge University Press 2011.

Table 15.1 Glossary of spinal terms

Spondyl(o)	Word element [Gr], vertebra; vertebral column. The term spondylosis is used to describe degenerative changes, commonly osteophytic projections encroaching on spinal or root canals, and spondylolisthesis to describe loss of vertebral alignment.
Myelopathy	Any functional disturbance and/or pathological change in the spinal cord, such as transverse myelopathy (extending across the spinal cord), central cord syndrome, anterior cord syndrome, posterior cord syndrome, Browne–Séquard syndrome.
Radiculopathy	Any functional disturbance and/or pathological change in a spinal nerve root.
Spinal stenosis	Reduction in the calibre of the spinal canal and hence the space available for the cord; due to disc protrusions, osteophytes, tumours and instability.
Instability	Instability of the spine is a spectrum of clinical situations, ranging from complete disruption to slowly worsening deformity. It is not easy to define, and the anaesthetic implications range from considerable to slight.
Subluxation	A significant structural displacement, visible on static imaging, such as subluxation of the atlanto-axial joint caused by rheumatoid arthritis, Down's syndrome or infection of the occipito-atlanto-axial complex. Can be anterior, posterior or vertical in direction. Rotatory subluxation of the atlas on the axis can occur in infection (Grisel's disease).

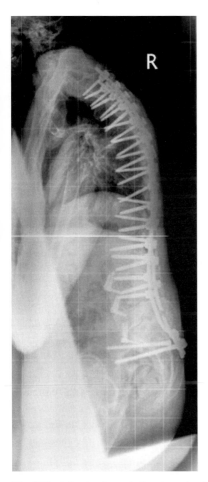

Fig. 15.1. Lateral radiograph showing extensive spinal fixation.

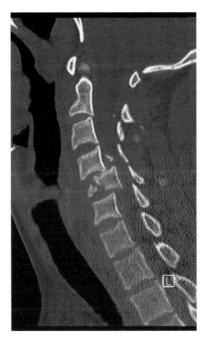

Fig. 15.2. CT scan showing disruption of the anterior column at C4/5/6.

Spine and spinal cord anatomy relevant to anaesthesia

Craniocervical junction

The anatomy of the spine will be familiar to most anaesthetists, but the special characteristics of the

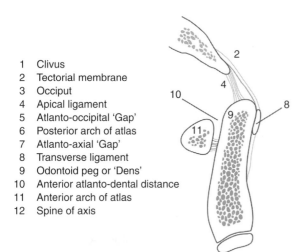

1   Clivus
2   Tectorial membrane
3   Occiput
4   Apical ligament
5   Atlanto-occipital 'Gap'
6   Posterior arch of atlas
7   Atlanto-axial 'Gap'
8   Transverse ligament
9   Odontoid peg or 'Dens'
10 Anterior atlanto-dental distance
11 Anterior arch of atlas
12 Spine of axis

Fig. 15.3. Diagram of the craniocervical junction or occipito-atlanto-axial complex.

occipito-atlanto-axial complex deserve particular study (Fig. 15.3).

The head weighs about 6 kg so the ligaments and joints of the craniocervical junction have to be powerful. The transverse portion of the cruciate ligament of the axis is said to be as strong as the cruciate ligament of the knee.

Airway management is influenced by craniocervical movement, as extension is required for both basic life support and direct laryngoscopy. In addition, mouth opening is limited if craniocervical extension is impaired. For example, persistent airway obstruction has been reported after fixation of the craniocervical junction in excess flexion. The range of motion between complete flexion and extension is normally about 24°, but in clinical practice it is very difficult to identify reduced craniocervical movement because of compensatory movement at lower levels. Curiously, a test of mouth opening such as the Mallampati score may be a better indicator of craniocervical rigidity than observation of craniocervical movement.

Spinal cord

In most individuals, the spinal cord descends to the level of L1/2 but in 2–3% as far as L2/3. The spinal cord is intolerant of retraction and, because of the varying anatomical structures that surround the spine, the implications of this (in terms of the simplicity of the surgical approach) on the most common indication for spine surgery, disc protrusion, are considerably different at different spinal levels. Lumbar disc protrusions can be approached posteriorly because the cauda equina can be retracted to allow extraction of disc fragments. However, at thoracic levels, the approach must be lateral, either through a thoracotomy or costo-transversectomy (removing the head of a rib), whereas at cervical levels the approach is usually anterior, although the oesophagus and great vessels are at risk. Lesions above C2 may require a mandibular or maxillary split for access.

The spinal cord derives its blood supply from anterior and posterior longitudinal arteries arising from the vertebral arteries, and radicular arteries arising from the aorta. The main vessels form a plexus around the cord, from which perforating vessels enter the cord. Spinal cord blood flow is believed to be governed by the same mechanisms that apply to cerebral blood flow. There are characteristic patterns of neurological impairment due to ischaemia, the commonest of which are the syndromes of central and anterior cord ischaemia (Fig. 15.4). Anterior cord syndrome is an incomplete spinal cord injury (SCI) due to ischaemia of the anterior regions of the cord. There is motor paralysis below the level of the lesion because of interruption of the corticospinal tract, and loss of pain and temperature sensation at and below the level because of interruption of the spinothalamic tract. Proprioception is retained. Central cord syndrome also results in incomplete SCI but with a disproportionately greater loss of motor power in the arms than the legs, as the axons supplying the legs are peripheral in the descending tracts. Sensory loss is variable below the lesion.

Vessel damage may occur at several sites during spine surgery. There is often a relatively large radicular

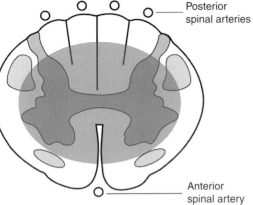

Central cord syndrome

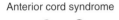

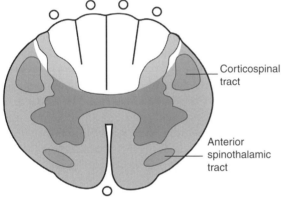

Anterior cord syndrome

Fig. 15.4. Diagram of the characteristic ischaemic areas in anterior and central cord syndromes.

Table 15.2 Medical Research Council (MRC) motor power grades

Grade 5	Normal movement
Grade 4	Movement against resistance, but weaker than the other side
Grade 3	Movement against gravity, but not against resistance
Grade 2	Movement only with gravity eliminated
Grade 1	Palpable contraction but no visible movement
Grade 0	No movement

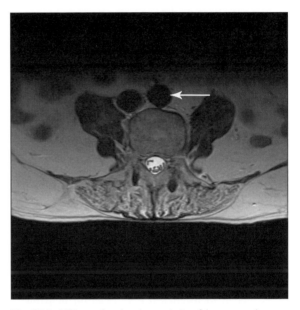

Fig. 15.5. MRI scan showing the proximity of the aorta and inferior vena cava to the spine (arrow). Surgeons can perforate the great vessels during discectomy, but bleeding into the disc space does not occur, probably because the disc annulus and the anterior longitudinal ligament seal the path.

vessel, known as the artery of Adamkiewicz, and damage to it results in significant risk of severe neurological dysfunction. Although the vertebral arteries are well protected, they are vulnerable to damage in cervical trauma and surgery as their course lies within the bone. The aorta and inferior vena cava lie in close approximation to the anterior of the spine and are vulnerable to damage during lumbar surgery (Fig. 15.5).

Spinal cord injury

Spinal cord injury is discussed in detail in Chapter 24. In summary, it can be complete or incomplete, with loss of motor, sensory and autonomic function below the level of the lesion in complete injuries. The commonest cause of incomplete SCI is central cord syndrome. Anterior and Brown–Séquard syndromes are well recognized, as is the cauda equina syndrome, which occurs

due to damage to the neuraxis below the conus of the spinal cord (see Chapter 24 for details). Motor power after SCI can be classified according to the Medical Research Council (MRC) grading scale (Table 15.2) or the American Spinal Injury Association (ASIA) neurological classification of SCI (Chapter 24).

Causation

Operations on the spine carry a risk of SCI, which increases with the complexity of the surgery and/or if a myelopathy is present pre-operatively. Spinal cord injury can also occur during non-spinal operations, presumably due to a combination of relative malposition and hypotension, although many patients are subsequently found to have a pre-existing but undiagnosed spinal abnormality such as canal stenosis. Spinal cord injury has also been described in conscious individuals with normal spines who have adopted, or been forced to adopt, an abnormal posture.

Trauma is the major cause of non-operative SCI and, although vertebral fracture or dislocation is frequently present, SCI can occur when there is no radiographic abnormality (spinal cord injury without radiographic abnormality – SCIWORA).

Demographics and associations

Youth, male sex and alcohol or drug intoxication are important risk factors for SCI, but there is also an association with falls in the elderly. There is a strong association between severe head or facial injury and SCI and, unsurprisingly, between the finding of a focal neurological deficit and SCI.

Autonomic consequences

Impairment and imbalance between sympathetic and parasympathetic supply (autonomic dysreflexia) can result in cardiovascular instability. Hypotension and bradycardia are common (but not invariable) in the acute phase and are often described as 'spinal shock'. Postural hypotension and instability of blood pressure can be a persistent problem. Autonomic dysreflexia can also cause dangerous hypertensive crises, often related to urological manipulation in patients with lesions above T6. Treatment is postural (sit the patient up), pharmacological (captopril or nifedipine) or anaesthetic (sevoflurane or isoflurane). Neuraxial block is an effective prophylactic measure during 'at-risk' procedures.

Prevention of secondary cord injury

Prevention of secondary SCI in the perioperative period is multifactorial.

Prevention of hypoxia

Hypoxia must be prevented. Possible aggravations of SCI by airway management manoeuvres are of secondary importance compared with the primacy of maintaining oxygen supply to a damaged cord. No method of intubation has been shown to be associated with improved outcome over another.

Spinal cord perfusion

Spinal cord perfusion must be maintained and a mean blood pressure of 85 mmHg has been recommended during the first week after SCI. Vasoconstrictor drugs may be needed to maintain perfusion pressure. Hypertension may be inappropriate because, in experimental models, cord swelling after trauma can be aggravated by severe hypertension. Fluid overload may also aggravate cord swelling and hypertonic (5%) saline has shown promising results in experimental reduction of cord swelling after trauma. Hyperglycaemia and hypoglycaemia should be avoided.

Immobilization

After suspected spinal injury, immobilization is a standard. While the concept does seem a priori to be sensible, it is also certain that it brings hazards. Immobilization methods may force the patient into a position they would not voluntarily adopt and cause ischaemic pain and tissue damage over pressure points. Cervical collars can increase intracranial pressure and contribute to airway obstruction in patients with obtunded consciousness. A Cochrane analysis found no evidence of improved outcome, and one study found a worse outcome in patients who were immobilized after blunt cervical injury. Manual in-line stabilization (MILS) is recommended during airway management, but there is no evidence that it is associated with improved outcome. As with cricoid pressure, MILS should be adjusted or released if necessary to achieve adequate ventilation.

Detection of injury

Observational studies have found late neurological impairment in patients without an early diagnosis of spinal injury. However, it is also accepted that a proportion (about 5%) of patients with a spinal injury will suffer a neurological deterioration despite all care. This can occur hours to weeks after the initial injury and is then called subacute, post-traumatic ascending myelopathy. The reasons for this are uncertain, but vertebral artery damage is common. This uncomfortable fact should be borne in mind whenever a patient with a history of a spinal injury requires anaesthesia.

'Clearing' the cervical spine

Twenty-five to 50% of patients with a traumatic cervical spine injury have an associated head injury, so the need to confirm or exclude cervical injury in an

Table 15.3 Criteria for confirming cervical spine stability following cervical trauma

Conscious patient	Unconscious patient
Alert, no distracting injuries	Plain radiographs are inadequate
No midline pain	The combination of plain films and CT scan is adequate to diagnose bony injury and ligamentous instability
Normal movement	
No neurological deficit	
	MR scans are not required for the exclusion of instability

unconscious patient is a common problem. There is local variation in practice but Table 15.3 summarizes the current recommendations in the UK. Some units dispense with plain films if the helical CT scan is satisfactory. MRI is required if there is focal neurological impairment, but the dangers inherent in transfer of a critically ill patient to an MRI scanner almost certainly exceed any benefit in patients with normal movement and a clear CT scan.

Pharmacological methods

High-dose methylprednisolone is controversial after SCI and is less used than previously. Many practitioners believe that convincing evidence of benefit that justifies an increased risk of infection, hyperglycaemia and psychosis is lacking (see Chapter 24). Magnesium is successful in experimental models but at doses that would not be tolerable in vivo.

Hypothermia

The debate about the possible benefit of 'moderate' (33°C) hypothermia after SCI continues. The advent of efficient intravascular cooling devices makes hypothermia an achievable goal, but whether any benefit exceeds the disadvantages of the intervention remains uncertain. As with traumatic brain injury, hyperthermia should be avoided.

Pre-operative assessment

There are specific issues that should be considered during the pre-operative assessment of patients undergoing spinal surgery.

Urgency

Few spinal cases can be classified as emergencies, although there are notable exceptions such as acute myelopathies or cauda equina syndromes due to haematomas or disc protrusions, and airway obstruction due to tissue swelling/haematoma after cervical spinal surgery.

Haemostatic function

Drugs that affect platelet function should be stopped if possible prior to spinal surgery. Aspirin or clopidogrel should be discontinued 7–10 days prior to surgery and non-steroidal anti-inflammatory drugs (NSAIDs) 48 h before. In emergency situations, it might be necessary to transfuse platelets. However, it is now clear that platelet inhibition is not always present in patients who are taking anti-platelet medication, and tests of platelet function that are entering clinical practice may distinguish those who need platelet supplementation from those who do not.

Assessment of symptoms and signs

It is wise to obtain the patient's description of laterality and, for comparison with post-operative observations, to assess and document motor power in the limbs using the MRC scale. Paresis suggests that a myelopathy or cauda equina lesion is present and that there might be denervation changes at the neuromuscular junction. Under such circumstances, suxamethonium should only be used if absolutely necessary.

Blood pressure

The patient's usual blood pressure should be ascertained and used to inform intraoperative-level blood pressure control. Those with suspect cord perfusion, such as patients with spinal stenosis, should not be allowed to be persistently hypotensive. There is recent evidence that elderly hypertensive patients may be at risk of a decline in neurocognitive function after spine surgery.

Post-operative ventilation

Some types of spinal surgery require overnight intubation or tracheostomy (see below) and patients with high-level myelopathy may require longer-term ventilatory support in the post-operative period.

Nutrition

Patients with a pre-operative swallowing difficulty or those who are likely to have prolonged difficulty swallowing post-operatively should be considered for a percutaneous endoscopic gastrostomy, as prolonged nasogastric intubation is associated with sinus infection. If a nasogastric tube is required in a patient who needs an awake intubation, it is sensible to pass it prior to intubation because it can be difficult and traumatic to intubate the stomach with a tracheal tube in place.

Airway assessment

The probability of serious airway difficulty is generally obvious from the end of the bed, but the following issues should also be considered when trying to predict difficult intubation:

- Conditions such as rheumatoid arthritis, ankylosing spondylitis, or iatrogenic problems such as halo-body or other cervical fixators, are well-known causes of difficulty and often necessitate special techniques such as awake intubation.
- Patients with disease of the craniocervical junction have a much higher prevalence of difficult laryngoscopy than those with disease below C3. It is generally difficult to identify restricted craniocervical movement by clinical examination of neck movement because of compensatory increased movement at lower cervical levels.
- Accurate prediction of airway difficulty in patients without 'end-of-the-bed' abnormality remains elusive. It is unlikely that a solution will be found, as the problem is essentially one of low prevalence. Unless a test can be devised that has nearly 100% specificity (negativity in health), even an extremely sensitive (positive in disease) test will result in an unacceptably high proportion of false-positive results if the prevalence is low.
- The Mallampati examination remains the most successful predictor of difficult direct laryngoscopy. Although its post-test probability is low (10–15%) when applied to a low-prevalence population (5%), this rises to around 50% in high-prevalence populations such as patients with rheumatoid arthritis. The relative success of the Mallampati score in spinal patients probably reflects the consequence of restricted mouth opening due to craniocervical stiffness.
- A combination of the Mallampati score and a thyromental distance of <6 cm has a likelihood ratio of about 9, which, while not suitable for screening, does offer some predictive power (pre-test probability × likelihood ratio = post-test probability).

- Poor separation of the posterior elements of the occiput, atlas and axis on lateral radiographs (the atlanto-occipital and atlanto-axial 'gaps' in Fig. 15.3) suggests poor craniocervical movement and is more predictive of difficult laryngoscopy than clinical tests.
- Although the advent of videolaryngoscopes means that it is nearly always possible to obtain a good view of the glottis, achieving intubation may still be difficult. It is not yet certain that alternatives to the combination of a Macintosh laryngoscope and a gum-elastic bougie represent a meaningful improvement over other, more complex, techniques.

Patient positioning

Careful patient positioning is crucial to maximize surgical access and prevent intraoperative nerve damage. The fact that the spinal cord descends to about L1/2 and is intolerant of retraction means that surgery on cervical and thoracic lesions anterior to the cord is conducted in the supine or lateral position. However, posterior decompressive and stabilizing procedures at these levels are performed in the prone position. The cauda equina is more tolerant of retraction, so that lumbar discs can be approached using the prone position. The sitting position is rarely used during spine surgery, but the increasing prevalence of gross obesity may re-popularize this position.

Damage to the ulnar nerve at the elbow is a serious complication. Pain and disability can be long-lasting, with 50% of affected patients having symptoms at 3 months, and some a year later. Perioperative ulnar nerve monitoring has demonstrated that conduction becomes abnormal in up to 6% of cases. Ulnar nerve damage is more common in male patients and those with extremes of body habitus. No position has been identified as being either safe or dangerous in this respect.

Patients with anterior AAS require a system that allows the head to move posteriorly while the upper cervical spine (C2 and below) is supported. A large doughnut ring is ideal in the supine position.

Hazards of the prone position

There are well-recognized hazards of the prone position.

Damage to the eyes and face

It is usually impossible to inspect the eyes and nose if surgery is performed above the lumbar region in the prone position, even with mirror systems such as the Prone View. Pressure damage can occur rapidly and serious consideration should be given to using a Mayfield skull pin fixation system to the skull so that the eyes and nose are not compressed. The nose is particularly vulnerable to pressure-induced ischaemic damage.

Serious eye damage can result from injury to the cornea due to drying (exposure keratopathy) if the eye is not properly taped shut. The eyes must also be protected from blood and cleaning fluids. The problem of post-operative visual loss (POVL) is discussed in detail later in this chapter.

Compression of the abdomen

Abdominal compression can result in both increased venous pressure and blood loss, and reduced ventilatory compliance. Hepatic ischaemia due to prolonged abdominal compression has also been described and has been the subject of an investigation by the National Patient Safety Agency in the UK.

Cardiovascular problems

These are unusual unless the abdomen is compressed, when the effect varies with the type of positioning system used. Cardiac massage can be performed in the prone position but is less efficient.

Regional anaesthesia

Lumbar surgery, particularly microdiscectomy, can be performed with intrathecal anaesthesia, although the block may recede if the dura is breached. Caution should be observed in attempting to insert an epidural catheter in a patient with spinal stenosis or a history of spinal surgery. Neuraxial block is an attractive option for non-spine surgery in patients with cervical disease that may make airway management or positioning difficult, for example, in patients with rheumatoid arthritis requiring joint arthroplasty. It is also believed to be an effective preventative measure against autonomic dysreflexia in patients with high cord injuries.

Intraoperative airway management

As the majority of patients undergoing spine surgery will be placed in the prone position, tracheal intubation remains the standard technique of airway control although a supra-glottic airway (SGA) has been employed in some circumstances. Suxamethonium should be avoided during tracheal intubation if myelopathy or myopathy might be present, because of the

risk of hyperkalaemia. Reinforced, kink-resistant endotracheal tubes are popular but not essential. The tube fixation technique must be resistant to wetting with cleaning solutions in high spinal surgery, and waterproof material, such as Bioclusive transparent dressing, is usually satisfactory.

There is no conclusive evidence in relation to the optimal airway management technique in patients with possible cervical instability. Manual in-line stabilization has been recommended, but there is no evidence of improved outcome with any technique. Practitioners should therefore use whatever technique is most suitable in their hands.

Double-lumen tubes or bronchial blockers may be required for thoracic spinal surgery. As thoracic discs or vertebral body lesions cannot be approached from behind, a thoracotomy may be required, and surgical access is more straightforward if the lung is deflated.

Tracheostomy is prudent in many cases of high anterior surgery or if a maxillotomy or mandibular split is required, as post-operative swelling can last for some days.

Post-operative airway obstruction

A post-operative haematoma capable of causing tracheal compression can occur after any anterior cervical operation and its treatment is immediate opening of the wound and evacuation of the haematoma. However, airway obstruction due to tissue swelling is much more likely, particularly after lengthy surgery (>5 h) or surgery at high spinal levels. It is also more common if a patient who has had anterior surgery is then placed prone for a prolonged posterior intervention (Fig. 15.6). This is true even if the posterior procedure is performed some days or even weeks after the anterior approach. Extubation should be delayed until the following day if combined anterior and posterior surgery is performed and considered if anterior surgery lasts 5 h or longer. Any past procedure or intervention (such as surgery or radiotherapy) on the head or neck should raise suspicion that the lymphatic drainage of the laryngopharynx may not be normal and that airway swelling after prone positioning is more likely.

Under such circumstances, the cause of the airway obstruction is pharyngolaryngeal oedema, not tracheal compression, as peri- and supra-glottic tissue swelling occludes the airway. The symptoms usually occur within 6 h, but diagnosis can be delayed because stridor and desaturation are late signs. Wanting to sit

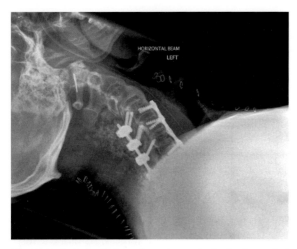

Fig. 15.6. Radiograph of anterior and posterior fixation for cervical spine fracture. Post-operative airway obstruction due to soft tissue swelling is likely and extubation should be delayed.

up and complaining of difficulty in breathing are constant features. The presence of a wound drain makes no difference to this complication.

Management

The immediate management of post-operative airway obstruction is opening of the wound, even though in most cases there is no haematoma. This is because relief of tissue pressure may critically improve airway patency. This fact is exemplified by a case report of airway obstruction due to extracapsular leaking of fluid during shoulder arthroscopy. In this case, initial rescue by direct laryngoscopy and intubation failed because of severe supra-glottic tissue swelling. However, a tracheostomy skin incision resulted in immediate improvement in the airway because of release of tissue pressure, and successful direct laryngoscopy and intubation.

The anaesthetist called upon to establish an airway in the presence of pharyngolaryngeal oedema is in an unenviable position. Folds of swollen pharyngeal tissue may make mask ventilation and direct laryngoscopy difficult or impossible, and preparations for emergency surgical tracheostomy should always be made. Awake flexible fibre-optic intubation has been successful in the author's experience but will not be suitable in the most acute cases. Because there is swelling of the pharyngeal soft tissues, airway collapse during inspiration often prevents a clear view of the cords, and the endoscopist must therefore advance the scope during expiration. Topical anaesthesia with lidocaine

may be useful but, because it is an irritant, its use has been associated with complete airway obstruction. The author has found that insertion of the endoscope into the trachea followed by a small dose of propofol (50–100 mg) allows the tube to be passed in these desperate patients.

The use of a videolaryngoscope to facilitate intubation of three patients with severe airway obstruction due to supra-glottic swelling has been reported. Topical anaesthesia (6 ml lidocaine 4%) was administered via an atomizer and a remifentanil infusion run at 3 ng ml^{-1}. Videolaryngoscopy and intubation were well tolerated. Inhalational induction of anaesthesia is often advanced as a safe technique in patients with airway obstruction, but the author has not known it to be successful in this situation. The issue of whether muscle relaxant drugs should be used also remains controversial. However, in the author's opinion, practitioners should use them whenever they feel that they will be helpful. Not using muscle relaxants is associated with difficult intubation, and there is a well-respected view that muscle relaxants permit intubation in patients who are impossible to ventilate via a face mask when not paralysed. One group observed that, in patients with stridor due to laryngotracheal stenosis, positive-pressure ventilation via a laryngeal mask airway (LMA) after propofol and atracurium induction resulted in better gas flows than in the same patients during awake spontaneous breathing. There is no doubt that direct or videolaryngoscopy will sometimes be difficult, but, provided the glottic reflexes are obtunded, a gum-elastic bougie can be placed or a tube passed. Successful intubation after rapid sequence induction followed by 'blind' gum-elastic bougie placement has been described in four patients with grossly distorted pharyngeal anatomy.

If laryngoscopy is unsuccessful, an SGA should be considered. Fibre-optic-guided intubation can be performed subsequently via the SGA, which is removed after intubation. This technique uses an Aintree catheter for intubation, or placement of a gum-elastic bougie through the tracheal tube, removal of the tube and SGA, and then railroading of another tube over the gum-elastic bougie.

Other causes of post-operative airway obstruction

There have been several reports of airway obstruction following craniocervical fixation, which appear to have been the result of fixation in excessive flexion.

Rheumatoid arthritis patients are at particular risk of post-operative airway obstruction because of exacerbation of cricoarytenoid arthritis by intubation. The smallest possible diameter tube should be used. Emergency reintubation for airway obstruction due to acute sialadenitis after prolonged surgery has been reported.

Unilateral laryngeal nerve damage occurs after anterior cervical surgery, but this does not cause airway obstruction. It is often asymptomatic, although patients may have a lowing cough and a weak voice. One prospective study found an incidence of 11.3%, diagnosed by laryngoscopy.

Major blood loss

Serious blood loss is a feature of some spinal procedures, notably scoliosis correction and tumour surgery (Fig. 15.7). Pre-operative radiological embolization of tumours can reduce operative bleeding. Facilities and portals for rapid blood infusion should always be available. Close cooperation with haematological colleagues is crucial so that blood products (red cells, platelets, fresh frozen plasma and factor concentrates) can be made available promptly. After four unit transfusion replacement with red cells, fresh frozen plasma and platelets should be in the ratio of 1:1:1.

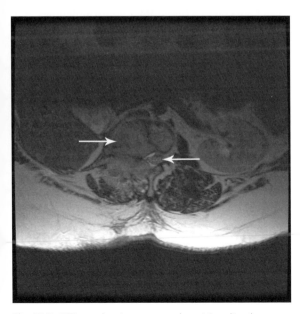

Fig. 15.7. MRI scan showing a tumour deposit invading the lumbar spine. The left arrow points to the tumour and the right to the cauda equina.

The most dramatic example of major blood loss associated with spinal surgery is damage to the aorta or inferior vena cava during lumbar discectomy. Surgeons are usually unaware that their rongeurs have perforated the great vessels because bleeding does not appear in the wound. Circulatory collapse is usually the first sign and mortality is very high. Damage to the iliac vessels can also occur, but the bleeding is usually less acute and the mortality rate correspondingly lower.

Monitoring the circulation is more difficult when the patient is prone. Central venous pressure monitoring is less accurate than in the supine position, but it nevertheless provides a useful trend to guide fluid management and the need for vasopressors. Cardiac output monitoring is increasingly practised, although oesophageal Doppler techniques are inconvenient when the patient is prone.

Aprotinin has been withdrawn, but tranexamic acid has been shown to reduce blood loss after spinal surgery. Induced hypotension does reduce blood loss and is controversial because of the risk of reduced spinal cord perfusion and concerns about its association with POVL. Hypotension may also cause an increased risk of post-operative cognitive impairment in elderly patients after spine surgery.

Minimizing the risk of perioperative spinal cord damage

Unsurprisingly, patients at greatest risk of perioperative SCI are those undergoing multilevel surgery with instrumentation as well as those with an established pre-operative myelopathy. It is important to realize that perioperative SCI is not confined to the cervical region but also occurs in the thoracic and lumbar (cauda equina) segments.

Airway management

The concept that airway management, and direct laryngoscopy in particular, is a cause of SCI has been described as a 'legend of anaesthesia'. There are many reports of SCI below the cervical level and the author of course does not attempt to implicate airway management as causative. However, when an SCI occurs in the cervical region, attention nearly always focuses on airway management and therefore on the anaesthetist. This may simply be an example of confusion between subsequence and consequence, as airway management is inevitably followed by alternative causations, such as prolonged minor malposition or inadequate spinal cord perfusion pressure.

There is neither a case report that unequivocally implicates airway management in the genesis of SCI nor any evidence of outcome difference with one airway management technique over another. However, absence of evidence does not prove that the phenomenon does not exist. In two studies of the effect of airway management in cadavers rendered grossly unstable, basic life support techniques (head tilt, jaw thrust) produced more disturbance at the unstable cervical spine sites than direct laryngoscopy. If this is true in vivo, it might be an argument for 'awake' intubation in patients with unstable necks. However, the quantity of vertebral displacement or angulation that occurs in a truly unstable spine during 'awake' intubation is not known, and might in fact be greater than during intubation under general anaesthesia. Surveys of anaesthetists have indicated that 'awake' flexible fibre-optic intubation is perceived as a good option in patients with suspected cervical instability, but the procedure is by no means always straightforward and has resulted in laryngeal damage and even complete airway obstruction necessitating an emergency surgical airway. In this author's view, it would not be in a patient's interests for an anaesthetist inexperienced in 'awake' endoscopy to attempt an 'awake' intubation on the grounds of suspected or actual cervical instability.

Laryngoscopy

Whether or not videolaryngoscopy is clinically superior to direct laryngoscopy is unknown. One study found no significant difference in cervical spine movement between GlideScope® videolaryngoscopy and direct laryngoscopy, despite not using the tactic of only exposing the glottis sufficiently to allow the introduction of a gum-elastic bougie. Nevertheless, videolaryngoscopy probably makes some intubations easier and it is of interest, irrespective of neurological considerations. Despite recent innovations, direct laryngoscopy with the Macintosh laryngoscope remains an accepted method of intubation for anaesthetists and emergency physicians.

Awake positioning

Prolonged abnormal spine positioning carries a small risk of neuraxial damage, even in patients with normal spines, and this risk is compounded in those with spinal disease. The majority of reports of SCI during

anaesthesia have involved patients with spinal canal stenosis (Fig. 15.8), not instability.

It is not possible to predict whether a particular position will be tolerable for the duration of surgery. Spinal cord monitoring techniques offer a potential guide to positional adequacy (see below), but 'awake' positioning has been suggested as an alternative. However, position-related SCI can still occur with awake positioning techniques because not even the patient can predict whether a position will still be tolerable some hours later. If awake positioning is undertaken, consideration must be given to where the dividing line between sedation and anaesthesia is to be drawn. In practice, this is not always clear cut and what is intended to be sedation can more closely resemble anaesthesia. Disinhibition and withdrawal of cooperation are possible, although unusual if the patient is properly prepared. In addition, some thought should be given to what action will be taken if a problem is suspected, as false positives have been described during awake positioning and the patient may not benefit from postponement of surgery.

Spinal cord monitoring

Sensory and motor evoked potentials have not been proved to improve outcome during spine surgery and both false-positive and false-negative results can occur. Sensory potentials have poorer sensitivity (52%) but higher specificity (100%) than motor potentials (100 and 96%, respectively) for cord damage. As evoked potentials are sensitive to hypotension, they also offer some guide to what level of blood pressure can be tolerated during surgery. For both sensory and motor evoked potentials, the best results are gained with propofol infusion, although sensory recordings can be elicited in the presence of low doses of volatile agents. Motor potentials are abolished by volatile agents and muscle-relaxant drugs, so propofol and remifentanil infusions are the most convenient anaesthetic technique. Sensory and motor evoked potential monitoring is discussed in detail in Chapter 8.

Blood pressure management

There is a tension between the possible improvement in operating conditions and reduction in blood loss obtainable with induced hypotension and reductions in spinal cord and optic nerve perfusion. Hypotension should be avoided if possible in all patients with known spinal cord compression. Unimpaired evoked

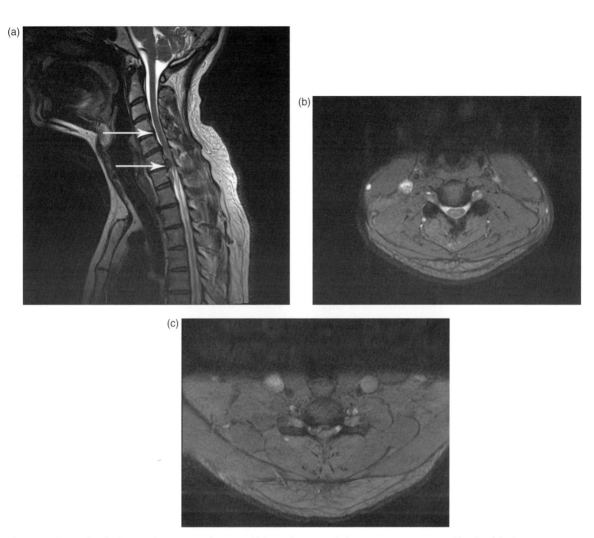

Fig. 15.8. T2-weighted MRI scans showing spinal stenosis. (a) Sagittal image with the upper arrow at a normal level and the lower arrow at an abnormal level. The abnormality could be disc or osteophyte. (b) Axial image showing a normal area where the cord is surrounded by cerebrospinal fluid (white) (upper arrow on the sagittal section). (c) Axial image showing an area of spinal stenosis causing cord compression (lower arrow on the sagittal section).

potentials are reassuring in terms of the adequacy of spinal perfusion, although false negatives can occur. Infusions of vasoconstrictors such as metaraminol or phenylephrine are often necessary to maintain adequate blood pressure during prolonged spine surgery.

Post-operative spinal haematoma

Age >60 years, pre-operative non-steroidal use, Rh-positive blood type, procedures involving more than five spinal levels, a haemoglobin falling to less that 10 g dl^{-1}, blood loss >1 l and, in the post-operative period, an international normalized ratio (INR) of >2 are independent associations with post-operative spinal haematoma.

Post-operative pain

Pain after spinal surgery can be severe and debilitating, and a multimodal approach to pain management is essential. Possible drugs include paracetamol, non-steroidal drugs, subanaesthetic doses of ketamine (0.5 mg kg^{-1} followed by 4 µg kg^{-1} min^{-1}), clonidine, dexamethasone, gabapentin, pregabalin and opioids. There has been concern that the use of non-steroidal drugs may inhibit bony fusion after spinal surgery, but current evidence suggests that treatment for 48 h is safe.

Epidural analgesia can be very effective, although pre-operative catheter placement can be difficult if the anatomy is abnormal. Intraoperative placement by the surgeon sounds simple, but, in practice, misplacement and failure occur relatively frequently. Staff education is important to avoid confusion between the effects of epidural local anaesthetic on motor power and complications such as intraspinal haematoma and intracranial spread of anaesthetic because of subdural catheter placement (note that intracranial spread does not occur with epidural placement, as the dura is inserted onto the foramen magnum). Epidural clonidine infusion has been shown to be effective and may avoid the possibility of staff attributing myelopathic symptoms to local anaesthetic effects.

Post-operative visual loss

The overall incidence of POVL after spine surgery is low, but, when it occurs, it is devastating for the patient. A retrospective study of all spine surgery in the USA found an overall incidence of 0.09%, with spine surgery for scoliosis correction having the highest rate (0.28%). Nearly all cases occur after the prone position and, curiously, it is common for patients not to report POVL immediately, possibly because they presume that the loss is a temporary peri-anaesthetic phenomenon.

Ophthalmological diagnoses

There are several causes of POVL:

1. *Ischaemic optic neuropathy (ION)*. This can be posterior when the optic nerve is damaged proximal to the eye, or anterior when the nerve is damaged as it enters the eye. Ischaemic optic neuropathy presents as painless, often bilateral, visual loss. The external appearances of both eyes are similar, although facial swelling is common after prolonged prone positioning. The retinal appearances can be normal in posterior ION, although the disc is swollen and there may be flame-shaped haemorrhages in anterior ION.
2. *Central retinal artery occlusion (CRAO)*. This is usually unilateral and presents with signs of external pressure with a swollen, proptosed eye, sometimes with ophthalmoplegia. Surprisingly, pain is not mentioned in published reports. The characteristic retinal appearances are 'cloudy swelling' due to retinal oedema, retinal pallor and a cherry-red spot at the fovea caused by well-

perfused sclera shining through the thinnest point of the retina.
3. *Non-ION, non-CRAO visual loss*.
4. *Cortical blindness*. This occurs due to damage to the visual cortex and is rare.

Causation

Central retinal artery occlusion is the rarest form of POVL and is often caused by external pressure on the eye. It can also be related to embolic obstruction in which case there are no external signs of pressure damage. The majority of reports of CRAO have involved the use of a horseshoe type of head rest, although it has been described with most types of head support apart from head-pin fixation.

The causation of ION and non-ION, non-CRAO visual loss remains uncertain, although these conditions might represent a form of compartment syndrome of the orbit. A striking finding of the American Society of Anesthesiologists' analysis of POVL was that the mean period in the prone position was 9.8 ± 3.1 h in 94% of cases of ION. Orbital swelling and increased intraocular pressure is common after even short periods in the prone position, and it is not difficult to imagine how the optic nerve can be compressed by oedematous and engorged orbital contents. The risk of ION is increased with prone position, age > 65 years, male sex, diabetes, hypotension, anaemia and duration of surgery. Patients who develop non-ION, non- CRAO visual loss are more likely to be hypertensive, have peripheral vascular disease and to have had a blood transfusion.

Prevention

It has been suggested that avoiding pressure on the eye, applying 10° of reverse Trendelenburg tilt during prone surgery, maintaining arterial pressure near the patient's baseline, avoiding large amounts of crystalloid infusion, keeping the haematocrit above 30 and staging surgery so that duration does not exceed 8 h might minimize the risk of POVL after spine surgery. An instructive account of a case of POVL can be found at http://www.rmf.harvard.edu/case-studies/specialty-reference/anesthesia/blindness-following-spine-surgery.aspx.

Preventing pressure on the eye

The most certain method of preventing pressure on the eye is to use a skull pin fixation device. However,

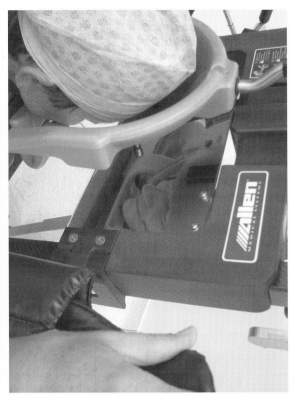

Fig. 15.9. An example of a mirror system that allows inspection of the eyes and nose during surgery in the prone position. See colour plate section.

this requires a skilled operator, as inadequate fixation, perforation of the skull and perforation of an eye have all been reported. Devices that allow inspection of the eye, such as the ProneView, during surgery in the prone position are attractive (Fig. 15.9). A high index of suspicion, amounting to virtual obsession, is required throughout surgery. The status of the eyes should be checked at regular intervals, although this is not always possible in practice and a safe frequency of checking is not agreed. A check should always be made if the position of the patient or table is changed.

Consent

The risk of POVL is not an issue that should be sprung on a patient on the day of surgery. In high-risk cases, a discussion must take place prior to admission to hospital.

Further reading

Awad, J. N., Kebaish, K. M., Donigan, J., Cohen, D. B. and Kostuik, J. P. (2005). Analysis of the risk factors for the development of post-operative spinal epidural haematoma. *J Bone Joint Surg Br* **87**, 1248–52.

Bhardwaj, A., Long, D. M., Ducker, T. B. and Toung, T. J. (2001). Neurologic deficits after cervical laminectomy in the prone position. *J Neurosurg Anesthesiol* **13**, 314–9.

Calder, I., Picard, J., Chapman. M., O'Sullivan, C. and Crockard, H. A. (2003). Mouth opening – a new angle. *Anesthesiology* **99**, 799–801.

Combes, X., Dumerat, M. and Dhonneur, G. (2004) Emergency gum elastic bougie-assisted tracheal intubation in four patients with upper airway distortion. *Can J Anaesth* **51**, 1022–4.

Crosby, E. T. (2006). Airway management in adults after cervical spine trauma. *Anesthesiology* **104**, 1293–318.

Donaldson, W. F. III, Heil, B. V., Donaldson, V. P. and Silvaggio, V. J. (1997). The effect of airway maneuvers on the unstable C1–C2 segment: a cadaver study. *Spine* **22**, 1215–18.

Edgecombe, H., Carter, K. and Yarrow, S. (2008). Anaesthesia in the prone position. *Brit J Anaesth*, **100**, 165–83.

Ewah, B. and Calder, I. (1991). Intraoperative death during lumbar discectomy. *Brit J Anaesth*, **66**, 721–3.

Harrop, J. S., Sharan, A. D., Vaccaro, A. R. and Przybylski, G. J. (2001). The cause of neurologic deterioration after cervical spinal cord injury. *Spine* **26**, 340–6.

Hauswald, M. and Braude, D. (2002). Spinal immobilization in trauma patients: is it really necessary? *Curr Opin Crit Care* **8**, 566–70.

Hebl, J. R., Horlocker, T. T., Kopp, S. L. and Schroeder, D. R. (2010). Neuraxial block in patients with preexisting spinal stenosis, lumbar disk disease, or priorspine surgery: efficacy and neurologic complications. *Anesth Analg* **111**, 1511–19.

Hindman, B. J., Palecek, J. P., Posner, K. L. *et al.* (2011). Cervical spine cord, root, and bony spine injuries. A closed claims analysis. *Anesthesiology* **114**, 782–95.

Kelleher, M. O., Tan, G., Sarjeant, R. and Fehlings, M. G. (2008). Predictive value of intraoperative neurophysiological monitoring during cervical spine surgery: a prospective analysis of 1055 consecutive cases. *J Neurosurg Spine*, **8**, 215–21.

Kheterpal, S., Martin, L., Shanks, A.M. and Tremper, K. K. (2009). Prediction and outcomes of impossible mask ventilation. A review of 50,000 anesthetics. *Anesthesiology*, **110**, 891–7.

Lewandrowski, K. U., McLain, R. F., Lieberman, I. and Orr, D. (2006). Cord and cauda equina injury complicating elective orthopaedic surgery. *Spine*, **31**, 1056–9.

Manoach, S. and Paladino, L. (2009). Laryngoscopy force, visualization and intubation failure in acute trauma:

should we modify the practice of manual in-line stabilization? *Anesthesiology* **110**, 6–7.

McCleod, A. D. M. and Calder, I. (2000). Direct laryngoscopy and cervical cord damage – the legend lives on. *Brit J Anaesth* **84**, 705–9.

Miller, S. M. (2008). Methylprednisolone in acute spinal cord injury: a tarnished standard. *J Neurosurg Anesthesiol* **20**, 140–2.

Miller, R. A., Crosby, G. and Sundaram, P. (1987). Exacerbated spinal neurological deficit during sedation of a patient with cervical spondylosis. *Anesthesiology* **67**, 844–6.

Morris, C. G., McCoy, E. P. and Lavery, G. G. (2004). Spinal immobilization for unconscious patients with multiple injuries. *BMJ* **329**, 495–9.

Nolan, J. P. and Wilson, M. E. (1993). Orotracheal intubation in patients with potential cervical spine injuries. An indication for the gum elastic bougie. *Anaesthesia* **48**, 630–3.

Patil, C. G., Lad, E. M., Lad, S. P., Ho, C. and Boakye, M. (2008). Visual loss after spinal surgery: a population-based study. *Spine* **33**, 1491–6.

Pradhan, B. B., Tatsumi, R. L., Gallina, J. *et al.* (2008). Ketorolac and spinal fusion: does the perioperative use of ketorolac really inhibit spinal fusion? *Spine* **33**, 2079–82.

Robitaille, A., Williams, S. R., Tremblay, M. H. *et al.* (2008). Cervical spine motion during tracheal intubation with manual in-line stabilization versus GlideScope® videolaryngoscopy. *Anesth Analg* **106**, 935–41.

Sagi, H. C., Beutler, W., Carroll, E. and Connolly, P. J. (2002). Airway complications associated with surgery on the anterior cervical spine. *Spine* **27**, 949–53.

Terao, Y., Matsumoto, S., Yamashita, K. *et al.* (2004). Increased incidence of emergency airway management after combined anterior-posterior cervical spine surgery. *J Neurosurg Anesthesiol* **16**, 282–6.

Wong, J., El Beheiry, H., Rampersaud, Y. R. *et al.* (2008). Tranexamic acid reduces perioperative blood loss in adult patients having spinal fusion surgery. *Anesth Analg* **107**, 1479–86.

Yocum, G. T., Gaudet, J. G., Teverbaugh, L. A. *et al.* (2009). Neurocognitive performance in hypertensive patients after spine surgery. *Anesthesiology* **110**, 254–61.

Chapter 16

Anaesthetic management of posterior fossa surgery

Tonny Veenith and Antony R. Absalom

Introduction

Anaesthesia for the posterior fossa provides a unique challenge for anaesthetists and neurosurgeons. The most common surgical procedures are excision of posterior fossa tumours, correction of congenital and acquired craniovertebral junction anomalies, and surgical procedures to relieve pressure on the brainstem.

Between 54 and 70% of all childhood brain tumours, and 15–20% of adult brain tumours, originate in the posterior fossa. In children <18 years, the majority of posterior fossa operations are for excision of tumours, of which the commonest are cerebellar astrocytomas, medulloblastomas and brainstem gliomas. The outlook for children with these tumours has improved since the advent of CT imaging of the brain, which enables early diagnosis and improved tumour excision during surgery. Improvements in mortality and morbidity following posterior cranial fossa surgery are also attributable to improved surgical and anaesthetic management.

Posterior cranial fossa anatomy

The base of the skull is divided into the anterior, middle and posterior cranial fossae. The posterior fossa is the largest and deepest and is densely packed with vital structures. The bony structures comprising the floor of the posterior fossa are the sphenoid, occipital and temporal bones, and the mastoid angles of the parietal bones. The occipital bone is separated superiorly from the parietal bone by the lambdoid suture, while the occipitomastoid suture separates the occipital bone and the mastoid part of the temporal bone. The posterior fossa is separated from the middle fossa centrally by the dorsum sellae of the sphenoid and laterally by the petrous temporal bones. It is limited posteriorly and inferiorly by the foramen magnum. The important structures occupying the posterior cranial fossa are the

cerebellum, pons and medulla oblongata. There are two reflections of the dura in the posterior cranial fossa – the tentorium cerebelli and the falx cerebelli. The falx cerebelli is a reflection of dura below the tentorium cerebelli, which separates the cerebellar hemispheres.

Venous sinuses in the posterior cranial fossa are formed by dural indentations lined with endothelium. The important ones are the right and left transverse sinuses, which form grooves on the bones of the posterior cranial fossa, and join the superior sagittal sinus and the straight sinus to form the confluence of sinuses (which causes a concavity in the skull below the occipital protuberance, known as the torcular Herophili). The confluence of sinuses drains into the left and right sigmoid sinuses, which leave the posterior fossa to continue as the internal jugular veins.

Openings in the floor of the posterior fossa that transmit important structures are the foramen magnum, the internal acoustic meatus (transmits facial and vestibulocochlear nerves), the condylar canal (hypoglossal nerve and a meningeal branch from the ascending pharyngeal artery) and the jugular foramen (internal jugular vein and glossopharyngeal, vagus and accessory nerves).

Types of posterior cranial fossa surgery

Excision of posterior fossa tumours

Posterior fossa tumours (Fig. 16.1) account for 20% of adult brain tumours, whereas the posterior fossa is the commonest location of brain tumours in children. Posterior fossa neoplastic lesions are often classified as arising from either the anterior or the posterior compartment. The reference point for this division is the fourth ventricle. Tumours of the anterior compartment

Core Topics in Neuroanaesthesia and Neurointensive Care, eds. Basil F. Matta, David K. Menon and Martin Smith. Published by Cambridge University Press. © Cambridge University Press 2011.

(a)   (b)   (c)

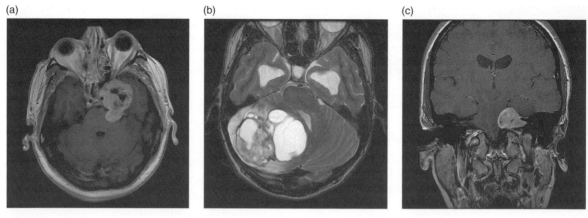

Fig. 16.1. (a) T2-weighted MRI image of a trigeminal neuroma; (b) T2-weighted MRI image of a cerebellar astrocytoma; (c) T1-weighted MRI of a vestibular schwannoma with gadolinium enhancement.

are further subdivided into intra-axial and extra-axial (i.e. arising from within and without the pia, respectively). The commonest intra-axial anterior compartment tumours are gliomas, whereas the common extra-axial anterior compartment tumours arise mainly from the cerebello-pontine angle (acoustic schwannoma, meningioma, epidermoid tumours, cysts, glomus tumours and metastases). Tumours of the posterior compartment are predominantly intra-axial tumours – most commonly cerebellar astrocytoma (common in children), medulloblastoma (second most common tumour in children), ependymoma, haemangioblastoma, lymphoma and metastases.

Histologically, all nervous system tumours can be broadly divided into three groups: primitive neuro-ectodermal tumours (PNETs, which occur in the brain, the sympathetic nervous system and the eye, e.g. medulloblastomas, pineoblastomas and ependymomas), glial tumours (which arise from the supportive tissue of the brain or glia, e.g. astrocytomas, ependymomas and gliomas) and metastatic tumours.

Procedures for vascular lesions (including aneurysms and arteriovenous malformations) and procedures to relieve cranial nerve compression by vascular structures

Aneurysms in the posterior fossa are rare but can arise from the vertebrobasilar system and the arteries of the posterior inferior cerebellar system. They can present with symptoms caused by general mass effects, or symptoms arising from direct compression of the cranial nerves. Commonly involved cranial nerves are the

VIIth and VIIIth, producing a picture resembling that of a cerebellopontine angle tumour.

Posterior fossa arteriovenous malformations (AVMs) are rare and are difficult to treat because of the proximity to vital brain structures. They represent 5–7% of all intracranial AVMs. More than half present following a haemorrhage. Initial presentation with headache or seizures is rare. They may be caused by congenital weakness of the vessel wall or an acquired lesion resulting from a head injury, or from closure of dural venous sinuses during surgery. The management options for posterior fossa AVMs are radiosurgery, surgical resection and endovascular obliteration.

Procedures for craniocervical abnormalities such as the Arnold–Chiari malformations

Craniovertebral junction anomalies are a group of unusual anomalies that include the occiput, atlas, axis and supporting ligaments that protect the medulla, spinal cord and lower cranial nerves. Their causes are numerous, the most common being Chiari anomalies, congenital bone diseases, metabolic diseases and genetic anomalies. Craniovertebral junction abnormalities are assessed by MRI of the brain and the spinal cord. The goal of surgical management is stabilization of the lesion. The surgical approach depends on the site of the lesion but is either transoral, transpalatopharyngeal, lateral or posterior.

Arnold–Chiari malformations (Fig. 16.2) were originally described by Chiari based on his experience of a series of autopsies in children with hydrocephalus. The estimated incidence is 1:1000 live births. The malformations can be classified into various types. Type I

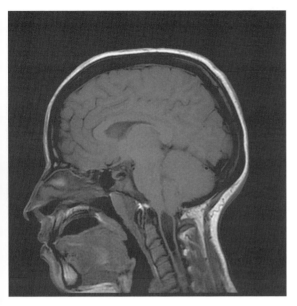

Fig. 16.2. T1-weighted MRI showing an Arnold–Chiari malformation and a large cervical spine syrinx.

is the commonest and involves herniation of the cerebellar tonsils, but not the brainstem, into the foramen magnum. Some patients are asymptomatic in early life and present in later life with headache and cerebellar signs. The condition is often a chance finding during radiological imaging for another condition.

Type II involves extension of the cerebellar tonsils and brainstem tissue into the foramen magnum and often is accompanied by a myelomeningocele, a form of spina bifida. In type III, part of the brain's fourth ventricle also may be herniated and, in rare cases, an occipital encephalocele forms. Type IV involves cerebellar hypoplasia, and parts of the skull and spinal cord may be exposed without any protection. The syndrome is caused by underdevelopment of the posterior fossa or an overgrowth of the supratentorial component. The commonest symptoms are headache, neck pain, weakness and paraesthesias of the hands, and fatigue. If the disease progresses, then management involves foramen magum decompression.

Evacuation of cerebellar haematomas, and decompressive craniectomy to relieve pressure on the brainstem

Haemorrhage (subarachnoid and intracerebral), infarction and neoplasia in the posterior fossa can cause an acute obstruction of cerebrospinal fluid (CSF) drainage pathways causing acute hydrocephalus.

In our institution, severe cerebellar infarction causing hydrocephalus and depressed levels of consciousness is initially managed with external ventricular drain (EVD) insertion and then with decompressive craniectomy if further deterioration occurs.

Anaesthetic challenges for posterior fossa procedures

Optimal patient positioning should facilitate surgical access without compromising patient safety. The important considerations are surgical access, securing and maintaining the airway, maintenance of adequate anaesthetic depth, haemodynamic stability and oxygenation. Also important are preservation of invasive monitors and intravenous catheters, and protecting the patient against pressure injuries to the skin, peripheral nerves and pressure sensitive organs such as eyes. Care should be taken to limit the 'blackout state' during which the patient is not monitored or connected to the breathing circuits during patient transfer or positioning on the operating table (current UK practice is to anaesthetize the patient in the anaesthetic room and then transfer to the theatre). The hazards during positioning can be reduced by meticulous planning, careful positioning and vigilance to facilitate early detection of complications.

The specific challenges in anaesthesia for posterior fossa procedures are caused by the following factors:

1. The vital structures within the posterior fossa, particularly the brainstem, cranial nerves and cerebellum.
2. The confined space of the posterior fossa.
3. The 'awkward' position and anatomy of the lesions complicating surgical access.
4. Relatively longer duration of surgery in extreme positions.
5. The potential for the development of hydrocephalus.

Patient positioning

Supine position with maximal rotation to the contralateral side

This position is used for access to the lateral structures of the posterior fossa. Depending on the site of the lesion, maximal lateral rotation may be required. Up to 45° can be achieved by lateral rotation, and anything beyond can be achieved by elevation of the ipsilateral shoulder by a roll or a pillow. This might not be possible in patients with impaired neck movement. It is usual to provide head-up tilt or reverse Trendelenburg positioning to improve venous drainage from the brain, but it should be remembered that each 2.5 cm increase in vertical height of the head above the level of the heart leads to a 2 mmHg reduction in cerebral perfusion pressure.

Lateral rotation is associated with reduced venous return from the brain, thereby theoretically increasing the chances for raised intracranial pressure (ICP). Extreme lateral rotation for a prolonged period can cause macroglossia, so a soft block should be placed to avoid injury by the teeth. To reduce the risk of brachial plexus stretch and injury, the use of a supporting pad under the ipsilateral shoulder is advisable.

Lateral position

The lateral position is suitable for unilateral procedures of the posterior fossa, as it improves surgical access by gravitational retraction of the cerebellum, and drainage of CSF and blood from the operating field. Drainage can be improved further by placing the table in a head-up position. The incidence of venous air embolism (VAE) is lower than with the prone position, and haemodynamic stability is better when compared with the supine and sitting position. The main problems associated with this position are peripheral nerve injury (stretch injures of the brachial plexus and pressure injuries of the nerves) and gravitational ventilation perfusion mismatch in the dependent lung. The dependent arm should be positioned carefully to avoid pressure-induced nerve injuries. Our current practice is to confirm the safety of the pressure points by a visual check after ensuring optimal surgical access.

Park-bench position

This is a variation of the lateral position and is so called as it resembles the posture of a person reclining on a park bench. It gives better access to the midline structures when compared with the lateral position. The patient is placed semi-prone with the head rotated and the neck flexed, resulting in the brow facing the floor. Disadvantages include peripheral nerve injuries, venous engorgement and macroglossia. If the reverse Trendelenburg position is used to improve surgical access, then the resulting haemodynamic effects should be countered by careful volume loading and judicious use of vasopressors.

Prone position

The prone position facilitates access to the posterior fossa, craniocervical junction and the upper spinal cord. The advantage of this position is the low incidence of air embolism and the easy and optimal surgical access. This position may not provide optimal surgical access in patients with restricted neck movements, and the major disadvantages are diaphragmatic splinting in obese patients, restricted airway access and incompatibility with effective cardiopulmonary resuscitation.

Extreme care and meticulous planning are required, as prone positing is logistically difficult both in the operating theatre and the intensive care unit, with a risk of dislodging the airway, venous catheters and the invasive monitoring. Horseshoe frames can cause pressure on the face and the orbit. In our institution, three-point fixation using the Mayfield head holder is preferred for head support. Care should be taken to avoid diaphragmatic splinting by leaving the chest free and partially support the abdomen and the pelvis. In our institution, this is achieved with a Wilson frame. This position can be combined with head elevation to optimize surgical access and assist with venous drainage, but this may cause hypotension (poorly tolerated in the elderly), and increase the risk of VAE.

Sitting position

The sitting position was introduced into clinical practice by De Martel in 1973. It has been declining in popularity since the 1980s due to the high incidence of complications. In the UK during the period 1981–1991, the number of neurosurgical centres using the sitting position routinely decreased by >50%. This position provides optimal surgical access to the craniovertebral junction and the posterior fossa, particularly midline structures and the cerebellopontine angle. It promotes drainage of blood and CSF, provides easy access to the airway and promotes favourable changes in ventilatory mechanics. This position has several potential life-threatening complications, which include VAE, postural cardiovascular effects compounded by general anaesthesia, quadriplegia, pneumocephalus, macroglossia and peripheral nerve injuries. It is contraindicated in patients with a risk of right-to-left shunt (such as patent foramen ovale, which has an incidence of 27.3% in autopsy studies). The sitting position is also contraindicated in patient with ventriculoatrial CSF shunts, as any air entering the cerebral ventricles during surgery may migrate into the atrium.

Physiological effects of the sitting position

There are several physiological effects of the sitting position on the body:

- *Cardiovascular system.* Awake subjects placed in the sitting position partially compensate for hypotension with an increase in the heart rate and the peripheral vascular resistance, but the capacity for compensation is limited in patients who are anaesthetized. The effects of reduced venous return and hydrostatic pooling are accentuated by advancing age and associated comorbidities.
- *Respiratory system.* There is an increase in the functional residual capacity of the lung in the sitting position, but the reduction in perfusion negates the effects on oxygenation. There is no evidence of improvement in pulmonary function after the sitting position.
- *Cerebral perfusion.* There is a reduction in global cerebral perfusion after placing the patient in the sitting position, increasing the risk of ischaemic damage.

Complications associated with the sitting position

There are a number of complications associated with the sitting position:

1. *Venous air embolism.* This is the entry of air into the peripheral or central vasculature. It is a recognized hazard of surgery in the sitting position and is caused by gravity and the negative pressure in the venous sinuses and veins of the skull and brain.

   The incidence of venous air embolism is high, approaching 100% in adults monitored by transoesophageal echocardiography. The incidence of VAE is thought to be lower in children because dural venous pressures are higher than in adults. In a large study, the incidence of VAE (defined by a fall in arterial carbon dioxide tension ($PaCO_2$)) was 9.3%. The addition of positive end-expiratory pressure (PEEP) causes an increase in right atrial pressure when compared with left atrial pressure, and this predisposes the development of a paradoxical air embolism (PAE) after a VAE.

   The clinical consequences of VAE are dependent on the rate of accumulation and the volume of air entrained. In adults, the lethal volume is thought to be between 200 and 300 ml, or 3–5 ml kg^{-1}. The air reaching the right atrium passes through the right ventricle and reaches the pulmonary vascular bed, causing an increase in the pulmonary vascular resistance, resulting in right heart strain and increased alveolar dead space (alveoli that are ventilated but not perfused), causing a reduction in end-tidal carbon dioxide ($EtCO_2$). The other postulated mechanisms are increased microvascular permeability, pulmonary hypertension related to the release of endothelin 1, and turbulent flow causing platelet aggregation and toxic free-radical damage. If the embolism is large (approximately 5 ml kg^{-1}), a gas air-lock scenario immediately occurs causing cardiac arrest.

   The commonest signs of VAE are tachypnoea, tachyarrhythmias, hypoxaemia, hypotension, wheezes on auscultation and a decrease in $EtCO_2$ with an increase in $PaCO_2$. In awake patients, the signs are continuous coughing, breathlessness, light-headedness, chest pain and a sense of impending doom. Any unexplained hypotension or decrease in $EtCO_2$ should trigger the suspicion of VAE. A PAE (5–10% of VAEs) usually produces signs and symptoms of myocardial and neurological symptoms of cerebral ischaemia.

   Monitoring for VAE relies on detecting the entrained air in the right heart using ultrasound techniques, or detecting the consequences of a pulmonary air embolism – appearance of nitrogen in the expired air in a nitrogen-free anaesthetic, a drop in $PaCO_2$ or PaO_2/oxygen saturation (SpO_2) or a rise in pulmonary artery pressures. A particular issue is the risk of systemic air embolism in the presence of a patent foramen ovale (PFO), as the increase in pulmonary artery pressures associated with a VAE will increase right-sided pressures and promote a right-to-left shunt across an existing or potential atrial septal defect. The incidence of a PFO in patients with a posterior fossa lesion is up to 27%, so there is case for identifying it in advance. Contrast-enhanced transcranial Doppler ultrasound is very sensitive for the diagnosis of a PFO, detecting its presence with an overall accuracy of 92.8%.

   The risk of VAE can be reduced by careful planning of the surgery, meticulous surgical technique and liberal use of bone wax, vigilance, avoidance of nitrous oxide (N_2O) and maximization of intravascular pressure. The treatment of VAE should be directed towards the prevention of further air entrapment by flooding the field with saline, putting the patient in the Trendelenburg position if acceptable, and transient jugular venous compression. The treatment is high-concentration oxygen, placing the patient in the left lateral decubitus position to reduce the gas-lock effect, attempted aspiration of air from the right atrium, haemodynamic support (with intravenous fluids, inotropes and anti-arrhythmic drugs) and cardiopulmonary resuscitation.

2. *Pneumocephalus.* Pneumocephalus occurs when air enters the brain or spaces around the brain after dural incision. If the volume of air is large, and this is accompanied by other factors that cause cerebral oedema, then tension pneumocephalus may occur. The latter is a life-threatening neurosurgical emergency, as it may cause brain herniation. Precipitants include post-operative cerebral oedema, re-expansion of the brain following mannitol administration and use of N_2O causing gas diffusion. The management is drainage of air via a burr hole, ventilation with 100% oxygen and avoidance of N_2O. The investigation of choice is a CT brain scan (which may show air under tension).

3. *Macroglossia and airway swelling.* This is caused by extreme neck flexion causing an obstruction of the lymphatic and venous drainage from the head. It can cause airway obstruction in children. Care should be taken to avoid trauma during oral airway and transoesophageal echo probe placement.

4. *Other complications.* These include cardiac arrhythmias caused by damage or oedema of the vital centres, post-operative respiratory depression, aspiration caused by involvement of cranial nerves, peripheral nerve injuries and spinal cord injury. Spinal cord injury may be caused by extreme flexion, causing a stretch of the spinal cord or reduced cord blood supply during the sitting position. The commonly injured nerves are the common peroneal and recurrent laryngeal nerves. These are caused by the stretch, compression or ischaemia of the nerve.

Pre-operative assessment for posterior fossa surgery

The basic principles for assessment of general health for any operation apply; this should include a detailed medical history in addition to questions about symptoms relating to the complications from the posterior fossa lesion. A review of the imaging of the brain should be performed for evidence for hydrocephalus or increased ICP. Symptoms and signs of cranial nerve palsies (such as impaired gag reflex or impaired cough) will indicate an increased risk of aspiration following the surgery. Localizing lesions for the brainstem and cerebellar signs (ataxia, nystagmus, staccato speech, etc.) should be sought. Craniovertebral junctional abnormalities can lead to instability of the spine or reduced neck movements, posing a challenge for securing the airway for the anaesthesia.

Children should be assessed for the complications of posterior cranial fossa tumours such as diabetes insipidus, dehydration and resulting electrolyte disturbances. Dehydration prior to surgery should be corrected with intravenous fluids. The pre-operative assessment should include consideration of the suitability of the proposed position for the surgery (which may be contraindicated for some patients, e.g. the sitting position in the presence of a PFO).

Monitoring during anaesthesia

Detection of venous air embolism

Monitoring for VAE should be instituted as appropriate for the surgery, patient and position. The various techniques available are listed below:

- Pre-cordial Doppler ultrasound is a sensitive non-invasive instrument for the diagnosis of VAE (it can detect 0.05 ml of air kg^{-1}). The probe should be placed at the second intercostal space on either side of the sternum or between the right scapula and the spine. A bubble test should be performed for the assessment of positioning prior to surgery. The major drawback is the interference with the use of cautery during surgery.

- Transoesophageal Doppler ultrasound is a very sensitive device for the diagnosis for the VAE (it can detect 0.02 ml of air kg^{-1} in the atrium). Treatment and preventative measures should be started if any small air embolism is detected.

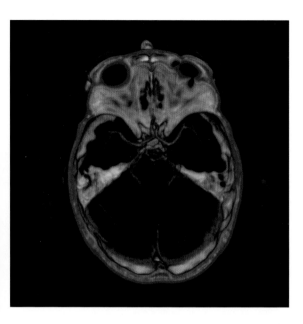

Fig. 1.2. CT angiogram of the circle of Willis.

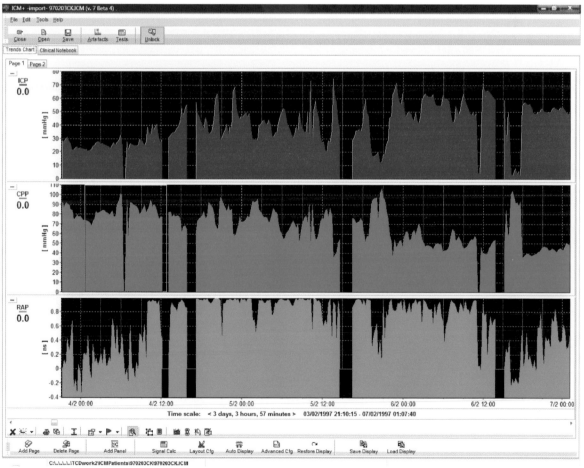

Fig. 4.7. Example of continuous recording of cerebral compensatory reserve using RAP index in a patient after traumatic brain injury: the entire period of recording covers approximately 4 days. During the initial period, even with elevation of intracranial pressure (ICP; mean 22 mmHg), RAP is low, indicating a good compensatory reserve. Later, ICP increases to 30–40 mmHg and is unstable, and RAP increases to +1, indicating a poor compensatory reserve. In the final period, ICP remains elevated, but cerebral perfusion pressure (CPP) decreases; RAP also decreases, indicating a final derangement of regulation of cerebrovascular tone. The patient died.

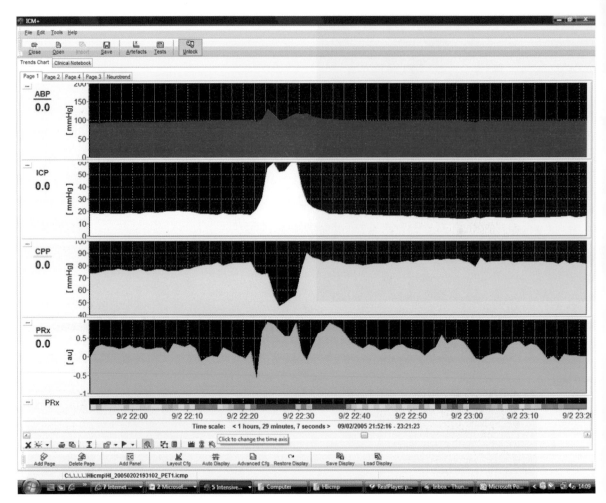

Fig. 4.8. Stable intracranial pressure (ICP) disturbed by a single plateau wave, which is associated with a decrease in cerebral perfusion pressure (CPP) and an increase in cerebrovascular pressure reactivity index (PRx), with the latter continuously monitored as a variable changing in time. On the bottom graph, green denotes good reactivity and red disturbed reactivity. Periods of disturbed reactivity extend for a period past the elevation of ICP, indicating that the ischaemic insult must have affected normal vascular tone for a longer period than the wave itself. ABP, arterial blood pressure.

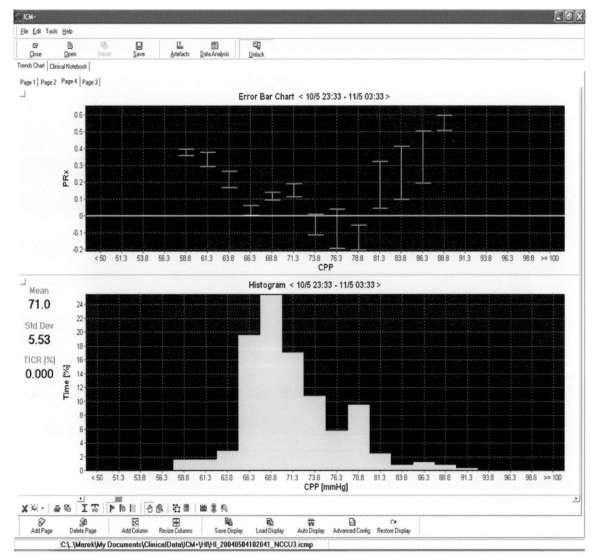

Fig. 4.9. Example of evaluation of 'optimal CPP'. This is a plot of pressure reactivity index (PRx) versus cerebral perfusion pressure (CPP) over a period of 4–6 h. The plot shows the typical U-shaped curve found in the presence of preserved autoregulation. The value of CPP associated with the lowest PRx is the 'optimal CPP'. The bottom graph shows a histogram of CPP over the same period of time. If the peak of the histogram is at the same CPP level as the bottom of the U-shaped curve in the top graph, it indicates that the current CPP is well matched to the optimal level. In this particular case, the optimal CPP was 76 and current modal CPP was 68 mmHg. According to the algorithm suggested by Steiner and colleagues, CPP should be slightly increased in the next step.

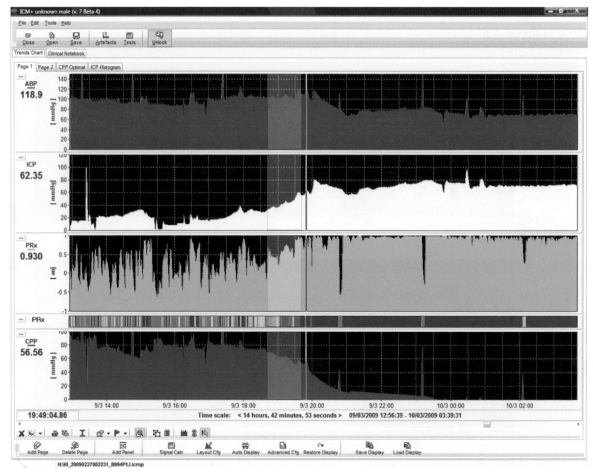

Fig. 4.10. Refractory intracranial hypertension. The second half of this graph shows intracranial pressure (ICP) increasing above 60 mmHg, while cerebral perfusion pressure (CPP) falls well below 40 mmHg. The patient died. The earlier part of the graph shows a rise in ICP from 20 to 40 mmHg, associated with a decrease in CPP below 50 mmHg. This period of progressive ICP elevation is preceded by a 60 min phase during which the pressure reactivity index (PRx) increases (note the change of colour of a bar from greenish to red within the critical period indicated by a grey background).

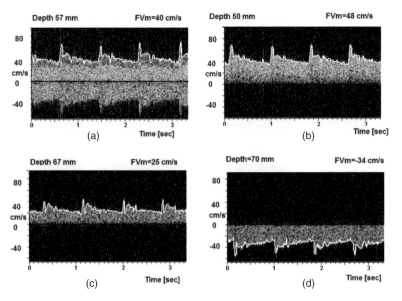

Fig. 5.7. Schematic representation of FV trace obtained from internal carotid artery bifurcation at 5.5–6.5 cm (a), the M1 segment of the middle cerebral artery in 3–6 cm (b), the posterior cerebral artery (P1) at 6–8 cm (c) and the anterior cerebral artery (A1) at 6–8 cm (d). Flow above the horizontal is towards the probe, while flow below the horizontal is away from the probe.

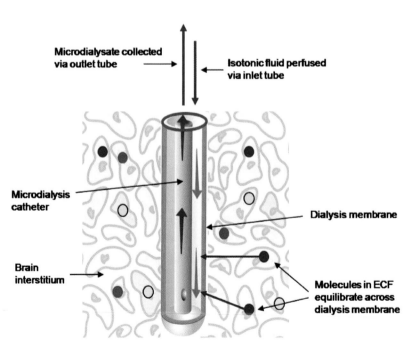

Fig. 7.1. Schematic representation of a microdialysis catheter in brain tissue. Fluid isotonic to the brain extracellular fluid (ECF) is pumped through the microdialysis catheter at a rate of 0.3 µl min^{-1}. Molecules at high concentration in the brain ECF equilibrate across the semi-permeable microdialysis membrane and can be analysed in the collected perfusate (the microdiasylate). (Reproduced with permission from Tisdall and Smith, 2006. *Brit J Anaesth* **97**, 18–25.)

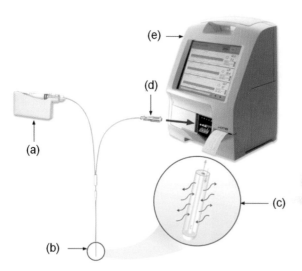

Fig. 7.2. Components of a clinical microdialysis system: (a) microdialysis pump; (b) microdialysis catheter; (c) microdialysis catheter tip showing exchange of molecules across the dialysis membrane; (d) microvial for collection of the microdialysate; (e) bedside analyser. (Reproduced with permission from CMA Microdialysis AB, Solna, Sweden.)

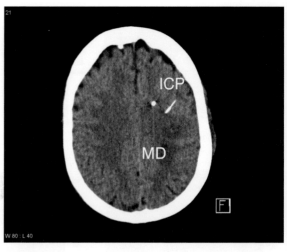

Fig. 7.3. Cranial CT scan showing the locations of an intracranial pressure monitor (ICP) and microdialysis catheter (MD). Microdialysis catheters have a small incorporated gold tip allowing their position to be clearly identified on a CT scan.

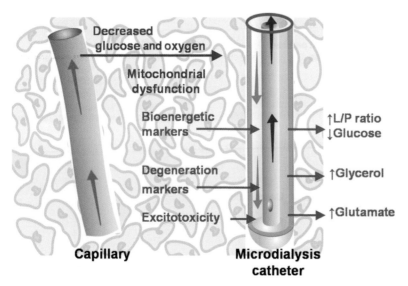

Fig. 7.4. Schematic representation of a blood capillary and microdialysis catheter in brain tissue. The concentration of substrate in the collected fluid (microdiasylate) is related to the balance between substrate delivery to, and uptake/excretion from, the brain extracellular fluid. L/P ratio, lactate to pyruvate ratio. (Reproduced with permission from Tisdall and Smith, 2006. *Brit J Anaesth* **97**, 18–25.)

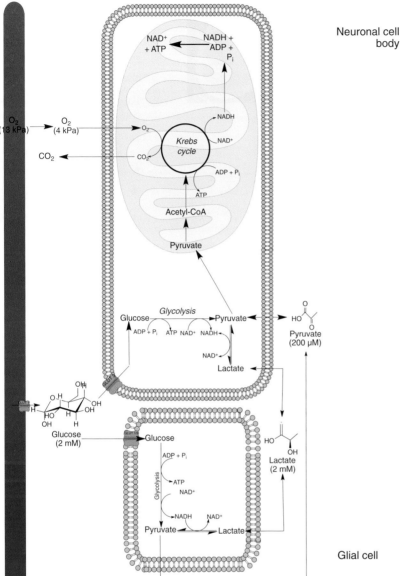

Fig. 7.5. Glucose metabolic pathways.

Neuronal cell body

Glial cell

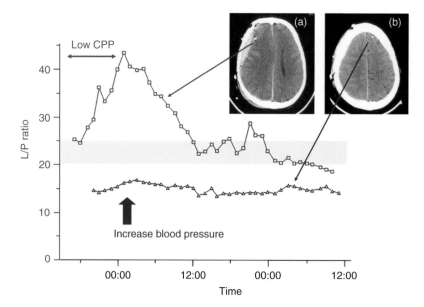

Fig. 7.6. Changes in lactate/pyruvate (L/P) ratio in 'at-risk' (a) and normal (b) brain tissue during a period of low and normal cerebral perfusion pressure (CPP). The normal range for the L/P ratio is shown by the shaded area. Note the rise in L/P ratio in the 'at-risk' tissue during a period of cerebral hypoperfusion but normal values measured by the catheter in normal brain. (Modified with permission from Tisdall and Smith, 2006. *Brit J Anaesth* **97**, 18–25.)

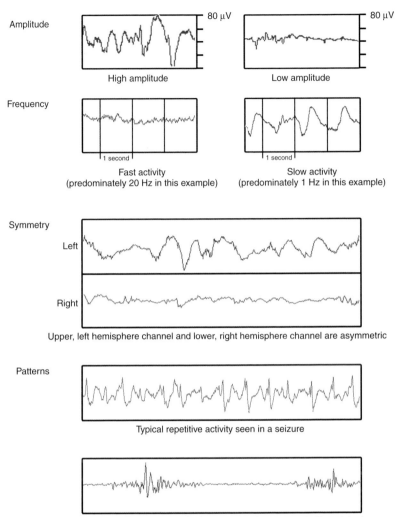

Amplitude

80 μV

High amplitude

80 μV

Low amplitude

Frequency

1 second

Fast activity
(predominately 20 Hz in this example)

1 second

Slow activity
(predominately 1 Hz in this example)

Symmetry

Left

Right

Upper, left hemisphere channel and lower, right hemisphere channel are asymmetric

Patterns

Typical repetitive activity seen in a seizure

A discontinuous 'burst-suppression' pattern seen in coma and with certain drugs

Fig. 8.4. Typical EEG traces and descriptors.

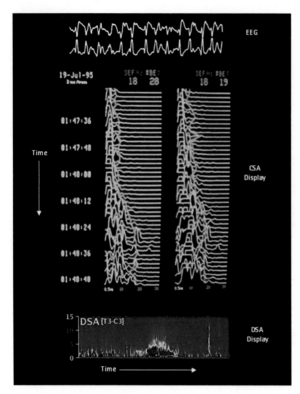

Fig. 8.7. EEG, compressed spectral array (CSA) and density spectral array (DSA) displays showing a seizure. A segment of the raw EEG during the seizure shown at the top and the spectral edge frequency (described in Table 8.4) is plotted on top of the CSA. At the bottom of the figure, a horizontal DSA display shows a seizure as the bright coloured area in the centre of the DSA.

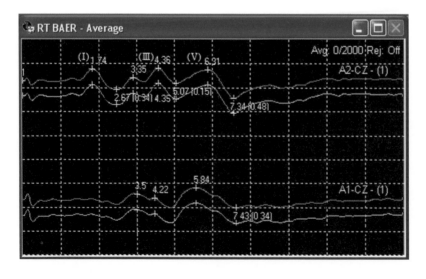

Fig. 8.9. Right brainstem auditory evoked response (BAER) recorded from ipsilateral A2–Cz and contralateral A1–Cz in a propofol-sedated patient. Waves I, III and V from the ipsilateral (to the stimulus) side are shown.

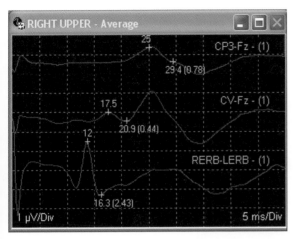

Fig. 8.10. Right upper-extremity somatosensory evoked potential (SSEP) recorded from Erb's point, C5 cervical spine and the left somatosensory cortex in a propofol-sedated patient. Note that the peripheral response (at the brachial plexus recorded at Erb's point) is delayed to 12 ms instead of the normal 9 ms. This delay shifts the subsequent peaks out by 3 ms and is most probably due to a peripheral neuropathy, but could also be due to a very long arm or a cold arm.

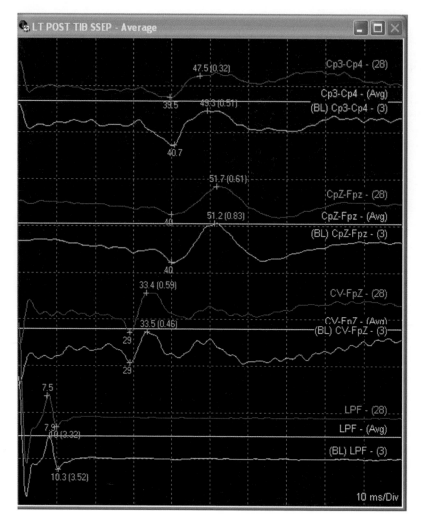

Fig. 8.11. Lower-extremity somatosensory evoked potential (SSEP), showing a peripheral response recorded from the popliteal fossa, a subcortical response recorded at the cervical spine and a cortical response recorded at the somatosensory cortex in a propofol-sedated patient.

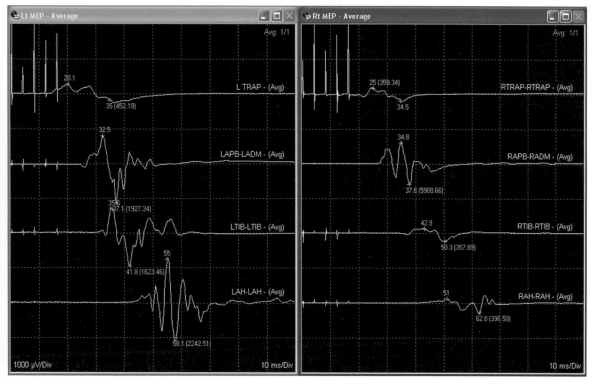

Fig. 8.12. Transcranial electrical motor evoked potentials (TceMEPs), recorded from left and right target muscles – the trapezius (TRAP) and abductor pollicis brevis (APB) in the upper extremities, tibialis anterior (TIB) in the lower extremities and abductor hallucis (AH) in the feet.

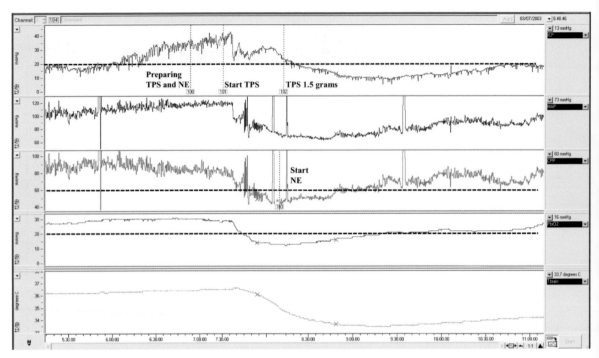

Fig. 9.1. Chart showing the changes in ICP, CPP, brain tissue oxygen tension (PbrO$_2$) and brain temperature (measured in the vicinity of a hypodense lesion) during barbiturate induction for the treatment of raised ICP. Thiopental effectively lowered ICP but induced a CPP reduction and an associated regional brain hypoxia that was corrected using norepinephrine. In this patient, these data showed the CPP threshold required to ensure an adequate brain oxygenation in a vulnerable area of the brain. TPS, thiopental; NE, norepinephrine.

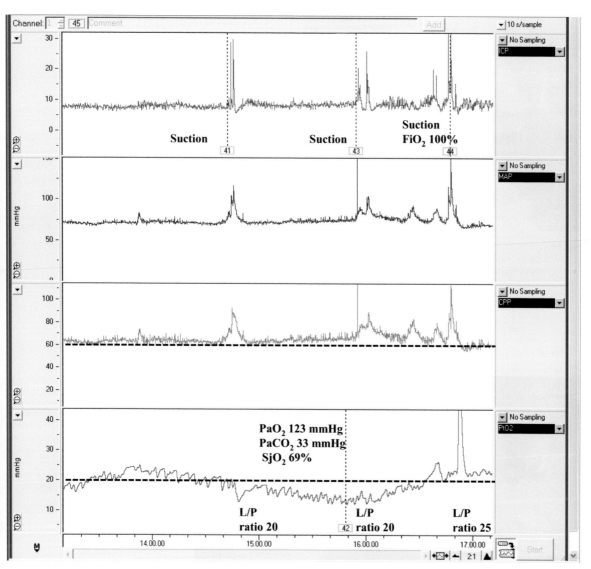

Fig. 9.2. Chart showing the occurrence of an episode of transient regional brain hypoxia (brain tissue oxygen tension ($PbrO_2$) measured in normal-appearing tissue) with no apparent cause and with spontaneous resolution. Cerebral perfusion pressure was stable and remained above the threshold of 60 mmHg, arterial partial pressure of oxygen (PaO_2)was adequate and $PaCO_2$ was in the range of mild hyperventilation. Jugular bulb oxygen saturation (SjO_2) was normal. The episode was followed by an increase in lactate/pyruvate (L/P) ratio measured in the corresponding area from 20 to 25. At follow-up CT scan, no ischaemic changes were observed in the monitored area. These data highlight the complexity of understanding the pathophysiology of regional oxygenation and integrating it with other physiological variables. FiO_2, fraction of inspired oxygen.

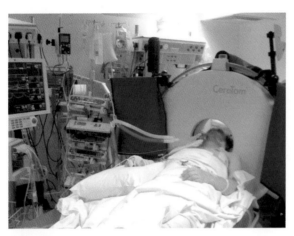

Fig. 10.1. Bedside CT. This patient sustained severe brain, chest and orthopaedic injuries following a road traffic accident. Using the CereTom mobile CT scanner (NeuroLogica Corporation, Danvers, MA, USA), imaging was obtained at the bedside without the need to transfer the patient to the radiology suite.

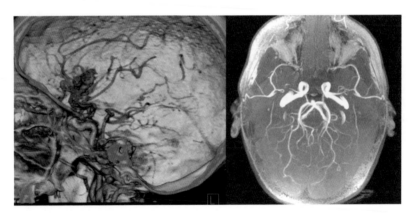

Fig. 10.11. CT and magnetic resonance angiography (MRA). The image in the left panel is from the same patient as shown in Fig. 10.10 and demonstrates the arteriovenous malformation within the region of the right Sylvian fissure. Further investigation using formal angiography was undertaken to delineate the arterial supply and venous drainage of the lesion. The image in the right panel was obtained using MRA and demonstrates a normal-appearing cerebral circulation.

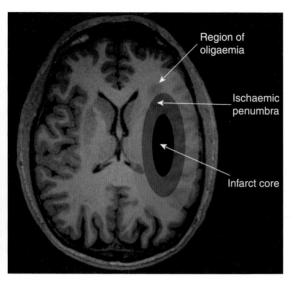

Fig. 10.12. Schematic demonstrating the ischaemic penumbra: ischaemic core of infarcted tissue (black), penumbral region of ischaemic brain tissue at high risk of cerebral infarction (purple) and the surrounding region of oligaemia (pink) above the threshold for cerebral injury following an acute vascular occlusion.

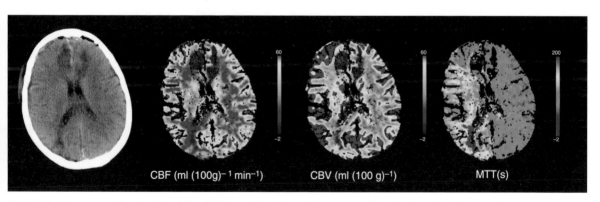

CBF (ml (100g)$^{-1}$ min^{-1})   CBV (ml (100 g)$^{-1}$)   MTT(s)

Fig. 10.13. Assessment of cerebral blood flow (CBF) using CT perfusion. This patient suffered a subarachnoid haemorrhage secondary to an anterior communicating artery aneurysm. The plain CT image on the left demonstrates hypodensity within the medial aspects of the frontal cortex in both hemispheres and also within the right occipital cortex. These areas have very low CBF and cerebral blood volume (CBV) suggestive of established infarction. In addition, there is a generalized reduction in CBF across the right hemisphere with an increase in CBV suggestive of cerebral ischaemia secondary to arterial vasospasm. This reduction of perfusion is most noticeable on the mean transit time (MTT) image, which clearly shows the delay in perfusion across the whole right hemisphere.

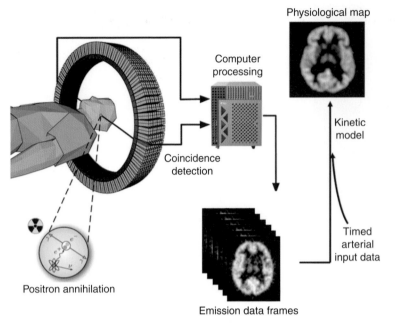

Physiological map

Fig. 10.14. Positron emission tomography (PET). The use of positron-emitting isotopes, incorporated into biological tracers, has enabled in vivo studies of human physiology in health and disease. These positron-emitting isotopes decay by emitting a positron, which is the positively charged anti-particle of the electron. The positron travels a short distance in tissue before it annihilates with an electron and causes the simultaneous release of two photons perpendicular to each other. As the photons are emitted simultaneously, *coincidence detection* occurs for each event through a cylindrical array of detectors. The large datasets acquired in PET require powerful computers to perform the data corrections and image reconstruction in a feasible timescale. The emission frames from the PET scanner and the arterial blood radioactivity data can be used to calculate absolute physiological parameters using appropriate kinetic models.

Computer processing

Coincidence detection

Kinetic model

Positron annihilation

Timed arterial input data

Emission data frames

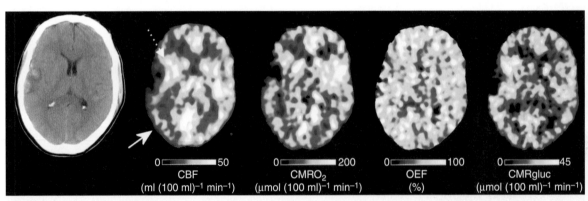

Fig. 10.15. Positron emission tomography (PET) imaging of regional metabolism following head injury. X-ray CT, PET cerebral blood flow (CBF), oxygen metabolism ($CMRO_2$), oxygen extraction fraction (OEF) and glucose metabolism (CMRglu) images obtained following early head injury. Note the right temporal haemorrhagic contusion with surrounding rim of hypodensity on the X-ray CT. The lesion core reflects infarcted brain with no or very low CBF. The pericontusional cerebral hemisphere displays variable pathophysiology. Immediately adjacent to the lesion core (dotted arrow), CBF is increased, $CMRO_2$ and OEF variable but glucose metabolism increased, while the right parietal occipital cortex (white arrow) demonstrates a decrease in CBF and $CMRO_2$ with an increase in OEF and variable glucose metabolism suggestive of regional cerebral ischaemia. The increase in CMRglu implies a switch to non-oxidative metabolism of glucose in order to meet underlying metabolic needs.

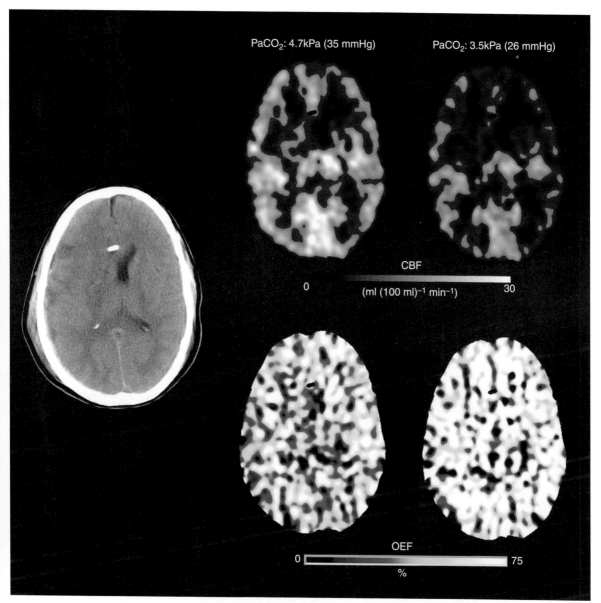

Fig. 10.16. Assessment of the efficacy of acute hyperventilation using positron emission tomography (PET) imaging. Structural CT following early head injury demonstrates a thin right subdural haematoma with underlying cerebral contusion, swollen hemisphere with effacement of the ipsilateral ventricle and midline shift. Greyscale PET cerebral blood flow (CBF) images were obtained at relative normocapnia (left panel) and hypocapnia (right panel). Voxels with a CBF <15 ml (100 ml)$^{-1}$ min^{-1} are picked out in red. Baseline intracranial pressure (ICP) was 21 mmHg and supports the use of hyperventilation to lower arterial carbon dioxide tension (PaCO$_2$) and improve ICP control. Hyperventilation did result in a reduction in ICP to 17 mmHg, but, in this individual, led to a substantial increase in the volume of hypoperfused brain. The PET oxygen extraction fraction (OEF) images show that the effect of the reduction in perfusion is a dramatic increase in OEF to levels consistent with cerebral ischaemia.

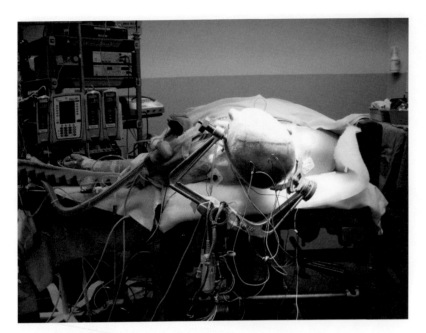

Fig. 11.1. Patient in the supine position with a slight head-up tilt. All pressure points are adequately padded and the eyes are protected.

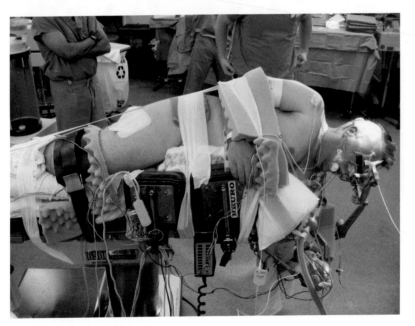

Fig. 11.2. This photograph shows a patient in the park-bench position. Once the patient is draped, the airway is not easily accessible. Therefore, securing the endotracheal tube and ensuring that the neck vessels are not obstructed is of paramount importance.

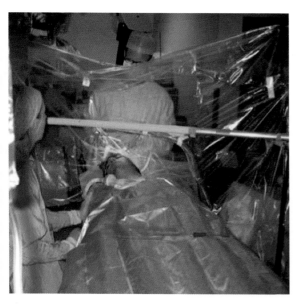

Fig. 12.2. Operating theatre arrangements for awake craniotomy. Note that the surgical drapes are placed to allow the anaesthetist access to the patient's airway and face for intraoperative testing and airway management.

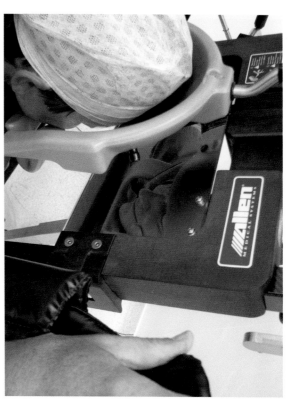

Fig. 15.9. An example of a mirror system that allows inspection of the eyes and nose during surgery in the prone position.

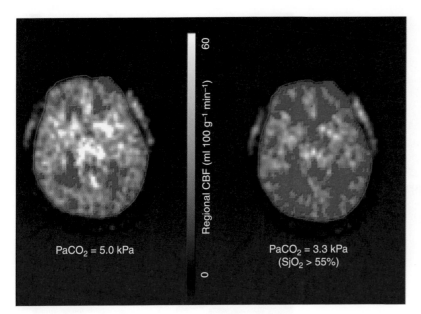

Fig. 21.6. Positron emission tomography imaging showing the effect of hyperventilation in the first 24 h following TBI on regional CBF. Even with an acceptable SjO_2, hyperventilation results in a marked increase in the volume of brain tissue (highlighted areas) below an ischaemic threshold (20 ml $(100\,g)^{-1}$ min^{-1}) due to vasoconstriction from hypocapnia.

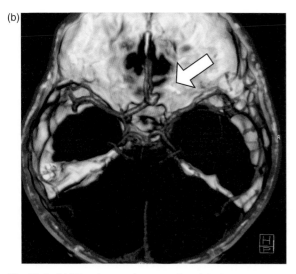

Fig. 22.1. (b) CT angiogram demonstrating a lobular aneurysm arising from the anterior communicating artery (arrow).

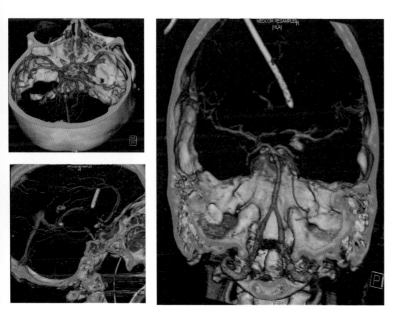

Fig. 22.2. Digital subtraction angiography showing an irregular and elongated (9 mm) aneurysm at the origin of the right posterior communicating artery. The aneurysm is directed posterolaterally, with a small lobule directed medially.

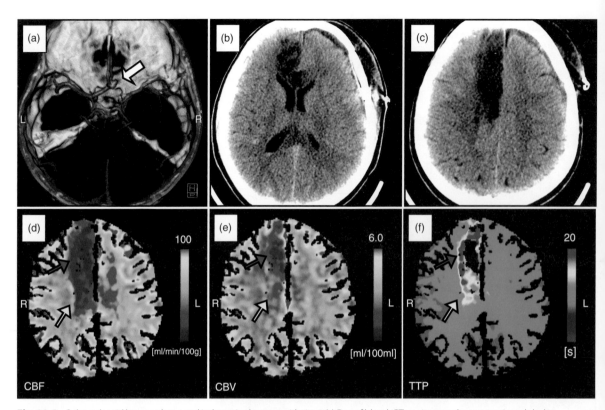

Fig. 22.3. Subarachnoid haemorrhage and ischaemic changes with time. (a) Day of bleed. CT angiogram demonstrating a lobular aneurysm arising from the anterior communicating artery (arrow). Both anterior cerebral arteries originate from the left side with hypoplasia of the right A1. (b, c) Day 10 post-bleed. Plain CT head showing extensive infarction of the right anterior cerebral artery territory involving the genu of the corpus callosum. (d–f) Day 11 post-bleed. CT perfusion showing an established infarct in the right anterior cerebral artery territory (reduced cerebral blood flow (CBF) and cerebral blood volume (CBV), grossly delayed time to peak; red arrows). There is a large, hypoperfused salvageable area extending into the left anterior cerebral artery territory (reduced CBF with maintained CBV and moderately delayed time to peak; yellow arrows).

- End-tidal carbon dioxide monitoring is convenient and available on most anaesthetic machines. A change of 2 mmHg $EtCO_2$ can be an indicator of VAE.
- End-tidal nitrogen detection is more sensitive than $EtCO_2$ as the warning appears approximately 60–90 s before the reduction of $EtCO_2$.
- A pulmonary artery catheter can detect rises in right heart pressures, but this is the most invasive of the monitoring tools available and is less sensitive than pre-cordial Doppler.
- Pulse oximetry, clinical vigilance, oesophageal stethoscopes and ECG changes are late and variable markers of air embolism but continue to be used in many centres.

Neurophysiological monitoring

Due to the concentration of the nerve structures in the brainstem, minor damage in the brainstem can cause devastating complications. Techniques used are sensory evoked potentials and brainstem auditory evoked potentials. These techniques monitor approximately 20% of the brainstem function during surgery and do not provide perfect real-time monitoring or detection of injury to specific tracts, as signal averaging over 40–60 s is required to elicit the signals. Brainstem auditory evoked potentials in response to auditory clicks played into the ears can be monitored by recording electrical signals from scalp electrodes. This technique is particularly important for cerebellopontine angle surgery and/or for microvascular decompression.

Brainstem mapping using a hand-held stimulator is used for the identification of safe entry zones for the surgeon. This is particularly important as oedema of the brainstem can make it difficult to identify the normal anatomical structures. This is done by stimulation of the brainstem to identify the anatomical position of important nuclei. Direct mapping of motor nuclei of the cranial nerves in the floor of the fourth ventricle can be achieved by placing a reference needle electrode in the exposed muscles and the monopolar electrode in the floor of the fourth ventricle. If there is an extension to the midbrain, cerebral peduncle mapping monitoring may be added to the battery of neurophysiological tests.

Continuous EMG monitoring of the VIth and VIIth cranial nerves enhances operative safety and facilitates aggressive monitoring during microvascular decompression, surgery for fourth ventricle tumours

and during acoustic neuroma surgery. Neuromuscular blocking agents should be avoided when monitoring the EMG.

Induction and maintenance of anaesthesia

The goals of induction are to maintain cerebral oxygenation and avoid any increase in ICP. Appropriate non-invasive monitoring (SpO_2, $EtCO_2$, ECG and depth of anaesthesia monitoring) should be instituted prior to induction. In patients with critically raised ICP, arterial line placement prior to induction will enable prompt treatment of any hypotension after induction or hypertension in response to laryngoscopy. Induction is achieved by administering a judicious dose of induction agent, an opiate and a muscle relaxant. After induction of anaesthesia, endotracheal intubation is performed with an appropriate-sized reinforced cuffed endotracheal tube. It is important to avoid hypertensive responses and coughing during laryngoscopy by administering additional doses of a short-acting opiate such as remifentanil and a hypnotic agent.

Further monitoring devices such as a temperature probe, urinary catheter, central venous catheters and arterial lines should be inserted if they have not been placed previously. Pre-cordial Dopplers should be placed for monitoring for VAE. Care should be taken to reduce venous pooling and a subsequent increase in ICP to a minimum during head-down position for the placement of central venous catheters. Head pin placement is a potent stimulant and should be performed after local anaesthesia and a bolus of a short-acting opiate such as remifentanil.

The aim of maintenance of anaesthesia is to reduce the ICP and to maintain haemodynamic stability. Anaesthesia can be maintained with either volatile agents or intravenous agents such as propofol. The choice of the anaesthetic agent is at the discretion of the individual anaesthetist. Propofol has the theoretical advantage that it reduces cerebral blood volume and ICP and preserves autoregulation and vascular reactivity. In healthy subjects, propofol reduces cerebral blood flow more than sevoflurane at equipotent concentrations. Rapid emergence after prolonged posterior fossa surgery can be facilitated by using short-acting drugs such as propofol and remifentanil.

Mechanical ventilation is essential for normocapnia and to avoid hypoxaemia during the surgery. It also reduces the incidence of VAE. Mild passive hypothermia is maintained during the surgery, with rewarming to a core temperature of 36°C prior to emergence to avoid shivering.

Normoglycaemia should be maintained throughout surgery and in the intensive care unit, as episodes of hyperglycaemia and hypoglycaemia are harmful.

Care in recovery room and intensive care management

Emergence from anaesthesia should be smooth. Coughing and straining should be avoided during endotracheal extubation. Rapid awakening assists with early post-operative neurological monitoring. If a decision is made to keep the patient sedated and ventilated post-operatively (for example because of pre-operative comorbidities or events such as failure of the return of gag reflex), an ICP monitoring probe should be used post-operatively, as deterioration of consciousness cannot be used for post-operative neurological monitoring. If the face is swollen causing airway compromise or there has been excessive manipulation of the brainstem causing impaired consciousness or gag reflex, then the patient should be kept ventilated until these improve.

Failure to recover from anaesthesia should prompt further investigations such as imaging of the brainstem to exclude any complications.

Conclusion

Posterior cranial fossa surgery provides a challenge for the anaesthetist and the surgeon. It is associated with many complications, several of which are unique to posterior fossa surgery. Meticulous planning and care throughout and after anaesthesia are required to limit these risks.

Further reading

Alden, T. D., Ojemann, J. G. and Park, T.S. (2001). Surgical treatment of Chiari I malformation: indications and approaches. *Neurosurg Focus* **11**, E2

American Society of Anesthesiologists (2000). Task Force on the Prevention of Perioperative Peripheral Neuropathies: Practice Advisory for the Prevention of Perioperative Peripheral Neuropathies. *Anesthesiology.* **92**, 1168–82.

Batjer, H. and Samson, D. (1986). Arteriovenous malformations of the posterior fossa: clinical presentation, diagnostic evaluation and surgical treatment. *Neurosurg Rev* **9**, 287–96.

Choi, I. S. and David, C. (2003). Giant intracranial aneurysms: development, clinical presentation and treatment. *Eur J Radiol* **46**, 178–94.

Da Costa, L. B. Jr, Thines, L., Dehdashti, A. R. *et al.* (2008). Management and clinical outcome of posterior fossa arteriovenous malformations – report on a single-center 15-year experience. *J Neurol Neurosurg Psychiatry* **80**, 376–9.

Elton, R. J. and Howell, R. S. (1994). The sitting position in neurosurgical anaesthesia: a survey of British practice in 1991. *Br J Anaesth* **73**, 247–8.

Enderby, G. E. (1954). Postural ischaemia and blood-pressure. *Lancet* **266**, 185–7.

Furuya, H., Suzuki, T., Okumura, F., Kishi, Y. and Uefuji, T. (1983). Detection of air embolism by transesophageal echocardiography. *Anesthesiology* **58**, 124–9.

Goodrich, J. T. (ed.) (2008). *Paediatric Neurosurgery,* 2nd edn. *Neurosurgical Operative Atlas.* New York: Thieme.

Hagen, P. T., Scholz, D. G. and Edwards, W. D. (1984). Incidence and size of patent foramen ovale during the first 10 decades of life: an autopsy study of 965 normal hearts. *Mayo Clin Proc* **59**, 17–20.

Harrison, E. A., Mackersie, A., McEwan, A. and Facer, E. (2002). The sitting position for neurosurgery in children: a review of 16 years' experience. *Br J Anaesth* **88**, 12–17.

Holbein, M., Béchir, M., Ludwig, S. *et al.* (2009). Differential influence of arterial blood glucose on cerebral metabolism following severe traumatic brain injury. *Critical Care* **13**, R13.

Kudo, H., Kawaguchi, T., Minami, H., *et al.* (2007). Controversy of surgical treatment for severe cerebellar infarction. *J Stroke Cerebrovasc Dis* **16**, 259–62.

Mammoto, T., Hayashi, Y. and Kuro, M. (1998). Incidence of venous and paradoxical air embolism in neurosurgical patients in the sitting position. Detection by transesophageal echocardiography. *Acta Anaesth Scand* **42**, 643–7.

Mangubat, E. Z., Chan, M., Ruland, S. and Roitberg, B. Z. (2008). Hydrocephalus in posterior fossa lesions: ventriculostomy and permanent shunt rates by diagnosis. *Neurol Res* **31**, 668–73.

Mathew, P., Teasdale, G., Bannan, A. and Oluoch-Olunya, D. (1995). Neurosurgical management of cerebellar hematoma and infarct. *J Neurol Neurosurg Psychiatry* **59**, 287–92.

Meier, R., Béchir, M., Ludwig, S. *et al.* (2008). Differential temporal profile of lowered blood glucose levels (3.5 to 6.5 mmol/l versus 5 to 8 mmol/l) in patients with severe traumatic brain injury. *Crit Care* **12**, R98.

Mirski, M. A., Lele, A. V., Fitzsimmons, L. and Toung, T. J. (2007). Diagnosis and treatment of vascular air embolism. *Anesthesiology* **106**, 164–77.

Morantz, R. A. and Walsh, J. W. (eds) (1993). *Brain Tumors, a Comprehensive Text*. New York: Informa Healthcare.

Novegno, F., Caldarelli, M., Massa, A. *et al.* (2008). The natural history of the Chiari Type I anomaly. *J Neurosurg Pediatr* **2**, 179–87.

Parízek, J., Mericka, P., Nemecek, S. *et al.* (1998). Posterior cranial fossa surgery in 454 children. Comparison of results obtained in pre-CT and CT era and after various types of management of dura mater. *Childs Nerv Syst* **14**, 426–38; discussion 439.

Parkin, D. M., Stiller, C. A., Draper, G. J. *et al.* (eds) (1988). *International Incidence of Childhood Cancer*. IARC Scientific Publications No. 87. Lyon: International Agency for Research on Cancer,.

Porter, J. M., Pidgeon, C. and Cunningham, A. J. (1999). The sitting position in neurosurgery: a critical appraisal. *Br J Anaesth* **82**, 117–28.

Pribram, H. F. W., Hudson, J. D. and Joynt. R. J. (1969). Posterior fossa aneurysms presenting as mass lesions. *Am J Roentgenol* **105**, 334–40.

Rozet, I. and Vavilala, M. S. (2007). Risks and benefits of patient positioning during neurosurgical care. *Anesthesiol Clin* **25**, 631–53.

Sakaki, T., Morimoto, T., Nakase, H., Kakizaki, T. and Nagata, K. (1996). Dural arteriovenous fistula of the posterior fossa developing after surgical occlusion of the sigmoid sinus. Report of five cases. *J Neurosurg* **84**, 113–18.

Sala, F., Manganotti, P., Tramontano, V., Bricolo, A. and Gerosa, M. (2007). Monitoring of motor pathways during brain stem surgery: what we have achieved and what we still miss? *Neurophysiol Clin* **37**, 399–406.

Smoker, W. R. and Khanna, G. (2008). Imaging the craniocervical junction. *Childs Nerv Syst* **24**, 1123–45.

Standring, S. (ed.) (2008). *Gray's Anatomy: the Anatomical Basis of Clinical Practice.*, 40th edn. Churchill Livingstone.

Stapf, C., Mohr, J. P., Pile-Spellman, J. *et al.* (2002). Concurrent arterial aneurysms in brain arteriovenous malformations with haemorrhagic presentation. *J Neurol Neurosurg Psychiatry* **73**, 294–8.

Stiller, C. A. and Nectoux, J. (1994). International incidence of childhood brain and spinal tumours. *Int J Epidemiol* **23**, 458–64.

Valiaveedan, S. S., Rath, G. P., Bithal, P. K., Ali, Z. and Prabhakar, H. (2008). Posterior fossa dermoid: yet another cause of difficult airway. *J Anesth* **22**, 446–8.

Voelker, R. (2009). Chiari conundrum: researchers tackle a brain puzzle for the 21st century. *JAMA* **301**, 147–9.

Wei, T. M., Lu, L. C., Ye, X. L., Li, S. and Wang, L. X. (2008). Impact of postures on blood pressure in healthy subjects. *Acta Clin Belg* **63**, 376–80.

Wilson, M., Davies, N. P., Brundle, M. *et al.* (2009). High resolution magic angle spinning ^{1}H NMR of childhood brain and nervous system tumours. *Mol Cancer* **8**, 6.

Anaesthesia for neurosurgery without craniotomy

Rowan M. Burnstein, Clara Poon and Andrea Lavinio

Transsphenoidal pituitary surgery

Neoplasms of the hypophysis represent approximately 10% of all brain tumours, and transsphenoidal pituitary surgery accounts for as much as one-fifth of all intracranial operations performed for primary brain tumours. In current practice, most sellar tumours are approached via the endonasal endoscopic approach, the classic sublabial approach being indicated only in a minority of patients for whom endonasal exposure may prove inadequate.

Patients with pituitary disease present with specific anaesthetic challenges. Common concerns relate either to the systemic effects of secreting adenomas, such as acromegaly and Cushing's disease – which will be discussed in detail – or the intracranial mass effect of large adenomas. Rapidly worsening visual impairment represents the main indication for emergency hypophysectomy and optic chiasm decompression.

Pituitary anatomy and physiology

The pituitary gland – or hypophysis – sits in the sella turcica (the Turkish saddle), a midline saddle-shaped depression in the sphenoid bone in the middle cranial fossa. The hypophysis is enveloped by the dura mater lining the sella and is covered by an open dural fold (diaphragma sellae). The hypophyseal stalk (infundibulum) runs through the opening of the diaphragma sellae, connecting the hypophysis and hypothalamus.

The pituitary gland is surrounded by a number of vital structures that may either be compressed by enlargement of the gland or damaged during surgical excision of pituitary tumours. The optic chiasm sits directly above the sella, and macroadenomas can compress the optic axons originating from the medial retina and crossing at the chiasm, typically causing temporal (or bitemporal) hemianopia. The cavernous sinuses, the internal carotid arteries, oculomotor nerve (III), trochlear nerve (IV), abducens nerve (VI) and the first two divisions of the trigeminal nerve (V) lie at both sides of the pituitary gland. Cranial nerve palsies (diplopia) are signs of lateral expansion of a pituitary tumour. The hypothalamus and third ventricle lie above the sella. Compression of these structures by large tumours can lead to headache, hypothalamic abnormalities, hydrocephalus and raised intracranial pressure (ICP).

Systemic signs and symptoms associated with pituitary disease may also be related to its endocrine physiology. The hypophysis is formed by two functionally distinct parts. The anterior pituitary gland (or adenohypophysis) comprises 80% of the hypophysis and synthesizes six hormones: growth hormone (GH), adrenocorticotropic hormone (ACTH), prolactin (PRL), thyroid-stimulating hormone (TSH), luteinizing hormone (LH) and follicle-stimulating hormone (FSH). These hormones are released from the anterior pituitary under the influence of hypothalamic releasing hormones (GH-releasing, gondatotropin-releasing, TSH-releasing and ACTH-releasing hormones) and inhibitory hormones (somatostatin or GH-inhibiting, and dopamine or PRL-inhibiting). Hypothalamic hormones are transported to the anterior pituitary by way of a special capillary system running in the hypophyseal stalk, the hypothalamic–hypophyseal portal system.

The posterior pituitary (neurohypophysis) is not a gland but a nervous structure with an endocrine function, being an intrasellar expansion of the hypothalamus capable of releasing hormones into the systemic circulation. The neurohypophysis contains hypothalamic axons originating from the supraoptic and paraventricular nuclei of the hypothalamus, and specialized glial cells called pituicytes. These hypothalamic nuclei synthesize oxytocin and antidiuretic hormone, which

Core Topics in Neuroanaesthesia and Neurointensive Care, eds. Basil F. Matta, David K. Menon and Martin Smith. Published by Cambridge University Press. © Cambridge University Press 2011.

are then secreted into the capillaries of the posterior hypophyseal circulation.

Pituitary disease

Pathology

The vast majority of intrasellar masses are pituitary adenomas, which can be locally invasive but do not metastasize. Pituitary adenomas are extremely common: their estimated prevalence in the overall population ranges from 14.4% in autopsy studies to 22.5% in radiological studies. Primary pituitary carcinomas and secondary metastases, the latter originating mostly from primary carcinoma of the lung, are rare. Other relatively uncommon pituitary masses include tumours of 'epithelial remnants' (craniopharyngiomas, chordomas), benign lesions (meningiomas, hamartomas, chondromas) and granulomatous/inflammatory lesions (sarcoidosis, tuberculomas, abscesses).

Pituitary adenomas are classified according to their size, immunohistochemistry and functional status (Fig. 17.1). According to their endocrine profile, adenomas are classified as 'functioning' (hormone-secreting) adenomas, or 'non-functioning' (non-secreting) adenomas. Frequent among secreting adenomas are GH-secreting adenomas and PRL-secreting adenomas. ACTH-, TSH-, FSH- and LH-secreting adenomas are relatively rare. So-called 'non-functioning' adenomas account for approximately one-third of all pituitary adenomas. However, although 'non-functioning' adenomas are devoid of clinically significant systemic endocrine effects, the majority stain positively by immunohistochemically for gonadotropin subunits (β-LH, β-FSH or α-subunit).

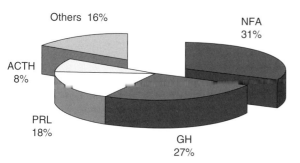

Fig. 17.1. Histology of surgically excised pituitary tumours – relative prevalence. NFA, non-functioning adenomas; GH, somatotrope adenomas; PRL, prolactinomas; ACTH, Cushing's disease; others, TSH-secreting and gonadotropin-secreting adenomas.

Adenomas can be further classified according to their size. Tumours >1 cm are classified as 'macroadenomas', while tumours <1 cm are classified as 'microadenomas'. With the exception of ACTH-secreting adenomas, which tend to be diagnosed early due to signs of hypercortisolism (Cushing's disease), the majority of all other adenomas – including secreting adenomas – tend to be diagnosed when their size exceeds 1 cm and are therefore classified as macroadenomas at the time of diagnosis. Non-functioning adenomas are, by definition, not associated with signs or symptoms of hormone excess, and they present with features relating to their mass effect.

With an increasing number of patients undergoing head CT or MRI for unrelated disorders (predominantly headache), more pituitary masses are being diagnosed in otherwise asymptomatic patients. While the incidental finding of a macroadenoma is a relatively rare occurrence, the prevalence of microadenomas in young and fit patients is surprisingly high. The prevalence of pituitary abnormalities detected by MRI in healthy volunteers varies from 0.3% for macroadenomas to 10% for microadenomas. These have a small risk of further enlargement, and surgery is not indicated in such cases. Non-secreting microadenomas are managed with a 'watchful wait' approach, repeating an MRI scan at 1 year. If the adenoma is not growing and is not hormonally active, no further imaging or laboratory testing is required, unless indicated by a worsening clinical picture.

Pituitary hyperplasia is also a common cause of pituitary enlargement. It is caused by excess secretion of hypophyseal releasing hormones stimulating pituitary growth and activity, and must be distinguished from pituitary adenoma. Pituitary hyperplasia can be observed in cases of primary hypothyroidism leading to reflex TSH-releasing hormone hyperproduction, or acromegaly secondary to ectopic (carcinoid) GH-releasing hormone (GHRH) secretion.

Worthy of mention here is the so-called empty sella syndrome, a rare condition that is characterized by a downward prolapse of the arachnoid through the diaphragm into the sella. Although there is no tumour, the sella is progressively enlarged by cerebrospinal fluid (CSF) pressure and the hypophysis is compressed against the posterior wall of the sella, causing panhypopituitarism.

Acromegaly

Acromegaly is a complex clinical condition caused by an excessive production of GH and characterized by an acquired progressive somatic disfigurement involving the face and extremities but also involving many other organs. The term (from the Greek *akros* meaning 'extremities' and *megas* meaning 'big') was introduced by Pierre Marie, a French neurologist who published the first description of the disease and its pathology in 1886. The term 'gigantism' refers to excessive production of GH beginning prior to pubertal closure of the epiphyseal plates.

The insidious progression of the disease typically leads to a late presentation and diagnosis. Acromegalic patients presenting for hypophysectomy are usually in their 40s and are presumed to have suffered from the disease for at least 4 years at the time of diagnosis. Most GH-secreting adenomas are therefore macroadenomas, and patients have well-established anatomical and physiological changes at the time of surgery. The clinical diagnosis is confirmed by MRI and biochemical tests. Diagnostic laboratory findings include increased serum GH concentrations that are not suppressed following an oral glucose load (oral glucose tolerance test) and an increased serum concentration of the major GH-dependent growth factor, insulin-like growth factor 1 (IGF-1). The excess GH originates from a monoclonal pituitary adenoma in >95% of acromegaly cases. In the case of a negative head MRI, other rare causes of acromegaly not related to pituitary adenomas include carcinoid tumours of the pancreas or lung-secreting GHRH, or genetic syndromes such as McCune–Albright syndrome.

Physical and facial appearances of acromegaly are characteristic. Hands and feet are broadened. Fingers are stubby. The nose is widened and thickened, the cheekbones are prominent, the forehead is bulging and the lips are bulky. Craniofacial changes include mandibular and maxillary overgrowth, prognathism, jaw thickening, teeth malocclusion and nasal bone hypertrophy. Systemic features of acromegaly include diffuse skin thickening and hyperhydrosis, periosteal bone growth and skeletal deformation resulting in rheumatological complications such as multiple peripheral arthropathy, spinal changes leading to significant kyphoscoliosis, and neuropathies, with carpal tunnel syndrome reported in up to 75% of cases. Prognatism, macroglossia, hypertrophy of the uvula and epiglottis, and calcinosis of the larynx may cause difficult laryngoscopy. Unanticipated difficulty with airway management is more than three times more common in acromegalic patients (9.1%) than in patients with non-functioning pituitary tumours. Hoarseness should

alert the physician to the possibility of laryngeal stenosis or recurrent laryngeal nerve injury. Cardiovascular manifestations (hypertension, myocardial hypertrophy), metabolic complications (diabetes in up to 56% of cases) and respiratory complications (sleep apnoea reported in up to 80% of cases) are also common. Overall, acromegaly is associated with increased mortality: 60% of patients die from cardiovascular disease, 25% from respiratory complications and 15% from cancer. Cardiac involvement is a GH-specific feature of acromegaly that occurs even in the absence of hypertension. It is initially asymptomatic and usually consists of hyperkinetic, concentric ventricular hypertrophy. Clinical symptoms such as dyspnoea and poor exercise tolerance, arrhythmias and/or conduction disorders (ventricular premature complexes are common) should be actively investigated as they may indicate congestive heart failure, especially in patients with other risk factors such as diabetes and sleep apnoea. Valve disorders can also contribute to the onset or aggravation of heart failure in patients with acromegaly. In contrast to myocardial hypertrophy, valve disorders persist even after effective treatment of acromegaly. Hypertension is due to endothelial dysfunction and chronic hypervolaemia, with a plasma volume 10–40% above normal due to increased renal sodium reabsorption at the distal tubule level. Sleep apnoea syndrome is also likely to contribute to the pathogenesis of hypertension. Respiratory complications of acromegaly are common, with sleep apnoea affecting the majority of patients. Hypercollapsibility of the pharyngeal walls and macroglossia cause obstructive apnoea, but up to one-third of patients are also reported to have central apnoea. Snoring, daytime sleepiness, morning fatigue and headache are common warning signs that should be documented and kept in consideration. Although subclinical hypoxaemia is sometimes present, no ventilation–perfusion mismatch has been demonstrated in acromegaly. A minority of patients will require prolonged nocturnal positive pressure ventilation for persistent sleep apnoea, despite successful treatment of acromegaly. Metabolic complications are related to insulin resistance, hyperinsulinism and increased blood glucose levels. Diabetes and glucose intolerance are diagnosed in up to 50% of cases.

Endoscopic transsphenoidal excision of pituitary adenoma is the first-line treatment for acromegaly. However, in one-third of cases, surgery fails to reduce GH and IGF-1 concentrations to normal levels. Negative prognostic factors include large tumour size and high pre-operative GH concentrations. When surgery fails to achieve good disease control, or when surgery is contraindicated, alternative options include stereotactic radiotherapy and/or pharmacological treatments, including somatostatin analogues (octreotide, lanreotide), dopamine agonists (cabergoline, bromocriptine), and GH-receptor antagonists (pegvisomant). Repeated transsphenoidal surgery is also considered if medical treatment is poorly tolerated or ineffective.

Cushing's disease

Cushing's disease is caused by an ACTH-secreting (corticotropic) pituitary adenoma, first described by Harvey Cushing in 1912. As ACTH controls the release of cortisol from the adrenal cortex, non-feedback-loop-controlled ACTH secretion by pituitary tumours causes excess cortisol secretion by the adrenal gland. Hypercortisolism leads in turn to central obesity, muscle wasting, skin atrophy (purple striae), diabetes, hypertension, cardiomyopathy, amenorrhoea, decreased libido, osteoporosis and psychiatric abnormalities. This broad collection of signs, symptoms and metabolic changes related to hypercortisolism is summarized in the definition of Cushing's syndrome. Although in the majority of cases Cushing's syndrome is caused by an ACTH-secreting pituitary adenoma (true Cushing's disease), other causes of Cushing's syndrome include ectopic ACTH production (lung carcinoids, pancreatic islet tumours), primary excess cortisol production from adrenal tumours and iatrogenic glucocorticoid excess. Nelson's syndrome refers to the aggressive and often invasive growth of an ACTH-secreting pituitary tumour following bilateral adrenalectomy in patients with Cushing's disease. The risk of patients with Cushing's disease developing Nelson's syndrome following bilateral adrenalectomy is high, ranging from 15 to 46%. Cushing's disease represents approximately 8% of pituitary adenomas presenting for surgical excision. As corticotropic adenomas tend to cause early signs and symptoms, ACTH-secreting tumours are the only pituitary tumours that are mostly diagnosed as microadenomas.

The patient's appearance is one of generalized obesity of the face, trunk and abdomen. A short and thick neck with a characteristic dorsocervical fat pad, and macroglossia are common predictors of difficult intubation. Although patients with Cushing's disease are statistically no more difficult to intubate than patients with non-functioning tumours, it must be pointed out that, when this is the case, there is a risk of a 'can't intubate, can't oxygenate' emergency, as Cushing's syndrome is also associated with multiple predictors of difficulty for bag-mask ventilation (obesity, obstructive sleep apnoea, decreased chest wall compliance). Airway access through the cricothyroid membrane can be difficult or impossible in patients with obesity of the neck.

Cushing's disease carries a fourfold risk of mortality, largely related to obesity, diabetes, hypertension and cardiovascular disease. Other significant morbidities in Cushing disease include hyperlipidaemia, coagulopathy, osteoporosis, depression, anxiety and cognitive impairment. Overt diabetes mellitus is diagnosed in one-third of all patients with Cushing's disease. As hyperglycaemia can aggravate ischaemic injury of the brain and spinal cord, blood glucose levels in excess of $180\,mg\,dl^{-1}$ ($10\,mmol\,l^{-1}$) should be treated with intravenous insulin perioperatively in all cases. The majority of patients with Cushing's disease have systemic hypertension, with a presenting diastolic blood pressure >130 mmHg in 10% of patients. Increased endogenous corticosteroids can cause hypertension by many different mechanisms, including increased cardiac output and increased hepatic production of angiotensinogen, which in turn activate the renin–angiotensin system causing sodium retention and plasma volume expansion. Glucocorticoids also reduce the synthesis of vasodilatory prostaglandins and increase the expression of angiotensinogen II, leading to increased sensitivity to endogenous vasoconstrictors such as angiotensin II, epinephrine and norepinephrine. This is relevant to anaesthetic management, as sensitivity to exogenous catecholamines may also be exaggerated. Left ventricular hypertrophy is often detected on 12-lead ECG and echocardiography. Echocardiography can reveal disproportionate hypertrophy of the intraventricular septum, with diastolic dysfunction in at least 40% of patients. Exercise tolerance is often limited by obesity, and congestive cardiac failure is not uncommon. As in the case of cardiomyopathy related to acromegaly, ECG and echocardiographic abnormalities often regress after curative adenomectomy. Obstructive sleep apnoea is common among patients with Cushing's disease. Polysomnographic studies indicate that one-third of patients with Cushing's disease have mild sleep apnoea, and about one-fifth of patients have severe sleep apnoea, suggesting higher risk of airway obstruction in the perioperative period. Sedative analgesics should be used with caution, and perioperative non-invasive positive-pressure ventilation may be indicated in selected cases. Patients suffering from Cushing's disease tend to have atrophic skin, and veins are often fragile and prone to bruising. In morbidly obese patients, venous cannulation can be extremely difficult. Such patients should be forewarned of the option of inhalational induction of anaesthesia. Although myopathy is common among patients with Cushing's disease, there is no specific contraindication or abnormal response to succinylcholine or non-depolarizing neuromuscular blockers. Osteoporosis is common, and particular care is needed when positioning the patient.

Effective surgical treatment restores normal cortisol levels and results in survival rates similar to those of the general population. Transsphenoidal selective adenomectomy is the treatment of choice, with partial or total hypophysectomy being surgical alternatives if the adenoma cannot be identified. Remission rates vary between 69 and 98%, with an acute surgical mortality rate of <2%. After failed transsphenoidal surgery for Cushing's disease, treatment options include repeated transsphenoidal surgery, radiotherapy, pharmacological therapy and bilateral adrenalectomies. The last option carries a significant risk of Nelson's syndrome. Selective adenomectomy and partial or total hypophysectomy have similar long-term remission rates. However, with increased removal of pituitary gland tissue, there is an increased rate of anterior and posterior pituitary failure.

Thyroid-stimulating hormone-producing adenomas

Thyrotropic adenomas represent <3% of all pituitary tumours and are a rare cause of hyperthyroidism. The clinical features of patients with TSH-producing adenomas are the same as those of patients with primary hyperthyroidism. Goitre is common, and symptoms include palpitations, tremor, weight loss, difficulty sleeping, heat intolerance and sweating. Patients are often initially misdiagnosed with more common causes of hyperthyroidism, such as Graves' disease. As a consequence, thyrotropic adenomas often remain unidentified and are allowed to grow for years, and tend to be large upon diagnosis. As for other hormonally active pituitary adenomas, medical therapy can help control symptoms but is rarely curative, and transsphenoidal hypophysectomy is the treatment of choice. Somatostatin analogues (octreotide) can suppress the production of TSH and reduce tumour size, while antithyroid medication (such as propylthiouracil 200–300 mg four times daily) reduce thyroid hormone secretion, controlling hyperthyroidism. If a β-blockade

is started (propranolol 30–60 mg three times daily) to control tremors or palpitation, it should be continued perioperatively.

Prolactinomas

Although PRL-secreting adenomas are the most commonly diagnosed pituitary tumour, the condition responds well to medical treatment and only a minority of patients are candidates for surgery. Patients with a prolactinoma are no more difficult to intubate than patients with non-functioning tumours, and hyperprolactinaemia does not have systemic effects that imply specific anaesthetic issues.

Prolactinomas are slow-growing adenomas and tend to remain stable in size for years. Symptoms are related to hyperprolactinaemia and suppressed gonadotropin secretion leading to menstrual disturbances, virilization and infertility in women, and gynaecomastia, loss of libido and oligospermia in men. Galactorrhoea is more evident and occurs mostly in women, so the diagnosis is made earlier, and PRL-secreting adenomas tend to be smaller at diagnosis in female patients.

Prolactin is secreted under the dominant inhibitory hypothalamic control of dopamine, and the vast majority of patients respond well to medical therapy with a dopamine agonist such as bromocriptine. However, medical treatment needs to be continued for life, and a minority of patients do not tolerate or do not respond to dopamine agonists. Transsphenoidal hypophysectomy is the second-line therapeutic option in such cases.

Craniopharyngiomas

Craniopharyngiomas were first described by Erdheim in 1904 as 'hypophysial duct tumours', but it was Cushing who later used the term 'craniopharyngioma' to define these benign tumours that develop along the pituitary stalk. Craniopharyngiomas originate from infundibular remnant nests of epithelium of Rathke's pouch, an embryonic precursor of the anterior pituitary.

Craniopharyngiomas represent 5% of all primary central nervous system (CNS) tumours diagnosed in childhood. They often have suprasellar extension and may be cystic and/or calcified. These features are helpful in differentiating craniopharyngiomas from pituitary adenomas on neuroimaging. Craniopharyngiomas present with symptoms of pituitary stalk compression, visual disturbances and hypopituitarism.

Transsphenoidal excision of a craniopharyngioma presents specific perioperative issues, caused by its tight adherence to vascular and cerebral structures, which can make surgery difficult. Although radical excision provides the best long-term remission, aggressive surgery is associated with significant incidence of complications, including profuse haemorrhage, CSF leak and hypopituitarism. Stereotactic radiotherapy, in the form of radiosurgery or fractionated stereotactic radiotherapy, is currently used in patients after limited surgery and achieves excellent long-term tumour control with minimal side effects.

Diagnosis and treatment

Diagnostic work-up: overview

Radiographic investigation of the sella turcica is considered obsolete and is rarely performed. MRI of the hypophysis is the neuroradiological technique of choice for imaging patients with pituitary adenomas. MRI distinguishes normal hypophysis from hyperplasia, adenomas and craniopharyngiomas.

Appropriate laboratory work-up for microadenomas diagnosed in otherwise asymptomatic patients (incidentalomas) includes PRL and IGF-1 levels, as PRL and GH hypersecretion are relatively common and can be clinically silent. Negative results rule out prolactinoma and acromegaly, and the absence of symptoms rules out other functioning adenomas, providing reassurance and improving the quality of life of anxious patients. Midnight salivary cortisol levels, low-dose dexamethasone suppression tests or 24 h urinary cortisol levels are not a required screening test and should be performed only in patients presenting with signs of hypercortisolism, such as central obesity, skin symptoms and myopathy. Similarly, TSH and thyroxine (T4) levels should be measured only in patients with signs of hyperthyroidism. There is no indication for routine assessment of FSH/LH in asymptomatic patients presenting with a small incidentaloma.

On the other hand, all patients presenting with macroadenomas should undergo a complete hormonal evaluation, as the increased intrasellar pressure and compression on the hypophyseal stalk can decrease pituitary perfusion and reduce the delivery of hypophyseal releasing hormones. Also, patients may become hyperprolactinaemic secondary to a loss of tonic inhibition of PRL secretion. Hypopituitarism is the most common feature of patients presenting with macroadenomas, and one or more anterior-pituitary deficiencies can be demonstrated in one-third of the cases. The clinical progression of hypopituitarism caused by macroadenomas is often slow and insidious; symptoms are non-specific and can be easily overlooked, explaining the indication for broad screening. The notable exception to the typical indolent progression of compressive hypopituitarism is the clinical syndrome diagnosed as pituitary apoplexy. The term 'pituitary apoplexy' is archaic and misleading, literally meaning 'pituitary seizure' (from the Greek *apoplèxia* meaning 'being struck down'). Pituitary apoplexy is instead an acute haemorrhagic infarction of the hypophysis resulting in a sudden, life-threatening failure of the hypophyseal–hypothalamic axis, optic chiasm compression and severe visual impairment, and midbrain compression resulting in dysautonomic disturbances, shock and unconsciousness. The risk of acute pituitary haemorrhagic infarction ('apoplexy') in patients with a macroadenoma was reported recently to be as high as 9.5% over 5 years.

In summary, in all cases of newly diagnosed macroadenomas, GH, PRL, LH/FSH, TSH and ACTH axes should be evaluated. Also, in addition to a full neurological examination with a particular focus on oculomotor and trigeminal abnormalities, formal visual-field testing is warranted for every patient diagnosed with a macroadenoma growing in proximity to the optic chiasm, as visual defects progress slowly – usually beginning from the superior temporal fields – and can be unnoticed by the patients.

Surgical indications

All macroadenomas have a tendency to grow and cause visual disturbances and/or hypopituitarism with time. Macroadenomas also carry a significant risk of pituitary infarction (pituitary apoplexy), and surgical hypophysectomy is indicated even for non-secreting, clinically silent macroadenomas, especially if the patient is young. The same considerations apply to other non-adenomatous tumours (such as craniopharyngiomas) that are growing or exerting mass effects.

Although medical treatment can help control symptoms in all hormonally active adenomas, medical therapy is considered to be a first-choice treatment only for prolactinomas, where dopamine agonists not only control symptoms but also normalize PRL and cause shrinking of the adenoma in >90% of patients. In all other cases of hormonally active adenomas, surgery is the only curative treatment, and the vast majority of cases are candidates for transsphenoidal hypophysectomy. As noted above, non-radical surgical treatment can be associated with stereotactic radiotherapy in order to spare healthy hypophysis and reduce complications in selected cases.

Surgical technique

The extracranial approach to the hypophysis was first described by Schloffer in 1906, who reported the excision of a pituitary tumour through the nose. The sublabial transseptal and transantral approaches to the hypophysis are nowadays adopted only in small children and for the excision of extremely large tumours, where the endonasal approach provides inadequate exposure of the mass. The majority of pituitary tumours, including those with suprasellar extension, are approached transnasally with the help a magnified endoscope. Direct transnasal transsphenoidal endoscopic-assisted pituitary surgery allows adequate excision of most pituitary masses, including those with suprasellar extension, and is associated with minimal cosmetic, dental and nasal complications. The endoscopic transsphenoidal approach is also associated with a shorter period of hospitalization and with a lower incidence of hypopituitarism and diabetes insipidus (DI).

A lumbar intrathecal catheter can be used to improve intraoperative visualization of pituitary tumours in selected cases with suprasellar extension. Injection of normal saline or Hartmann's solution in the lumbar subarachnoid space through the lumbar catheter increases CSF pressure, producing a pressure gradient that can dislocate the tumour towards the surgical field, facilitating surgery. A three-way stopcock connected to a pressure transducer can be used to monitor lumbar CSF pressure intraoperatively during CSF-volume manipulation. Particular care in lumbar catheterization should be taken in patients with large tumours or signs of raised ICP, as inadvertent CSF withdrawal at the time of lumbar drain insertion poses a risk of downward brain herniation.

The patient is positioned supine on the operating table, with a 30° head-up tilt. Local anaesthetic with vasoconstrictor is instilled into each nostril to improve surgical conditions and to minimize hypertensive responses to surgical stimulation, and the tumour is accessed through the sphenoidal air sinuses for endoscopic excision. During excision, the anaesthetist may be required to inject saline in the lumbar catheter to improve visualization of the tumour.

After successful resection of the tumour, a Valsalva manoeuvre is used to test for CSF leaks. In the case of a significant CSF leak, the neurosurgeon will seal the sella with autologous fat, usually harvested from the patient's thigh. After completion of surgery, nasal packs are inserted to remain in place for 48–72 h post-surgery.

Complications

The most frequent complication of transsphenoidal pituitary surgery is hypopituitarism: the reported rate of anterior pituitary failure ranges from 2 to 41%, but is <20% in most published series. The incidence of permanent DI following pituitary surgery ranges from 3 to 9%. Other reported complications include CSF leaks (0–8%), meningitis (0–3%), new neurological deficits (0–2%), post-operative haematomas (0–6%), thrombo-embolic events (0–4%) and wound or nasoseptal complications (0–4%). Blood loss is usually minimal, but major haemorrhage can occur if there is surgical damage of cavernous sinuses or the carotid artery. Massive haemorrhage is an unusual but potentially fatal complication of transsphenoidal surgery.

Anaesthetic management

Pre-operative anaesthetic assessment

Routine clinical examination includes a formal neurological evaluation. Signs and symptoms of raised ICP and neurological deficits should be documented. As increased retro-orbital fat deposition is present in one-third of patients with Cushing's disease, exophthalmos should also be documented on the anaesthetic chart, and extra care in eye protection is warranted to prevent corneal abrasions.

The upper airway should be evaluated for predictors of difficult intubation, especially in acromegaly and Cushing's disease. Awake, fibre-optic-assisted intubation is the most prudent option if difficulties with face-mask ventilation and problematical airway access through the cricothyroid membrane are anticipated. Obesity and a history of obstructive sleep apnoea should be taken into account, and arrangements for a high-dependency bed and perioperative non-invasive positive-pressure ventilation should be made in advance in such cases. Nasal packing should be explained pre-operatively, as the patient needs to be prepared to breathe orally after surgery and until the removal of nasal packs.

Pre-operative laboratory evaluation should include coagulation and a complete blood count to assess the presence of clotting abnormalities and anaemia. Electrolytes, creatinine, urea and glycaemia should be assessed for pre-operative hyponatraemia (DI), hypo-kalaemia, renal failure and diabetes. Women presenting with amenorrhoea should have a pregnancy test before elective surgery. Patients with hypopituitarism should receive hormone replacement therapy with hydrocortisone and/or thyroxine, as guided by laboratory studies and discussed with the endocrinologist. Transsphenoidal hypophysectomy poses a minor surgical stress, and most patients on maintenance glucocorticoid therapy (usually 30–50 mg hydrocortisone daily) do not require extra perioperative steroid cover during the perioperative period. If a β-blockade is established, it should be continued perioperatively.

Transfusions are rarely required except for large tumours with suprasellar extension and for craniopharyngiomas, which have a higher risk of blood loss due to meningeal adherences. The risk of haemorrhagic complications should be discussed pre-operatively with the surgeon. If pre-operative volume expansion is indicated, avoid hypotonic crystalloids (dextrose). There is no indication for routine prophylactic phenytoin. Antibiotic prophylaxis is indicated.

Induction and maintenance of anaesthesia

The fundamental principles of anaesthesia for pituitary surgery are very similar to those for other supratentorial surgical procedures. In contrast to most neuroanaesthetic procedures, the anaesthetist can be required to *increase* ICP in order to facilitate exposure and surgical excision of the pituitary tumour. This can be done safely in patients with small adenomas and no signs of intracranial hypertension. Ventilation is manipulated to achieve mild hypercapnia, and isotonic crystalloids can be infused through a lumbar catheter to increase CSF pressure with no adverse effects. Nitrous oxide is best avoided. During surgery, air may be injected transsphenoidaly to favour surgical exposure or to improve fluoroscopic visualization of the tumour. Nitrous oxide poses the risk of an untoward expansion of the pneumoencephalic bubble.

Our anaesthetic technique of choice is target controlled infusion (TCI) total intravenous anaesthesia (TIVA). Invasive arterial blood pressure is indicated in all patients, as transsphenoidal surgery is often associated with significant episodes of hypertension. Central venous monitoring is not routinely indicated. Visual evoked potential (VEP) monitoring has been advocated in the past for surgery close to the visual pathways. However, polysynaptic cortical waveforms such as those detected by VEP monitoring are more sensitive to the effects of anaesthetic depth than to the effects of surgery, resulting in a failure of the technique to improve post-operative visual acuity. Strong evidence supporting routine use of VEP monitoring for transsphenoidal pituitary surgery is lacking.

Osteoporosis may occur in up to 50% of patients presenting with Cushing's disease and almost 20% of patients may have pathological fractures. Positioning should therefore be particularly careful in such cases. Some degree of head-up positioning reduces venous engorgement, with venous air embolism being a theoretical risk discussed extensively elsewhere.

The mucosal surfaces of the nose are infiltrated with local anaesthetic and a vasoconstrictor such as epinephrine solution to reduce bleeding and facilitate dissection. Epinephrine can sometimes cause hypertension, which can usually be managed by increasing the depth of anaesthesia. A total spinal anaesthetic after inadvertent local anaesthetic injection through the cribriform plate at this stage is an extremely remote risk.

A mean arterial blood pressure between 60 and 80 mmHg at the highest point of the skull maintains cerebral perfusion with minimal oozing in the surgical field. Large respiratory volumes are sometimes required to control carbon dioxide in acromegaly. Ventilation and CSF volume can be manipulated as detailed above to facilitate tumour visualization. Hypotonic fluids are best avoided. Intraoperative fluids are administered based on starvation, insensitive losses and urinary output in catheterized patients. Blood loss is usually <100 ml.

After successful excision of the tumour, a Valsalva manoeuvre is performed to detect CSF leaks. After completion of surgery in patients with obstructive sleep apnoea, the surgeon should place a nasopharyngeal airway before the nose is packed. Transitional analgesia is provided with morphine (50 μg kg^{-1} IV), paracetamol (1 g IV) and non-steroidal anti-inflammatory drugs (NSAIDs), unless contraindicated.

Post-operative management

Neurological complications are rare and the post-operative course is usually smooth. Post-operative neurological examination should be focused on worsening visual acuity, scotomas and cranial nerve palsies. Any of these findings should trigger surgical re-exploration of the hypophysis or urgent CT.

Patients should be questioned regarding rhinorrhea or the feeling of fluid leaking down the back of their throat. Some degree of nasal discharge is common, and the suspicion of CSF leak can be confirmed by sending the fluid for a β_2-transferrin assay, which is a highly sensitive and specific test for CSF.

Given the high risk of post-operative nausea and vomiting in patients undergoing transsphenoidal pituitary surgery, and the theoretical detrimental effects of vomiting on ICP, routine pharmacological prophylaxis is indicated. Dexamethasone does not interfere with post-operative serum cortisol assays and has anti-oedemogenic properties, and is a useful anti-emetic alongside serotonin 5-hydroxtryptamine receptor (5-HT$_3$) antagonists (ondansetron) and histamine H1 receptor antagonist (cyclizine), which may be prescribed on an 'as required' basis.

Post-operative headache is relatively common, and adequate analgesia is warranted for all patients. However, narcotics and benzodiazepines should be used with extreme caution, especially in patients with a history of obstructive sleep apnoea. In such patients, a nasal airways catheter inserted through the nasal packing can be very helpful, facilitating non-invasive positive-pressure ventilation if required. Post-operative hypertension is relatively common despite adequate analgesia, and may only resolve after nasal packs are removed. Traditionally, patients with Cushing's disease were prescribed prophylactic steroids to prevent post-operative adrenal insufficiency. In current practice, steroids are withheld and cortisol levels are tested every 6 h after surgery, in order to document disease remission. Hydrocortisone should be administered only if cortisol levels are below 2 μg dl^{-1} and in the presence of signs of adrenal insufficiency.

Disorders of water balance

Antidiuretic hormone (ADH), also known as arginine vasopressin (AVP) or argipressin, is a peptide hormone synthesized in the hypothalamus and stored in vesicles in the posterior pituitary, from where it is released into the systemic circulation. Physiologically, ADH is secreted in response to dehydration. The main effect of ADH is to cause the kidneys to concentrate and reduce the volume of urine (antidiuretic effect), thus retaining free water, diluting plasma and decreasing its osmolarity.

Disturbances in osmoregulation resulting in polyuria and abnormalities of serum sodium concentration are common and should be monitored, even after selective transsphenoidal surgery for pituitary adenomas. The physiological control of ADH secretion can be impaired with two opposite mechanisms: insufficient ADH secretion leading to DI, and excessive ADH secretion leading to the syndrome of inappropriate anti-diuretic hormone secretion (SIADH).

Diabetes insipidus

If the ADH-synthesizing hypothalamic nuclei are damaged during surgery, the patient will lose his or her ability to secrete ADH and to retain water. Free water is subsequently lost in large volumes with urine (hypotonic polyuria), while the plasma becomes more and more concentrated (hyperosmolar hypernatraemia). This condition goes under the definition of DI, which literally means 'hypotonic polyuria'. Polyuria aside, DI has nothing in common with diabetes mellitus, and glucose metabolism is normal. The pathogenesis of DI is insufficient antidiuresis secondary to the inability of the brain to synthesise and secrete ADH (neurogenic DI). A similar clinical scenario, not relevant to perioperative management of patients undergoing pituitary surgery, can be caused by the inability of the kidney to respond to ADH (nephrogenic DI). Nephrogenic DI can be caused by renal amyloidosis, polycystic kidney disease, lithium toxicity, etc.

Diabetes insipidus is a common – but fortunately transitory in most cases – complication of transsphenoidal surgery. Early post-operative DI is diagnosed in >30% of patients, while persisting DI – resulting from widespread destruction of the paraventricular and supraoptic nuclei – affects approximately 1 in 20 patients. Diabetes insipidus presents on the first or second day following surgery, with sudden profuse polyuria, often in excess of 500 ml h^{-1}. Urine is dilute (specific gravity 1.001–1.005) and hypo-osmolar (U$_{Osm}$ <280 mOsm l^{-1}). If the patient is alert and has free access to water, compensatory polydipsia will limit volume contraction and hypernatraemia. However, in fragile patients with inadequate access to fluids or impaired thirst mechanisms, as in the case of most elderly patients, failure to promptly recognize and treat DI can lead to hypovolaemic shock, severe hypernatraemia, coma and death.

The treatment of DI is based on ADH replacement with its synthetic analogue desmopressin (1-deamino-8-D-arginine vasopressin, or DDAVP). Apart from hypernatraemia (serum Na >145 mmol l^{-1}) and rapidly increasing serum sodium concentration, indications for treatment include the inability of the patient to match urinary output with fluid intake, resulting in progressive hypovolaemia and nocturia interfering with sleep.

In the acute setting, the subcutaneous and intranasal routes of administration are preferred (DDAVP 1 µg SC or IN). Although polyuria resolves quickly with negligible haemodynamic effects, electrolytes (urinary and serum), urine output and fluid balance should be monitored closely at this stage. As DI is transient in the majority of cases, often only a single dose of DDAVP is required. In the minority of patients with persistent DI, DDAVP treatment needs to be continued – often for life – and may be administered orally. The oral starting dose of DDAVP is usually 100 µg. Parenteral DDAVP administration is used as required during the titration of oral DDAVP.

To avoid the unnecessary risk of hyponatraemia, it is of paramount importance that treatment with DDAVP is commenced only in patients with confirmed DI. Polyuria, urine gravity <1.005 and hypernatraemia should all be confirmed before administering DDAVP. Physiological polyuria is common in the perioperative period and is often secondary to generous intravenous fluid administration, but urine is concentrated (urine gravity >1.005) and hypernatraemia is uncommon. Administration of DDAVP in such cases leads to excessive antidiuresis, inappropriate free-water retention and hyponatraemia.

Syndrome of inappropriate anti-diuretic hormone secretion

Physiologically, ADH secretion is finely tuned by hypothalamic and periventricular osmoreceptors. Following pituitary surgery, such delicate regulatory mechanisms are often impaired, and delayed inappropriate (excessive) secretion of ADH is observed in up to 25% of cases. In SIADH, free water intake exceeds free water excretion, urine is relatively concentrated and plasma becomes progressive diluted, leading to hyponatraemia (serum Na <135 mmol l^{-1}) and serum hypo-osmolarity (P_{OSM} <280 mOsm l^{-1}). Despite worsening hyponatraemia, excess ADH continues stimulating reabsorption of free water and urinary sodium concentration remains high (U_{Na} >40 mEq l^{-1}). Thus, SIADH is characterized by hyponatraemia and eu- or hypervolaemia, and should therefore be distinguished from the so-called cerebral salt-wasting syndrome (CSWS), a less-understood disease featuring hyponatraemia and dehydration (hypovolaemia) due to excessive renal sodium excretion resulting from a centrally mediated process. While aggressive fluid replacement is the cornerstone of CSWS treatment, SIADH is treated with fluid restriction. Although fluid restriction is effective in the majority of SIADH cases, in the subgroup of patients presenting with severe, symptomatic hyponatraemia (headache, nausea and vomiting, seizures, coma), hypertonic saline infusions should be considered to help correct serum sodium. The use of hypertonic solutions should be cautious and sodium correction must be slow (<1 mEq h^{-1}) in order to prevent pontine myelinolysis.

Ventriculoperitoneal shunts and allied procedures

Cet enfant a de l'eau dans la tete, dit le vulgaire; Cet enfant est hydrocephale, dit gravement le medicin, repetant litteralment par un mot grec ce qui dit l'ignorant dans sa propre langue. Mais quelle est cette eau? D'ou vient-elle?

F. Magendie (1842)

Hydrocephalus comprises a miscellaneous group of disorders of CSF dynamics leading to an excessive accumulation of CSF within the brain, resulting in ventricular dilation and increased ICP (Table 17.1). Prior to the introduction of techniques to bypass the normal means of draining CSF, hydrocephalus had an extremely poor prognosis. Children with congenital hydrocephalus suffered disabling neurological sequelae and rarely reached adulthood. The prognosis of hydrocephalus was greatly improved by the introduction of silicone ventricular shunts, designed by John Holter, in collaboration with Eugene Spitz, in 1956. Holter realized that the available technology was clumsy, and developed the first functional silicone shunt in order to treat his own son, Casey, who was born with spina bifida and congenital hydrocephalus in 1955.

A ventricular shunt is a system of two silicone catheters connected by means of a one-way valve. The purpose of a shunt is to divert CSF from the lateral ventricles of the brain to high-capacitance bodily cavities such as the peritoneum, cardiac atrium or pleura, where CSF can be reabsorbed. Lumbar shunts serve a similar purpose, diverting CSF from the lumbar subarachnoid space to the pleura or peritoneum. The main clinical difference between ventricular shunts and lumbar shunts is that lumbar shunts are contraindicated in 'non-communicating' (obstructive) forms of hydrocephalus, where cranio-caudal pressure gradients could cause downward herniation of the brain as CSF is shunted from the lumbar subarachnoid space.

Table 17.1 Hydrocephalus: definitions and classification

Each row in the table compares and contrasts commonly used terms and concepts: hydrocephalus vs. ventriculomegaly, congenital vs. acquired hydrocephalus, non-communicating vs. communicating hydrocephalus, and hydrocephalus resulting from excessive CSF production vs. impaired CSF reabsorption.

Hydrocephalus	**Ventriculomegaly**
The category comprises miscellaneous abnormalities in production, flow or reabsorption of CSF, resulting in ventricular dilatation and increased ICP.	The term describes ventricular enlargement, which can be secondary to cerebral atrophy (*ex vacuo* hydrocephalus). Shunting is *not* indicated in such cases.
Congenital hydrocephalus	**Acquired hydrocephalus**
Typically non-communicating. Spina bifida, myelomeningocele, stenosis of the cerebral aqueduct, Arnold–Chiari malformation, arachnoid cysts, vascular malformations.	CNS infections, subarachnoid haemorrhage, traumatic brain injury, tumours compressing or obstructing CSF pathways.
Non-communicating hydrocephalus	**Communicating hydrocephalus**
'Obstructive' hydrocephalus. CSF pathways are blocked by tumours, blood clots or malformations. Absolute contraindication to lumbar shunting. Third ventriculostomy is a surgical option.	CSF reabsorption impaired at subarachnoid granulations (bulk flow theory) or reduced brain compliance (hydrodynamic theory). Ventricular and lumbar shunting can be indicated.
Pathogenesis: excessive CSF production	**Pathogenesis: impaired CSF reabsorption**
Choroid plexus papilloma (very rare).	Vast majority of cases. Includes communicating and non-communicating forms of hydrocephalus.

CNS, central nervous system; CSF, cerebrospinal fluid; ICP, intracranial pressure.

Cerebrospinal fluid shunting is carried out in a wide range of age groups, ranging from neonates (congenital hydrocephalus) to adults (post-traumatic, post-haemorrhagic and post-infective hydrocephalus, and idiopathic intracranial hypertension) and the elderly (normal pressure hydrocephalus, NPH).

Hydrocephalus

Hydrocephalus comprises a miscellaneous group of disorders of CSF dynamics leading to an excessive accumulation of CSF within the brain, resulting in ventricular dilation and increased ICP. If hydrocephalus ensues before cranial sutures are fused, cranial fontanelles become tense and bulging, sutures are splayed and cranial circumference tend to increase abnormally.

It is of paramount important to stress the difference between the terms hydrocephalus and ventriculomegaly. These terms should not be used interchangeably. The term 'ventriculomegaly' describes the finding of ventricular enlargement on brain imaging and is not a specific feature of hydrocephalus. Ventriculomegaly is a common anatomical feature of brain atrophy following ischaemic and traumatic brain injury, or in senile dementia. In such cases, CSF compensates the intracranial space freed by a shrinking brain, causing the ventricles and cerebral sulci to appear enlarged.

The CSF pressure is low and there is no indication for shunting. At the other end of the spectrum, patients with long-standing hydrocephalus and shunt obstruction can present with *slit ventricles*, despite impaired CSF reabsorption and increased ICP.

The aetiology and pathogenesis of hydrocephalus vary widely. Impaired CSF reabsorption of different aetiology is by far the most common cause of hydrocephalus, while excessive CSF secretion caused by choroid plexus papillomas is a rare causal mechanism. Disturbed cerebral venous outflow is thought to play a significant role in the pathogenesis of idiopathic intracranial hypertension (IIH), and reduced brain compliance is probably involved in the pathogenesis of NPH.

Hydrocephalus can be categorized as congenital or acquired. Congenital hydrocephalus is present at birth and is often associated with developmental defects. It is typically non-communicating (obstructive) and requires urgent surgical treatment. The incidence of infantile hydrocephalus is estimated at 1–5 cases per 1000 live births. Acquired hydrocephalus occurs after the development of the brain and ventricles. It is a more heterogeneous category, including obstructive and non-obstructive forms of hydrocephalus.

Pathogenetic classification subdivides hydrocephalus into communicating and non-communicating forms. The term 'communicating' refers to the free flow and transmission of CSF pressure from the ventricles to the subarachnoid space. Non-communicating (obstructive) hydrocephalus is due to narrowing or obstruction of the normal CSF flow pathways within the brain. Non-communicating hydrocephalus causes a significant increase in ICP and usually has an acute presentation. It can be congenital (commonly associated with CNS malformations such as myelomeningocele) or acquired (caused by tumours compressing the aqueduct or intraventricular clots). Communicating forms of hydrocephalus have a much less intuitive pathogenesis. Communicating hydrocephalus is caused by 'functional disorders' of CSF reabsorption in the presence of patent CSF pathways. Communicating forms of hydrocephalus, such as NPH, typically have an indolent and chronic clinical presentation. Normal pressure hydrocephalus is a clinical syndrome presenting with the classic triad of gait difficulties, urinary incontinence and mental decline, as first described by Hakim and Adams in 1965. Although in NPH vasogenic CSF pressure waves can be prominent, baseline CSF pressure is usually normal, and – clinically – patients do not present with the typical signs and symptoms of increased ICP. The pathogenesis of communicating hydrocephalus is a matter of intense debate. The classical bulk flow theory suggests that communicating hydrocephalus is caused by a CSF reabsorption deficit at the arachnoid villi. More recently, hydrodynamic theories have been used to explain the features of communicating hydrocephalus. According to the hydrodynamic concept, communicating hydrocephalus is caused by decreased cerebral compliance resulting in increased systolic pressure transmission into the brain parenchyma. The increased systolic pressure distends the brain towards the skull while simultaneously compressing the periventricular region against the ventricles, which are fluid filled and therefore not compressible. Irrespective of the theoretical framework, ventricular shunting corrects the mechanistic CSF dynamics disorder of communicating hydrocephalus in both theoretical scenarios. On the other hand, the indication of a third ventriculostomy in communicating hydrocephalus has a rationale only in the context of the hydrodynamic theory.

Although not strictly classified as hydrocephalus, IIH is a disturbance of CSF dynamics that responds to ventricular or lumbar shunting, and is defined as a persistent increase in ICP in the absence of any intracranial lesions. The term IIH, introduced by Buchheit in 1969, corresponds to the former term 'pseudotumour cerebri'; the term 'benign intracranial hypertension' should be avoided, as permanent visual defects are serious and not infrequent complications of this condition. Idiopathic intracranial hypertension is a relatively rare disease, but a rapidly increasing incidence is being reported due to a global increasing incidence of obesity.

Testing cerebrospinal fluid dynamics and shunt valve performance in vivo

Brain imaging can be misleading in the diagnosis of hydrocephalus. While the enlargement of cerebral ventricles is not necessarily of hydrocephalic nature – as in the aforementioned case of atrophic ventriculomegaly – even the finding of slit ventricles does not strictly exclude hydrocephalus and shunt malfunction.

Moreover, while shunting dramatically improves CSF dynamics, changes in ventricular size are often subtle or absent, even in shunt responders. In this context, it is often difficult to decide whether a patient needs a shunt or a shunt revision simply on the basis of brain imaging. However, it is possible to measure CSF outflow resistance and shunt valve performance with a simple bedside infusion test. Comprehensive computerized tools for evaluation of shunts are commercially available.

Computerized infusion tests can be used to estimate the resistance to CSF outflow (R_{OUT}) preoperatively (lumbar infusion studies, only in communicating hydrocephalus), intraoperatively (via ventricular reservoir, prior to shunting) and post-operatively (via shunt antechamber or ventricular reservoir). Preoperatively or intraoperatively, the finding of increased resistance to CSF outflow ($R_{OUT} > 13$ mmHg ml^{-1} min^{-1}) indicates a need for shunting. Post-operatively, the technique is used to detect shunt malfunction (including posture-related overdrainage and shunt obstruction) indicating a need for shunt revision. Infusion tests can be performed in awake or in anaesthetized patients (Fig. 17.2). In communicating hydrocephalus, access to the subarachnoid space is usually obtained via two lumbar needles that are connected to an infusion pump and to a pressure transducer via a stiff saline-filled tube. The CSF pressure, zeroed at the level of external acoustical meatus, yields a measure of ICP. In communicating hydrocephalus, the lumbar access is substituted by two 27G needles connected to the shunt antechamber or, intraoperatively, to the ventricular reservoir,

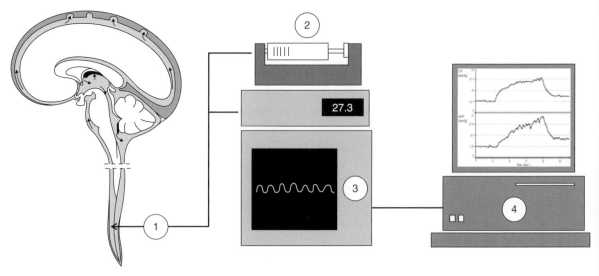

Fig. 17.2. Infusion tests. In communicating hydrocephalus, access to the subarachnoid space is usually obtained via two lumbar needles (1) that are connected to an infusion pump (2) and to a pressure transducer (3) via a stiff saline-filled tube. The cerebrospinal fluid (CSF) pressure, zeroed at the level of external acoustical meatus, yields a measure of intracranial pressure (ICP). The response of ICP to the infusion of fluid can be plotted (4) to provide information about CSF dynamics. In communicating hydrocephalus, the lumbar access is substituted by two 27G needles connected to the shunt antechamber or, intraoperatively, to the ventricular reservoir, providing a direct measure of ICP.

providing a direct measure of ICP. Although infusion studies are listed as part of the management of hydrocephalus by recent NPH guidelines, individualized CSF dynamics assessment is not yet common practice. Computerized CSF infusion studies provide a quantitative diagnosis of shunt malfunction, comparing the in vivo findings with the expected performance of the specific shunt model. Such tests can also be performed on outpatients, avoiding unnecessary admissions and significantly reducing the need for revisions.

Surgical technique and shunt valves

For ventricular shunts, the distal catheter is positioned in the peritoneum, right cardiac atrium or, less commonly, the pleura. For ventriculoperitoneal shunts, a high abdominal incision is made, and the distal catheter is tunnelled subcutaneously from the scalp to the peritoneal cavity using a long, hollow, metal rod (tunnelling device). For ventriculopleural catheters, a thoracic incision is made, and the distal catheter is tunnelled from the scalp to the pleural cavity. For ventriculoatrial shunt systems, the route to the caval system is established by a lateral, right-sided neck dissection and isolation of the external jugular vein, in which the distal catheter is advanced into the superior vena cava.

Lumbar shunts are indicated in communicating hydrocephalus and IIH. For lumbar–peritoneal shunts, the distal catheter is threaded subcutaneously through the tunnelling device from the lumbar incision to the peritoneal cavity. For lumbar–pleural catheters, a thoracic incision is made, and the distal catheter is tunnelled from the lumbar wound to the pleural cavity.

Shunt valves can be 'flow regulating' or 'pressure regulating'. Flow-regulating shunt valves maintain a constant CSF drainage flow over a wide range of CSF pressures (e.g. constant drainage of 0.3–0.5 ml min^{-1} – approximating physiological CSF production rate – for CSF pressures of 5–30 mmHg). Pressure-regulating shunt valves open when the pressure difference across the valve exceeds a predefined value. More recently, programmable shunt valves allow the opening pressure to be modified non-invasively. Programmable shunt valves are 'ball-on-spring' valves, which can be programmed by adjusting the tension of the spring with a magnetic rotor. The valves are programmed transcutaneously with a special programming tool, which is a purpose-designed strong external magnet.

Shunt systems may be accessorized with CSF reservoirs and/or 'gravitational' devices. Reservoirs are small silicone devices connected to the ventricular catheter proximal to the shunt valve. Reservoirs can be palpated under the skin and provide transcutaneous access to the CSF using hypodermic needles, allowing CSF sampling for microbiology and CSF pressure monitoring.

Overdrainage of CSF may cause disabling symptoms, including dizziness or visual disturbances, as the patient stands up. Gravitational devices are anti-siphoning devices that prevent overdrainage of CSF. They are a built-in feature in some of the most recent devices.

Anaesthetic management for shunt surgery

Pre-operative assessment includes the standard age-specific anaesthetic work-up and interview. Specific issues related to increased ICP, including decreased level of consciousness, increased risk of aspiration, dehydration and electrolyte impairment are discussed in detail elsewhere. Sedative pre-medication is best avoided.

Invasive blood pressure monitoring is usually not necessary. Induction may be undertaken using either intravenous agents or volatile agents. Rapid sequence induction can be indicated in patients with impaired consciousness or at risk of aspiration. Ketamine is best avoided for its detrimental effects on ICP.

Intubation should be undertaken using an armoured endotracheal tube as the patient positioning predisposes to kinking of standard tubes. The patient is positioned supine for ventricular shunts and in the lateral recumbent position for lumbar shunts. A warming air blanket is used to maintain normothermia. Anaesthesia is maintained with TIVA or a volatile agent, and ventilation is controlled to normocarbia.

Systemic antibiotics should be administered at induction to prevent shunt infection, regardless of the patient's age and the type of shunt valve used. Further antibiotic prophylaxis following the first 24 h is not indicated.

The advancement of the tunnelling device under the skin is the most stimulating part of surgery. Pre-emptive infiltration of the skin with local anaesthetic may be used to minimize autonomic responses to the manoeuvre. In the case of pleural shunts, positive-pressure ventilation is discontinued for a few seconds, allowing for some degree of pneumothorax in order to facilitate the advancement of the intrapleural catheter. After satisfactory positioning of the catheter, local anaesthetic may be injected into the pleural space for post-operative analgesia. Valsalva manoeuvres and end-expiratory positive pressure is delivered to favour adequate re-expansion of the lung before closure of the chest wall. Post-operative pain for ventriculoperitoneal and ventriculoatrial shunting procedures is mild to moderate, and satisfactory analgesia can usually be achieved with a combination of paracetamol and NSAIDs, with additional opiates 'as required' for breakthrough pain. In the case of pleural shunts, chest pain can be severe, and oral opiates are usually required in the first 48–72 h post-operatively.

Spinal anaesthesia, and sedation for MRI in patients with shunts

Patients with shunts frequently present for general anaesthesia for unrelated surgical conditions. The most common anaesthetic dilemmas in these patients relate to spinal anaesthesia and sedation for MRI.

Although there is no formal contraindication to performing a spinal anaesthetic in patients with CSF shunts, many anaesthetists refrain from using a spinal technique in this population, mostly for concerns related to the risk of shunt contamination and CNS infection. However, the risk of infection following a spinal anaesthetic is of theoretical concern, with literature showing that the incidence of meningitis after spinal anaesthetic or lumbar puncture is the same as in the general population. Concern that dural CSF leakage following a spinal anaesthetic in patients with a ventricular shunt could compromise shunt function is also unfounded. If reservoirs or shunt antechambers are not readily accessible for CSF sampling in febrile shunted patients, lumbar punctures are performed as a routine investigation by neurosurgeons in this patient group without any subsequent adverse effect on shunt performance.

The majority of published cases of the use of regional anaesthesia in patients carrying ventricular shunts have been reported in the obstetric literature for labour analgesia and Caesarean section anaesthesia. The use of spinal anaesthesia has also been reported to be safe and effective for elective abdominal and perineal surgery in paediatric case series. The use of strict aseptic technique and antibiotic prophylaxis in shunted patients seem to be adequate precautions to ensure uneventful spinal anaesthesia. Pre-operatively, signs of systemic infection should be excluded, and normal functioning of the ventriculoperitoneal shunt should be ascertained in consultation with a neurosurgeon.

As small magnets are used in all types of programmable shunt valves, the safety of MRI scanning is frequently raised for patients with ventriculoperitoneal shunts. The main risks for a patient with an implanted programmable shunt are related to the resetting of the valve, heating and dislodgement of the implant during

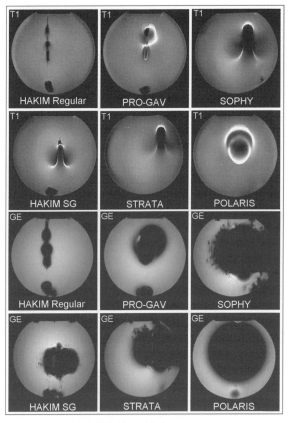

Fig. 17.3. Tesla MRI gradient echo (GE) and T1-weighted spin echo sequences (T1) revealing shunt valve-generated artefacts. The slice with the greatest artefact area is shown. Ghost diameter, 20 cm.

the imaging procedure. Moreover, shunt valves can generate considerable artefacts, thus invalidating the imaging procedure itself (Fig. 17.3). Imaging artefacts produced during MRI scans by programmable shunts vary and need to be checked on an individual basis, based on the shunt model and the diagnostic indication for imaging. Heating of the valves during MRI scanning is negligible for all commercially available models. Some models are resistant to inadvertent reprogramming during MRI, while others are promptly reset by exposure to weak magnetic fields. Checking the valve setting after MRI sequences should be considered a mandatory safety precaution in all patients carrying such shunts.

Anaesthesia for neuroendoscopic surgery

Aside from pituitary surgery, third ventriculostomy is the most widely performed neuroendoscopic procedure. Other conditions lend themselves to neuroendoscopic intervention. These include biopsy or tumour retrieval, removal or fenestration of cysts, shunt placement and endoscopic strip craniectomy. The advantages of undertaking such procedures endoscopically include accurate localization of intracranial lesions, especially when located in eloquent areas of the brain, access to regions not normally accessible by conventional surgery and reduction of surgical damage to healthy brain. There is also the potential to undertake tissue sampling prior to definitive treatment for a number of conditions. As there is minimal disruption to normal tissue, procedures tend to be shorter, with the possibility of early recovery and early hospital discharge.

Third ventriculostomy

Endoscopic neurosurgery was first performed by Lespinasse in 1910 when he used a cystoscope to coagulate the choroid plexus in a case of hydrocephalus. Third ventriculostomy is commonly used to treat non-communicating hydrocephalus and is particularly used in patients with aqueduct stenosis, although a range of other conditions can also be managed this way. Contraindications to the procedure include abnormal ventricular anatomy, intraventricular haemorrhage and meningitis.

Third ventriculostomy involves accessing the horn of the lateral ventricle to undertake fenestration of the floor of the third ventricle. This creates a communication between the ventricular system and the basal cisterns, creating a path for CSF reabsorption that bypasses the aqueduct of Sylvius. A number of methods are used to create the hole, including using the scope itself, blunt probes or lasers. Once the hole has been formed, a balloon catheter is passed through the hole and expanded to dilate the opening. Maintaining CSF flow through the opening is fundamental to maintaining patency and therefore ensuring success of the procedure.

Procedure-specific complications include damage to the wall of the third ventricle (hypothalamus), which may occur if the procedure is undertaken in patients with smaller ventricles. A number of other critical structures are located in the vicinity of the ventriculostomy, most notably the basilar artery, as well as midbrain structures. Cranial nerve palsies, SIADH, altered memory status and confusion have all been described. Venous bleeding is usually controlled with simple irrigation. Intraventricular clots may cause problems with

CSF flow, necessitating further endoscopic diversion procedures. The procedure itself requires the use of irrigation fluid, which in turn may cause acute rises in ICP. In small children in particular, the volumes of irrigation fluid used can also result in hypothermia unless adequately warmed. A range of arrhythmias has been described during these procedures including bradycardias and cardiac arrest. When successful, the need for an artificial shunt is eliminated, the success rate comparing favourably with that for shunts in children.

Anaesthetic considerations

The considerations for anaesthesia for third ventriculostomy and other neuroendoscopic procedures are similar to those for any patient with raised ICP. The procedure itself is undertaken in the supine, head-up position. Standard monitoring and anaesthesia are used. Invasive monitoring is not normally indicated. Occasionally, the head may be fixed in a frame. Intraoperative arrhythmias and bradycardia in particular are common. This may respond to repositioning of the endoscope or removal of irrigation fluid but does also occasionally require pharmacological treatment. Post-operative analgesic requirements are mild to moderate, and opiates are rarely required beyond the recovery room.

Stereotactic neurosurgery and functional neurosurgery

The word 'stereotactic' is a mongrel word from the Greek *stereo* meaning 'three-dimensional' and the Latin *tactus* meaning 'to touch'. Neurosurgical stereotactic techniques comprise methods for locating surgical targets within the brain relative to an external frame of reference, therefore assisting accurate navigation to a region without direct visualization. Its history can be traced back to animal studies by Sir Victor Horsley and Robert Clarke in the early 1900s. Modern stereotactic neurosurgery was pioneered by Lars Leksell, who invented a navigation apparatus suitable for clinical use, which is still in use today.

Frame-based versus frameless stereotactic navigation

Navigation to any surgical area of interest requires the establishment of an external reference system from which target location can be deduced by subsequent imaging. The technique can be broadly classified into frame-based and frameless methods. The frame-based technique utilizes a rigid stereotactic frame firmly attached to the patient's skull to establish such an external reference. The frame is held in place by pins that penetrate the outer layer of the skull. With the frame in situ, the patient's head is imaged with either MRI or CT. Based on the radiological data, the coordinates of the area of interest and the most appropriate surgical approach can be planned.

Frameless stereotaxy is a recent technique aiming to reduce trauma and to improve surgical access to the patient. Special markers (fiducials) are pasted onto the patient's scalp before imaging. In the subsequent surgical procedure, the patient's head (together with the fiducials) is secured to the operating table with a neuronavigation reference attachment. Using a special probe or pointer, the fiducials on the patient's head are cross-referenced with those on the MR images, which will be used to direct the procedure and provide real-time interaction with MRI.

The utilization of stereotaxy is expanding and the technique is invaluable in procedures such as biopsies of deep-seated targets, treatment of functional disease by target lesioning or stimulation, and delivery of radiation in tumours or vascular malformations.

Anaesthetic implications for stereotactic surgery

Application of the rigid head frame for surgery imaging is often well tolerated by patients using local anaesthesia, with or without sedation. The choice of whether or not this is done under general anaesthesia is often dictated by the invasiveness of the subsequent surgical intervention, the relationship of the operative site to critical structures or brain regions, and the degree and type of intraoperative neuromonitoring, specifically in deep brain stimulation procedures. In addition, there are a number of specific anaesthetic issues warranting special attention when deciding on the technique to be used.

A significant portion of the head frame is positioned over the nose and mouth and close to the patient's shoulders. This can hinder access to the patient's airway. For this reason, instruments that are required to release the frame should be readily available for as long as the head frame is in situ. Continuous observation of airway adequacy is crucial. If general anaesthesia is necessary for the subsequent surgical intervention, endotracheal intubation is best performed before the frame is applied.

Great care is given to patient positioning. The back portion of the frame can be close to the patient's shoulder and decrease mobility of the head and neck. Poor head and back position can result in neuropraxia and local trauma, especially if the patient is under sedation or general anaesthesia and unable to notify any discomfort.

Deep brain stimulation and anaesthesia

The evolution of deep brain stimulation (DBS) can be traced back to the initial use of intraoperative electrical stimulation for target exploration prior to lesioning in patients with movement disorders, particularly but not exclusively in Parkinson's disease. Deep brain stimulation provides advantages over the traditional ablative procedures such as thalamotomy and pallidotomy as it is non-destructive, reversible and adjustable.

Thalamic stimulation was first developed for tremor control. Subsequently, ventralis intermedius nucleus (Vim), subthalamic nucleus (STN) and internal globus palludus (GPi) stimulation were also investigated. The effect of stimulation on various nuclei differs. Ventralis intermedius nucleus stimulation provides good tremor relief in Parkinson's disease but little improvement of other symptoms such as akinesia, rigidity, bradykinesia and drug-induced dyskinesia. Stimulation of the GPi and in particular STN, on the other hand, can relieve most cardinal motor features of Parkinson's disease, including rigidity, tremor, bradykinesia, gait disturbances and motor fluctuations, and levodopa-induced dyskinesia in advanced Parkinson's disease. Currently, the STN is the preferred target in this disease. Following its success in Parkinson's disease, the indications and applications for DBS have extended into other disorders such as essential tremor, dystonia, epilepsy, chronic pain and psychiatric disorders. The exact mechanism of action of the success of neurostimulation, however, remains unclear.

Surgical technique

The DBS hardware commonly employed has four main components:

1. Multicontact intracranial quadripolar electrodes designed to be surgically inserted into the deep brain unilaterally or bilaterally via a burr hole.
2. A plastic ring and cap seated onto the burr hole to fix the electrodes.
3. A single- or dual-channel internal pulse generator (IPG) with battery unit.
4. An extension cable tunnelled subcutaneously from the cranial area to the chest or abdomen, connecting the DBS electrode(s) to the IPG.

The installation of the whole system is a two-stages process: the insertion of electrode(s) into the target area(s) of the brain, followed by internalization of extension cable and implantation of the IPG. Successful outcome relies on accurate insertion of electrodes. Frequently, this is achieved using a combination of methods including:

1. *Stereotactic, frame-based imaging to identify the target nuclei and establish stereotactic coordinates.* A frame-based stereotactic technique is used. The frame is usually applied under local anaesthesia, except for uncooperative patients or those with severe dystonia. With the stereotactic frame in place, MRI is performed to identify target nuclei and allow surgical planning to establish external coordinates for electrode insertion. In subjects with contraindication to MRI assessment, CT can also be used. The use of frameless stereotaxis in place of the frame-based technique has also been reported with the potential to provide better patient tolerability and ease of surgical planning. However, experience with a frameless stereotactic approach remains limited, mostly due to concerns regarding the accuracy of the method.

2. *Electrophysiological guidance with the use of microelectrode recording.* Due to brain shift during patient positioning and loss of CSF through the burr hole, and because of the intrinsic inaccuracies of current frame-guided navigation techniques, stereotactic navigation is not flawless. To further fine tune the location of the electrode, many centres utilize an electrophysiological mapping technique known as microelectrode recording (MER). A microelectrode is passed along the calculated trajectory to 10–15 mm above the target, then slowly advanced in 50 to 100 μm increments while its tip records and amplifies neuronal discharges along its path. Specific brain structures can be identified based on their unique patterns of firing. This allows feedback of the actual trajectory and fine adjustments of position before inserting the final electrode.

3. *Macrostimulation testing on an awake patient to observe symptoms improvement and side effects of neurostimulation.* Finally, if the patient is awake, intraoperative macrostimulation through the deep brain electrode helps to confirm clinical improvement and assess side effects during neurostimulation. When the team is satisfied with the electrode location, it is secured and the burr hole can be closed off. A second electrode may be inserted in the contralateral side if bilateral deep brain stimulation is planned. The electrode insertion is routinely followed by radiological confirmation.

Internalization of electrodes and IPG implantation can be performed under general anaesthesia either immediately or as second-stage surgery. The electrode is connected to the external cable, which is tunnelled subcutaneously in the scalp and at the side of the neck to a pulse generator implanted in the chest or abdomen. Currently, there is no evidence favouring the best timing of this stage. The decision is dependent on the patient's condition, team preference and local hospital logistics. Oedema around freshly implanted electrodes leading to the so-called 'microlesion effect' may interfere with assessment of clinical symptoms post-operatively. For this reason, most centres do not initiate stimulation until 2–4 weeks following lead implantation.

Anaesthetic management

Pre-operative evaluation

The pre-operative preparation starts with careful patient selection, as this is a major determinant of successful outcome. The decision to operate should be based on an individualized risk-to-benefit assessment, balancing the risk of the procedure against the perceived improvement in quality of life. The level of patient disability, likelihood of improvement following DBS, risk factors for complications, general life expectancy and the patient's motivation should all be taken into account. This is best accomplished using a multidisciplinary approach addressing medical, neurological, anaesthetic, psychiatric and social issues by a team consisting of neurologists, neurosurgeons, anaesthetists, neuropsychologists and nurses.

Deep brain stimulation can be considered for Parkinson's disease when the patient develops moderate to severe motor fluctuation, medication-induced dyskinesia, refractory tremor or intolerance to medications. The disabling symptoms and their response to medications should be identified. Patients who do not improve significantly with levodopa are unlikely to improve with surgery. For patients with dystonia, DBS may benefit those with primary or secondary dystonia suffering from significant disability despite optimal medical management.

Patients are evaluated based on their general physical condition (in particular, cardiopulmonary comorbidities) and psychiatric and cognitive function. There is no specific age limit for DBS, but it is a factor affecting how the patient will cope with the surgical procedure and behave post-operatively. Older patients may have only modest motor improvement and have increased incidence of intraoperative delirium and cognitive dysfunction after STN stimulation.

The severity of the underlying conditions poses significant concerns to anaesthetists. Besides motor problems, patients with long-standing Parkinson's disease can have autonomic dysfunction, increased aspiration risk, sleep apnoea, impaired respiratory reserve and impaired cough due to respiratory muscle dysfunction. Many have significant physiological or psychological comorbidities that can be age- or disease-related. Patients with dementia may be unable to tolerate and cooperate with the awake procedures typically employed in DBS insertion and may have trouble accurately observing and communicating their symptoms after the procedure, complicating the post-operative titration of stimulation parameters and medication.

Medical conditions that can substantially increase the surgical risk, such as poorly controlled hypertension and coagulopathy, should be identified and optimized before surgery. Polypharmacy is frequent in patients with Parkinson's disease and there is a risk of perioperative drug interactions. Children with debilitating dystonia are often malnourished and hypovolaemic. Contractures can cause skeletal deformity. Developmental delay and communication difficulties are common.

Pre-operative assessment helps to determine the optimal mode of anaesthesia. If an awake technique is contemplated, the patient should be motivated and able, physically and cognitively, to remain attentive and cooperative while undergoing a stressful procedure and testing requiring several hours of immobilization. A history of claustrophobia, psychiatric disorder or previous sedation failure warrants special attention. Regardless of the original anaesthetic plan, meticulous airway assessment is imperative to assess the risk of airway compromise and to assist in formulating a plan should intervention be required at any stage.

Patients are usually admitted the evening before surgery. A standard pre-operative fasting regimen is implemented. Anti-parkinsonism medication is often withheld to render the patients in an 'off-drug' state for intraoperative neurological testing, but such abrupt withdrawal of medication may result in significant patient discomfort and side effects. Pre-medication should be used judiciously, as many agents can interfere with patients' cooperation and tremor interpretation.

Anaesthetic techniques

The anaesthetic priorities during deep brain electrode insertion are (i) to provide optimal surgical conditions and patient comfort during the procedure, (ii) to facilitate intraoperative monitoring and target localization and (iii) to rapidly diagnose and treat any complications. Various anaesthetic techniques have been described. These include local anaesthesia with or without conscious sedation on an awake patient and methods that involve general anaesthesia, either throughout the entire procedure or temporarily as in an asleep–awake–asleep technique. Currently, there is no consensus regarding which technique is superior, and most centres have developed their own practice to address their team preference, local hospital setting and each patient's individual needs. Certainly, general anaesthesia provides the highest degree of patient comfort and physiological control but may render many of the available intraoperative tests difficult or impossible. Teams who wish to perform MER and macrostimulation have to balance the conflicting interests of improving patient comfort through sedation and minimizing pharmacological interferences.

Awake technique

This technique is frequently employed. Clinical improvement and side effects of stimulation can readily be observed. This also avoids the emergence excitation and its associated haemodynamic fluctuations. Patients with less post-operative nausea and vomiting can also resume oral anti-parkinsonism medication earlier.

Intravenous access and monitoring is established first. Standard monitoring such as ECG, non-invasive arterial blood pressure and pulse and oxygen saturation can be challenging in the presence of a severe movement disorder. The degree of any additional monitoring is dictated by the patient's comorbidities. Capnography and respiratory rate monitoring are particularly helpful. Patients with labile blood pressure may benefit from invasive monitoring for enhanced titration of antihypertensive infusions. Positioning must be done patiently with frequent patient feedback to ensure comfort. Attention to thermal control improves tolerability. Patients should be encouraged to void before surgery and urinary catheterization is undesirable particularly in males, where a sheath catheter is a good alternative. Excessive fluid administration is discouraged to prevent bladder distension. Draping should allow access to the patient's face, arms and legs while maintaining a sterile surgical site. Attention to detail, good patient communication, patient reassurance and motivation are all necessary. Antibiotics are typically administered before incision. The scalp may be anaesthetized at sites of incision and pin attachments. A combined supraorbital and greater occipital nerve block is a good alternative.

To increase patient tolerability, some centres use intravenous sedation for the incisions and bony opening until electrophysiological mapping begins. Cerebral subcortical areas are extremely sensitive to γ-aminobutyric acid (GABA) receptor-mediated medications. The use of gabaminergic sedative medication, even in small doses, has been shown to affect the quality of MER. An ideal sedative agent should have no or at least a readily reversible effect on subcortical activity to allow MER and clinical testing. Benzodiazepines should be avoided as they can abolish MER and induce dyskinesia. Propofol has been used with success, although it is not yet clear to what extent propofol interferes with MER, and it is known to cause dyskinetic effects and abolish tremor. Although it is titratable with a rapid onset and offset, its pharmacokinetic behaviour in patients with Parkinson's disease may differ from that of the population from which the target-controlled infusion models were developed. When it is used as part of the asleep–awake–asleep technique, delayed awakening can be a problem after cessation and use of the bispectral index (BIS) to titrate the anaesthetic depth does not seem to offer any advantage regarding times to arousal, total propofol consumption and cardiopulmonary stability.

In a number of centres, dexmedetomidine is the sedative agent of choice. Dexmedetomidine reliably produces conscious sedation mediated through activation of α_2-adrenoreceptors in the locus coeruleus, a key modulator for arousal, sleep and anxiety. This, together with minimal respiratory depression, makes it an attractive agent to use in 'awake' functional neurosurgery. Low-dose infusion of this drug (0.3–$0.6\,\mu g$ $kg^{-1}\,h^{-1}$) provides sedation from which patients are easily arousable and cooperative with verbal stimulation, allowing sophisticated cognitive tests to be successfully carried out. It has also been shown to attenuate the haemodynamic and neuroendocrine responses to headpin insertion in patients undergoing craniotomy and to significantly reduce the concomitant use of antihypertensive medication. Even in the setting of a compromised cerebral circulation, there is, so far, no evidence of adverse effects on cerebral haemodynamics, and several animal studies have even suggested a neuroprotective effect. Dexmedetomidine does not ameliorate clinical signs of Parkinson's disease and it seems that, at least in low-dose infusion, anxiolysis can be achieved with no effect on MER.

The awake technique may initially seem deceptively simple, but it is important to realize that the procedure can impose significant stress to patients. In a retrospective questionnaire interview of patients who underwent DBS electrode insertion, almost all recalled physical pain and psychological suffering during the procedure. Besides sedation, various measures have been implemented to improve patient tolerance, including intrathecal hydromorphone to alleviate lower back pain, intraoperative physiotherapy, local massage and respiratory exercises.

General anaesthesia

Although conscious sedation has been used successfully in some children, general anaesthesia may be necessary in others and in adults who cannot tolerate the awake technique, either due to concurrent psychiatric problems, dystonia or severe anxiety with associated hypertension. The decision for general anaesthesia is best made before surgery after careful pre-operative assessment, as the presence of a stereotactic head frame can complicate airway management, and any unplanned conversion to general anaesthesia in the midst of the procedure carries significant risk. The airway should be secured before head frame insertion, as access to the airway is restricted afterwards.

Concerns developed over whether the procedure performed under general anaesthesia would render MER impossible, and whether the lack of intraoperative assessment would result in a higher risk of suboptimal electrode placement. Current evidence suggests that MER is possible under a light level of general anaesthesia with careful titration of desflurane and propofol. A study by Maltete on post-operative outcome in patients who underwent bilateral STN electrode placement found that residual motor disability and the intensity of stimulation appeared to be slightly higher in patients operated on under general anaesthesia with propofol, implying that STN stimulation was less precise in the absence of intraoperative clinical assessment. However, this result was not reproduced in other investigations. A cohort study also failed to demonstrate any definite influence of the type of anaesthesia on surgical outcome. Furthermore, continued advancement in neuroimaging is likely to bring about improvements in target localization under general anaesthesia. Recently, the placement of DBS electrodes under general anaesthesia using a skull-mounted aiming device under interventional MRI has been reported. The technique eliminates the use of the traditional stereotactic frame and possibly the need for any intraoperative recording or testing and may become a future alternative method in patients who are unable to tolerate awake surgery.

Regardless of the anaesthetic technique employed, vigilance is necessary, as complications do occasionally occur. Monitoring in the recovery area should include frequent assessment of neurological status, good blood pressure control, attention to respiratory status and prompt treatment of any pain or nausea. If anti-parkinsonism medications have been withheld, they should be resumed as soon as possible to avoid motor fluctuations and deterioration in neurological and respiratory function.

Intraoperative anaesthetic-related complications

There is only limited data on the incidence of intraoperative anaesthetic complications during DBS. Overall, intraoperative complications are reported to occur in 5–16% of patients.

Hypertension is a common intraoperative problem, usually related to poor pre-operative control, patient distress or anxiety during the procedure. If necessary, α- or β-blockers or calcium-channel antagonists may be used. A venous air embolism can occur at any time during the burr hole procedure both in the supine and in the semi-sitting position.

Potential loss of airway is an important consideration with the awake technique, especially if sedation is used. The stereotactic head frame makes airway access difficult. A gradual shift of the body with neck flexion often occurs during surgery and may slowly compromise the airway. Oversedation can lead to both

Table 17.2 Summary of devices that may potentially interfere with a neurostimulator

Device	Potential interactions	Precaution(s)
ECG	Deep brain stimulation (DBS) may directly produce ECG artefacts Severe tremor after DBS deactivation can lead to ECG artefacts	Bipolar stimulation of neurostimulator may minimize ECG artefacts
Short-wave diathermy	Induces heating of DBS electrodes leading to brain damage	Use of short-wave diathermy is contraindicated
Phaecoemulsification	No interference reported	
Electrocautery	Potential thermal injury to brain Reprogramming and damage of DBS	Switching off pulse generator may decrease damage to neurostimulator Use of battery-operated heat-generating pulse generator Use the lowest diathermy energy in short irregular pulses Re-interrogate DBS system after surgery
Pacemakers	Cross-interference between the two devices	Bipolar DBS and bipolar pacemaker stimulation can decrease interference Interrogation of the two devices before and after surgery
External defibrillator and internal cardioverter–defibrillator (ICD)	Tissue heating around the brain target Reprogramming and damaging of DBS	Position external defibrillator paddle as far away from neurostimulator as possible, perpendicular to the lead system Bipolar DBS + ICD electrodes can minimize interference Interrogation of DBS + ICD device after defibrillation
Peripheral nerve stimulator	No interference reported	
Electroconvulsive therapy (ECT)	No interference reported	Place ECT electrodes away from DBS hardware
MRI	Electrode heating leading to brain damage DBS reprogramming and damage MRI image artefacts	Follow safety MRI guidelines Limit MRI exposure

obstructive and central apnoea and further aggravate this situation. It is important to note that, while dexmedetomidine is known to cause minimal respiratory depression in healthy volunteers and patients without respiratory disease, it can still produce upper airway obstruction. Prompt laryngeal mask airway insertion and even head frame disengagement can be life-saving during an airway crisis.

Seizure is the most common neurological complication and patients with multiple sclerosis undergoing DBS may be at particularly high risk. Most periprocedural seizures occur during test stimulation and are often self-limiting and focal in nature. However, generalized tonic clonic seizures do occasionally occur, and hence all indwelling catheters should be secured to prevent inadvertent dislodgement, and anticonvulsants should always be readily available. Post-ictal airway patency must be ensured.

Haemorrhage, although rare, can be devastating. The only consistent factor associated with the occurrence of haematoma is hypertension. The number of MER penetrations is, at most, weakly correlated with the occurrence of haematoma in the absence of hypertension.

Other changes in neurological status such as confusion, speech deficit or limb weakness can occur both during and after the procedure. The aetiology ranges from patient fatigue, medication withdrawal, seizures and intracranial bleeding to pneumoencephalus and can be difficult to determine in the midst of the procedure. Akinetic crisis due to acute drug withdrawal has been reported.

There is little information on the management of patients with existing deep brain stimulators who present for unrelated surgeries. The potential exists that the neurostimulator may interfere with other monitoring and therapeutic equipment with possible severe consequences. Table 17.2 summarizes the current knowledge on possible interference.

Further reading

Abuabara, A. (2007). Cerebrospinal fluid rhinorrhoea: diagnosis and management. *Med Oral Pathol Oral Cir Bucal* **12**, E397–400.

Ali, Z., Prabhakar, H., Bithal, P. K. and Dash, H. H. (2009). Bispectral index-guided administration of anesthesia for transsphenoidal resection of pituitary tumors: a comparison of 3 anesthetic techniques. *J Neurosurg Anesthesiol* **21**, 10–15.

Arita, K., Tominaga, A., Sugiyama, K. *et al.* (2006). Natural course of incidentally found nonfunctioning pituitary adenoma, with special reference to pituitary apoplexy during follow-up examination. *J Neurosurg* **104**, 884–91.

Baru, J. S., Bloom, D. A., Muraszko, K. and Koop, C. E. (2001). John Holter's shunt. *J Am Coll Surg* **192**, 79–85.

Bauchet, L., Rigau, V., Mathieu-Daude, H. *et al.* (2009). Clinical epidemiology for childhood primary central nervous system tumors. *J Neurooncol* **92**, 87–98.

Beric, A., Kelly, P. J., Rezai, A. *et al.* (2001). Complications of deep brain stimulation surgery. *Stereotact Funct Neurosurg* **77**, 73–8.

Blomstedt, P. and Hariz, M. I. (2010). Deep brain stimulation for movement disorders before DBS for movement disorders. *Parkinsonism Relat Disord* **16**, 429–33.

Burton, C. M. and Nemergut, E. C. (2006). Anesthetic and critical care management of patients undergoing pituitary surgery. *Front Horm Res* **34**, 236–55.

Chanson, P. and Salenave, S. (2008). Acromegaly. *Orphanet J Rare Dis* **3**, 17.

Chevrier, E., Fraix, V., Krack, P. *et al.* (2006). Is there a role for physiotherapy during deep brain stimulation surgery in patients with Parkinson's disease? *Eur J Neurol* **13**, 496–8.

Czosnyka, Z. H., Czosnyka, M. and Pickard, J. D. (2002). Shunt testing in-vivo: a method based on the data from the UK shunt evaluation laboratory. *Acta Neurochir Suppl* **81**, 27–30.

Deflandre, E., Bonhomme, V. and Hans, P. (2008). Delta down compared with delta pulse pressure as an indicator of volaemia during intracranial surgery. *Br J Anaesth* **100**, 245–50.

Eger, E. I. II, Lampe, G. H. and Wauk, L. Z. *et al.* (1990). Clinical pharmacology of nitrous oxide: an argument for its continued use. *Anesth Analg* **71**, 575–85.

Ezzat, S., Asa, S. L., Couldwell, W. T. *et al.* (2004). The prevalence of pituitary adenomas: a systematic review. *Cancer* **101**, 613–9.

Fukushima, T. and Maroon, J. C. (1998). Repair of carotid artery perforations during transsphenoidal surgery. *Surg Neurol* **50**, 174–7.

Greitz, D. (2007). Paradigm shift in hydrocephalus research in legacy of Dandy's pioneering work: rationale for third ventriculostomy in communicating hydrocephalus. *Childs Nerv Syst* **23**, 487–9.

Gross, R. E., Krack, P., Rodriguez-Oroz, M. C., Rezai, A. R. and Benabid, A. L. (2006). Electrophysiological mapping for the implantation of deep brain stimulators for Parkinson's disease and tremor. *Mov Disord* **21** (Suppl. 14), S259–83.

Hall, W. A., Luciano, M. G., Doppman, J. L., Patronas, N. J. and Oldfield, E. H. (1994). Pituitary magnetic resonance imaging in normal human volunteers: occult adenomas in the general population. *Ann Intern Med* **120**, 817–20.

Hensen, J., Henig, A., Fahlbusch, R. *et al.* (1999). Prevalence, predictors and patterns of post-operative polyuria and hyponatraemia in the immediate course after transsphenoidal surgery for pituitary adenomas. *Clin Endocrinol* **50**, 431–9.

Holdaway, I. M. and Rajasoorya, C. (1999). Epidemiology of acromegaly. *Pituitary* **2**, 29–41.

Jane, J. A. Jr and Laws, E. R. Jr (2001). The surgical management of pituitary adenomas in a series of 3,093 patients. *J Am Coll Surg* **193**, 651–9.

Johnson, J. O., Jimenez, D. F. and Tobias, J. D. (2002). Anaesthetic care during minimally invasive neurosurgical procedures in infants and children. *Paediatric Anaesthesia* **12**, 478–88.

Johnson, M. D., Miocinovic, S., McIntyre, C. C. and Vitek, J. L. (2008). Mechanisms and targets of deep brain stimulation in movement disorders. *Neurotherapeutics* **5**, 294–308.

Johnson, R. D., Qadri, S. R., Joint, C. *et al.* (2010). Perioperative seizures following deep brain stimulation in patients with multiple sclerosis. *Br J Neurosurg* **24**, 289–90.

Kachko, L., Platis, C. M., Livni, G. *et al.* (2006). Spinal anesthesia in infants with ventriculoperitoneal shunt:

report of five cases and review of literature. *Paediatr Anaesth* **16**, 578–83.

Kamenicky, P., Viengchareun, S., Blanchard, A. *et al.* (2008). Epithelial sodium channel is a key mediator of growth hormone-induced sodium retention in acromegaly. *Endocrinology* **149**, 3294–305.

Keegan, M. T., Atkinson, J. L., Kasperbauer, J. L. and Lanier, W. L. (2000). Exaggerated hemodynamic responses to nasal injection and awakening from anesthesia in a Cushingoid patient having transsphenoidal hypophysectomy. *J Neurosurg Anesthesiol* **12**, 225–9.

Kelly, D. F. (2007). Transsphenoidal surgery for Cushing's disease: a review of success rates, remission predictors, management of failed surgery, and Nelson's Syndrome. *Neurosurg Focus* **23**, E5.

Kenney, C., Simpson, R., Hunter, C. *et al.* (2007). Short-term and long-term safety of deep brain stimulation in the treatment of movement disorders. *J Neurosurg* **106**, 621–5.

Kern, E. B., Pearson, B. W., McDonald, T. J. and Laws, E. R. Jr (1979). The transseptal approach to lesions of the pituitary and parasellar regions. *Laryngoscope* **89** (Suppl. 15), 1–34.

Krauss, J. K., Akeyson, E. W., Giam, P. and Jankovic, J. (1996). Propofol-induced dyskinesias in Parkinson's disease. *Anesth Analg* **83**, 420–22.

Larson, P. S. (2008). Deep brain stimulation for psychiatric disorders. *Neurotherapeutics* **5**, 50–8.

Lavinio, A., Czosnyka, Z. and Czosnyka, M. (2008). Cerebrospinal fluid dynamics: disturbances and diagnostics. *Eur J Anaesthesiol Suppl* **42**, 137–41.

Lavinio, A., Harding, S., Van Der Boogaard, F. *et al.* (2008). Magnetic field interactions in adjustable hydrocephalus shunts. *J Neurosurg Pediatr* **2**, 222–8.

Law, J. A. (2008). Relying on just a few predictors of easy airway management may bite back! *Anesth Analg* **106**, 668; author reply 9.

Lefaucheur, J. P., Gurruchaga, J. M., Pollin, B. *et al.* (2008). Outcome of bilateral subthalamic nucleus stimulation in the treatment of Parkinson's disease: correlation with intra-operative multi-unit recordings but not with the type of anaesthesia. *Eur Neurol* **60**, 186–99.

Maltete, D., Navarro, S., Welter, M. L. *et al.* (2004). Subthalamic stimulation in Parkinson disease: with or without anesthesia? *Arch Neurol* **61**, 390–2.

Mann, J. M., Foote, K. D., Garvan, C. W. *et al.* (2009). Brain penetration effects of microelectrodes and DBS leads in STN or GPi. *J Neurol Neurosurg Psychiatry* **80**, 794–7.

Minniti, G., Esposito, V., Amichetti, M. and Maurizi Enrici, R. (2009). The role of fractionated radiotherapy and radiosurgery in the management of patients with craniopharyngioma. *Neurosurg Rev* **32**, 125–32.

Moro, E., Lozano, A. M., Pollak, P. *et al.* (2010). Long-term results of a multicenter study on subthalamic and pallidal stimulation in Parkinson's disease. *Mov Disord* **25**, 578–86.

Nemergut, E. C. and Zuo, Z. (2006). Airway management in patients with pituitary disease: a review of 746 patients. *J Neurosurg Anesthesiol* **18**, 73–7.

Nemergut, E. C., Dumont, A. S., Barry, U. T. and Laws, E. R. (2005). Perioperative management of patients undergoing transsphenoidal pituitary surgery. *Anesth Analg* **101**, 1170–81.

Nomikos, P., Buchfelder, M. and Fahlbusch, R. (2005). The outcome of surgery in 668 patients with acromegaly using current criteria of biochemical 'cure'. *Eur J Endocrinol* **152**, 379–87.

Osamura, R. Y., Kajiya, H., Takei, M. *et al.* (2008). Pathology of the human pituitary adenomas. *Histochem Cell Biol* **130**, 495–507.

Ostrem, J. L. and Starr, P. A. (2008). Treatment of dystonia with deep brain stimulation. *Neurotherapeutics* **5**, 320–30.

Poon, C. C. and Irwin, M. G. (2009). Anaesthesia for deep brain stimulation and in patients with implanted neurostimulator devices. *Br J Anaesth* **103**, 152–65.

Ratilal, B., Costa, J. and Sampaio, C. (2008). Antibiotic prophylaxis for surgical introduction of intracranial ventricular shunts: a systematic review. *J Neurosurg Pediatr* **1**, 48–56.

Richards, H. K., Seeley, H. M. and Pickard, J. D. (2005). IIIrd ventriculostomy: data from the UK Shunt Registry. *Cerebrospinal Fluid Res* **2** (Suppl. 1), S52.

Ritchie, C. M., Sheridan, B., Fraser, R. *et al.* (1990). Studies on the pathogenesis of hypertension in Cushing's disease and acromegaly. *Q J Med* **76**, 855–67.

Rozet, I. (2008). Anesthesia for functional neurosurgery: the role of dexmedetomidine. *Curr Opin Anaesthesiol* **21**, 537–43.

Saito, K., Kuwayama, A., Yamamoto, N. and Sugita, K. (1995). The transsphenoidal removal of nonfunctioning pituitary adenomas with suprasellar extensions: the open sella method and intentionally staged operation. *Neurosurgery* **36**, 668–75; discussion 75–6.

Schulz, U., Keh, D., Barner, C., Kaisers, U. and Boemke, W. (2007). Bispectral index monitoring does not improve anesthesia performance in patients with movement disorders undergoing deep brain stimulating electrode implantation. *Anesth Analg* **104**, 1481–7.

Schwalb, J. M. and Hamani, C. (2008). The history and future of deep brain stimulation. *Neurotherapeutics* **5**, 3–13.

Serhal, D., Weil, R. J. and Hamrahian, A. H. (2008). Evaluation and management of pituitary incidentalomas. *Cleve Clin J Med* **75**, 793–801.

Shah, S. and Har-El, G. (2001). Diabetes insipidus after pituitary surgery: incidence after traditional versus endoscopic transsphenoidal approaches. *Am J Rhinol* **15**, 377–9.

Shipley, J. E., Schteingart, D. E., Tandon, R. and Starkman, M. N. (1992). Sleep architecture and sleep apnea in patients with Cushing's disease. *Sleep* **15**, 514–18.

Silverberg, G. D., Mayo, M., Saul, T. *et al.* (2008). Continuous CSF drainage in AD: results of a double-blind, randomized, placebo-controlled study. *Neurology* **71**, 202–9.

Skau, M., Brennum, J., Gjerris, F. and Jensen, R. (2006). What is new about idiopathic intracranial hypertension? An updated review of mechanism and treatment. *Cephalalgia* **26**, 384–99.

Smielewski, P., Lavinio, A., Timofeev, I. *et al.* (2008). ICM+, a flexible platform for investigations of cerebrospinal dynamics in clinical practice. *Acta Neurochir Suppl* **102**, 145–51.

Trombetta, C., Deogaonkar, A., Deogaonkar, M. *et al.* (2010). Delayed awakening in dystonia patients undergoing deep brain stimulation surgery. *J Clin Neurosci* **17**, 865–8.

Vance, M. L. (2003). Perioperative management of patients undergoing pituitary surgery. *Endocrinol Metab Clin North Am* **32**, 355–65.

Vernooij, M. W., Ikram, M. A., Tanghe, H. L. *et al.* (2007). Incidental findings on brain MRI in the general population. *N Engl J Med* **357**, 1821–8.

Williams, A., Gill, S., Varma, T. *et al.* (2010). Deep brain stimulation plus best medical therapy versus best medical therapy alone for advanced Parkinson's disease (PD SURG trial): a randomised, open-label trial. *Lancet Neurol* **9**, 581–91.

Yamada, K., Goto, S., Kuratsu, J. *et al.* (2007). Stereotactic surgery for subthalamic nucleus stimulation under general anesthesia: a retrospective evaluation of Japanese patients with Parkinson's disease. *Parkinsonism Relat Disord* **13**, 101–7.

Young, M. L. and Hanson, C. W. III. (1993). An alternative to tracheostomy following transsphenoidal hypophysectomy in a patient with acromegaly and sleep apnea. *Anesth Analg* **76**, 446–9.

Chapter 18

Overview of neurointensive care

Martin Smith

Introduction

Critical care medicine has evolved rapidly over the last two decades, with therapeutic and technological advances leading to improved outcome in a wide variety of life-threatening conditions. This is particularly the case for neurological disorders where improved understanding of the pathophysiology of neurological injury, in association with advances in monitoring and imaging techniques, has led to the introduction of more effective and individualized treatment strategies that have translated into improved outcomes. In parallel, neurointensive care has developed as a subspecialty of intensive care medicine dedicated to the treatment of critically ill patients with primary and secondary neurological disease. This chapter will review the history, evolution and organization of neurointensive care units and emphasize the key role that neurointensive care teams play in delivering improved outcomes for patients.

History of neurointensive care

The origins of neurointensive care date back to the poliomyelitis epidemics of the 1940s and 1950s when specialized teams established the principles of prolonged mechanical ventilation and high-intensity nursing support in dedicated wards. In the 1970s and 1980s, advances in neurosurgery and neuroanaesthesia allowed more complex interventions that brought the need for close monitoring and management in the post-operative period. Areas of neurosurgical wards, staffed by neurosurgical teams, became the early neurosurgical intensive care units (ICUs). Thereafter, neurointensive care expanded to include the management of patients with a broader range of neurological disorders such as traumatic brain injury (TBI), subarachnoid haemorrhage (SAH), intracranial

haemorrhage, elevated intracranial pressure (ICP), neuromuscular respiratory failure, status epilepticus and the medical complications of brain injury. The management of critically ill patients with neurosurgical and neurological disease were thus combined into a single specialist unit where neurointensivists, neurologists, neurosurgeons and their teams provide comprehensive management for complex and life-threatening disorders of the central nervous system (CNS). More recently, neurointensive care has embraced the management of conditions, such as acute ischaemic stroke, that were not traditionally seen as part of its role. Its primary challenge now is the resuscitation and treatment of patients with massive traumatic and vascular brain injuries that were previously assumed to be unsalvageable.

Key to the success of neurointensive care is an appreciation that not only is the CNS, and particularly the injured brain, greatly influenced by systemic physiological perturbations but that brain injury itself can adversely affect non-neurological organ systems. Neurointensive care has therefore evolved from its original single-system focus on the CNS to a multisystem speciality providing all aspects of a patient's care.

Neuromonitoring

The monitoring of critically ill neurological patients has become increasingly complex. Besides the close monitoring and assessment of cardiac and respiratory functions common to all critically ill patients, modern neurointensive care utilizes a host of neurological monitoring techniques to identify or predict the occurrence of secondary insults and guide therapeutic interventions. The benefits of neuromonitoring can be summarized as follows:

Core Topics in Neuroanaesthesia and Neurointensive Care, eds. Basil F. Matta, David K. Menon and Martin Smith. Published by Cambridge University Press. © Cambridge University Press 2011.

1. Monitoring temporal changes in the pathophysiology of brain injury and its response to treatment.
2. Early detection of secondary adverse events.
3. Guiding individualized, patient-specific therapy.
4. Avoiding unnecessary, and potentially harmful, treatment interventions.

The role of the clinical examination in the assessment of neurological status should not be underestimated. The Glasgow Coma Scale (GCS) provides a standardized, internationally recognized method for evaluating a patient's global neurological status by recording their best eye opening, motor and verbal responses to physical and verbal stimuli (see Chapter 32). As the GCS is a global assessment of neurological function, it provides no information about focal deficits. Localizing signs such as pupil responses and limb weaknesses provide useful additional information and should be recorded alongside the GCS. The Medical Research Council (MRC) grading scale is widely used to assess motor response (see Chapter 15).

Although serial clinical assessment performed by an experienced nurse is the simplest and most effective neurological monitor, clinical evaluation has several limitations. It is unable to detect changes in patients who are receiving sedative drugs and provides a qualitative rather than quantitative assessment of neurological function. Various cerebral monitoring techniques have been developed in an attempt to overcome these disadvantages and are discussed elsewhere in this book.

Developments in multimodality monitoring have allowed a move away from rigid physiological target setting towards an individually tailored, patient-specific approach to management. Multimodal monitoring also allows cross-validation between different monitoring variables, improved artefact rejection and greater confidence in making treatment decisions. In addition, it gives clinicians confidence to withhold potentially dangerous therapy in those without evidence of brain ischaemia/hypoxia or metabolic disturbance. The wealth of data generated by multimodal monitoring provides a challenge in terms of data integration, analysis and accessibility, but software applications that provide clinically relevant information at the bedside have recently become available.

Variations in monitoring practice

Despite the widespread availability and relative simplicity of many neuromonitoring techniques, there is considerable variation in their placement and in the application of monitoring-guided therapeutic strategies. This is the case even for ICP monitoring, the indications for which are the subject of expert consensus guidance. In a 2002 study from the USA, ICP monitors were placed in only 58% of patients who fulfilled the established criteria for monitoring, but therapies to reduce raised ICP were routinely applied in patients who were not monitored. Recent audits suggest that around 75% of neurointensive care units in developed countries now use ICP monitoring after TBI, compared with 9–28% of non-specialist units that care for head-injured patients. Although a recent systematic review conducted by the Cochrane collaboration concluded that there is no evidence that ICP monitoring improves outcome in comatose brain-injured patients, there is a large body of clinical evidence supporting its use to detect expanding intracranial mass lesions, guide therapeutic interventions and assess prognosis after TBI. It is now widely accepted as a relatively low-risk, high-yield and value-for-money intervention in severe head injury and is being increasingly used in other conditions.

Principles of neurointensive care

Critically ill neurological patients require meticulous general intensive care support as well as interventions targeted to their neurological disorder. The overall goals of neurointensive care are to resuscitate and support the acutely ill patient, minimize secondary neurological injury, and prevent or treat systemic (non-neurological) complications.

Evolving practice

Many developments over the last decade have changed the way that acute disorders of the CNS are viewed and treated. For example, the intensive care management of brain injury has undergone extensive revision as evidence accumulates that long-standing and established practices are not as efficacious or innocuous as previously believed. Traditional therapies such as fluid restriction and hyperventilation have been called into question and are no longer recommended, and newer or reinvented therapies, such as therapeutic hypothermia and decompressive craniectomy, remain controversial. The sole goal of identifying and treating intracranial hypertension has been superseded by a focus on the prevention of secondary cerebral ischaemic insults using a multifaceted physiological neuroprotective

Table 18.1 Summary of intensive care management of patients with brain injury

Respiratory	PaO_2 >13 kPa and $PaCO_2$ 4.5–5.0 kPa
	PEEP (<15 cmH$_2$O) to maintain oxygenation
	Strategies to minimize risk of pneumonia
Cardiovascular	MAP >90 mmHg
	Normovolaemia
	Vasopressors/inotropes
ICP and CPP management (after TBI)	ICP <20 mmHg and CPP 50–70 mmHg
	Sedation/analgesia
	20–30° head-up tilt
	Volume expansion plus norepinephrine to maintain CPP
Treatment of intracranial hypertension	Osmotic therapy (mannitol or hypertonic saline)
	Moderate hyperventilation
	Moderate hypothermia
	Cerebrospinal fluid drainage
	Barbiturates
	Decompressive craniectomy
Miscellaneous	Normoglycaemia
	Pyrexia treatment
	Enteral nutrition
	Thromboembolic prophylaxis
	Seizure control

CPP, cerebral perfusion pressure; ICP, intracranial pressure; MAP, mean arterial pressure; PaCO$_2$, arterial partial pressure of carbon dioxide; PaO$_2$, arterial partial pressure of oxygen; PEEP, positive end-expiratory pressure.

strategy. This usually incorporates a systematic, step-wise approach to maintenance of adequate cerebral perfusion and oxygenation, and control of raised ICP. As there is considerable pathophysiological heterogeneity after brain injury, some commonly used interventions may be ineffective, unnecessary or even harmful in some patients at certain times. The importance of individualized therapy, guided by multimodal monitoring, cannot therefore be overemphasized. The general principles of the intensive care management of brain injury are shown in Table 18.1.

The scope of practice

As neurointensive care has evolved, its case mix has broadened and, in parallel, the severity of cases admitted to neurointensive care units has increased.

Traumatic brain injury

Consensus guidance for the management of TBI has been available for many years and the most comprehensive, from the Brain Trauma Foundation, has recently been revised. Because of the lack of class 1 data from randomized controlled trials, the majority of the recommendations are at the level of options based on class 2 or 3 data, i.e. from small prospective or retrospective studies, observational studies or case series. Despite the paucity of high-quality evidence, there is a consensus that rigorous and continuous monitoring and management of TBI on the neurointensive care unit is associated with improved outcome.

The intensive care management of TBI is complex and requires a coordinated approach. In addition to brain-targeted therapy, general intensive care principles, including optimization of cardiorespiratory variables, glycaemic control, management of pyrexia and early enteral nutrition, are of key importance. The details of the intensive care management of TBI are discussed in detail in Chapter 21.

Cerebral ischaemia is the dominant factor determining secondary brain injury, and recent studies characterizing its incidence and mechanisms have demonstrated that the ischaemic burden is correlated with outcome after TBI. Prevention and treatment of cerebral ischaemia using ICP- and cerebral perfusion pressure (CPP)-guided treatment strategies is a major focus of the intensive care management of TBI. However, recent evidence suggests that brain resuscitation based on control of ICP and CPP alone does not prevent cerebral ischaemia/hypoxia in all patients. Measurement of ICP and CPP in association with monitors of the *adequacy* of cerebral perfusion, such as brain tissue oxygenation and biochemistry, provides a more complete picture of the injured brain and its response to treatment. There is preliminary evidence to suggest that treatment targeted towards maintenance of adequate brain tissue oxygen tension, in addition to ICP and CPP, might be associated with improved outcome after TBI.

A study from the Trauma Audit and Research Network confirmed that 33% of 22,216 patients presenting with severe TBI in the UK between 1989 and 2003 were not treated in a neurosurgical centre at any stage in their management. This was associated with a 26% increase in mortality and a 2.15-fold increase (95% confidence interval (CI) 1.77–2.60) in the case-mix adjusted odds of death compared with treatment in a neurosurgical centre. Underprovision of specialized neurointensive care beds is the reason why many head-injured patients continue to be managed in non-neurosurgical units in many parts of the world. As a consequence, referral practices are dominated in many areas by the need for operative neurosurgical intervention at presentation so that those requiring urgent intracranial surgery are prioritized for transfer to a neurointensive care unit. However, many patients with severe TBI have evidence of raised ICP in the absence of surgical lesions, and suffer morbidity and mortality equal to those with such lesions. Furthermore, patients with no surgically remedial lesion often require complex therapeutic interventions to control ICP and CPP, and outcome is improved when these are delivered within the context of specialist neurointensive care. It is therefore illogical that these are the patients who are still most likely to be managed in non-neuroscience units. It can also never be certain that a patient with severe TBI will not require urgent neurosurgical intervention at some stage, and delay in providing such treatment is a major preventable cause of mortality and morbidity.

Subarachnoid haemorrhage

Patients with aneurysmal SAH require complex treatment and extended monitoring. Management is targeted at securing the ruptured aneurysm, optimizing cardiovascular variables, detecting and treating cerebral vasospasm and managing medical complications. These treatment strategies call for interdisciplinary collaboration between neurosurgeons, neuroradiologists, neurointensivists and specialist nurses, and the neurointensive care unit is the focal point of these combined efforts. Multidisciplinary clinical collaborations, in association with technological advances, have reduced the overall mortality rate after aneurysmal SAH from around 50% to 20% over the last two decades. The advent of less invasive interventions for securing a ruptured aneurysm has allowed effective treatment of sicker patients and, as a result, many more World Federation of Neurological Surgeons (WFNS) grade 4 and 5 SAH patients are being admitted to neurointensive care units. Although such patients have substantial comorbidities and are at increased risk of developing intracranial and systemic complications, there is accumulating evidence that aggressive cardiopulmonary and neurological resuscitation, in association with early aneurysm control and advanced monitoring and management in a neurointensive care unit, offers the best potential for achieving good outcomes.

Intracerebral haemorrhage

Intracerebral haemorrhage is the most devastating form of stroke, with high rates of mortality and morbidity. Aggressive treatment, including monitoring and management of cardiorespiratory variables and ICP, in addition to meticulous blood pressure, fluid balance and glycaemic control, improves outcome after intracranial haemorrhage. There is substantial evidence that management of patients in a specialist neurointensive care unit is also associated with improved outcomes. One study analysed data collected prospectively by Project Impact (a data collection tool developed by the Society of Critical Care Medicine) from 42 participating ICUs over a 3-year period and found that not being in a neurointensive care unit was associated with an increased hospital mortality rate (odds ratio 3.4) after acute intracranial haemorrhage. In another study, mortality and hospital discharge status were significantly improved following treatment of intracranial haemorrhage in a neurointensive care unit compared with a similar cohort of patients treated 2 years earlier in a general ICU in the same institution. In this study, patients treated in the neurointensive care unit also had shorter hospital stays and lower total costs of care than a national benchmark.

Ischaemic stroke

Early studies confirmed that patients cared for by dedicated stroke teams in stroke units have better outcomes, and integrated multidisciplinary services for stroke patients are now commonplace. More recent studies have demonstrated that input from a specialized neurointensive care team can bring additional outcome benefits in critically ill stroke patients. In a retrospective case note review of 400 patients with acute ischaemic stroke admitted to a neurointensive care unit over a 3-year period, the introduction of a neurointensive care multidisciplinary team was associated with decreased ICU and hospital lengths of stay and a significantly greater proportion of patients being discharged home rather than to a long-term care facility (47 vs. 36%, respectively).

Recent advances in stroke management include intra-arterial thrombolysis, neurointerventional techniques for mechanical clot extraction or lysis, and decompressive craniectomy for malignant middle cerebral artery infarction. In most comprehensive stroke centres, the neurointensive care unit has become the focal point for coordinating these urgent, high-intensity and complex interventions, and for managing intracranial and systemic complications.

Hypoxic brain injury

Although overall survival rates following cardiac arrest remain low, approximately one-third of patients admitted to an ICU after cardiac arrest survive to hospital discharge. However, there is considerable variation in post-cardiac arrest treatment and patient outcome between institutions, despite good evidence that targeted interventions applied after the return of spontaneous circulation significantly increase the chances of survival with good neurological outcome. The neurointensive care unit is the optimal location for the management of comatose cardiac arrest survivors because many of the interventions that increase the chances of a good neurological recovery are identical to those that are widely applied in brain-injured patients generally.

Primary neurological disease

Specialist neurointensive care units are also concerned with the management of primary neurological illness and its consequences. These include myasthenia gravis, Guillain–Barré syndrome, encephalopathies, CNS infections and status epilepticus. Management is directed towards specific treatments of the primary condition and also to the management of ensuing complications, such as profound neuromuscular weakness-related ventilatory failure, autonomic derangements and bulbar insufficiency. The management of these conditions is discussed in detail in Chapter 26. Many neurological patients remain dependent on intensive care support for very long periods of time, resulting in significant psychological demands on the patient, their carers and the neurointensive care unit multidisciplinary team.

Systemic complications

Injured brains cause impairment of systemic organs systems and, because non-neurological organ dysfunction and failure are independent contributors to morbidity and mortality after brain injury, they represent potentially modifiable risk factors. However, their management presents significant challenges because the optimum treatment for the failing systemic organ system can have potentially adverse effects on the injured brain and vice versa. These issues are discussed in detail in Chapter 19. Brain-injured patients cared for by specialist neurointensive care teams suffer fewer significant non-neurological complications compared with those managed in general ICUs.

Protocol-guided management

Protocol-guided treatment improves clinical outcome in all areas of medicine and is effective in reducing mortality and improving outcome after brain injury.

In a UK study published in 2002, the establishment of an evidence-based management protocol aimed at control of ICP and CPP after TBI resulted in a significant reduction in mortality compared with historic controls, from 59.6 to 40.4%. Furthermore, 66% of patients with raised ICP in the absence of a mass lesion, and 60% of those who required complex interventions to optimize ICP and CPP, had a favourable outcome. A US study that included all categories of head injury admitted to an ICU compared outcomes after the introduction of a standardized treatment protocol with two previous time periods – one before the availability of a neurointensive care unit and the other after the establishment of a basic neurointensive care unit without protocolized treatment strategies. There was a decrease in mortality from 40 to 27 to 2.8% in the three time periods, respectively, in association with an increase in the incidence of good functional outcome in survivors from 40 to 68 to 84%. In another US study, management in a level I centre was associated with better outcome after severe head injury than outcome in a level II centre, but it was significantly improved in both following the introduction of standardized treatment protocols.

Inevitably, the majority of studies examining the introduction of protocolized management strategies have used historic control groups, and these limit interpretation to some extent because of the unknown impact of the temporal differences in outcome that might have resulted from unrelated changes in technology, patient management, personnel and organization. Both practical and ethical issues are likely to prevent randomized controlled trials in this area, but a UK study published in 2004 attempted to deal with this issue. In this study, the introduction of an evidence-based management protocol significantly reduced ICU mortality from around 20 to 13.5% and overall hospital mortality from 24.5 to 20.8% in patients with severe TBI. These improvements occurred despite an increase in the median age and APACHE II score of the patient population after implementation of the protocol. Although historic controls were also used in this study, the mortality of patients with non-neurological disease admitted to the same (mixed) ICU did not change significantly over the same period. This strongly suggests, although it does not prove, that the benefits to the head-injured patients was related to the introduction of the protocol-driven management paradigm, rather than because of other changes.

Despite the available evidence and guidance, there is considerable variation in the implementation of established neurointensive care management strategies. Several studies have confirmed that units that aggressively monitor, and therefore presumably aggressively manage, ICP after severe head injury have better outcomes than those that do not. However, such studies do not confirm whether aggressive management per se improves outcome or whether the implementation of complex monitoring and management strategies are proxy markers for units that provide an integrated approach to management and higher standards of care overall. Although the application of protocol-guided monitoring and management after head injury increases resource usage, the improvements in outcome are likely to justify the increased cost of the treatment episode. For example, a study from the Centers for Disease Control and Prevention in the USA demonstrated that a significantly greater proportion (66 vs. 35%) of patients with severe TBI had a good outcome when their management was based on Brain Trauma Foundation guidelines. Extrapolation of these findings suggests that widespread implementation of guideline-based management would result in cost savings of US$250 million per year in the USA alone.

Notwithstanding the multiple evidence that aggressive ICP- and CPP-targeted treatment after head injury is beneficial, there is some suggestion that it is associated with increased levels of therapy intensity but not necessarily with improved outcome. A Dutch study published in 2005 compared 333 patients with severe TBI managed in two head-injury centres. One provided supportive intensive care (mean arterial pressure >90 mmHg and other therapeutic interventions directed by clinical observations and CT findings) without ICP monitoring, whereas the other provided protocol-driven intensive care, guided by ICP monitoring, to maintain ICP <20 mmHg and CPP >70 mmHg, according to Brain Trauma Foundation guidelines. Hospital mortality was similar in the two centres (34 vs. 33%) and the odds ratio for a more favourable outcome following ICP- and CPP-targeted therapy was 0.95 (95% CI 0.62–1.44). However, intensity of treatment,

assessed by the use of sedatives, vasoactive drugs, mannitol and barbiturates, was greater in the centre providing ICP-guided care, and the median time on mechanical ventilation was also significantly longer (12 days vs. 5 days). In this study, statistical uncertainty allowed for the possible benefit of ICP monitoring and management, but the authors calculated that this potential benefit would be rather small, with a number needed to treat of 16. In another European head-injury study published in 2008, patients who received ICP monitoring and management had a tendency to lower raw and risk-adjusted mortality rates than those who were not monitored, but this difference was not statistically significant. As in the Dutch study, the use of ICP monitoring and management was associated with increased treatment intensity, including higher vasopressor use, and did not show a significant association with neurological outcome at discharge from hospital.

Although the Dutch study has been criticized, it is of some interest that ICP-guided treatment in this study failed to control ICP within its target range (<20 mmHg) in more than one-quarter of patients. This raises the important question whether continuation of ICP- and CPP-guided treatment, with its associated side effects, is warranted if it is clearly not achieving its aim. Shifting the CPP target downwards is likely to be more beneficial than continuing to increase vasopressor support in patients without evidence of brain tissue ischaemia/hypoxia or metabolic disturbance. The concept of individualized CPP management, targeting a patient-specific CPP rather than a generic target, is gaining acceptance and is likely to reduce the incidence of treatment-related complications (see Chapter 19).

Benefits of neurointensive care units

A consensus is emerging that treatment in dedicated neurointensive care units is beneficial for patients with neurological disease generally but particularly for those with acute brain injury. Several studies have shown that neurointensive care units, staffed by dedicated neurointensivists, not only save lives and improve outcome but that they are also associated with better resource utilization compared with management of critically ill neurological patients in a general ICU. The potential benefits of neurointensive care are likely to be multifactorial and are summarized in Table 18.2. The fact that protocol-guided brain resuscitation within the context of excellent general critical care reduces mortality and

Table 18.2 Aspects of neurointensive care that contribute to improved outcome

Delivery of individualized, protocol-guided care
Multimodal brain monitoring-guided treatment strategies
Dedicated, specialist multidisciplinary team including specialist neuroscience critical care nurses and therapists
Supervision of management by dedicated neurointensivists
Rapid access to neurosurgical services
Increased expertise from higher caseload
Awareness of the interplay between the injured brain and systemic organ systems:
• Improved control of systemic physiology
• Greater understanding of the causes and treatment of non-neurological organ system dysfunction and failure

improves outcome after brain injury is clearly a major contributor to these benefits, but the advantages of specialized neurointensive care must surely extend beyond this single issue.

Caseload

Specialization attracts a greater caseload and this is likely to increase expertise. In an Austrian study of 1856 patients with severe TBI, those admitted to units treating more than 30 cases per year had lower mortality compared with those admitted to medium (10–30 cases per year) and small (<10 cases per year) centres. Compared with large units, the odds ratio for hospital mortality was 1.85 (95% CI 1.42–2.40) for patients managed in medium-sized units and 1.91 (95% CI 1.24–2.93) for those managed in small units. Analysis of data collected as part of the National Acute Brain Injury Study: Hypothermia also examined inter-centre differences in physiological and treatment variables during the intensive care management of head-injured patients included in the parent study. There were no significant differences in the incidence or severity of intracranial hypertension between units, but there were significant differences in the maintenance of arterial blood pressure and CPP targets, and in the use of vasopressors and mannitol. Specialist units admitting larger numbers of head-injured patients performed better. Two US studies also showed that mortality after SAH is significantly reduced in high-volume centres that provide access to specialized multidisciplinary

neurocritical care. Finally, among 4674 post-cardiac arrest patients admitted to ICUs in 39 hospitals in the USA, age- and severity of illness-adjusted institutional mortality ranged from 46 to 68%, with the lowest mortality rates occurring in ICUs treating a higher volume of post-cardiac arrest survivors.

The neurointensive care team

It is well recognized that the organization of ICU teams can directly affect patient outcome and resource utilization. In particular, staffing units with critical care physicians is associated with positive outcome benefits. In a systematic review of 26 observational studies of staffing models in general medical and surgical ICUs, high-intensity staffing (full-time presence of an intensivist or closed ICU) was associated with a reduced mortality in 94% of studies compared with low-intensity staffing (no full-time intensivist). There was also reduced hospital length of stay in all the studies that controlled for case mix. Similar findings have recently been confirmed in neurointensive care. In one study, the appointment of a full-time neurointensivist was associated with a 51% reduction in neurointensive care unit mortality, a 12% shorter hospital length of stay and 57% greater odds of being discharged to home or a rehabilitation unit rather than to a long-term care facility. The presence of a neurocritical care team is also an independent predictor of decreased hospital mortality and reduced costs of care.

It is difficult to pinpoint exactly why neurointensive care teams influence patient outcome, but a major contributor is likely to be that a dedicated team provides standardized diagnosis and management of the most common problems, and explicit goal setting related to the prevention of secondary brain insults by control of ICP, CPP, arterial blood pressure, blood glucose and temperature. Round-the-clock provision of dedicated and experienced neurointensive care teams not only facilitates the application of individualized treatment strategies but also ensures that such therapies are applied in a timely and consistent fashion. In a US study, a significantly higher proportion of specialist centres had treatment guidelines in place than non-specialist centres (78.4 vs. 53.7%) and adherence to such guidelines was also much higher in specialist units.

A crucial component of the neurocritical care team is its nursing staff. Neuroscience critical care nurses not only need the skills held by their general ICU counterparts but must also become proficient at the neurological examination to a much greater degree of sophistication and precision. Despite advances in neuromonitoring techniques, the neurocritical care nurse remains the most important neurological monitor and is able to detect subtle changes in neurological status and identify deterioration early. The bedside nurse is also in a unique position to make sure that everyone is aware of local management protocols and that they are followed. Acute rehabilitation plays a major role in securing improved long-term outcome after neurological illness, and intervention from neurophysiotherapists is likely to occur earlier and more reliably in a specialist than in a general unit.

Management of systemic physiological variables

Neurointensivists and their teams focus on the interplay between the brain and other organ systems and integrate all aspects of neurological and medical management into a single care plan. The neurocritical care team is familiar with the unique aspects of the primary disease processes and also with the effects of interventions on the injured brain. For example, blood pressure control is more aggressive in neurointensive care units compared with general units, resulting in a lower incidence of systemic (often iatrogenic) hypotension. Other physiological derangements, such as fever, hyperglycaemia, anaemia, sodium disturbances and delirium, have specific consequences in the context of acute brain injury and require different management strategies than in general intensive care. Neurointensive care clinicians have a clear understanding of the pathophysiological basis of the systemic complications of brain injury, and balance treatment strategies to minimize adverse effects on the underlying brain injury.

Therapeutic nihilism

Because of the availability of less invasive and more effective treatments, patients with severe brain injury who would previously have been considered unsalvageable are increasingly being offered treatment. There is considerable evidence that early aggressive intervention on the neurointensive care unit can result in excellent outcomes in substantial numbers of such patients, and recent attention has focused on the major role that therapeutic nihilism can have on determining outcome when severely brain-injured patients are cared for by non-specialist teams.

Despite maximal intervention, some patients will have a poor outcome, and it is essential that aggressive early treatment is linked to compassionate end-of-life care if a satisfactory degree of clinical improvement does not occur within an appropriate timescale. The confidence to withdraw treatment after a failed trial of early maximal intervention means that the usual justification for withholding treatment in the acute phase (i.e. survival with a devastating neurological injury) becomes irrelevant. This ensures that patients have access to care that might allow them to recover beyond initial expectations but also that decisions to withhold or withdraw support are made by those with sufficient expertise.

Training

Neurointensivists must be trained and experienced in general intensive care and, conversely, neurointensive care is a vital part of the training of general intensivists. In October 2005, neurointensive care gained formal recognition by the United Council of Neurological Subspecialties (UCNS) in the USA. Subsequently, this has led to accreditation of neurointensive care training programmes and certification of neurointensive care physicians in the USA. This has been a major milestone in the recognition of neurointensive care as a subspecialty of intensive care medicine and, although there is no similar recognition in other countries, there are clearly opportunities to extend UCNS neurointensive care training standards outside the USA. Importantly, expertise in neurointensive care involves procedural skills, proficiency with standard (systemic) monitoring and management, as well as specialized neuromonitoring techniques and interventions. Training programmes should therefore be split between neurological diseases and conditions, and medical diseases and conditions that commonly complicate acute neurological illness. Further information is available at http://www.ucns.org/go/subspecialty/neurocritical/certification.

Research

Although improved outcomes can be achieved by applying consistently what we have learned through research, there are limited data to guide most interventions on the neurointensive care unit. Over the years, numerous drugs with promising neuroprotective effects in the laboratory have been evaluated in large clinical studies and failed to offer outcome benefits to patients. In contrast, the effectiveness of many of the basic treatment algorithms and physiological interventions that are routinely applied during the critical care management of brain injury have not been evaluated in large studies. While there is always reluctance to subject long-standing clinical practices to rigorous investigation, there is no doubt that well-conducted studies are required to determine optimal strategies for many neurointensive care interventions.

There are many challenges to conducting research in critically ill neurological patients, particularly in the heterogeneous brain injury population. In order to be successful, future trials will need to be targeted to subgroups of patients with a specific pathology and an intermediate prognosis; the outcome of those who will inevitably fair well or badly is unlikely to be modified by the intervention being tested. In addition, blinding of treatment interventions, prevention of protocol violations and treatment cross-overs remain problematic. Clinical equipoise is also an issue, as the firmly held biases of some clinicians are likely to prevent randomization to reference or investigational therapy. For example, it is unlikely that experts in neurotrauma would support the notion that ICP monitoring is no better than no monitoring, and a randomized controlled trial of ICP-guided therapy, coordinated through the Traumatic Coma Data Bank, has previously been proposed but not funded. The ethical issues of such a study have in any case been questioned, and the prospect of embarking on a study of a technique that is considered by many experts to be indispensable is limited, not least because accepted treatments and decision-making in TBI are driven by protocols guided by ICP monitoring.

Despite these issues, neurointensivists and their teams are establishing excellent track records for the coordination of complex, multicentre randomized controlled studies. Ongoing studies in 2010 include those investigating brain tissue oxygenation-guided therapy and decompressive craniectomy after TBI, therapeutic hypothermia for control of ICP and the indications for surgery after intracranial haemorrhage. The UK-based Risk Adjustment in Neurocritical Care (RAIN) study is a prospective validation of risk prediction models for adult patients with acute TBI designed to evaluate the optimum location for management of TBI and the comparative costs of neurointensive care. It is anticipated that these and other studies will provide an evidence base for many of the interventions that are currently provided on an empirical basis during neurointensive care.

Summary

The management of critically ill neurological patients is complex and requires a coordinated and stepwise approach that includes clinical assessment, monitoring and individualized multifaceted management strategies to minimize secondary neurological injury. Improved understanding of the pathophysiology of the injured brain has allowed new diagnostic, prognostic and treatment modalities to be incorporated into routine management strategies. The complex treatment modalities applied in brain-injured patients call for interdisciplinary collaboration between neurointensivists, neurosurgeons, neurologists, specialist nurses and therapists, and the neurointensive care unit serves as the focal point for these efforts. Although there is substantial evidence that patients managed in specialist neurointensive care units have better outcomes than those managed in general units, it is important that we continue to strive to determine exactly why this is the case.

Further reading

Bleck, T. P. (2009). Historical aspects of critical care and the nervous system. *Crit Care Clin* **25**, 153–64.

Bulger, E. M., Nathens, A. B., Rivara, F. P. *et al.* (2002). Management of severe head injury: institutional variations in care and effect on outcome. *Crit Care Med* **30**, 1870–6.

Cremer, O. L., van Dijk, G. W., van Wensen, E. *et al.* (2005). Effect of intracranial pressure monitoring and targeted intensive care on functional outcome after severe head injury. *Crit Care Med* **33**, 2207–13.

Diringer, M. N. and Edwards, D. F. (2001). Admission to a neurologic/neurosurgical intensive care unit is associated with reduced mortality rate after intracerebral hemorrhage. *Crit Care Med* **29**, 635–40.

Elf, K., Nilsson, P. and Enblad, P. (2002). Outcome after traumatic brain injury improved by an organized secondary insult program and standardized neurointensive care. *Crit Care Med* **30**, 2129–34.

Fakhry, S. M., Trask, A. L., Waller, M. A. *et al.* (2004). Management of brain-injured patients by an evidence-based medicine protocol improves outcomes and decreases hospital charges. *J Trauma* **56**, 492–9.

Hemphill, J. C. III, Newman, J., Zhao, S. and Johnston, S. C. (2004). Hospital usage of early do-not-resuscitate orders and outcome after intracerebral hemorrhage. *Stroke* **35**, 1130–4.

Hesdorffer, D. C. and Ghajar, J. (2007). Marked improvement in adherence to traumatic brain injury guidelines in United States trauma centers. *J Trauma* **63**, 841–7.

Komotar, R. J., Schmidt, J. M., Starke, R. M. *et al.* (2009). Resuscitation and critical care of poor-grade subarachnoid hemorrhage. *Neurosurgery* **64**, 397–410.

Mauritz, W., Steltzer, H., Bauer, P., Dolanski-Aghamanoukjan, L. and Metnitz, P. (2008). Monitoring of intracranial pressure in patients with severe traumatic brain injury: an Austrian prospective multicenter study. *Intensive Care Med* **34**, 1208–15.

Mayer, S. A. (2006). Neurological intensive care: emergence of a new specialty. *Neurocrit Care* **5**, 82–4.

Menon, D. (2004). Neurocritical care: turf label, organizational construct, or clinical asset? *Curr Opin Crit Care* **10**, 91–3.

Mirski, M. A., Chang, C. W. and Cowan, R. (2001). Impact of a neuroscience intensive care unit on neurosurgical patient outcomes and cost of care: evidence-based support for an intensivist-directed specialty ICU model of care. *J Neurosurg Anesthesiol* **13**, 83–92.

Patel, H. C., Menon, D. K., Tebbs, S. *et al.* (2002). Specialist neurocritical care and outcome from head injury. *Intensive Care Med* **28**, 547–53.

Patel, H. C., Bouamra, O., Woodford, M. *et al.* (2005). Trends in head injury outcome from 1989 to 2003 and the effect of neurosurgical care: an observational study. *Lancet* **366**, 1538–44.

Pronovost, P. J., Angus, D. C., Dorman, T. *et al.* (2002). Physician staffing patterns and clinical outcomes in critically ill patients. *JAMA* **288**, 2151–62.

Provencio, J. J., Bleck, T. P. and Connors, A. F. Jr (2001). Critical care neurology. *Am J Respir Crit Care Med* **164**, 341–5.

Rincon, F. and Mayer, S. A. (2007). Neurocritical care: a distinct discipline? *Curr Opin Crit Care* **13**, 115–21.

Smith, M. (2004). Neurocritical care: has it come of age? *Br J Anaesth* **93**, 753–5.

Sorani, M. D., Hemphill, J. C. III, Morabito, D., Rosenthal, G. and Manley, G. T. (2007). New approaches to physiological informatics in neurocritical care. *Neurocrit Care* **7**, 45–52.

Stocchetti, N., Penny, K. I., Dearden, M. *et al.* (2001). Intensive care management of head-injured patients in Europe: a survey from the European brain injury consortium. *Intensive Care Med* **27**, 400–6.

Suarez, J. I. (2006). Outcome in neurocritical care: advances in monitoring and treatment and effect of a specialized neurocritical care team. *Crit Care Med* **34**, S232–8.

Suarez, J. I., Zaidat, O. O., Suri, M. F. *et al.* (2004). Length of stay and mortality in neurocritically ill patients: impact of a specialized neurocritical care team. *Crit Care Med* **32**, 2311–17.

Teig, M. and Smith, M. (2010). Where should patients with severe traumatic brain injury be managed? All patients should be managed in a neurocritical care unit. *J Neurosurg Anesthesiol* **22**, 357–9.

Varelas, P. N., Conti, M. M., Spanaki, M. V. *et al.* (2004). The impact of a neurointensivist-led team on a semiclosed neurosciences intensive care unit. *Crit Care Med* **32**, 2191–8.

Varelas, P. N., Eastwood, D., Yun, H. J. *et al.* (2006). Impact of a neurointensivist on outcomes in patients with head trauma treated in a neurosciences intensive care unit. *J Neurosurg* **104**, 713–19.

Chapter

19

Systemic complications of neurological disease

Magnus Teig and Martin Smith

Introduction

Non-neurological complications are common after brain injury and their importance as independent contributors to morbidity and mortality are well recognized. They arise from neurogenic causes, such as the catecholamine and neuroinflammatory response associated with brain injury, or as a complication of brain-directed therapies. Coincidental injuries may also adversely affect systemic organ systems in brain-trauma patients. Non-neurological complications represent potentially modifiable risk factors. This chapter will review the aetiology of systemic complications in critically ill neurological patients, identify options for their prevention and treatment, and consider their effects on outcome.

More than 80% of patients suffer dysfunction of at least one non-neurological organ system after traumatic brain injury (TBI), with multiple organ dysfunction occurring in 60%. Organ failure develops in around 35% of patients. Cardiovascular and respiratory dysfunction and failure occur most frequently, with renal and hepatic failure occurring rarely (Fig. 19.1). Non-neurological organ dysfunction is independently associated with

higher hospital mortality and worsened neurological outcome in survivors. Overall, the odds ratios for poor outcome and mortality are 1.53 and 1.63, respectively, for single non-neurological system failure after TBI, although acute lung injury (ALI) has been associated with a doubling of mortality in some studies.

Non-neurological complications are also common after aneurysmal subarachnoid haemorrhage (SAH) (Table 19.1), with dysfunction and failure of at least one systemic organ system occurring in 80 and 26% of patients, respectively. Around 23% of deaths after SAH are directly related to systemic complications, which is similar to the mortality associated with vasospasm (23%) and rebleeding (22%). Mortality increases from 31% for single system failure to >90% when two or more non-neurological organ systems fail. Multiple systemic complications are independent predictors of poor outcome after SAH (Table 19.2). Specific scoring systems of non-neurological organ dysfunction have superior predictive power after SAH compared with more general scoring systems, such as APACHE II. The Subarachnoid Haemorrhage Physiological Derangement Score (SAH-PDS) generates a score of 0–8 by

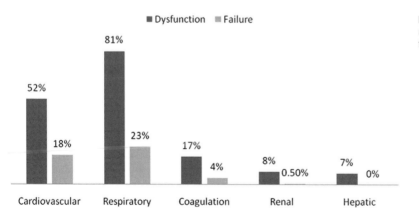

Fig. 19.1. The incidence of non-neurological organ dysfunction and failure after severe head injury.

Core Topics in Neuroanaesthesia and Neurointensive Care, eds. Basil F. Matta, David K. Menon and Martin Smith. Published by Cambridge University Press. © Cambridge University Press 2011.

Table 19.1 Non-neurological complications after subarachnoid haemorrhage

Complication	Total SAH population affected (%)	SAH patients with poor outcome (dead or severely disabled) affected (%)
Fever	54	75
Anaemia	36	48
Hyperglycaemia	30	48
Hypertension	27	35
Pneumonia	20	33
Hypotension	18	36
Hypernatraemia	18	34
Pulmonary oedema	15	25
Hyponatraemia	15	17

Table 19.2 Outcome effects of common systemic complications after subarachnoid haemorrhage

Complication	Odds ratio for poor outcome
Hypernatraemia (serum sodium >150 mmol l^{-1})	8.1
Hypotension (systolic blood pressure <100 mmHg treated with vasopressors)	7.1
Stunned myocardium syndrome (elevated cardiac troponin I and ECG changes)	6.2
Fever (>38.3°C)	4.4
Hyperglycaemia (blood glucose >11.0 mmol l^{-1})	4.2
Pulmonary oedema	4.2
Anaemia (haemoglobin concentration <9 mg dl^{-1})	2.5

Table 19.3. Subarachnoid Haemorrhage Physiological Derangement Score (SAH-PDS)

Physiological derangement	Score
Alveolar–arterial oxygen gradient >16.5 kPa	3
Serum bicarbonate < 20 mmol l^{-1}	2
Serum glucose > 10 mmol l^{-1}	2
Mean arterial blood pressure < 70 or >130 mmHg	1
Maximum score	**8**

The risk of poor outcome rises linearly from 18 to > 80% as the score rises from 0 to 8.

injury. These include catecholamine- and inflammatory-related effects, as well as endocrine and coagulation abnormalities. This section will outline the sequelae of brain injury that are related to endogenous catecholamine release, activation of adrenoceptors and neuroinflammation. Neuroendocrine and electrolyte disturbance, and other causes of non-neurological organ dysfunction, will be considered later in the chapter.

Brain injury-related catecholamine release is the primary driver of neurogenic systemic complications. Plasma concentrations of norepinephrine, epinephrine and dopamine can rise to 1200, 145 and 35 times the normal levels, respectively, after SAH and may remain high for up to 10 days. The catecholamine surge is driven by the central neuroendocrine axis, which massively increases sympathetic outflow and activates the adrenal glands. It has been suggested that the catecholamine surge is a 'protective' mechanism designed to maintain cerebral perfusion in the presence of intracranial hypertension. However, it also has an adverse impact on many organ systems, with particularly important effects on the cardiovascular and respiratory systems (Fig. 19.2).

classifying organ dysfunction in four variables measured in the first 24 h after presentation (Table 19.3). The risk of poor outcome rises linearly from 18 to >80% as the score rises from 0 to 8.

Neurogenic causes of systemic organ dysfunction

Several central nervous system (CNS)-driven changes contribute to systemic organ dysfunction after brain

Neurogenic stunned myocardium syndrome

Severe brain injury can be associated with a reversible cardiac myopathy that has been termed neurogenic stunned myocardium (NSM) syndrome. It is characterized by ECG changes, reversible left ventricular (LV) dysfunction and release of biomarkers of cardiac injury in the absence of a defect in coronary perfusion. Neurogenic stunned myocardium may cause minimal clinical effects

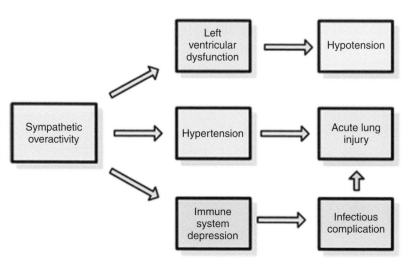

Fig. 19.2. Cardiorespiratory effects of the brain injury-related catecholamine surge (Reproduced from Lim and Smith, 2007, with permission).

but, in severe cases, can lead to cardiogenic shock and pulmonary oedema. The development of NSM can be rapid; animal studies confirm electromicroscopic evidence of cardiac myocyte damage within 4 h of SAH.

It was previously assumed that brain injury-related cardiac abnormalities were associated with coronary artery disease/spasm or myocardial ischaemia secondary to hypertension and tachycardia. However, normal angiographic findings in patients with significant ECG and echocardiography abnormalities indicated that this was not the case. Animal and human studies have subsequently confirmed that NSM is caused by excessive norepinephrine release from myocardial sympathetic nerve terminals, resulting in a physiological myocardial denervation in the presence of normal coronary perfusion. This causes a typical histological picture – myocardial contraction band necrosis – that is characterized by focal myocytolysis, myofibrillar degeneration, hypercontracted sarcomeres and irregular cross-band formation. In animal models of intracranial hypertension, the development of contraction band necrosis is not prevented by bilateral adrenalectomy, thus confirming that the mediator of cardiac injury is released locally in the heart. Although classically associated with SAH, the histological changes of NSM have also been demonstrated in patients with TBI, as well as other conditions such as near-drowning, fatal status asthmaticus and phaemochromocytoma. The pattern of the histological injury corresponds with ventricular regional wall motion abnormalties (RWMA) and is most dense in subendocardial regions of the heart, with relative apical sparing.

Systemic catecholamine effects

The catecholamine surge causes an initial hyperdynamic response characterized by hypertension and tachycardia. Intense systemic arterial vasoconstriction increases cardiac afterload, which results in increased myocardial workload and oxygen demand. Sympathetic over-stimulation within the myocardium leads to coronary vasoconstriction and, because there is no simultaneous increase in myocardial oxygen delivery, subendocardial ischaemia may ensue. This can lead to impaired ventricular function, hypotension and cardiogenic pulmonary oedema.

Although hypotension in isolated head injury is uncommon, neurogenic hypotension can occur and is associated with a higher mortality than haemorrhagic hypotension. The exact aetiology is unclear but is likely to be related to disruption of brainstem centres for haemodynamic control as it is particularly common in diffuse axonal injury.

Neurogenic pulmonary oedema

Neurogenic pulmonary oedema (NPO) is brain injury-related pulmonary oedema that develops in the absence of primary cardiac failure or significant volume overload. It is associated with TBI and SAH, as well as with other neurological problems including epileptic seizures, intracerebral haemorrhage (ICH), stroke or an abrupt rise in intracranial pressure (ICP) from any cause. Clinically, it is characterized by interstitial and alveolar oedema, decreased lung compliance, increased pulmonary shunt and profound hypoxaemia. Neurogenic pulmonary

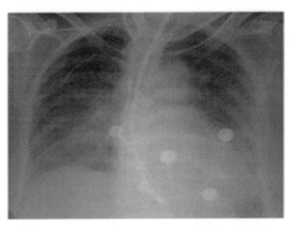

Fig. 19.3. Typical chest radiograph findings of neurogenic pulmonary oedema in a patient with subarachnoid haemorrhage showing bilateral pulmonary congestion. (Modified from Tanabe *et al.,* 2008, with permission.)

oedema is usually bilateral (Fig. 19.3), although unilateral oedema has been described. Onset is generally acute, occurring within seconds or minutes after brain injury, although NPO can develop anytime during the first 14 days after injury.

The mechanism of NPO is controversial but is likely to be related to neurogenic-mediated catecholamine release that leads to both hydrostatic and permeability oedema. Activation of α- and β-adrenoceptors causes systemic vasoconstriction and a fluid shift to the relatively lower-resistance pulmonary beds. Thus, the development of NPO requires the presence of a normal circulating volume. A massive, but not necessarily prolonged, pulmonary vasoconstriction results in increased pulmonary intravascular hydrostatic pressure and transudation of plasma fluid into the extravascular space. The increased extravascular lung water leads to reduced pulmonary compliance and an increase in the alveolar–arterial oxygen difference. The sympathetic surge may also damage pulmonary capillary endothelium because of direct injury from sustained increases in hydrostatic pressure as well as via central mechanisms, including release of brain cytokines and adhesion molecules that alter its barrier function. In some patients, this leads to the development of permeability oedema with high protein content oedema fluid. Ventricular dysfunction induced by NSM may also contribute to brain injury-associated pulmonary oedema and, because the two are frequently associated, the cardiac contribution to NPO is probably under-recognized.

Neurogenic ventilation–perfusion mismatch

Some brain-injured patients with moderate to severe hypoxaemia have no radiographic evidence of pulmonary oedema. Thus, it has been postulated that respiratory failure can occur because of a neurogenic ventilation–perfusion mismatch in the absences of interstitial or alveolar oedema. The aetiology of this abnormality is unknown but might include hypothalamic-mediated redistribution of pulmonary blood flow, an increase in dead space secondary to pulmonary microembolism and depletion of lung surfactant because of excessive sympathetic stimulation.

Neuroinflammation

Although the brain was previously believed to be immunologically inert, recent evidence confirms that brain injury, particularly TBI and SAH, activates an intense inflammatory response. A cascade of immunologically active mediators is released from the brain into the systemic circulation and this contributes to the development of systemic organ dysfunction.

Cells of the CNS are an abundant source of inflammatory mediators and brain injury induces the production and activation of complement, cytokines, adhesion molecules and other multifunctional peptides. Central nervous system expression of pro-inflammatory cytokines and complement components leads to recruitment of peripheral inflammatory cells (neutrophils and monocytes/macrophages) across a modified blood–brain barrier (BBB), which further enhances the established neuroinflammation. Cerebrospinal fluid interleukin-8 (IL-8) concentration is elevated to levels 300 times above baseline after severe TBI, a concentration similar to that seen in bacterial meningitis. The passage of central inflammatory mediators into the systemic circulation results in a systemic inflammatory response syndrome (SIRS) characterized by fever, neutrophilia, muscle breakdown, altered amino acid metabolism, production of hepatic acute-phase reactants and altered endothelial permeability. Systemic inflammatory response syndrome is an important mediator of systemic organ system dysfunction and failure after brain injury. The extent of neuronal damage, and therefore neurological outcome, is also worsened by the inflammatory response because of direct immunologically mediated damage to

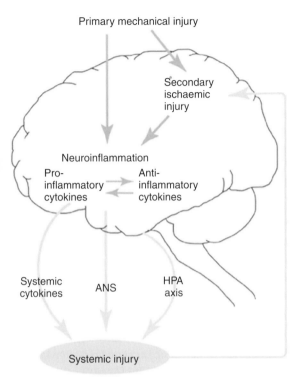

Fig. 19.4. The mechanism of systemic complications after traumatic brain injury. Primary mechanical injury and secondary ischaemic/reperfusion injury induces an acute neuroinflammatory reaction that can lead to systemic organ injury via three interrelated mechanisms: (i) overspill of intracranial cytokines into the systemic circulation; (ii) the autonomic nervous system (ANS); and (iii) the hypothalamic–pituitary–adrenal (HPA) axis. (Reproduced from Lim and Smith, *Anaesthesia*, **62**:474–482 with permission).

the injured brain and also because of reduced cerebral oxygenation and perfusion as a result of SIRS-related cardiorespiratory failure.

The complex interaction between the brain and immune system, including the systemic effects of neuroinflammation, is mediated via neuroendocrine pathways including the hypothalamic–pituitary–adrenal axis and autonomic nervous system (Fig. 19.4). The latter detects the presence of inflammatory stimuli and modulates cytokine production via an inflammatory reflex system. Under normal circumstances, the vagus nerve inhibits acute inflammation via decreased production of pro-inflammatory cytokines – failure of this system results in increased systemic inflammation. The presence of sympathetic nerve fibres in the lymphoid organs, together with the expression of adrenoreceptors on immune cells, suggests a role also for the sympathetic nervous system as an immune modulator. Intracranial hypertension results in IL-10 release from

peripheral monocytes and the resultant immuno-depression can be blocked by systemic β-adrenergic blockade.

The overall immunosuppressive effect of TBI is multifactorial. Endogenous catecholamines lead to selective suppression of cellular immunity through immunoinhibitory cytokines, and the stress-induced hypermetabolic response may also contribute to the immunocompromised state. Severe brain injury is also associated with suppression of cell-mediated immunity by a variety of mechanisms. Defective T-lymphocyte function affects antibody production because of their key role in the control of B lymphocytes. Corticosteroids released as part of the initial stress response are profoundly immunosuppressive, inhibiting many functions of lymphocytes and macrophages, reducing the production of cytokines and other inflammatory mediators, and attenuating some of their effects on target tissues. The overall effect of these different mechanisms is depression of the immune system and suppression of cell-mediated immunity. T-helper-cell suppression occurs within 24 h of isolated head injury, and function does not return to normal for at least 3 weeks.

This early immunosuppression correlates with the high rate of infection, particularly pneumonia, in the acute phase after TBI. Granulocyte colony-stimulating factor (GCSF) has modulatory effects on neuroinflammation and there has been interest in its use to improve immune function after TBI. Animal and clinical trials suggest that GCSF might reduce the incidence of sepsis and pyrexia, but it remains to be seen whether this will influence neurological outcome after TBI.

Cardiovascular complications

The clinical syndrome of NSM includes a transient metabolic acidosis, widespread ECG changes, reversible LV RWMA and, in severe cases, cardiogenic shock, pulmonary oedema and death. Neurogenic stunned myocardium is more common in women than in men and its severity is related to the severity of the brain injury.

Cardiovascular dysfunction often resolves spontaneously after a variable period and the importance of pro-active intervention, including treatment of the underlying brain injury and general supportive critical care, during episodes of instability cannot be overestimated. A systemic review including 2690 patients from 25 studies (16 prospective) demonstrated that markers of cardiac damage and dysfunction after SAH are

Table 19.4 ECG changes after subarachnoid haemorrhage

ECG abnormality	Reported incidence (%)
ST segment changes	15–51
Inverted or isoelectric T waves	12–92
QTc prolongation	11–66
Prominent U waves	4–47
Sinus bradycardia	16
Sinus tachycardia	8.5

associated with an increased risk of mortality, delayed ischaemic neurological deficit (DIND) and worsened neurological outcome in survivors. However, the effect of such complications on overall mortality is relatively small. A meta-analysis published in 2005 identified them as the cause of death in only three out of 979 patients.

ECG changes

ECG abnormalities have been recognized after SAH for more than 50 years, but they also occur after TBI and other intracranial pathologies. In SAH, the overall incidence of ECG abnormalities ranges from 49 to 100% (Table 19.4). ST segment changes and QTc prolongation are the most common and can be difficult to distinguish from an acute coronary event (Fig. 19.5). Prolongation of the QTc interval is particularly associated with TBI and the degree of prolongation with the severity of the injury. Both ST abnormalities and QTc changes occur within the first few days after the injury and, although they are usually transient, may persist for up to 8 weeks in some patients. Although the frequency of ECG abnormalities is related to the severity of the neurological injury, in themselves they do not appear to contribute significantly to mortality or morbidity.

As well as changes in ECG morphology, rhythm disturbances can also occur. Most are benign and include sinus tachycardia and premature atrial and ventricular contractions, although clinically significant arrhythmias, such as atrial fibrillation and atrioventricular dissociation, can be seen. However, serious arrhythmias, such as torsades de point and ventricular fibrillation, are rare.

ECG changes are believed to occur as a result of the increase in sympathetic activity following posterior hypothalamic ischaemia at the time of brain injury. There is often little association between ECG changes and the presence of elevated cardiac enzymes (see below).

A 12-lead ECG should be recorded in all brain-injured patients on admission and repeated at 24 h intervals until any abnormalities have resolved. Continuous three-lead ECG monitoring on the neurointensive care unit allows early diagnosis of malignant arrhythmias. Although standard therapies, including correction of electrolyte disturbances, should be provided, management of the underlying intracranial pathology is the most effective way to prevent and treat ECG abnormalities. There is no evidence that treatment guided by morphological ECG changes improves outcome after brain injury, although anti-arrhythmic agents offer short-term benefit during periods of haemodynamic instability while intracranial hypertension is brought under control. The presence of minor ECG changes should not delay definitive treatment, but it can sometimes be necessary to delay neurosurgical intervention in those with significant ECG abnormalities associated with elevations in cardiac enzymes or ventricular dysfunction, when there is an increased risk of malignant arrhythmias.

Sudden cardiac death

Most neurogenic arrhythmias are innocuous but others carry a poor prognosis and may progress to sudden cardiac death. This is a rare event, although its true incidence is uncertain because it may be the cause of pre-hospital mortality in some patients. The exact mechanism is also unclear, but severe QTc prolongation, driven by abnormalities in the insula, may be responsible. Drugs that prolong the QTc interval should be avoided in the acute phase, and the introduction of QTc interval-modifying antipsychotic drugs has been proposed as a potential cause of malignant arrhythmias during the rehabilitation period.

Biomarkers of cardiac injury

Cardiac troponin I (cTnI) is elevated in 20–40% of patients after TBI. It usually peaks in the first 24–36 h after injury and resolves within 5–10 days. The degree of elevation of cTnI has prognostic significance after SAH and is associated with a significantly increased risk of DIND, poor functional outcome and death. In one study, the mortality rate increased from 27 to 48 to >70% if peak cTIn was <2 μg l^{-1}, 2–9.5 μg l^{-1} and >9.5 μg l^{-1} respectively. In patients with a highly positive cTnI response (>1.0 μg l^{-1}), 54% develop LV dysfunction after SAH compared with 10 and 2% of those

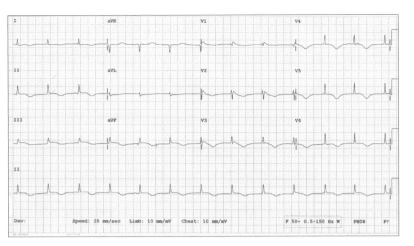

Fig. 19.5. Typical ECG changes after subarachnoid haemorrhage. Note the deep T-wave inversion and prolonged QTc interval.

with mildly positive (cTnI 0.1–1.0 μg l⁻¹) and negative responses, respectively. The degree of elevation in cTnI is also related to an increased risk of pulmonary complications – pulmonary oedema occurs in 79% of patients with a highly positive response but in only 29% of those with no cTnI rise.

The creatine phosphokinase–myocardial fraction (CK-MB) is also elevated after brain injury but is not as good a predictor for cardiac dysfunction as cTnI. Elevations in CK-MB are associated with RWMAs but not with ECG changes. B-type natriuretic peptide (BNP) is released from the heart after myocardial infarction and congestive cardiac failure, but elevated levels are also found after SAH. Levels of BNP increase soon after the ictus and return to baseline withinin 1–2 weeks. The aetiology of BNP release after brain injury is controversial but may be related to hypothalamic hypoxic injury and catecholamine-induced myocardial damage. Whatever the cause, elevated BNP is associated with the classic features of NSM, pulmonary oedema and both systolic and diastolic ventricular dysfunction.

Ventricular dysfunction

The typical echocardiographic findings in patients with NSM include decreased LV contractility, hypokinesia and low ejection fractions (EFs). The majority of RWMAs involve the basal and middle ventricular portions of the anteroseptal and anterior walls, with relative apical sparing (Fig. 19.6). These changes reflect the distribution of sympathetic nerves rather than specific vascular territories in line with the known aetiology of NSM. Left ventricular dysfunction occurs in around

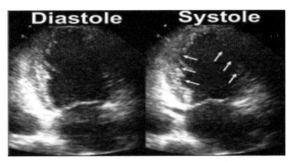

Fig. 19.6. Echocardiogram of a patient with Hunt and Hess grade 3 subarachnoid haemorrhage showing midventricular wall motion abnormalities (arrows) in the apical two-chamber view. Wall motion score was 1.9 and ejection fraction 30%. (Modified from Tanabe *et al.*, 2008, with permission.)

18% of patients after SAH, usually within 3 days of the ictus, but the degree of dysfunction is often mild. In a cohort of 300 patients, mean LV EF was 53 ± 13% and <50% in only 8% of patients. Although RWMAs are usually temporary, they can be associated with a higher mortality after SAH.

Left ventricular apical ballooning (LVAB), often referred to as Takotsubo cardiomyopathy, is characterized by transient, virtually global LV dysfunction consisting of apical and mid-ventricular akinesia with relative sparing of the basal segment. It is a well-recognized response to sudden physical or emotional stress and occurs predominantly (90% of reports) in females. Left ventricular apical ballooning generally has a benign prognosis – only 1% of reported cases died and those who survive almost always recover fully. Conversely, although it is a rare cause of ventricular dysfunction after SAH and TBI, LVAB is associated with increased mortality in the context of brain injury.

287

Diastolic dysfunction is not well investigated after brain injury but may be more common than previously believed. In one study, 71% of 223 patients had some degree of diastolic dysfunction and this was an independent predictor for the development of pulmonary oedema.

Differentiation between neurogenic myocardium and acute coronary syndromes

It is important for the clinician to be able to differentiate between stunned myocardium and acute coronary syndromes, but this is not always straightforward because of the common clinical and diagnostic features. Angiography is the definitive diagnostic tool but is rarely indicated in this high-risk patient population. In any case, the presence of significant coronary artery disease does not exclude coincidental NSM. A neurogenic cause of cardiovascular dysfunction after brain injury is therefore usually a diagnosis of exclusion. Factors favouring NSM include widespread ECG changes in isolation, modest elevation in serum cTnI concentration, inconsistency between echocardiographic and ECG findings, inconsistency between cTnI and LV EF (cTnI < 2.8 μg l^{-1} in association with EF < 40%) and spontaneous resolution of cardiac abnormalities.

Blood pressure control

The initial brain injury-related catecholamine surge results in hypertension and tachycardia. Studies from the 1970s demonstrated that β-adrenergic blockade reduces myocardial injury and improves neurological outcome following SAH, but its effect after TBI is unknown. Sympathetic blockade is in any case considered to be impractical because of its potential adverse effects on blood pressure and cerebral perfusion pressure (CPP). However, three retrospective cohort studies have demonstrated that patients pre-exposed to β-blockers have significantly reduced mortality after TBI despite being older and more severely injured. In one study, there was a mortality reduction from 10.8 to 5.1% and the relative risk of death was 0.29 for patients exposed to β-blockers. The exact mechanism through which β-blockade might mediate this effect is unknown but is likely to include cardioprotection in patients with NSM through limitation of myocardial oxygen demand by reduction in heart rate, stroke volume and blood pressure. Neuroprotective effects from

β-blockade might also accrue through decreased cerebral blood flow and metabolism, but this is speculative. Further studies must address the role of β-blockade after TBI and should identify the optimal type/dose and safety profile. Furthermore, it is important to establish whether post-injury treatment produces similar effects to pre-exposure. Other sympathomimetic therapies, such as magnesium sulfate and clonidine, have been investigated, but there is no clinical evidence to support their use after brain injury.

The initial hyperdynamic phase is often followed by hypotension because of unopposed peripheral vasodilation, ventricular dysfunction and cardiac arrhythmias. Hypotension usually responds to fluid resuscitation and standard vasopressor/inotropic support. Norepinephrine offers predictable augmentation of blood pressure and CPP after TBI and is widely used. Refractory hypotension may be treated with vasopressin although there is some concern that it might cause cerebral vasoconstriction and worsen ischaemic injury. Dobutamine normalizes the cardiac index and improves cerebral oxygenation in the presence of NSM-related low cardiac output states after SAH.

Regional wall motion abnormalities after SAH are associated with higher vasopressor requirement and this association is intriguing. Neurogenic stunned myocardium and associated events often result in hypotension and this is usually treated with vasopressors. In this context, high-dose vasopressor use is presumably a marker for more severe disease. However, sympathomimetic drugs increase myocardial oxygen demand and, if the myocardium is already compromised by NSM, vasopressors might themselves increase myocyte necrosis and worsen myocardial damage. Thus, if exogenous as well as endogenous catecholamines cause or worsen NSM, high-dose vasopressors would presumably be dangerous after brain injury and it would then be necessary to find alternative means to support cerebral perfusion. Current data cannot resolve this issue, which warrants further investigation. In the meantime, a careful balance must be struck between the need to support blood pressure and CPP and the risks of exogenous catecholamine-induced injury.

Pulmonary complications

Pulmonary complications are common after brain injury. Respiratory dysfunction and failure occur in around 80 and 23% of patients, respectively, after TBI.

Non-evacuated mass lesions are associated with a five-fold increase in the incidence of ALI and diffuse axonal injury with a tenfold increase. The mortality rate in TBI patients with ALI is 38% compared with around 20% in those without respiratory failure.

Pulmonary aspiration

Brain-injured patients are at significant risk of pulmonary aspiration because of decreased consciousness and an unprotected airway. In one study, 40% of patients with severe TBI had gross signs of pulmonary aspiration during pre-hospital intubation and 73% of them went on to develop pneumonia. Aspiration of gastric contents after brain injury increases the overall odds of developing early-onset pneumonia by a factor of 5.5.

Pneumonia

Pneumonia is the commonest non-neurological complication of severe brain injury. It occurs in 40–65% of patients after TBI, with those with the severest injury being most at risk. It aggravates secondary brain injury because of its association with fever, hypotension, hypoxaemia and hypercapnoea and is therefore an important modifiable risk factor. Pneumonia is associated with a significantly longer duration of mechanical ventilation, and intensive care unit (ICU) and hospital lengths of stay, but not increased hospital mortality, after brain injury. Patients who develop pneumonia are also more likely to require a tracheostomy and develop multiple organ dysfunction and failure.

Early-onset pneumonia, developing within the first 5 days after injury, is most common and causative organisms include *Staphylococcus aureus*, *Haemophilus influenzae* and *Streptococcus pneumoniae*. Risk factors for the development of early-onset pneumonia include bacterial colonization of the upper airway, pulmonary aspiration and barbiturate infusion. Late-onset pneumonia, developing after 5 days, is a typical ventilator-associated pneumonia (VAP) associated with Gram-negative and multidrug-resistant bacteria. In a single-centre study, 45% of ventilated patients with severe TBI developed VAP. Patients with multiple trauma are at higher risk than those with isolated head injury (risk ratio 1.7, 95% confidence interval (CI) 0.9–3.1). Minimizing the risk of pneumonia after brain injury is a key part of intensive care management strategies, and the application of ventilator care bundles is now commonplace and reduces the incidence of VAP. The use of head-up positioning (also useful for lowering ICP), meticulous oral hygiene,

regular oropharyngeal suctioning and early enteral feeding are important elements.

As early tracheal colonization is a risk factor for the development of pneumonia after brain injury, there has been interest in the use of prophylactic antibiotics to reduce its incidence. A small single-centre study comparing treatment of 3 days of intravenous ampicillin/sulbactam with standard (no antibiotic) care in patients with TBI and SAH was terminated early because of a significantly reduced incidence of early-onset pneumonia in the treatment group (39.5 vs. 57.9%). However, there was a tendency towards a greater likelihood of multidrug-resistant organisms as the causative agent in late-onset pneumonia in the patients who had received prophylactic antibiotics. Many other studies have also demonstrated this increased risk of colonization with resistant pathogens, as well as increased risk of opportunistic infections such *Clostridium difficile* colitis, following prophylactic antibiotics.

Nasal carriage of *Staphylococcus aureus* brings a fivefold increase in the risk of pneumonia after severe TBI and topical eradication would intuitively appear to be an attractive alternative to prophylactic systemic antibiotics. However, although topical mupirocin is a highly effective eradication therapy, it does not reduce the incidence of pneumonia.

Neurogenic pulmonary oedema

General approaches to the management of pulmonary oedema, including fluid restriction and diuretic therapy, are not appropriate in many patients with brain injury. In NPO, catecholamine-induced redistribution of blood into the pulmonary circulation results in an underfilled systemic circulation, and diuretics may exacerbate this acutely hypovolaemic state and adversely affect cerebral perfusion. Positive end-expiratory pressure (PEEP) may be used to optimize oxygenation and reduce extravascular lung water acutely after NPO, but pharmacological intervention is seldom required as the oedema tends to be self-limiting. In resistant cases, the β-adrenergic agonist dobutamine can be effective in improving oxygenation and reversing NPO because of beneficial effects on myocardial function and reduction of systemic and pulmonary vascular resistance.

Respiratory arrhythmias

Abnormal breathing patterns are common after brain injury. Many patients significantly hyperventilate with low tidal volumes in the early recovery period, and this is often associated with other respiratory arrhythmias, including periods of hypoventilation, that, together with a reduced cough reflex, can lead to alveolar atelectasis and basal consolidation. These issues should be taken into account when designing respiratory weaning programmes in brain-injured patients.

Mechanical ventilation in brain-injured patients

The concept of ventilator-induced pulmonary injury has changed the approach to the ventilatory management of patients with ALI and acute respiratory distress syndrome (ARDS). ARDSnet guidance (http://www.ardsnet.org/) recommends low tidal volume ventilation (6 ml kg^{-1} ideal body weight) and the avoidance of peak inspiratory pressure >30 cmH$_2$O to minimize the risk of ventilator-induced pulmonary injury.

The link between high tidal volumes, barotrauma and the development of ALI/ARDS is as true for brain-injured patients as the general ICU population. In a prospective observational study in patients with severe TBI, those ventilated with a 'high' tidal volume (average of 10.4 ml kg^{-1}) had a 5.4 times greater likelihood of developing ALI/ARDS than those ventilated with a protective strategy (tidal volume <6 ml kg^{-1}). The patients who developed ALI/ARDS had a significantly greater length of ICU stay (25 vs. 20 days) and higher mortality (28 vs. 22%) than those who did not. However, the extension of lung-protective ventilation strategies to patients with brain injury is challenging because some aspects conflict with brain-protective therapy. Permissive hypoxaemia and hypercapnia are key components of protective ventilation strategies but the ARDSnet arterial partial pressure of oxygen (PaO$_2$) target of 7.5–10 kPa may be too low in the context of brain injury where consensus guidance recommends that PaO$_2$ should be maintained at >13.0 kPa. Permissive hypercapnia should also be avoided in patients with intact cerebrovascular reactivity when elevated PaCO$_2$ may lead to rises in ICP.

Although the use of several standard ventilator strategies has been questioned in brain-injured patients, their potential disadvantages have probably been overemphasized. High levels of PEEP may compromise cerebral venous outflow by increasing intrathoracic pressure, and this has led to the classic teaching of no or low-level PEEP after brain injury to minimize rises

in ICP. This is incorrect because the effect of PEEP on ICP depends crucially on its effect on the lungs. When PEEP results in significant alveolar recruitment, ICP is likely to be reduced because of improved systemic oxygenation. On the other hand, if PEEP does not increase lung volumes, ICP might increase because of the associated rise in arterial partial pressure of carbon dioxide (PaCO$_2$). Clinical studies demonstrate that, with adequate volume resuscitation, PEEP <12–15 cmH$_2$O has minimal effect on ICP and CPP and, as described above, may actually reduce ICP because of improved systemic and therefore cerebral oxygenation. A PEEP of 5 cmH$_2$O is applied in all ventilated patients during neurointensive care and at higher levels in those in whom oxygenation is problematic. Concerns that inverse-ratio ventilation might impair cerebral venous outflow and increase ICP also appear to be unfounded. In one study, pressure control inverse-ratio ventilation had similar effects on ICP and CPP to volume-cycled ventilation.

Many patients with brain injury and ALI can be managed safely using lung-protection ventilation strategies without compromising the injured brain. However, in those with refractory intracranial hypertension and ALI, a ventilation strategy that maximizes oxygenation while balancing the risks to the lungs and the injured brain should be identified individually for each patient. Further research is needed to determine optimal ventilation strategies in this challenging group of patients.

Haematological complications

Haematological complications, particularly coagulopathy, occur in 20–36% of patients after brain injury.

Coagulopathy

Severe TBI initially induces a hypercoagulable state that can precipitate microclot formation in the brain and other organs and contribute to secondary cerebral and systemic injury. Activation of the coagulation system overwhelms physiological inhibitory mechanisms and leads to increased secondary fibrinolysis and consumptive coagulopathy. Disseminated intravascular coagulation is present in 24–35% of patients with abnormal clotting studies after TBI and is associated with higher mortality and worsened neurological outcome in survivors. Markers associated with fibrinolytic activity, such as fibrinogen degradation products, D-dimers and α$_2$-plasmin inhibitor-plasmin complex, are correlated with the severity of TBI and these markers are more sensitive than routine coagulation tests in predicting patients at risk of poor outcome.

Correction of coagulopathy minimizes intracranial haemorrhagic complications after brain injury and, as the ischaemic brain drives ongoing coagulopathy, multiple doses of fresh frozen plasma may be required to achieve consistent haemostasis. Thrombocytopaenia may predict progressive haemorrhage in patients with intracerebral contusion, and it has been suggested that a platelet threshold of $<100 \times 10^9\,l^{-1}$ should be the trigger for platelet transfusion.

Anaemia

Anaemia is relatively common after brain injury and can be related to blood loss from associated injuries, from a direct neurogenic effect on erythropoesis or as a result of the complex interaction between SIRS and red cell consumption. Anaemia requiring red cell transfusion is a poor prognostic sign after SAH and associated with a 1.8-fold increase in the risk of death. It is unclear whether it is the anaemia itself that leads to the poor outcome or whether it is simply a marker of the severity of the underlying brain injury.

Targets for haemoglobin levels in general intensive care patients have recently been revised downwards following evidence that mortality rates are higher in patients managed with a transfusion target threshold $>10.0\,g\,dl^{-1}$ compared with those with a threshold of $>7.0\,g\,dl^{-1}$. The optimum haemoglobin level after brain injury remains controversial but is likely to be $>7.0\,g\,dl^{-1}$. A recent microdialysis study identified signs of cellular bioenergetic distress in patients with poor-grade SAH when the haemoglobin concentration was $<9.0\,g\,dl^{-1}$.

Fever

Up to three-quarters of patients on the neurointensive care unit develop clinically relevant pyrexia. Over half of the fever episodes are infection related and the rest occur secondary to the brain injury-related neuroinflammatory response. Neuroinflammation-driven fever has been identified in around 33% of brain-injured patients overall but is more common after SAH than after TBI. It generally occurs earlier (<3 days) than fever from an infectious cause (>4 days), and its severity and duration are proportional to the severity of neurological insult.

Both high and low admission brain temperature is associated with increased mortality after TBI, and increased brain temperature with worsened neurological outcome in survivors. Brain temperature is higher than systemic temperature, and, because the correlation is not linear or absolute, there is an increasing trend towards monitoring brain temperature during neurointensive care. Aggressive fever control should be applied routinely.

Neuroendocrine dysfunction

The brain controls multiple endocrine systems via the hypothalamic–pituitary axis (HPA). As the mechanisms regulating pituitary and adrenal function are located within the hypothalamus and brainstem, acute brain injury has significant potential to disrupt various neuroendocrine responses. Most often the disruption is transient, but in some cases there is permanent loss of endocrine function.

Pathophysiology of neuroendocrine dysfunction

Endocrine failure after brain injury is related to multiple mechanisms. There may be direct injury to the HPA in TBI or ischaemic injury during episodes of high ICP. Reduced neuronal input from cortical and brainstem sites may secondarily affect the HPA, and brain injury-induced release of substances such as somatomedin and catecholamines may further alter HPA hormone release. Primary endocrine gland failure may also occur, most commonly because of systemic infective complications – up to 60% of septic ICU patients have some degree of adrenal insufficiency (AI). Several drugs and direct trauma to the endocrine glands are also causes of endocrine dysfunction, but these are not specific to brain injury.

The blood supply to the HPA is complex and the site of a watershed phenomenon. The anterior lobe of the pituitary gland is particularly vulnerable, and anterior hypopituitarism is common after brain injury. Spasm of small feeding arteries arising from the circle of Willis has also been described as a cause of HPA ischaemia after SAH. Imaging reveals the presence of vascular insults to the HPA in 50% of brain-injured patients, although no abnormalities are identified in 6% of patients with confirmed pituitary dysfunction. Post-mortem studies identify structural abnormalities of the HPA in more than two-thirds of patients dying from severe TBI. Anterior pituitary abnormalities are most common, with isolated hypothalamic and posterior pituitary lesions reported in 43 and 40% of cases, respectively.

Incidence

The incidence of anterior pituitary failure after brain injury is reported variously as between 1 and 35%. This wide variation reflects the number of hormones assayed, the use of stimulation tests and the variable times since the brain injury in different studies. A single-centre study identified pituitary dysfunction in 37.5, 57.1 and 59.3% of patients with mild, moderate and severe TBI, respectively, with more than one hormone pathway affected in around 20% of cases. Posterior lobe dysfunction is less common than anterior dysfunction, occurring in 20–25% of patients. It is usually transient, although central diabetes insipidus (CDI) persists long term in around 6% of cases. A recent systematic review of 19 studies including 1137 patients demonstrated that the pooled prevalence of hypopituitarism in the chronic phase after TBI and SAH was 27.5% (95% CI 22.8–28.9%) and 47% (95% CI 37.4–56.8%), respectively.

The extent of abnormal adrenal function after brain injury is not clear, although in one study 53% of patients with moderate or severe TBI had at least transient AI. Those developing AI were younger, more severely injured and had a higher frequency of secondary adverse insults including hypotension and hypoxaemia.

Sick euthyroid syndrome is well recognized in many acute illnesses and is characterized by low tri-iodothyronine (T_3), low or normal tetra-iodothyronine (T_4), normal thyroid stimulating hormone (TSH) and elevated reverse T_3 (rT_3). Such changes usually return to normal during recovery and hormone replacement does not appear to alter the clinical course. 'Central' hypothyroidism occurs in 10–15% of patients after TBI but is often diagnosed late or mistaken for sick euthyroid syndrome.

Diagnosis

Recent consensus statements aim to increase the awareness of endocrine failure after brain injury and encourage routine endocrine evaluation during the acute and rehabilitation periods. Most patients develop symptoms of hypopituitarism soon after injury, but around 15% of cases are not diagnosed for up to 5 years. Clinical features that should prompt the consideration of endocrine failure after brain injury include:

- Prolonged unresponsiveness, particularly if not predicted by the severity of the underlying brain injury.
- Hypotension requiring vasopressor support.
- Hyponatraemia.
- Hypoglycaemia.
- Polyuria.
- CT evidence of lesions (oedema, haemorrhage or infarction) in the region of the hypothalamus.
- Skull base fracture in the presence of cranial nerve defects.

Many of these features occur as a result of other TBI-related pathological processes, so a high index of clinical suspicion is essential. It has thus been suggested that routine endocrine screening, including measurement of serum cortisol levels, should be undertaken in all brain-injured patients receiving heavy sedation and high-dose vasopressor support.

Although serum cortisol is the primary investigation for assessing adrenal status, the serum concentration for diagnosis of AI is controversial. TBI-induced stress increases basal cortisol concentration and obliterates the circadian rhythm. However, the cortisol response for a given degree of injury cannot be predicted and, in any case, might change with time. Furthermore, a triphasic response, comprising an initial increase lasting around 2 days, followed by a 3-day period of low levels and a final phase of increased cortisol, has also been described in some patients. A random cortisol concentration lower than 15–18 µg dl^{-1} is usually recommended as an appropriate threshold for diagnosis of AI, although higher levels up to 25–36 µg dl^{-1} have been suggested as being more appropriate after brain injury. The magnitude of the serum cortisol response to adrenocorticotrophin hormone (ACTH) stimulation is widely used in the diagnosis of adrenal failure and identifies patients as 'responders' or 'non-responders'. Although also controversial after TBI, a rise in serum cortisol concentration >9 µg dl^{-1} above baseline is considered necessary to confirm adequate adrenal responsiveness.

In the presence of low levels of circulating thyroid hormones after TBI, low levels of serum TSH, and failure of TSH release in response to thyrotropin-releasing hormone, are diagnostic of HPA dysfunction. Specific HPA assays or stimulation tests may be required to distinguish primary gland dysfunction from HPA failure, particularly if complex hormone replacement is indicated. Advice from an endocrinologist should always be sought early.

Endocrine replacement therapy

With the exception of replacement of cortisol and anti-diuretic hormone (ADH) in clinically relevant AI and CDI, current evidence does not support other endocrine replacement in the acute phase after brain injury.

Although high-dose steroids have adverse effects after TBI, proven adrenal failure requires replacement therapy. Low-dose steroid replacement (200–300 mg hydrocortisone per 24 h in divided doses) in ACTH 'non-responders' has been widely applied in sepsis-related AI, and similar regimens have also been recommended after TBI. The dose should be reduced to maintenance levels of 10–20 mg every 8 h as soon as clinical status allows. Supplemental mineralocorticoid therapy is only indicated for primary adrenal failure or if there is significant and resistant hyponatraemia.

Delayed diagnosis

Traumatic brain injury-related endocrine dysfunction is present in around 40% of patients during the rehabilitation phase. The late signs of HPA failure are easily mistaken for the neuropsychological and psychiatric sequelae of TBI, and their diagnosis is often missed or delayed. There are no studies that link endocrine insufficiency to outcome in the chronic phase of TBI, but appropriate replacement therapy can be beneficial in reversing some psychological symptoms and memory loss.

Sodium disturbances

The CNS plays a major role in the regulation of sodium and water homeostasis, so sodium disturbances are common after brain injury. They can lead to serious complications and adverse outcomes, which can be minimized by a systematic approach to recognition, diagnosis and treatment of the sodium imbalance.

Hyponatraemia

Hyponatraemia is defined as a serum sodium concentration <135 mmol l^{-1} and occurs in up to 15% of the general adult hospital inpatient population. It is more common after brain injury and in pituitary disease, especially in those patients who are critically ill.

It usually develops between 2 and 7 days after injury and is associated with mortality increases of up to 60%. Hyponatraemia is related to three general mechanisms – impairment of water excretion, excessive water intake and an increase in urinary sodium excretion. These all increase body water content relative to sodium, thereby reducing the serum sodium concentration. After brain injury, hyponatraemia related to impaired water excretion results from inappropriate elevations of ADH, also known as arginine vasopressin (AVP). Brain injury-related hyponatraemia is most commonly associated with normo- or hypovolaemia and the cause of the low serum sodium can be determined by the associated volume status. In most cases, hyponatraemia is associated with hypotonicity, creating a gradient across the BBB, favouring entry of water into the brain and the development of cerebral oedema.

Iatrogenic hyponatraemia usually results from the administration of inappropriately hypotonic fluids, often in the post-operative period when ADH levels are raised because of the stress response to surgery. After brain injury, hyponatraemia occurs most frequently because of the syndrome of inappropriate ADH secretion (SIADH) or cerebral salt-wasting syndrome (CSWS). Important drug-related causes include anticonvulsant drugs (particularly carbamazepine) and diuretics (particularly thiazides).

Syndrome of inappropriate antidiuretic hormone secretion

The pathophysiology of SIADH is not fully understood. ADH release is related to the threshold of the thirst response and this is lower in patients with SIADH. There is also loss of control of ADH release so that plasma ADH concentration is unaffected by continued fluid administration/intake or by osmotic stimulus. The concentration of ADH is therefore inappropriately high in the context of the production of small volumes of concentrated urine. The most common neurological causes of SIADH are SAH, TBI, brain tumour, meningitis and encephalitis. The diagnostic features include the following:

- Serum sodium <135 mmol l^{-1}.
- Serum osmolality <280 mmol kg^{-1}.
- Urine sodium >18 mmol l^{-1}.
- Urine osmolality > serum osmolality.
- Normal thyroid, adrenal and renal function.
- Absence of peripheral oedema or dehydration.

Cerebral salt-wasting syndrome

Cerebral salt-wasting syndrome is characterized by renal loss of sodium that occurs secondary to a centrally mediated process and results in polyuria, natiuresis, hyponatraemia and hypovolaemia. It is predominantly associated with SAH and TBI but has also been described after brain tumour, ischaemic stroke and tuberculous meningitis. It usually occurs in the first week and resolves spontaneously within 2–4 weeks. The exact incidence is uncertain because many cases of CSWS are mistakenly diagnosed as SIADH (see below).

Following its first description in 1950, CSWS has been related to disruption of hypothalamo–renal pathways. The precise pathophysiology is unclear, but raised levels of atrial natriuretic peptide (ANP) and BNP are likely to mediate, at least in part, the natiuresis and hyponatraemia associated with brain injury. There is an initial elevation of ANP following SAH, but this rise is not correlated with the degree of hyponatraemia and ANP levels subsequently fall. Elevated BNP levels have been correlated with raised ICP and urinary sodium excretion. The increased sympathetic activity after brain injury results in increased renal perfusion pressure and this may worsen the natiuresis and hyponatraemia.

The biochemical criteria for the diagnosis of CSWS are as follows:

- Low serum sodium concentration (may be normal)
- High or normal serum osmolality
- High or normal urine osmolality
- Increased haematocrit, urea, bicarbonate and albumin as a consequence of hypovolaemia.

However, these criteria are often inconclusive, and analysis of urinary sodium levels can be of assistance. Urinary sodium concentration is usually low ($<20\,mmol\ l^{-1}$) in hypovolaemic patients, but, in CSWS, urinary sodium levels are high. This finding is not necessarily diagnostic because urinary sodium concentration is also raised in SIADH. However, in CSWS, total daily urine sodium excretion is greater than intake, whereas it is usually equal to intake in SIADH, i.e. overall sodium balance is negative in CSWS and generally neutral in SIADH.

Differentiating between syndrome of inappropriate antidiuretic hormone secretion and cerebral salt-wasting syndrome

It is important to distinguish between SIADH and CSWS because the treatment of the two conditions

Table 19.5 Biochemical and water changes in the syndrome of inappropriate ADH secretion (SIADH) and cerebral salt-wasting syndrome (CSWS)

Change	SIADH	CSWS
Plasma volume	Raised	Lowered
Sodium balance	Positive/equal	Negative
Water balance	Positive	Negative
Serum sodium	Low	Low
Serum osmolality	Lowered	High/normal
Urine sodium	High	High
Urine osmolality	High	Normal/high

Normal values: serum osmolality $278–305\,mmol\ kg^{-1}$, serum sodium $135–145\,mmol\ l^{-1}$, urine osmolality $350–1000\,mmol\ kg^{-1}$, urine sodium $20–60\,mmol\ l^{-1}$ or $100–250\,mmol$ per $24\,h$.

is diametrically opposed. Because biochemical criteria may fail to differentiate CSWS from SIADH, the diagnosis is based on a careful clinical examination (Table 19.5).

Measurement of isolated serum and urine sodium concentrations is insufficient, and the key to diagnosis lies in the accurate assessment of volume status and overall sodium balance. The presence of dehydration and volume depletion in CSWS is the key feature differentiating it from SIADH. Daily weight offers useful information, and examination of mucous membranes, skin turgor, capillary refill time, jugular venous pressure and cardiovascular variables (particularly orthostatic blood pressure changes) should also be undertaken. A thorough review of fluid balance charts will also demonstrate an overall negative balance in CSWS. Volume status can be difficult to assess clinically and may rarely also be a confounding factor. Hypovolaemia has been identified in some patients fulfilling the diagnostic criteria for SIADH because the volume depletion of CSWS may cause a secondary rise in ADH. However, under such conditions, the correct diagnosis is CSWS rather than SIADH. Levels of ADH are therefore not particularly helpful in confirming the diagnosis because they can be raised in both SIADH and CSWS. However, in the latter, the elevated ADH is an appropriate response to hypovolaemia.

Clinical features of hyponatraemia

The brain is the organ most susceptible to a sudden decrease in serum sodium concentration and the symptoms of hyponatraemia are therefore primarily neurological. Water moves freely across cell membranes along an osmotic gradient and a reduction in serum sodium concentration leads to entry of water into brain cells and consequent cerebral oedema. In acute hyponatraemia, cerebral oedema is very common and results in raised ICP, reduced brain perfusion and, if unchecked, brainstem herniation and death. Patients with mild hyponatraemia (130–135 mmol l^{-1}) are usually asymptomatic, whereas a serum sodium concentration of 125–130 mmol l^{-1} is associated with nausea, vomiting and other non-specific symptoms such as dizziness and gait problems. More severe hyponatraemia (<125 mmol l^{-1}) causes more serious neurological symptoms, including agitation and confusion. When serum sodium concentration falls below 115 mmol l^{-1}, the arbitrary definition of severe hypopnatraemia, there is great risk of cerebral oedema, seizures, coma and death.

A slow and gradual decline in serum sodium concentration provides sufficient time for the completion of compensatory mechanisms within the brain so that the degree of cerebral oedema is limited. The severity of symptoms and signs therefore depends not only on the degree of the hyponatraemia but also on the rapidity of the fall in the serum sodium concentration. Chronic hyponatraemia (developing over more than 48 h) may therefore be asymptomatic, even when the decrease in serum sodium concentration is relatively large. In contrast, in patients with acute hyponatraemia, the rapid decline in serum sodium concentration overwhelms the adaptive mechanisms, and severe symptoms, such as seizures and coma, are common. Untreated acute severe hyponatraemia is associated with high rates of morbidity and mortality

Treatment of hyponatraemia

In the context of brain injury, an expectant and supportive treatment strategy is best in asymptomatic patients, as sodium disturbances are often transient and self-limiting. However, prompt treatment is always indicated in those with acute symptomatic hyponatraemia in order to minimize the risk of neurological complications and death. Except in a life-threatening emergency, the underlying cause of the hyponatraemia should be identified before treatment is initiated. Correction of hyponatraemia can itself lead to neurological sequelae and these risks should be minimized by gradual correction of sodium deficits (see below). Treatment should always be targeted to the point of alleviation of symptoms rather than to an arbitrary serum sodium value. The optimal treatment

of hyponatraemia is controversial, reflecting different estimates of the comparative risks of the disorder and its treatment.

Specific treatment of SIADH

As SIADH is often a self-limiting disease in patients with brain injury, treatment should only be initiated in symptomatic patients or if the serum sodium is significantly low or falling rapidly. Electrolyte-free water restriction, initially to 1000–1500 ml day^{-1}, forms the mainstay of treatment and usually results in a slow rise in serum sodium of 1.5 mmol l^{-1} day^{-1}. This degree of fluid restriction may be unpleasant for conscious patients and may worsen cardiovascular instability and increase the risk of cerebral hypoperfusion in critically ill brain-injured patients. Hypertonic saline (1.8%) has a limited place in the treatment of SIADH and should be restricted to severe acute hyponatraemia, particularly after SAH, when fluid restriction is associated with an increased incidence of cerebral ischaemia. Hypertonic saline infusion should be discontinued when serum sodium reaches 120–125 mmol l^{-1} and further management continued with fluid restriction.

Pharmacological treatment is an option when the diagnosis of SIADH is certain. Different classes of drugs are effective through different mechanisms:

1. Furosemide and other diuretics increase water excretion – simultaneous saline or salt administration is often required to compensate for the associated sodium loss.
2. Demeclocycline and lithium inhibit the renal responses of ADH – demeclocycline is the least toxic and initial daily doses of 900–1200 mg should be reduced to 600–900 mg after therapeutic effect is achieved, usually after 3 days to 3 weeks.
3. ADH-receptor antagonists, such as conivaptan and lixivaptan, inhibit the binding of ADH to renal receptors, thereby inducing aquaresis, the electrolyte-sparing excretion of free water.

Specific treatment of CSWS

The primary treatment of CSWS is volume and sodium resuscitation. The optimal saline solution is controversial, but, as a general rule, 0.9% saline is indicated in the first instance. In acute symptomatic hyponatraemia, hypertonic (1.8 or 3%) saline is recommended, with consideration of the concomitant administration of furosemide to minimize the risks of fluid overload. Central venous administration is required for 3% saline. It is of note that, in some patients, administration of sodium may actually increase the natiuresis and associated water loss and worsen the clinical status in CSWS. Once normovolaemia and normonatraemia have been restored, ongoing losses should be replaced with either intravenous saline, or water and sodium tablets, until there is resolution of the CSWS. Close monitoring of serum sodium concentration, and sodium and fluid balance, should continue during this period. In some cases, CSWS may be refractory to standard therapy and fludrocortisone (0.1–0.4 mg daily) may limit the sodium loss by increasing sodium reabsorption from the renal tubule. Fludrocortisone may cause hyperkalaemia, and serum potassium should be closely monitored.

Dangers of correction of hyponatraemia

It is essential to correct hyponatraemia slowly as brain cells can be damaged by rapid osmotic shifts. Myelinolysis is the most serious complication and affects mainly pontine and extrapontine structures. It occurs after a rapid increase in sodium levels and is characterized by mutism, dysarthria, lethargy and, in extreme cases, pseudobulbar palsy and spastic paraparesis. The risk of myelinolysis can be minimized by gradual correction of the serum sodium concentration at a rate of no greater than 0.5 mmol l^{-1} h^{-1} or 8–10 mmol l^{-1} day^{-1}.

Hypernatraemia

Hypernatraemia is defined as a serum sodium concentration of >145 mmol l^{-1}. It occurs less commonly than hyponatraemia, with an incidence of around 1% in the general inpatient hospital population and 9% in the general intensive care setting. Hypernatraemia is usually related to inadequate free water intake or excess water loss and only rarely with excessive salt intake. With the exception of CDI, hypernatraemia can only be maintained if access to water is denied or thirst is impaired. Hypernatraemia is often a paraphenomenon indicating the severity of the underlying disease process. Specific causes of hypernatraemia are listed in Table 19.6. Brain injury-associated hypernatraemia is most commonly related to the overzealous use of osmotic diuretics such as mannitol or the development of CDI. Moderate hypernatraemia cause a variety of

Table 19.6 Causes of hypernatraemia

Effect	Causes
Decreased extracellular fluid volume	Poor thirst/reduced water intake

	Intrarenal water loss:
	• Diabetes insipidus:
	  ○ Central
	  ○ Nephrogenic
	• Osmotic diuresis (e.g. mannitol)
	• Diuretics
	• Extrarenal water loss:
	• Respiratory tract
	• Gastrointestinal tract
	• Fever

Increased extracellular fluid volume	Iatrogenic – administration of sodium-containing fluids
	Mineralocorticoid excess: • Primary hyperaldosteronism • Cushing's syndrome • Exogenous

non-specific symptoms including weakness and irritability, whereas serum sodium levels >160 mmol l^{-1} are associated with changes in conscious level and seizures.

Central diabetes insipidus

The overall incidence of CDI in a neurosurgical unit has been reported as 3.7%. One-third of cases were related to SAH, one third to TBI and one-sixth each to pituitary surgery and ICH. The prevalence of CDI in patients with severe TBI is 20% in the acute phase and 9.6% in the chronic phase. Refractory CDI has a high mortality after TBI (around 70% in one study) and is often associated with severe, pre-terminal cerebral oedema. It is therefore a common finding after brainstem death and has particular relevance in the management of the brain dead organ donor (see Chapter 30). Pituitary stalk haematoma is a rare complicating factor of TBI, and MRI has been recommended for patients in whom the CDI is out of proportion to the severity of the head injury.

Central diabetes insipidus results from a failure of ADH release from the HPA leading to an impairment of the ability to concentrate urine and the production of a large volume of dilute urine. This inappropriate loss of water leads to an increase in serum sodium concentration and osmolality, and a state of clinical dehydration. The anatomical and pathophysiological basis of CDI is relatively well understood. Damage to the hypothalamus above the median eminence may lead to permanent CDI, whereas below this level, or after disturbance of the posterior lobe of the pituitary gland, it leads to transient CDI because ADH can subsequently be released from nerve fibres ending in the median eminence.

Diagnosis

In conscious patients, the classic symptoms of polyuria, polydipsia and thirst makes CDI relatively easy to diagnose, although hyperglycaemia, with its similar symptomatology, should be excluded. It is easy to differentiate between simple dehydration and CDI, even though thirst is often an unreliable or absent sign in brain-injured patients. Dehydration is associated with low urine volume (in the absence of renal failure), whereas CDI results in high urine output, sometimes in excess of $6 \, l \, day^{-1}$. Other causes of high urine volume in brain-injured patients, including osmotic diuretics and triple-H therapy (hypervolaemia, hypertension and haemodilution), should be excluded.

In the context of brain injury, the diagnosis of CDI is made in the presence of:

- Increased urine volume (>3000 ml per 24 h)
- High serum sodium (>145 mmol l^{-1})
- High serum osmolality (>305 mmol kg^{-1})
- Abnormally low urine osmolality (<350 mmol kg^{-1}).

While waiting for these laboratory tests, a simple, but not totally reliable, bedside test of urine specific gravity may be of assistance. A urine specific gravity <1.005 is suggestive of CDI in the presence of high urine output and high serum sodium concentration. Plasma ADH level can distinguish between nephrogenic and neurogenic CDI, but confirmation of the diagnosis ultimately comes with the observation of the response to synthetic ADH.

Treatment

There are two aims in the management of CDI – replacement and retention of water, and replacement of ADH. Conscious patients are able to increase water intake themselves and this is often sufficient treatment if the CDI is self-limiting. In unconscious patients, enteral water (via a nasogastric tube) or intravenous 5% dextrose are suitable fluid-replacement regimens. In some cases, saline solutions may aggravate renal water loss, as urine concentration cannot be achieved in the absence of vasopressin. Excessive fluid input is a risk in unconscious patients and treatment should be guided by accurate assessment of volume status. If urine output >250 ml h^{-1} is maintained, synthetic ADH, usually in the form of 1-deamino-8-D-arginine vasopressin (DDAVP), should be administered. Small titrated doses given intranasally (100–200 μg) or intravenously (0.4 μg) minimize the risk of overprolonged action and can be repeated if necessary to obtain the desired clinical effect.

Over-rapid correction of hypernatraemia can have serious side effects, including pulmonary and cerebral oedema. Serum sodium should generally be reduced no quicker than 10 mmol l^{-1} day^{-1}, although more rapid correction is probably safe in those in whom the hypernatraemia developed over a period of only a few hours.

Glucose disturbance

Brain-injured patients frequently develop hyperglycaemia. In a single unit's SAH population, hyperglycaemia >11.0 mmol l^{-1} occurred in 30% of patients and was a significant predictor of poor outcome. The total burden of hyperglycaemia was strongly associated with disability and loss of high-level functional independence but less so with 3-month mortality. After ischaemic stroke, the incidence of poor outcome is threefold higher in diabetic patients compared with those without glycaemic disturbance. Hyperglycaemia is also associated with poor outcome after TBI.

Hyperglycaemia exacerbates secondary ischaemic injury and worsens neurological outcome by several mechanisms including hyperosmolality, lactic acidosis, alterations in neuronal pH and increases in excitatory amino acids. The overall effect is of increased cellular oxidative stress and subsequent energy failure-related neuronal damage.

The optimal targets for systemic glycaemic control after brain injury are not established, but there is accumulating evidence that 'tight' control with insulin infusion might result in cerebral hypoglycaemia in a substantial number of patients (see Chapter 7). Current evidence suggests that systemic glucose levels <10 mmol l^{-1} should not be treated. Hypoglycaemic episodes and large swings in systemic glucose levels should be avoided.

Complications of brain-directed treatment

Brain-directed therapies may adversely affect non-neurological organ function, and the balance between these potentially opposing interests can be a major challenge during the neurointensive care management of brain injury.

Cardiovascular support

Current management of brain injury focuses on maximizing cerebral oxygenation and perfusion using multifaceted, physiological neuroprotective strategies. Induced hypertension with fluid and vasopressors/inotropes has been advocated to maintain CPP after TBI, but, in one study, this was associated with a five-fold increase in the occurrence of ALI in patients managed with a higher CPP threshold (70 vs. 50 mmHg). Subsequent analysis of these data strongly indicated a link between excessive fluid resuscitation and administration of exogenous catecholamines and the development of symptomatic ALI. Triple-H therapy is widely used after SAH, but it can also exacerbate the cardiopulmonary complications of SAH and lead to intracranial complications such as worsening of cerebral oedema, increased ICP and intracranial haemorrhage.

Therapeutic hypothermia

Although moderate hypothermia has not been shown equivocally to improve outcome in clinical trials of TBI, it is an effective means of reducing ICP resistant to other therapies and is widely incorporated into ICP management protocols. Hypothermia suppresses both cellular and humoral immunity and is associated with an increased risk of infection, particularly pneumonia, and other systemic complications including hypokalaemia, hypomagnesaemia, coagulopathy and cardiac arrhythmias. Relatively short periods of hypothermia (34°C for 48 h) are relatively safe, but there are significant increases in inflammatory markers, such as C-reactive protein and white blood count, during and after rewarming. The decrease in serum potassium and magnesium concentrations during hypothermia often requires electrolyte supplementation and there is a risk of rebound, clinically significant, hyperkalaemia and hypermagnesaemia if rewarming is too rapid. Hypothermia should therefore only be applied within the context of strict management protocols with close attention to the prevention of side effects.

Pharmacological therapies

Many pharmacological brain-directed interventions can result in direct or indirect adverse effects on the injured brain.

Osmotic agents

Mannitol is widely used in the management of raised ICP. An intact BBB is a prerequisite for mannitol administration, as cerebral oedema may be worsened in the presence of deranged BBB function or by prolonged mannitol administration. Mannitol has itself been implicated in BBB failure by causing transient shrinkage of barrier endothelial cells and disruption of tight junctions. The doses of mannitol used in clinical practice vary, but doses >1.0 g kg^{-1} should not be used because of the high incidence of side effects and no improved efficacy compared with lower doses. The side effects of mannitol include initial fluid overload, subsequent hypotension, metabolic acidosis and electrolyte imbalance, all of which can adversely affect the injured brain. In particular, repeated administration may result in unacceptably high serum osmolality (>320 mOsm l^{-1}) and associated neurological and renal complications, including renal failure.

Hypertonic saline is an effective alternative to mannitol and has proven efficacy in controlling ICP resistant to mannitol. It is associated with fewer side effects. In particular, the large intravascular volume shifts seen with mannitol are absent, and renal complications occur less frequently.

Sedative agents

Sedation and analgesia are crucial components of the management of brain injury but are not without risk.

Propofol

Propofol is widely used as a sedative agent because it reduces ICP and has profound cerebral metabolic suppressive effects and a pharmacological profile that allows easy control of sedation levels and rapid wake-up. Propofol has well-recognized adverse effects on blood pressure and cardiac output, but these can generally be managed with fluid and vasopressor support. More severe complications in brain-injured patients include sudden cardiovascular collapse and propofol infusion syndrome (PRIS).

Propofol infusion syndrome is characterized by unexplained metabolic acidosis and elevated creatinine kinase, rhabdomyolysis and widespread ECG changes.

It is generally associated with high-dose or long-term propofol use but can also occur as an idiosyncratic response. It is more common when high-dose propofol is administered simultaneously with a vasopressor, a common combination in critically ill brain-injured patients. In one study of 50 patients with severe TBI, PRIS occurred in 6%, but such a high incidence has not been reported elsewhere. This might be related to underdiagnosis because the metabolic and ECG consequences of PRIS can be difficult to differentiate from those associated with NSM.

The exact aetiology of PRIS is unclear, but impaired utilization of fatty acids within the mitochondria is a likely cause. Propofol inhibits several cellular enzymatic processes and results in reduced entry of long-chain free fatty acids into the mitochondria. In addition, uncoupling of specific oxidative complexes in the mitochondrial respiratory chain leads to failure of medium- and short-chain fatty acid metabolism and subsequent cellular energy failure. Cardiac and peripheral myocytolysis, rhabdomyolysis and acute renal failure follow. Early warning signs of PRIS include unexplained lactic acidosis, lipaemia and ECG changes and, if these occur, propofol infusion should be discontinued immediately. To minimize the risk of PRIS, it is recommended that a propofol infusion rate of 4 mg kg^{-1} h^{-1} should not be exceeded.

Barbiturates

Barbiturates effectively lower ICP by a variety of mechanism, including reduction of cerebral metabolic rate and reduced CBF, inhibition of free radicals and reduction of lipid peroxidation. There is no good evidence that they improve outcome, and high-dose barbiturate therapy is therefore reserved for refractory intracranial hypertension. Hypotension is a frequent complication of treatment and is associated with an increased requirement for inotropic/vasopressor support to maintain CPP. The long half-life of barbiturates results in drug accumulation and delayed recovery leading to difficulty with early clinical assessment when the drug is discontinued or in the diagnosis of brainstem death. Barbiturates are also immunosuppressive and associated with increased risk of pneumonia and other infections after brain injury.

Associated injuries

Traumatic brain injury may be associated with other injuries that can adversely affect outcome. Road traffic accidents, assault and falls are more frequently associated with non-neurological injury. Coincidental pulmonary contusional injury may contribute to ALI and poor gas exchange. Multiple trauma, long-bone fractures and massive blood transfusion all predispose to ALI and multiple organ failure.

Conclusions

Non-neurological organ dysfunction and failure are common after brain injury because of the dynamic interaction between the injured brain and systemic organ systems. Catecholamine and neuroinflammatory effects play key roles in the generation of systemic complications, which may also arise because of complication of brain-directed treatments or co-incidental injuries.

Non-neurological organ dysfunction and failure are independent contributors to morbidity and mortality and therefore present potentially modifiable targets for treatment. However, the management of non-neurological organ dysfunction and failure presents a significant challenge because optimum treatments for failing systemic organ systems can have adverse effects on the injured brain and vice versa. Large-scale studies are required to determine whether prevention, early recognition and treatment of non-neurological organ system dysfunction results in improved outcome after brain injury.

Further reading

Acquarolo, A., Urli, T., Perone, G. et al. (2005). Antibiotic prophylaxis of early onset pneumonia in critically ill comatose patients. A randomized study. *Intensive Care Med* **31**, 510–16.

Banki, N. M., Kopelnik, A., Dae, M. W. et al. (2005). Acute neurocardiogenic injury after subarachnoid hemorrhage. *Circulation* **112**, 3314–19.

Boddie, D. E., Currie, D. G., Eremin, O. and Heys, S. D. (2003). Immune suppression and isolated severe head injury: a significant clinical problem. *Br J Neurosurg* **17**, 405–17.

Bondanelli, M., De Marinis, L., Ambrosio, M. R. et al. (2004). Occurrence of pituitary dysfunction following traumatic brain injury. *J Neurotrauma* **21**, 685–96.

Bronchard, R., Albaladejo, P., Brezac, G. et al. (2004). Early onset pneumonia: risk factors and consequences in head trauma patients. *Anesthesiology* **100**, 234–9.

Claassen, J., Vu A, Kreiter, K. T. et al. (2004). Effect of acute physiologic derangements on outcome after subarachnoid hemorrhage. *Crit Care Med* **32**, 832–8.

Cohan, P., Wang, C., McArthur, D. L. et al. (2005). Acute secondary adrenal insufficiency after traumatic brain injury: a prospective study. *Crit Care Med* **33**, 2358–66.

Contant, C. F., Valadka, A. B., Gopinath, S. P., Hannay, H. J. and Robertson, C. S. (2001). Adult respiratory distress syndrome: a complication of induced hypertension after severe head injury. *J Neurosurg* **95**, 560–8.

Frontera, J. A., Parra, A., Shimbo, D. *et al.* (2008). Cardiac arrhythmias after subarachnoid hemorrhage: risk factors and impact on outcome. *Cerebrovasc Dis* **26**, 71–8.

Kleindienst, A., Brabant, G., Bock, C., Maser-Gluth, C. and Buchfelder, M. (2009). Neuroendocrine function following traumatic brain injury and subsequent intensive care treatment: a prospective longitudinal evaluation. *J Neurotrauma* **26**, 1435–46.

Kumar, S., Selim, M. H. and Caplan, L. R. (2010). Medical complications after stroke. *Lancet Neurol* **9**, 105–18.

Lepelletier, D., Roquilly, A., Demeure dit latte D *et al.* (2010). Retrospective analysis of the risk factors and pathogens associated with early-onset ventilator-associated pneumonia in surgical-ICU head-trauma patients. *J Neurosurg Anesthesiol* **22**, 32–7.

Lim, H. B. and Smith, M. (2007). Systemic complications after head injury: a clinical review. *Anaesthesia* **62**, 474–82.

Lowe, G. J. and Ferguson, N. D. (2006). Lung-protective ventilation in neurosurgical patients. *Curr Opin Crit Care* **12**, 3–7.

Macmillan, C. S., Grant, I. S. and Andrews, P. J. (2002). Pulmonary and cardiac sequelae of subarachnoid haemorrhage: time for active management? *Intensive Care Med* **28**, 1012–23.

Maramattom, B. V., Weigand, S., Reinalda, M., Wijdicks, E. F. and Manno, E. M. (2006). Pulmonary complications after intracerebral hemorrhage. *Neurocrit Care* **5**, 115–19.

Mascia, L., Zavala, E., Bosma, K. *et al.* (2007). High tidal volume is associated with the development of acute lung injury after severe brain injury: an international observational study. *Crit Care Med* **35**, 1815–20.

Naidech, A. M., Kreiter, K. T., Janjua, N. *et al.* (2005). Cardiac troponin elevation, cardiovascular morbidity, and outcome after subarachnoid hemorrhage. *Circulation* **112**, 2851–6.

Otterspoor, L. C., Kalkman, C. J. and Cremer, O. L. (2008). Update on the propofol infusion syndrome in ICU management of patients with head injury. *Curr Opin Anaesthesiol* **21**, 544–51.

Powner, D. J., Boccalandro, C., Alp, M. S. and Vollmer, D. G. (2006). Endocrine failure after traumatic brain injury in adults. *Neurocrit Care* **5**, 61–70.

Robertson, C. S., Valadka, A. B., Hannay, H. J. *et al.* (1999). Prevention of secondary ischemic insults after severe head injury. *Crit Care Med* **27**, 2086–95.

Tanabe, M., Crago, E. A., Suffoletto, M. S. *et al.* (2008). Relation of elevation in cardiac troponin I to clinical severity, cardiac dysfunction, and pulmonary congestion in patients with subarachnoid hemorrhage. *Am J Cardiol* **102**, 1545–50.

Tung, P., Kopelnik, A., Banki, N. *et al.* (2004). Predictors of neurocardiogenic injury after subarachnoid hemorrhage. *Stroke* **35**, 548–51.

Wartenberg, K. E. and Mayer, S. A. (2006). Medical complications after subarachnoid hemorrhage: new strategies for prevention and management. *Curr Opin Crit Care* **12**, 78–84.

Wartenberg, K. E. and Mayer, S. A. (2010). Medical complications after subarachnoid hemorrhage. *Neurosurg Clin N Am* **21**, 325–38.

Wartenberg, K. E., Schmidt, J. M., Claassen, J. *et al.* (2006). Impact of medical complications on outcome after subarachnoid hemorrhage. *Crit Care Med* **34**, 617–23.

Young, N., Rhodes, J. K., Mascia, L. and Andrews, P. J. (2010). Ventilatory strategies for patients with acute brain injury. *Curr Opin Crit Care* **16**, 45–52.

Zaroff, J. G., Rordorf, G. A., Ogilvy, C. S. and Picard, M. H. (2000). Regional patterns of left ventricular systolic dysfunction after subarachnoid hemorrhage: evidence for neurally mediated cardiac injury. *J Am Soc Echocardiogr* **13**, 774–9.

Zygun, D. (2005). Non-neurological organ dysfunction in neurocritical care: impact on outcome and etiological considerations. *Curr Opin Crit Care* **11**, 139–43.

Zygun, D. A., Kortbeek, J. B., Fick, G. H., Laupland, K. B. and Doig, C. J. (2005). Non-neurologic organ dysfunction in severe traumatic brain injury. *Crit Care Med* **33**, 654–60.

Zygun, D. A., Zuege, D. J., Boiteau, P. J. *et al.* (2006). Ventilator-associated pneumonia in severe traumatic brain injury. *Neurocrit Care* **5**, 108–14.

Post-operative care of neurosurgical patients

Christoph S. Burkhart, Stephan P. Strebel and Luzius A. Steiner

Indications for post-operative admission

After neurosurgical procedures, the rate of complications is high. In retrospective studies, a 13–27% rate of major complications has been reported. To avoid, detect and treat complications, specialized care and specific monitoring have to be provided for neurosurgical patients in the early post-operative phase. Often, this care and monitoring is provided in an intensive care unit (ICU). However, only a small fraction of post-operative neurosurgical patients require medical interventions in the ICU beyond the first 4–12 h, e.g. intracranial haemorrhage (ICH) occurs typically during the first 4 h after surgery.

Specific aspects in the post-operative care of neurosurgical patients that will influence the decision to admit a neurosurgical patient to an ICU include the need for tight blood pressure control, delayed recovery and respiratory dysfunction. After long surgical procedures (>6 h), complicated surgery, surgery for large tumours, cerebral arteriovenous malformation (AVM) resection, major intraoperative bleeding and a pre-operative altered level of consciousness, delayed recovery, possibly including prolonged mechanical ventilation in an ICU, may be necessary. Respiratory dysfunction after brain surgery may occur for several reasons. Firstly, cranial nerve dysfunction interfering with airway patency may occur after procedures in the posterior fossa, at the base of the skull or after carotid endarterectomy. Secondly, brainstem compression by post-operative haematoma or acute obstructive hydrocephalus may lead to irregular respiratory patterns or apnoea. Thirdly, mechanical airway obstruction may occur due to macroglossia, secondary to venous obstruction after posterior fossa surgery, or due to oedema and haematoma after carotid endarterectomy

or upper spinal surgery. Moreover, comorbidities irrespective of the type of neurosurgical procedure may necessitate observation or treatment in an ICU.

The indications for post-operative admission to an ICU, a high-dependency unit or a specialized neurosurgical ward will vary from institution to institution depending on local structures and characteristics of the available units. Therefore, we prefer to suggest minimal monitoring requirements after neurosurgical procedures rather than indications for ICU admission. Table 20.1 summarizes such suggested minimal monitoring requirements. However, as there are hardly any data on this topic in the literature, these requirements represent suggestions only and need to be adapted to the specific needs and comorbidities of individual patients.

Monitoring strategies

Besides frequent standardized neurological assessment and scoring, systemic and specific neuromonitoring are important tools to identify patients who are deteriorating post-operatively. Any delay in identifying such patients and in treating the underlying cause may have detrimental effects on outcome.

Systemic monitoring

In neurosurgical patients, cardiovascular disturbances such as hypotension, hypertension, dysrhythmias and myocardial failure are common. They can be caused by central neurogenic effects on the heart, by the consequence of medical or surgical therapy, or by pre-existing disease. In traumatic brain injury (TBI), hypoxia and hypotension are the two most important systemic factors responsible for secondary cerebral insults. This may be applicable to other forms of brain injury including those experienced by neurosurgical patients.

Core Topics in Neuroanaesthesia and Neurointensive Care, eds. Basil F. Matta, David K. Menon and Martin Smith. Published by Cambridge University Press. © Cambridge University Press 2011.

Table 20.1 Suggested minimal monitoring requirements for post-operative neurosurgical patients

Procedure	Minimal duration of intensive clinical neurological evaluation (every 1–4 h)	Consider continuous intra-arterial blood pressure measurement	Consider continuous ECG monitoring	Additional monitoring to be considered
Craniotomy excluding posterior fossa surgery	4–6 h	Yes	Yes	ICP
Posterior fossa surgery	12–24 h	Yes	Yes	
Intracranial vascular procedures (SAH, malformation)	24 h	Yes	Yes	TCD, ICP
Haematoma evacuation	12 h	Yes	Yes	ICP, CT
Carotid surgery	12 h	Yes	Yes	TCD
Spinal surgery				
Minor spinal surgery	4 h	No	No	
Major spinal surgery	6–12 h	Yes	Yes	
Epilepsy surgery	6 h	Yes	Yes	
Implantation of stimulation devices				
Cerebral	6 h	Yes	Yes	
Spinal	4 h	No	No	
Interventional vascular procedures				
Carotid artery	12 h	Yes	Yes	TCD
Intracranial	24 h	Yes	Yes	

Continuous measurement of oxygen saturation (SpO_2) by pulse oxymetry must be used in all post-operative neurosurgical patients. ICP, intracranial pressure; SAH, subarachnoid haemorrhage; TCD, transcranial Doppler.

Consequently, cardiovascular and respiratory monitoring are compulsory in these patients.

Cardiovascular monitoring

Continuous ECG monitoring is routinely used in most post-operative neurosurgical patients. It allows detection of arrhythmias that may occur in patients with any form of brain injury, especially in patients with subarachnoid haemorrhage (SAH) where ECG changes are present in up to 80%.

Haemodynamic disturbances are common in post-operative neurosurgical patients. While non-invasive blood pressure measurements every 15 min may be sufficient in some settings (e.g. after minor spinal surgery), direct intra-arterial blood pressure measurements to facilitate tight blood pressure control must be used in most neurosurgical patients including those undergoing major spinal surgery. An arterial cannula also provides convenient access for sampling of arterial blood for arterial blood gas (ABG) analysis and other laboratory tests. Usually, arterial blood pressure is measured with the pressure transducer referenced to the level of the right atrium. However, this practice may lead to overestimation of cerebral perfusion pressure (CPP) if the head is elevated and intracranial pressure (ICP) is referenced to the level of the foramen of Monroe. Therefore, both transducers should be placed at the level of the external auditory meatus when CPP is being used as a therapeutic target.

Pulmonary artery catheters or other cardiac output monitors are not routinely used in post-operative neurosurgical patients, but may be indicated in selected groups of patients, e.g. those who are treated with triple-H therapy (hypervolaemia, hypertension and haemodilution) for vasospasm after SAH, or in patients with neurogenic pulmonary oedema or pre-existing severe cardiac disease.

Respiratory monitoring

Post-operative monitoring of oxygenation and carbon dioxide elimination is mandatory, as the injured brain is particularly vulnerable to hypoxaemia and hypercapnia, both of which can precipitate intracranial hypertension. Continuous measurement of oxygen saturation (SpO_2) by pulse oximetry must be used in all post-operative neurosurgical patients. Monitoring of ABGs is frequently used in post-operative neurosurgical patients. Cerebral blood flow (CBF) and cerebral blood volume are very dependent on the arterial partial pressure of carbon dioxide ($PaCO_2$). Patients with low intracranial compliance are at risk of developing raised ICP with vasodilation caused by a rise in $PaCO_2$. End-tidal carbon dioxide ($ETCO_2$) may not be a reliable substitute for $PaCO_2$. The correlation between the two methods may be poor, and the $PaCO_2$–$ETCO_2$ gradient may not be stable over time. Therefore, $PaCO_2$ rather than $ETCO_2$ should be monitored whenever possible.

Temperature

Brain temperature is typically 0.5–0.8°C higher than core temperature. Temperature should be measured regularly, as an elevated body temperature may not only be a sign of infection but is itself associated with poor outcome in patients with cerebral ischaemia. Furthermore, neurosurgical patients may be permitted to become somewhat hypothermic in the operating room as mild hypothermia may protect the brain from ischaemic injury. Slow, controlled rewarming of these patients is important in order to prevent cerebral damage and shivering.

Laboratory testing

Apart from ABGs, close monitoring of glucose, sodium and coagulation parameters is necessary in neurosurgical patients.

Hyperglycaemia occurs often in post-operative neurosurgical patients due to high circulating levels of catabolic hormones stimulating gluconeogenesis and reducing glucose tolerance. Hyperglycaemia increases morbidity and mortality in patients with TBI, SAH or spinal cord injury. However, tight glycaemic control (4.4–6.1 mmol l^{-1}) is controversial in these patients. Hypoglycaemic episodes are not uncommon, and increased mortality has been reported in ICU patients with this regimen. A less restrictive target for systemic glucose control (6–10 mmol l^{-1}) has recently been suggested in patients with brain injury and in post-operative neurosurgical patients.

Sodium is the principal determinant of total extracellular volume. Disorders of sodium balance are common in post-operative neurosurgical patients. The syndrome of inappropriate secretion of antidiuretic hormone (SIADH), diabetes insipidus and cerebral salt-wasting syndrome (CSWS) may develop in neurosurgical patients. Hyponatraemia can lead to brain oedema by transmembrane water equilibration across the blood–brain barrier. Manifestations include nausea, vomiting, weakness, disorientation, lethargy, coma and seizures. Hyponatraemia with decreased total body sodium content is caused by renal or nonrenal losses of sodium. Severe hypernatraemia occurs in patients with diabetes insipidus or after osmotically induced loss of water. Clinically, an increased volume of hypotonic urine is present. If hypernatraemia develops abruptly, brain tissue dehydration occurs, leading to restlessness, seizures and hyperreflexia.

Thromboplastin is abundant in brain tissue and plays an important role in the initiation of coagulopathy in patients with brain injury. Furthermore, patients with large intraoperative blood loss, as may be the case in major spinal surgery or resection of meningiomas, may receive large amounts of fluids or packed red blood cells. These patients are also at increased risk for developing coagulation abnormalities and may develop post-operative intracranial or spinal haematoma. Finally, it is important to realize that considerable doses of heparin are used during neuroradiological interventions such as implantations of endovascular stents or coils. Many patients arrive in the ICU with a significantly prolonged activated partial thromboplastin time (aPTT). Coagulation testing and controlled correction of coagulation abnormalities are important in patients after neurosurgical procedures and may prevent haemorrhagic complications.

Further laboratory parameters may be helpful in neurosurgical patients such as plasma troponin levels as an indicator of evolving myocardial infarction in patients with ECG abnormalities.

Neuromonitoring

Clinical scores

Often clinical deterioration is the first sign of a potentially fatal complication such as a rise in ICP, vasospasm, developing intracerebral haematoma and systemic complications. This underlines the importance of standardized repeated neurological assessment to detect such a clinical deterioration as early as possible.

Standardized scoring systems facilitate quantitative reporting of the neurological status and are indispensable if the neurological status needs to be compared with earlier assessments. The most popular score is the Glasgow Coma Scale (GCS), despite the fact that it was not developed for this purpose. It is widely used to estimate the level of consciousness, not only in critically ill patients. Recently, a new coma scale has been introduced: the Full Outline of UnResponsiveness (FOUR Score). It addresses some of the shortcomings of the GCS by including brainstem reflexes and respiration, allowing detection of subtle neurological changes and thus further classification of deeply comatose patients.

To identify post-operative delirium, specific scores such as the Confusion Assessment Method (CAM, CAM-ICU) or the Intensive Care Delirium Screening Checklist (ICDSC) are available. It is recommended such a score is determined once every shift. Furthermore, sedation scores such as the Richmond Agitation–Sedation Scale (RASS) should be used regularly in patients who are sedated in the ICU.

Intracranial pressure

Several methods for ICP monitoring are available, with intraventricular catheters and intraparenchymal probes being the most widely used. An advantage of intraventricular catheters, which are considered to be the 'gold standard' for ICP measurement, is the possibility of drainage of cerebrospinal fluid (CSF) in the treatment of ICP. However, a major disadvantage is the risk of infection increasing over time with the catheter in place. The rationale for monitoring ICP is the finding that increased ICP is a predictor of poor outcome in brain-injured patients. While guidelines from the Brain Trauma Foundation define indications for ICP monitoring in patients with TBI, the indications in post-operative patients are less clear. Up to 18% of patients have a post-operative sustained ICP elevation after elective supratentorial or infratentorial surgery. Especially with repeat surgery, a long duration of intracranial surgery (>6h) and after resection of meningiomas and gliomas, patients are at increased risk for developing increased ICP. In patients after SAH, the incidence and perhaps the relevance of raised ICP are possibly underestimated. However, data showing a clear relationship between ICP monitoring and improved outcome are required before ICP monitoring can be recommended in patients with aneurismal SAH. After ICH, some patients with suspected intracranial hypertension and a decreasing level of consciousness might require invasive ICP monitoring, although its added value beyond clinical or radiological monitoring has not yet been proven. Currently, the decision to monitor ICP in post-operative neurosurgical patients must be based on the individual patient's history and experience of the responsible team.

Cerebral blood flow

Inadequate CBF can contribute to brain ischaemia and result in post-traumatic secondary brain insults after brain injury. Therefore, monitoring of CBF may be useful in brain-injured patients. However, post-operative CBF monitoring is not performed routinely in neurosurgical patients due to a lack of data suggesting an impact on outcome in addition to technical and logistical limitations. Transcranial Doppler may be used for detection and serial monitoring of cerebral vasospasm in patients after SAH.

Brain oxygenation and metabolic monitoring

There are currently no data supporting the use of invasive brain tissue oxygenation or cerebral metabolic monitoring with microdialysis in post-operative neurosurgical patients. Near-infrared spectroscopy (NIRS) may be a non-invasive alternative to monitor cerebral oxygenation. The tissue oxygenation measured by the absorption of near-infrared light gives a continuous measure of cerebral tissue oxygen saturation. However, thresholds for this method are unclear, and the clinical use of NIRS in neurosurgical patients remains limited.

EEG

Post-operative neurosurgical patients are at increased risk of seizures, especially after evacuation of intracerebral or chronic subdural haematomas; surgical procedures for abscess and SAH; and after resection of AVMs, gliomas and meningiomas. The overall incidence of seizures in neurosurgical patients is estimated to be 17%. Whereas overt seizures are easily recognized, non-convulsive seizures and non-convulsive status epilepticus may be clinically undetectable in comatose patients. Not only overt seizures but also non-convulsive seizure activity can aggravate brain damage. Therefore, early detection and immediate treatment is mandatory. Performing an EEG in patients with altered level of consciousness that cannot be otherwise explained is therefore recommended. Continuous EEG monitoring or simplified EEG tracings can be used if required (see also Chapter 8).

Imaging

Brain imaging by CT and MRI offers important information on the patient's brain. However, it only represents the situation at a particular point in time and cannot be used as a monitor. Positron emission tomography (PET) offers measurements of CBF and cerebral oxygen and glucose metabolisms. Accepted indications for post-operative PET imaging are, however, lacking. Imaging generally necessitates intrahospital transport. While imaging can yield invaluable information, it is important to remember that transport of critically ill patients is associated with complications.

Blood pressure control

Both hypo- and hypertension can affect the injured brain and lead to poor outcome. Even short periods of hypotension may compromise cerebral perfusion and oxygenation. Hypertension during emergence from anaesthesia and during the early post-operative phase is associated with a higher incidence of post-operative ICH after intracranial surgery. Therefore, tight blood pressure control is vital in post-operative neurosurgical patients. Blood pressure derangements may be caused by central neurogenic effects on the heart, by changes in systemic vascular resistance due to circulating or local factors, or by dysfunction of brainstem pressor and depressor centres due to direct injury or neurohumoral stimulation. Concomitant medical therapy and pre-existing disease may further affect blood pressure control.

It is important to remember that not all hypertensive episodes require prompt and aggressive normalization of blood pressure. In many neurological emergencies, hypertension is due to the Cushing reflex and is a modulating factor rather than the primary inciting cause of central nervous system injury. The level to which elevated blood pressure should be lowered depends on several factors, and there are no absolute thresholds. Post-operatively, acute hypertensive episodes may be caused by insufficient analgesia, ischaemia, intracranial hypertension, ICH and pre-existing arterial hypertension.

Antihypertensive drugs

In the post-operative care of neurosurgical patients, adequate analgesia is important not only for patient comfort but also to avoid hypertension. If after sufficient pain control and exclusion of other common causes of post-operative hypertension, such as bladder distension or shivering, hypertension persists, blood pressure can be controlled by administration of antihypertensive drugs. Esmolol, labetalol, nicardipine, enalaprilat, urapidil and fenoldopam have no significant effect on CBF and are appropriate and effective for blood pressure control in neurosurgical patients. An overview of antihypertensive drugs commonly used in neurosurgical or neurological patients is presented in Table 20.2. Esmolol is a short-acting, relatively cardioselective β-blocker. Its rapid onset of action and short half-life make it especially useful in managing hypertension during emergence and extubation. Urapidil may increase ICP in patients with intracranial hypertension, whereas in patients with normal intracranial compliance, it has only little effect on ICP. Other drugs such as calcium-channel blocking agents, nitroglycerine and sodium nitroprusside are cerebral vasodilators that increase CBV. Their use may increase ICP and disturb cerebrovascular autoregulation. They are therefore avoided in neurosurgical patients.

Vasopressors

The first intervention for hypotension caused by shock or hypovolaemia is a series of fluid challenges with isotonic or hypertonic fluids. Crystalloids and colloids may be used. Modern hydroxyethyl starch preparations (e.g. HAES 130/0.4) are relatively safe and probably have less of an impact on coagulation. If hypotension is not caused by hypovolaemia, restoration of cerebral perfusion can be achieved by administration of phenylephrine, norepinephrine or dopamine. The decision of which vasopressor to use has to be based on the baseline cardiovascular state of the patient and on the intended goal of therapy. In the injured brain, the effect of various pressors on CBF may be unpredictable and depends on various factors including a possibly disturbed cerebrovascular autoregulation or a dysfunctional blood–brain barrier. The profile and dosage of vasopressors commonly used in neurosurgical and neurological patients are presented in Table 20.3.

Blood pressure management in special situations

Intubation, emergence and extubation

If intubation is necessary in the ICU, a sufficient anaesthetic dose should to be used to avoid acute

Table 20.2 Antihypertensive agents

Agent	Mechanism	Dose	Onset (min)	Duration of action (min)	Side effects	Cautions
Esmolol	β_1-Antagonist	500 µg kg^{-1} bolus, 50–300 µg kg^{-1} min^{-1} infusion	1–2	10–30	Hypotension, bradycardia, nausea, bronchospasm	Asthma, COPD, LV failure, second or third-degree AV block
Labetalol	α_1-, β_1-, β_2-Antagonist	5–80 mg boluses up to maximum 300 mg; 0.5–2 mg min^{-1} infusion	5–10	180–360	Bradycardia, nausea, vomiting, dizziness, bronchospasm, hypotension, hepatic injury	Asthma, COPD, LV failure, second- or third-degree AV block
Enalaprilat	ACE inhibitor	0.625 mg bolus, then 1.25–5 mg every 6 h	15–30	360–720	Hypotension, headache, cough	Acute MI, hypersensitivity
Nicardipine	L-type calcium-channel blocker	5–15 mg h^{-1} infusion	5–10	30–240	Reflex tachycardia, nausea, flushing, headache	Severe AS, LV failure, cardiac ischaemia
Fenoldopam	DA1 agonist	0.1–0.3 mg kg^{-1} min^{-1} infusion	5–15	30–240	Tachycardia, nausea, headache, flushing	Glaucoma, liver disease
Urapidil	α_1-Antagonist	5–25 mg bolus, then 5–30 mg h^{-1} infusion	2–10	360	Nausea, vertigo, headache	Aortic stenosis

ACE, angiotensin-converting enzyme; AS, aortic stenosis; AV, atrioventricular; COPD, chronic obstructive pulmonary disease; LV, left ventricle; MI, myocardial infarction.
Adapted from Rose and Mayer (2004).

hypertension potentially resulting in cerebral oedema and bleeding. Incremental doses of esmolol may still be necessary to control blood pressure. However, hypotension may also develop, and a selection of vasoactive drugs should be prepared prior to the administration of anaesthetics. Hypertension during emergence from anaesthesia for intracranial surgery and in the early post-operative period is common. Total intravenous anaesthesia using propofol and remifentanil may possibly reduce the incidence of these hypertensive episodes during emergence. Nevertheless, in addition to sufficient analgesia, the administration of boluses of short-acting antihypertensive drugs such as esmolol, labetalol or urapidil may be necessary to control blood pressure during emergence and extubation. Some patients will require blood pressure control with a continuous infusion of an antihypertensive drug. Table 20.2 shows possible regimens. In patients with increased ICP, coughing during extubation should be prevented.

The use of a remifentanil infusion during extubation may decrease coughing. In some patients, intravenous lidocaine (1 mg kg^{-1}) may also be effective.

After carotid endarterectomy

After carotid endarterectomy, many patients experience carotid sinus dysfunction resulting in hypo- or hypertension. In the case of hypotension, patients are at increased risk of stroke and myocardial infarction, whereas hypertension may cause cerebral hyperaemia and haemorrhage. Efforts should be made to maintain blood pressure in the normal pre-operative range (see also Chapter 13).

Subarachnoid haemorrhage and cerebral vasospasm

Aneurysmal SAH and rebleeding are accompanied by a high rate of mortality and morbidity. Blood pressure control in these patients requires special consideration and is discussed in Chapters 13 and 22.

Table 20.3. Vasopressors

Agent	Mechanism	Dose	Onset (min)	Duration of action (min)	Side effects	Cautions
Phenylephrine	α_1-agonist	50–100 µg bolus; 40–180 µg min^{-1}	Immediate	10–15	Myocardial ischaemia, tachycardia, headache, nausea	Tachyarrhythmias, CAD, thyroid disease
Norepinephrine	α_1-, β_1-agonist	2–40 µg min^{-1}	Immediate	<10	Tachycardia, limb ischaemia	Myocardial ischaemia, sulfa hypersensitivity
Dopamine	DA1 agonist	1–2.5 µg kg^{-1} min^{-1}	1–2	<10	Tachycardia, nausea, headache, chest pain, dyspnea, ischaemic limb necrosis	Tachyarrhythmias, CAD, sulfa hypersensitivity
	α_1 DA1 agonist	2.5–10 µg kg^{-1} min^{-1}				
	α_1, β_1, DA1 agonist	>10 µg kg^{-1} min^{-1}				

CAD, coronary artery disease.
Adapted from Rose and Mayer (2004).

Arteriovenous malformation correction

Cerebral hyperaemia after obliteration of a cerebral AVM may result in haemorrhage or severe oedema in approximately 10% of cases. These hyperaemic complications are thought to result from 'normal perfusion pressure breakthrough'. This widely accepted concept assumes that brain areas previously accustomed to low intravascular pressure are perfused with 'normal' perfusion pressure after AVM resection. Tight blood pressure control in the range of 90–110 mmHg of systolic pressure is used to prevent this problem after AVM resection (see also Chapter 13).

Intracerebral haemorrhage

In the case of ICH, high blood pressure may cause haematoma growth while low blood pressure might exacerbate ischaemia in perihaematoma brain tissue. Current recommendations limit mean arterial blood pressure (MAP) to 130 mmHg in patients with a history of hypertension before craniotomy and to 100 mmHg after craniotomy. In all cases, systolic blood pressure should be maintained above 90 mmHg or CPP above 70 mmHg.

Acute ischaemic stroke

Current guidelines for management of blood pressure during the acute and subacute phases of ischaemic stroke are not consistent. Withholding antihypertensive therapy for acute ischaemic stroke may be acceptable unless the patient is scheduled for thrombolysis, concomitant hypertensive organ damage is present or the blood pressure is excessively high (systolic blood pressure >220 mmHg or diastolic blood pressure >120 mmHg). For patients undergoing intravenous thrombolysis, systolic blood pressure should be <185 mmHg and >110 mmHg before starting thrombolytic therapy.

Traumatic brain injury

Restoring cerebral perfusion to minimize cerebral ischaemia is a key element in all algorithms for the treatment of patients with TBI. Blood pressure management plays an important role in achieving this goal. For further information, see Chapter 21.

The suggested blood pressure management in selected post-operative complications is summarized in Table 20.4.

Management of common complications

Neurological complications

The overall incidence of neurological complications after intracranial and spinal procedures is 3–7%. However, this rate may be much higher after certain surgical procedures and in some patient groups. The history of the patient and the type of surgery performed

Table 20.4 Blood pressure management in selected situations

Condition	Phase	Target (mmHg)	Recommended medications
Intracerebral haemorrhage (Broderick *et al.*, 1999)	Acute phase	MAP ≤130	Esmolol, labetalol, nicardipine IV
	Post-craniotomy	MAP ≤100	Esmolol, labetalol, nicardipine IV
Subarachnoid haemorrhage (Miller *et al.*, 1995)	All cases for 21 days	SBP ≥100	Nimodipine, labetalol, esmolol, nicardipine
	Pre-repair	SBP ≤160	Nimodipine, labetalol, esmolol, nicardipine
	Symptomatic vasospasm	Raise SBP to maximum 200–220	Phenylephrine, norepinephrine, dopamine
Severe traumatic brain injury (Brain Trauma Foundation, 2007)	Acute phase	SBP ≥90	Phenylephrine, norepinephrine, dopamine
	ICU phase (ICP monitor)	CPP ≥60 and CPP ≤90	Phenylephrine, norepinephrine, dopamine Esmolol, labetalol, nicardipine
Traumatic spinal cord injury (Ackerman and Traynelis, 2002)	For the first 7 days	SBP ≥90	Phenylephrine, norepinephrine, dopamine
Spinal cord infarction (Ackerman and Traynelis, 2002)	Within several hours of onset	SBP ≥95 and lumbar drainage of CSF to maintain CSF pressure ≤10 cm	Phenylephrine, norepinephrine, dopamine
Acute ischaemic stroke (Adams *et al.*, 2003)	Outside tPA window	BP ≤220/120	Esmolol, labetalol or nicardipine IV, candesartan PO
	IV thrombolysis	BP ≤185/110 before and ≤180/105 after tPA	Esmolol, labetalol or nicardipine IV

BP, blood pressure; CPP, cerebral perfusion pressure; ICP, intracranial pressure; ICU, intensive care unit; MAP, mean arterial pressure; SBP, systolic blood pressure; tPA, tissue plasminogen activator.
Adapted from Rose and Mayer (2004).

will provide important insights into the problems that may arise. After resection of intra-axial brain tumours, neurological complication rates as high as 25% have been reported, commonly including motor and sensory deficits as well as coma. One of the first signs of any neurological complication may be an altered level of consciousness. In 61% of patients with post-operative haematoma, a decreased level of consciousness is present. This underlines the need for repeated neurological assessment using a standardized scoring system.

Decreased level of consciousness

A decreased level of consciousness is one of the most common clinical symptoms in intensive care, and the differential diagnosis is complex. Delayed diagnosis and treatment of a decreased level of consciousness may lead to significant morbidity and mortality,

increased cost, prolonged length of stay in the ICU and extended overall hospital stay.

Consciousness can be divided into wakefulness and awareness. The former includes arousal, alertness and vigilance, while the latter is the sum of cognitive and emotional functions. Disorders of wakefulness are always accompanied by impaired awareness. Cerebral structures implicated in wakefulness are the ascending reticular activating system (ARAS) and the descending corticoreticular pathways. The cerebral cortex of both hemispheres, associated white-matter tracts, subcortical nuclei and descending corticofugal systems are responsible for awareness. Although the distinction between wakefulness and awareness is important for the understanding of the pathophysiology of altered consciousness, in our experience, the distinction between the two is of limited clinical importance in

Table 20.5 Aetiology of an altered level of consciousness

Diffuse or toxic/metabolic encephalopathies	Supra- or infratentorial focal lesions
Hypotension/hypertension	Post-operative bleeding
Hypoglycaemia	Elevated intracranial pressure
Hypercapnia	Ischaemic stroke
Hypoxia	Perforator stroke
Electrolyte and osmolality abnormalities	Vasospasm
Seizures	Retraction injury
Delirium	Tension pneumocephalus
Drugs/toxins and withdrawal	Cerebrospinal fluid hypotension
Hypo-/hyperthermia	Hyperperfusion syndrome
Meningitis/encephalitis	Basilar artery occlusion
Sepsis	
Hypothyroidism	
Renal and hepatic failure	
Psychosis	

the evaluation of patients with post-operatively altered levels of consciousness. The causes of a decreased level of consciousness can be divided roughly into toxic/metabolic encephalopathies and focal lesions (Table 20.5). In patients with new focal signs, a CT scan should be performed whenever time permits, and the neurosurgical team should be informed as early as possible. The management of selected complications that typically present with a decrease in consciousness and focal signs are presented below. In patients without focal signs, the decision to perform a CT scan must be based on the patient's history and clinical presentation, and on the judgement of the treating physician. Consider MRI for suspected posterior fossa lesions and early detection of ischaemia. Do not delay imaging while waiting for laboratory results.

Post-operative delirium is a disorder of awareness. It is characterized by a global disturbance of cognition, a fluctuating course and sleep–wake cycle disturbances, and should be distinguished from disorders of wakefulness. The clinical presentation of the different forms of delirium can be classified as hyperactive, hypoactive and mixed subtypes. Elderly patients are at increased risk for developing post-operative delirium after neurosurgical procedures (20% by post-operative day 3), especially when pre-existing dementia or diabetes mellitus are present. Delirium can be caused or precipitated by a wide variety of conditions (Table 20.6). Treatment of delirium is primarily supportive; frequent reassurance and presentation of orienting information including date, time, location and names of hospital personnel, use of visual and hearing aids, and limiting physical restraints play an important role. Symptomatic treatment should be provided not only to agitated patients but also to those with a hypoactive subtype of delirium. Symptomatic treatment is frequently provided with haloperidol, a typical antipsychotic dopaminergic antagonist, administered intravenously in incremental doses of 0.5–1 mg every 10–15 min. However, haloperidol and other typical antipsychotic drugs lower the seizure threshold and can potentially precipitate seizures. While atypical antipsychotic drugs such as quetiapine or risperidone are not approved for the symptomatic treatment of delirium, they may be as effective as haloperidol and have a much smaller effect on the seizure threshold.

Intracranial haemorrhage

In patients with a decreasing level of consciousness, new pupillary abnormalities or new focal signs after intracranial surgery, an intracranial haematoma must be rapidly ruled out. An increased risk for developing intracranial haematoma has been described for patients with coagulopathy, those using antiplatelet agents (aspirin and non-steroidal anti-inflammatory drugs) and anticoagulants, after high intraoperative blood loss and after surgery for meningiomas. If an intracranial haematoma is suspected, a CT scan should be performed rapidly whenever possible to establish or rule out the diagnosis. Coagulation abnormalities should be corrected promptly. Surgical re-exploration and evacuation of the haematoma may be necessary, and early consultation with neurosurgeons is essential.

Table 20.6 Precipitating factors in delirium

Type	Factors
Neurological	Head injury Increased intracranial pressure Vascular: • Subarachnoid haemorrhage • Stroke (infarction and intracerebral haemorrhage) • Venous thrombosis • Subdural haemorrhage Infection Non-convulsive status epilepticus Postictal state
Systemic	Underlying dementia Psychogenic disturbances Infections (e.g. urinary tract, pulmonary) Metabolic disorders: • Hypoxia • Hypoglycaemia, hyperglycaemia • Hyponatraemia, hypernatraemia • Hypercalcaemia • Porphyria • Thiamine deficiency (Wernicke's encephalophathy) • Fluid-balance disorders Endocrine • Hypothyroidism • Hyperthyroidism • Cushing's • Hyperparathyroidism • Hepatic failure • Renal failure • Anaemia • Hypothermia
Extrinsic	Drugs • Narcotics • Steroids • Tricyclic antidepressants • Furosemide • Benzodiazepines Pain Bladder catheter use, urinary retention, constipation Intensive care unit admission Alcohol and/or drug withdrawal

Adapted from Johnson (2001).

Cerebral vasospasm

A further important cause of a decreased level of consciousness, possibly in combination with new focal deficits, is cerebral vasospasm. Vasospasm may occur in all patients with subarachnoid haemorrhage. However, the clinical significance is only well documented in patients suffering from aneurismal SAH. Delayed cerebral ischaemic deficits caused by vasospasm complicate SAH in 20–30% of patients initially surviving SAH. Treatment and blood pressure management in patients presenting with vasospasm is controversial and is discussed further in Chapter 22.

Post-operative ischaemic stroke

After carotid endarterectomy, occlusion of the operated carotid artery or perioperative embolic events may cause cerebral ischaemia. If a new focal deficit is present post-operatively, immediate diagnostic evaluation should be performed to differentiate ischaemic stroke from carotid artery occlusion from ICH, which may also occur after carotid endarterectomy (see below). Surgical re-exploration may be necessary.

After stenting of symptomatic intracranial stenosis, perforator stroke is reported with an incidence rate of 3%. Treatment is supportive. The use and dosage of heparin should be discussed with the team performing the intervention.

A further cause of new focal lesions includes retraction injuries. Maintaining retraction on the brain during surgery for adequate exposure can cause brain damage by compression of blood vessels and impairing oxygen delivery to the retracted areas. The incidence of the resulting retraction injuries varies considerably depending not only on surgical technique and duration of retraction but also on the region operated on. In skull base surgery, a rate of 10% has been described. Clinically, brain contusion or infarction after retraction may present as aphasia, hemiparesis, numbness or visual-field defects depending on the region of the brain affected. There is no specific treatment for these lesions.

In all patients with post-operative ischaemic stroke, elevated body temperature and hyperglycaemia should be treated promptly.

Cerebral hyperperfusion

After carotid endarterectomy, 1–3% of patients develop dramatic increases in CBF and present with ipsilateral headache, hypertension, seizures and focal neurological deficits. This constellation of symptoms is known as hyperperfusion syndrome, and the increase in CBF can lead to cerebral oedema and ICH or SAH if left untreated. Hypertension must be treated aggressively.

Post-operative seizures

Neurosurgical patients are at high risk of developing post-operative seizures, especially within the first week after surgery. The overall incidence is 15–20% and is highest during the first 48 h after surgery. Overt seizures rarely pose diagnostic problems, whereas clinically undetectable non-convulsive seizures and non-convulsive status epilepticus may occur in some patients. Therefore, performing an EEG – with continuous EEG monitoring if required and available – is recommendable in patients with inconspicuous imaging results who remain comatose post-operatively, or in patients with altered levels of consciousness that cannot be otherwise explained. There is no proof of the efficacy of anti-epileptic agents in preventing the onset of post-operative epilepsy. However, prophylactic administration of phenytoin, carbamazepine, valproate or phenobarbital may reduce the risk of seizures during the first post-operative week by up to 50%. In patients not experiencing seizures, tapering and discontinuing anticonvulsants after the first post-operative week seems to be appropriate.

For patients who develop post-operative seizures, several drugs are available for treatment. Initially, lorazepam (e.g. boluses of 1–4 mg) or another benzodiazepine is frequently used; if ineffective, propofol or thiopentone are acceptable alternatives. For long-term therapy, phenytoin, carbamazepine or valproate may be used. However, valproate may cause a dysfunction of platelets. The role of newer drugs such as levetiracetam has yet to be defined in post-operative neurosurgical patients. Early consultation with a neurologist to optimize and monitor treatment is recommended.

Cerebrospinal fluid hypotension

Mild CSF hypovolaemia after violation of the dura by dural puncture or minor operative procedures involving opening of the dura during intracranial or spinal surgery may present with postural headache, vertigo, nausea and visual complaints. Acute alterations in mental status and signs of transtentorial herniation 2–4 days after intraoperative CSF drainage, e.g. spinal drainage for aneurysm surgery, may be due to CSF hypotension ('brain sag'). If a CT scan is performed, effacement of the basal cisterns with an oblong brainstem can be

seen. The symptoms are reversible after placement of the patient in the Trendelenburg position.

Cerebrospinal fluid leak

Cerebrospinal fluid leaks need to be closed surgically to avoid meningitis. Continuous nasal discharge after transsphenoidal surgery may be a sign of a CSF leak and should be addressed by analysis for τ-transferrin (tau-transferrin, t-transferrin) or β-trace protein. If a CSF leak is confirmed, treatment consists of surgical repair of the leak.

Cranial nerve palsies

Transsphenoidal surgery may be complicated by cranial nerve palsy or a visual field defect due to the proximity of cranial nerves II–VI to the pituitary gland. If this complication occurs, the patient is brought back to the operation room for re-exploration either directly or after a CT scan or MRI has been performed. However, a new lateral rectus weakness with impaired ocular abduction may represent a false localizing sign due to pressure on the abducens nerve and signify raised ICP.

Spinal haematoma

After spinal procedures such as laminectomy and spinal cord decompression, a haematoma at the operative site may present as a progressive decrease in neurological function. Difficulties with bowel and bladder function may be a sign of lumbar haematoma. MRI provides the best means of investigating patients presenting with such symptoms. If spinal haematoma is present, emergent surgical re-exploration has to be performed in order to avoid permanent neurological sequelae.

If a transthoracic or transabdominal approach is used for spinal cord decompression and stabilization, it is important to consider whether the patient has a pneumothorax requiring drainage with a chest tube. It is also important in the haemodynamically unstable patient to consider the possibility of bleeding from injury to the aorta or common iliac blood vessels, which may require volume resuscitation and surgical re-exploration. As in all neurosurgical patients with post-operative bleeding, correction of any coagulation abnormalities is essential.

Systemic complications

Respiratory dysfunction

Cranial nerve dysfunction interfering with airway patency can occur after procedures in the posterior fossa, at the base of the skull, or after carotid endarterectomy. Brainstem compression by post-operative haematoma or acute obstructive hydrocephalus can lead to irregular respiratory patterns or apnoea. Mechanical airway obstruction can occur due to macroglossia secondary to venous obstruction after posterior fossa surgery or due to oedema or haematoma after carotid endarterectomy or anterior cervical spine surgery. Where there is clinical evidence of airway compromise, careful observation of swallowing should be performed before extubation is attempted. Reintubation, often technically difficult, must be anticipated, and trained staff as well as equipment for the management of a difficult airway should be available when such patients are extubated.

In patients with severe brain injuries, SAH, stroke or spinal cord injury, neurogenic pulmonary oedema may occur in up to 50% of cases. Systemic vasoconstriction in response to the sympathetic storm associated with an acute event results in translocation of blood to the pulmonary circuit. Overdistension of the pulmonary vascular bed results in capillary leak and the development of neurogenic pulmonary oedema. It typically resolves within 1–2 days and is addressed by supportive therapy. Mechanical ventilation may be necessary. Other forms of pulmonary oedema, especially cardiac causes, have to be excluded before making the diagnosis.

Diabetes insipidus, syndrome of inappropriate antidiuretic hormone secretion and cerebral salt-wasting syndrome

Transient or permanent disturbances of sodium levels are common in neurosurgical patients. Diabetes insipidus, SIADH and CSWS may occur, and osmotic diuretics such as mannitol may lead to renal loss of sodium and water. Management of sodium disorders may include replacement or restriction of sodium and water, as well as replacement of antidiuretic hormone and is described in Chapter 19.

Infection and elevated body temperature

Fever and leucocytosis are common in patients after neurosurgical procedures and are frequently not a sign of infection but rather a stress response. The incidence of surgical site infections in neurosurgery is low. After craniotomy, a rate of 4% has been reported. However, such infections may lead to intracranial infections, ventriculitis and meningitis. In the case of surgical site infection, antibiotic therapy and surgical

re-exploration are options for treatment. Antibiotic prophylaxis before neurosurgical procedures is routinely performed in most centres, and has been shown to reduce the rates of post-operative infection after craniotomy and after surgical introduction of intracranial ventricular shunts but not for basilar skull fractures. Patients with post-operative CSF leaks have an increased risk for wound infection.

Pulmonary and non-pulmonary infections are common complications in critically ill patients. Pneumonia can develop in patients with acute neurological disease because of secretion retention or aspiration in patients who cannot protect their airway. Prolonged bladder catheterization may be complicated by urinary tract infection. Maxillary sinusitis develops in 20–40% of patients with nasotracheal intubation, and such nosocomial sinusitis needs to be considered in septic ventilated patients. If present, it should be treated appropriately to reduce the occurrence of ventilator-associated pneumonia. Acute otitis media is seen in about 17% of head-injured patients intubated either nasotracheally or orotracheally.

Elevated body temperature, irrespective of its cause, should be normalized in post-operative neurosurgical patients using paracetamol, metamizole or, if there are no concerns with regard to platelet dysfunction, non-steroidal anti-inflammatory drugs. Physical cooling may also be used. However, shivering may be a relevant problem limiting the use of external cooling.

Hyperglycaemia

Hyperglycaemia must be treated aggressively in all neurosurgical patients. Typically, subcutaneous or intravenous injections of boluses of insulin provide insufficient glycaemic control. We suggest using intravenous infusions of insulin. Currently, there are no clear thresholds for glycaemic control in neurosurgical patients. Recommendations vary from tight glycaemic control (4.4–6.1 mmol l^{-1}) to a threshold of 10 mmol l^{-1}. We suggest that unit-specific guidelines are used defining a threshold that seems acceptable to the responsible clinicians.

Post-operative pain

Post-operative pain is an important issue in neurosurgical patients and may still be undertreated. Fear of side effects of analgesic drugs, lack of standardized protocols and controversy regarding the choice of the anaesthetic regimen for intracranial surgery may be the reason for the reluctance to use adequate analgesia. Scalp infiltration by long-acting local anaesthetics provides a useful basis for post-operative analgesia. If paracetamol fails to achieve sufficient pain control, opiates may be used safely to treat pain after craniotomy provided that they are titrated and adequate monitoring is used. Apart from intravenous morphine, patient-controlled morphine analgesia can be used without an increase in patient morbidity, side effects or compromising neurological assessment. Non-steroidal anti-inflammatory drugs are often avoided in the early post-operative phase because they potentially increase the incidence of intracranial haematoma due to their anti-platelet effect. Alternatively, metamizole may be used before opiates are administered.

Post-operative nausea and vomiting

Post-operative nausea and vomiting (PONV) is one of the most frequent side effects in the post-operative period and is common in neurosurgical patients. Post-operative retching or vomiting causes arterial hypertension and elevates ICP. Thus, PONV not only has a negative impact on the patients' subjective well-being but can also cause major medical complications in neurosurgical patients and delay discharge. For prevention of PONV, the administration of 5-hydroxytryptamine 3 receptor (5-HT$_3$) antagonists intraoperatively is effective, safe and acceptable. Tropisetron 2–5 mg IV or ondansetron 4–8 mg IV can be used for this purpose. Alternatively, droperidol 0.625–1.25 mg IV can be administered. In this small dose, the effects of droperidol on the QT interval are negligible. Treatment of established PONV has not been investigated in post-craniotomy patients. In other groups of patients, administration of 5-HT$_3$ antagonist and droperidol has been recommended. Propofol (up 20 mg IV administered as needed) can be used as a rescue therapy. If patients have already received dexamethasone during the neurosurgical procedure, increasing the dose to treat PONV is not recommended because there is a ceiling effect in the dose range of 5–8 mg.

Stress ulceration

In patients with intracranial disease, especially in TBI, gastrointestinal stress ulcers occur frequently and may lead to clinically significant bleeding, especially with concurrent administration of steroids. Prophylactic administration of antacids, H$_2$ antagonists or sucralfate is effective.

Intrahospital transfer of critically ill neurosurgical patients

Adverse effects of intrahospital transfer may occur in up to 70% of transports. Hypotension and arrhythmias due to inadvertent hypoventilation or hyperventilation, hypertension due to inadequate sedation while shifting the patient, deterioration of gas exchange leading to a fall in oxygen saturation, and an increase in ICP may occur during transport. Furthermore, disconnection of nasogastric or chest tubes and dislocation of the endotracheal tube or disconnection from the ventilator may occur. Problems related to the monitoring include ECG lead disconnection, monitor power failure and disconnection of intravenous or intra-arterial lines. If the patient has to be transferred, standards of intensive monitoring and respiratory care should be maintained during transport and the patient should be accompanied by a minimum of two persons, one of them a critical care nurse. For patients with unstable physiology, a physician is required to accompany the patient. Standard equipment includes monitoring of ECG, pulse oxymetry, blood pressure and respiratory rate, airway management equipment, sufficient gas supply, drugs for resuscitation and intravenous fluids, and a portable ventilator for patients requiring mechanical ventilation.

Further reading

Ackerman, L. L. and Traynelis, V. C. (2002). Treatment of delayed-onset neurological deficit after aortic surgery with lumbar cerebrospinal fluid drainage. *Neurosurgery* **51**, 1414–21.

Adams, H. P. Jr, Adams, R. J., Brott, T. *et al.* (2003). Guidelines for the early management of patients with ischemic stroke: a scientific statement from the Stroke Council of the American Stroke Association. *Stroke* **34**, 1056–83.

Andrews, R. J. and Bringas, J. R. (1993). A review of brain retraction and recommendations for minimizing intraoperative brain injury. *Neurosurgery* **33**, 1052–63.

Asgari, S., Rohrborn, H. J., Engelhorn, T., Fauser, B. and Stolke, D. (2003). Intraoperative measurement of cortical oxygen saturation and blood volume adjacent to cerebral arteriovenous malformations using near-infrared spectroscopy. *Neurosurgery* **52**, 1298–304.

Barker, F. G. II (2007). Efficacy of prophylactic antibiotics against meningitis after craniotomy: a meta-analysis. *Neurosurgery* **60**, 887–94.

Basali, A., Mascha, E. J., Kalfas, I. and Schubert, A. (2000). Relation between perioperative hypertension and intracranial hemorrhage after craniotomy. *Anesthesiology* **93**, 48–54.

Brain Trauma Foundation (2007). Guidelines for the management of severe traumatic brain injury. *J Neurotrauma* **24** (Suppl. 1), S1–106.

Broderick, J. P., Adams, H. P. Jr, Barsan, W. *et al.* (1999). Guidelines for the management of spontaneous intracerebral hemorrhage: a statement for healthcare professionals from a special writing group of the Stroke Council, American Heart Association. *Stroke* **30**, 905–15.

Bruder, N. J. (2002). Awakening management after neurosurgery for intracranial tumours. *Curr Opin Anaesthesiol* **15**, 477–82.

Devlin, J. W., Fong, J. J., Fraser, G. L. and Riker, R. R. (2007). Delirium assessment in the critically ill. *Intensive Care Med* **33**, 929–40.

Eberhart, L. H. J., Morin, A. M., Kranke, P. *et al.* (2007). Prevention and control of postoperative nausea and vomiting in post-craniotomy patients. *Best Pract Res Clin Anaesthesiol* **21**, 575–93.

Finfer, S., Chittock, D. R., Su, S. Y. *et al.* (2009). Intensive versus conventional glucose control in critically ill patients. *N Engl J Med* **360**, 1283–97.

Foy, P. M., Copeland, G. P. and Shaw, M. D. (1981). The incidence of postoperative seizures. *Acta Neurochi (Wien)* **55**, 253–64.

Glantz, M. J., Cole, B. F., Forsyth, P. A. *et al.* (2000). Practice parameter: anticonvulsant prophylaxis in patients with newly diagnosed brain tumors. Report of the Quality Standards Subcommittee of the American Academy of Neurology. *Neurology* **54**, 1886–93.

Howell, S. J. (2007). Carotid endarterectomy. *Br J Anaesth* **99**, 119–31.

Jiang, W. J., Srivastava, T., Gao, F. *et al.* (2006). Perforator stroke after elective stenting of symptomatic intracranial stenosis. *Neurology* **66**, 1868–72.

Johnson, M. H. (2001). Assessing confused patients. *J Neurol Neurosurg Psychiatry* **71** (Suppl. 1), i7–12.

Komotar, R. J., Mocco, J., Ransom, E. R. *et al.* (2005) Herniation secondary to critical postcraniotomy cerebrospinal fluid hypovolemia. *Neurosurgery* **57**, 286–92.

Korinek, A. M. (1997) Risk factors for neurosurgical site infections after craniotomy: a prospective multicenter study of 2944 patients. The French Study Group of Neurosurgical Infections, the SEHP, and the C-CLIN Paris-Nord. Service Epidemiologie Hygiene et Prevention. *Neurosurgery* **41**, 1073–9.

Magni, G., La Rosa, I., Gimignani, S. *et al.* (2007) Early postoperative complications after intracranial surgery: comparison between total intravenous and balanced anesthesia. *J Neurosurg Anesthesiol* **19**, 229–34.

Miller, J. A., Dacey, R. G. Jr and Diringer, M. N. (1995) Safety of hypertensive hypervolemic therapy with phenylephrine in the treatment of delayed ischemic deficits after subarachnoid hemorrhage. *Stroke* **26**, 2260–6.

Nemergut, E. C., Dumont, A. S., Barry, U. T. and Laws, E. R. (2005) Perioperative management of patients undergoing transsphenoidal pituitary surgery. *Anesth Analg* **101**, 1170–81.

Nemergut, E. C., Durieux, M. E., Missaghi, N. B. and Himmelseher, S. (2007) Pain management after craniotomy. *Best Pract Res Clin Anaesthesiol* **21**, 557–73.

Oddo, M., Schmidt, J. M., Mayer, S. A. and Chiolero, R. L. (2008) Glucose control after severe brain injury. *Curr Opin Clin Nutr Metab Care* **11**, 134–9.

Pfister, D., Strebel, S. P. and Steiner, L. A. (2007) Postoperative management of adult central neurosurgical patients: systemic and neuro-monitoring. *Best Pract Res Clin Anaesthesiol* **21**, 449–63.

Prakash, A. and Matta, B. F. (2008) Hyperglycaemia and neurological injury. *Curr Opin Anaesthesiol*, **21** 565–9.

Robertson, C. S., Contant, C. F., Gokaslan, Z. L., Narayan, R. K. and Grossman, R. G. (1992) Cerebral blood flow, arteriovenous oxygen difference, and outcome in head injured patients. *J Neurol Neurosurg Psychiatry* **55**, 594–603.

Rose, J. C. and Mayer, S. A. (2004) Optimizing blood pressure in neurological emergencies. *Neurocritic Care* **1**, 287–99.

Sawaya, R., Hammoud, M., Schoppa, D. *et al.* (1998) Neurosurgical outcomes in a modern series of 400 craniotomies for treatment of parenchymal tumors. *Neurosurgery* **42**, 1044–55.

Smith, M. and Elwell, C. (2009) Near-infrared spectroscopy: shedding light on the injured brain. *Anesth Analg* **108**, 1055–7.

Steiner, T., Kaste, M., Forsting, M. *et al.* (2006) Recommendations for the management of intracranial haemorrhage – part I: spontaneous intracerebral haemorrhage. The European Stroke Initiative Writing Committee and the Writing Committee for the EUSI Executive Committee. *Cerebrovasc Dis* **22**, 294–316.

Waydhas, C. (1999) Intrahospital transport of critically ill patients. *Crit Care* **3**, R83–9.

Wijdicks, E. F., Bamlet, W. R., Maramattom, B. V., Manno, E. M. and McClelland, R. L. (2005) Validation of a new coma scale: the FOUR score. *Ann Neurol* **58**, 585–93.

Zetterling, M. and Ronne-Engstrom, E. (2004) High intraoperative blood loss may be a risk factor for postoperative hematoma. *J Neurosurg Anesthesiol* **16**, 151–5.

Chapter 21

Traumatic brain injury

Ari Ercole and David K. Menon

Introduction

Despite public health measures and improvements in therapy, traumatic brain injury (TBI) remains a leading cause of death and disability in young individuals. Approximately 1.4 million patients suffer a head injury in the UK each year, and about 2500 of these are severe as defined by a post-resuscitation Glasgow Coma Score (GCS) of 8 or less (Table 21.1). The epidemiology of TBI in high-income countries is changing with the effects of improvements in road safety being offset by increases in fall-related injuries in an ageing population. Nevertheless, the direct and indirect socio-economic burden of TBI is profound, as the majority of victims are potentially economically active, and serious, life-long disability is common.

Care of patients with TBI has evolved with improvements in pre-hospital medicine, neuroimaging and access to multidisciplinary expertise through the development of specialist neurotrauma services, together with advances in our understanding of the underlying pathophysiology. Although survival has generally improved, there is enormous variability in inpatient case fatality rate for all head injuries (including for severe head injury, which ought to represent a more homogeneous subgroup of patients) from US and UK centres. Conversely, good outcomes, defined as a Glasgow Outcome Scale of 1 or 2 (Table 21.2) vary from <50 to nearly 70%. Identification of the cause of such variability is important if overall outcome is to improve.

Pathogenesis and pathophysiology

Brain tissue is particularly vulnerable to traumatic insult due to its high specific metabolic requirements and limited energy reserve. In health, oxygen delivery by cerebral blood flow (CBF) is efficiently matched to the cerebral metabolic rate for oxygen ($CMRO_2$) over a range of normal cerebral perfusion pressures (CPPs). After traumatic injury, a reduction in CPP due to either systemic arterial hypotension or increased intracranial pressure (ICP), and/or pathological changes in tissue architecture and function, may lead to a reduction in global or regional oxygen delivery. Furthermore, normal autoregulatory mechanisms may fail in injured brain or when oxygen delivery becomes critically low for a given $CMRO_2$.

The impact of TBI may be conceptually divided into *primary* and *secondary injuries*. The primary injury occurs as an immediate result of the head trauma and, although clearly a determinant of outcome, is generally not regarded as treatable. Subsequent secondary injury occurs as a result of hypoxia or ischaemia and may be equally important in determining the ultimate clinical outcome. Care of the neurotrauma patient is focused on preventing, or at least limiting, the secondary neurological injury.

At the moment of impact, the head is subjected to a variety of external forces governed, according to Newton's second law, by the size and direction of the acceleration and/or deceleration experienced. From this, it follows that mechanisms of injury involving high-speed impacts with rigid objects are associated with particularly large forces. It is the magnitude and time course of these forces that determines the nature of the injuries sustained (Fig. 21.1). As the intracranial contents are not uniformly dense and have inhomogeneous and anisotropic viscoelastic properties, the brain experiences a complex spatiotemporally varying combination of tensile, compressive and shearing strains, which can lead to an equally complex pattern of structural lesions, which may be focal or diffuse. Furthermore, sudden forces applied to the skull may initiate pressure waves that are focused by the approximately spherical cranial cavity giving rise to damage to

Core Topics in Neuroanaesthesia and Neurointensive Care, eds. Basil F. Matta, David K. Menon and Martin Smith. Published by Cambridge University Press. © Cambridge University Press 2011.

Table 21.1 Glasgow Coma Scale for adults

Parameter	15-Point adult scale	Score[a]
Eye opening	Spontaneous	4
	To sound	3
	To pain	2
	None	1
Best verbal response	Orientated	5
	Confused	4
	Inappropriate words	3
	Incomprehensible sounds	2
	None	1
Best motor response	Obeys commands	6
	Localizes pain	5
	Flexion (withdrawal)	4
	Flexion (abnormal)	3
	Extension	2
	None	1

[a] The best score achieved in each domain is recorded.

Table 21.2 Glasgow Outcome Scale

Score	Outcome
1	Good recovery
2	Moderate disability
3	Severe disability
4	Vegetative state
5	Dead

Many studies dichotomize the scale to 'good outcome' (1 and 2) and 'poor outcome' (3–5).

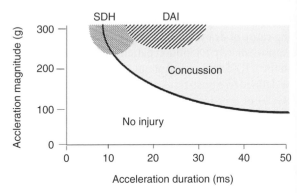

Fig. 21.1. Effect of the duration and magnitude of acceleration/deceleration on the type of injury produced in the brain. DAI, diffuse axonal injury; SDH, subdural haematoma.

deep structures or leading to contracoup lesions well away from the point of impact. Injury occurs not only at a macroscopic and cellular level but also at a subcellular level, resulting in initial widespread neuronal dysfunction. At the same time, macroscopic contusions and vascular disruption leading to axial or extra-axial haematomas will be associated with temporally evolving microscopic and ultramicroscopic changes such as ischaemia, astrocyte swelling with microvascular compromise and disruption of the blood–brain barrier (BBB).

A range of inflammatory and cytotoxic processes lasting hours or days may be triggered depending on the lesion (Fig. 21.2). Localized excitatory neurotransmitter accumulation leads to activation of N-methyl-D-aspartate (NMDA) receptors resulting in necrotic or apoptotic cell death mediated by calcium/calmodulin-dependent enzymes such as nitric oxide synthetase and calcineurin.

Increased production of pro-inflammatory cytokines (such as interleukin-6 (IL-6)) and anti-inflammatory cytokines (such as IL-10), is seen along with adhesion molecule upregulation, resulting in early neutrophil influx and later recruitment of lymphocytes and macrophages and the transformation of

microglial cells into dendritic antigen-presenting cells (Fig. 21.3). These mononuclear cells may contribute to the later stages of a prolonged inflammatory response that may be associated with the laying down of amyloid. Indeed, head injury is a recognized risk factor for both amyloid deposition in the brain and the development of Alzheimer's disease. Furthermore, the risk of these outcomes is related to the individual's apolipoprotein E (ApoE) genotype. The presence of the ApoE-ε4 variant is not only implicated in the development of Alzheimer's disease but is also directly associated with poor outcome and cognitive function after TBI. Indeed, it is becoming increasingly clear that outcome after TBI is in part genetically determined, with a number of polymorphisms in genes involved with vascular function, immune response and catecholamine metabolism having already been identified as significant.

Cerebral perfusion after traumatic brain injury

The varied consequences of a single structural pathology are well reflected by the sequential changes in

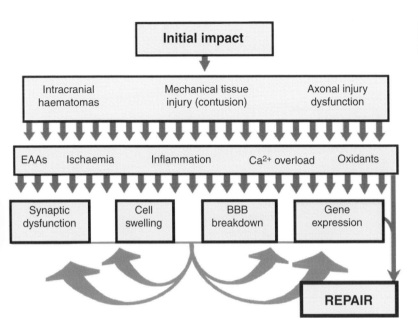

Fig. 21.2. Sequential activation of injury processes in traumatic brain injury. EAAs, excitatory amino acids.

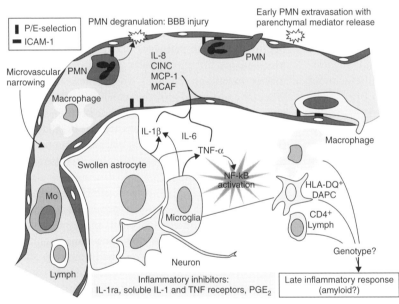

Fig. 21.3. Induction of inflammatory responses following acute brain injury: tumour necrosis factor alpha (TNF-α), interleukin-1β (IL-1β) and IL-6 are secreted by astrocytes and microglial cells, with later production of chemokines including IL-8, cytokine-induced neutrophil chemotactic factor (CINC), monocyte chemoattractant protein-1 (MCP-1) and monocyte chemotactic and activating factor (MCAF), which attracts monocytes and macrophages. Leucocytes attracted by these chemokines subsequently interact with adhesion molecules such as P- and E-selectin and intracellular adhesion molecule-1 (ICAM-1). The initial cellular response is mainly polymorphonuclear (PMN); later cellular responses predominantly involve invading macrophages and CD4+ lymphocytes. These cells, along with microglia-derived HLA-DQ+ tissue macrophages with the morphology of dendritic antigen-presenting cells (DAPCs) may be responsible for a sustained inflammatory response, the magnitude of which may show genetic polymorphism. Tumour necrosis factor alpha also produces activation of the nuclear factor NF-κB, which has wide ranging effects. BBB, blood–brain barrier; Mo, monocyte. (Adapted from Menon, 1999, with permission.)

cerebrovascular physiology that are observed following head injury (Fig. 21.4). Classically, CBF is thought to show triphasic behaviour after injury. In the first 12 h or so after TBI (phase I), global CBF is observed to fall, as microvascular dysfunction may limit the ability of the injured brain to autoregulate for CPP values below 60–70 mmHg. Indeed, regional CBF may fall to ischaemic levels. Between 12 and 24 h post-injury (phase II),

CBF increases and may become supranormal. While many reports refer to this phenomenon as hyperaemia, the absence of consistent reductions in cerebral oxygen extraction suggest preservation of flow–metabolism coupling, suggesting that hyperperfusion is a more appropriate description, at least in some cases. Cerebral blood flow values begin to fall again several days after head injury (phase III). In some patients,

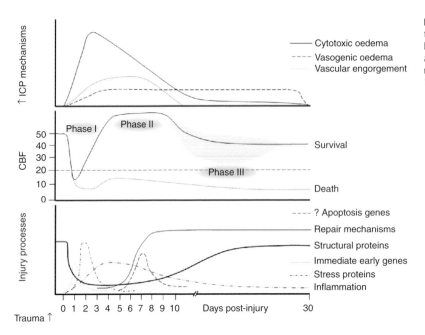

Fig. 21.4. Time line of contributions to intracranial pressure (ICP), triphasic behaviour of cerebral blood flow (CBF) and their underlying pathophysiological mechanisms. (Modified from Bullock, 1997).

these reductions in CBF may be associated with marked increases in large vessel flow velocity measured by transcranial Doppler (TCD) ultrasound, suggesting vasospasm (secondary to traumatic subarachnoid haemorrhage (SAH)) as a possible mechanism.

These haemodynamic responses also define the vascular contribution to ICP elevation over time (Fig. 21.4). Immediately after head injury, there is no vascular engorgement, and while a transient BBB leak has been reported immediately after impact in experimental animals, this phenomenon is too short lived to be clinically appreciated. Apart from surgical lesions (e.g. intracranial haematomas), ICP elevation during this phase is commonly the consequence of cytotoxic oedema; ischaemia results in uncompensated intracellular cation accumulation in neurons and astrocytes, with water following the resulting osmotic disturbance. From the second day post-injury, increases in CBF and cerebral blood volume (CBV) make vascular engorgement an important contributor to intracranial hypertension. The integrity of the BBB appears to become compromised between the second and fifth days. Ionic and macromolecular osmotic and hydrostatic gradients then give rise to a vasogenic oedema with extravasation of proteinaceous ultrafiltrate leading to brain swelling. The nature of this limited disruption of the BBB is complex, and numerous processes have been proposed including endothelial cell retraction, uncoupling of tight junctions and proteolytic breakdown of basement membrane. Activation and/or upregulation of a number of molecular pathways occurs after ischaemia. Mechanisms for extracellular proteolysis (involving matrix metalloproteinases), angiogenesis (involving vascular endothelial growth factor) and inflammation (involving thrombin and nitric oxide synthetase) have all been implicated. A more catastrophic breakdown of capillary integrity with cellular extravasation may also take place. Such *haemorrhagic conversion* is also a complex process, resulting from oxidative stress as a result of prolonged ischaemia and aggravated by reperfusion. Unfortunately for the clinician, patients are very heterogeneous, with different mechanisms responsible for intracranial hypertension operating concurrently at any given time point. However, the framework above does provide a useful basis on which to select initial 'best-guess' therapy in an individual patient, especially when data from multimodality monitoring and advanced imaging are also available to help guide therapeutic choices.

In health, ICP represents the equilibrium pressure at which cerebrospinal fluid (CSF) production and absorption are in balance. The production of CSF remains constant as long as CPP remains adequate. Absorption of CSF through the arachnoid granulations is a passive process and increases with the increase in CSF pressure.

The intracranial contents are rigidly confined within the skull. Small increases in volume from cerebral oedema, vascular congestion or the presence of an intracranial space-occupying lesion can initially be compensated for by translocation of CSF into the spinal subarachnoid space or a reduction in cerebral venous volume. Once this mechanism is exhausted, or if CSF drainage is impaired, ICP will necessarily rise rapidly with further increases in intracranial contents. This leads to the concept of a pressure–volume compliance curve. As CPP is determined by the difference between mean arterial pressure (MAP) and ICP, a high ICP will lead to cerebral ischaemia. Prolonged rises in ICP are associated with a poor prognosis, and vigorous treatment should be instituted if ICP exceeds 20–25 mmHg for >5 min or so.

Arterial carbon dioxide tension ($PaCO_2$) is one of the most potent regulators of cerebral haemodynamics. Cerebral blood flow increases linearly by about 25% per kPa increase in $PaCO_2$ over the range of 3–10 kPa. The effect of $PaCO_2$ on CBV is less pronounced, changing by about 10% per kPa in the healthy individual. However, in the injured brain, the relationship between $PaCO_2$, CBV and ICP is less predictable. The CBV constitutes only around 5% of the total intracranial volume, but, as the brain is situated in an enclosed space, even a small change in CBV can have a profound effect on ICP, particularly in patients with reduced intracranial compliance.

Hypoxaemia is also a potent cerebral vasodilator capable of overriding any vasoconstriction from hypocapnia. However, due to the shape of the oxygen–haemoglobin dissociation curve, arterial oxygen content is initially well preserved for PaO_2 in the physiological range. Consequently, CBF remains fairly constant until a PaO_2 threshold around 7–8 kPa, below which arterial vasodilation causes CBF to increase very rapidly. In healthy volunteers, this corresponds to only modest reductions in oxygen saturation (SpO_2) with SpO_2 <90%.

There is substantial evidence that hyperoxia is capable of inducing cerebral vasoconstriction, which may variably reduce blood flow by 10–27% in healthy volunteers. The physiology of this hyperoxic vasoreactivity is less well defined and appears to depend on other factors such as $PaCO_2$, vascular disease and injury.

Systemic effects of head injury

In addition to the effects of extracranial trauma, TBI itself is a multisystem disorder with profound systemic complications. Respiratory, cardiovascular, haematological, electrolyte and neuroendocrinological dysfunction may occur with important implications for treatment and outcome.

Immediate or delayed hypoxia is common after TBI and is associated with poor neurological outcome. The causes of hypoxaemia after traumatic injury may include the following:

- Airway obstruction.
- Abnormal respiratory patterns as a result of cerebral hemispheric or basal ganglia damage.
- Neurogenic alterations in residual functional capacity and ventilation/perfusion matching.
- Acute neurogenic pulmonary oedema.
- Aspiration pneumonia/pneumonitis due to impaired airway reflexes, and subsequent acute respiratory distress syndrome.
- Direct lung trauma, pneumothorax or tracheobronchial injury.

Systemic haemodynamic disturbances may be observed after TBI. Increased sympathetic activation occurs as a reflex response to raised ICP, after brainstem compression or medullary ischaemia. This can give rise to severe hypertension, cardiac dysrhythmias, acute ECG abnormalities, myocardial ischaemia and even necrosis. The presence of these cardiovascular changes may complicate the management of the head-injured patient with cerebral hypoperfusion, as the use of inotropes to preserve cerebral perfusion may simultaneously worsen the myocardial ischaemia. On the other hand, the presence of intracranial pathology may prohibit the use of venodilators because of their cerebral vasodilatory effects. Increased levels of circulating catecholamines and cortisol may also give rise to hyperglycaemia, which, if untreated, is known to worsen neurological outcome. The stress response is also associated with an increased risk of gastric ulceration and gastrointestinal bleeding.

Coagulation disturbances are seen in TBI patients, not only as a result of haemorrhage from extracranial injuries but also as a direct result of the brain injury itself. Release of brain tissue thromboplastin and platelet activation by damaged cerebral endothelium may independently activate the coagulation cascade, resulting in intravascular coagulation and coagulation factor depletion. Fibrin deposition on cerebral endothelium has been observed and may impair oxygen diffusion and worsen cerebral tissue hypoxia. Severe coagulopathy is a predictor of poor outcome.

Hyponatraemia may contribute to cerebral oedema and lower the threshold for seizures. It may arise after TBI either due to disordered antidiuretic hormone (ADH) secretion out of proportion to serum osmolarity (syndrome of inappropriate antidiuretic hormone hypersecretion, SIADH) or due to enhanced renal sodium losses through cerebral salt wasting (cerebral salt-wasting syndrome, CSWS), thought to be mediated by elevated levels of brain natriuretic peptide. While hypernatraemia is commonly iatrogenic, secondary to hyperosmolar therapy for raised ICP, it may also occur due to hypothalamic/pituitary axis dysfunction leading to diabetes insipidus.

Thermoregulatory dysfunction is known to occur after TBI. A primary, non-infectious, post-traumatic hyperthemia is not uncommon, and may have several mechanisms. An altered thermoregulatory set point may arise either as a regulated hypothalamic response to inflammatory cytokines or through physical damage to thermoregulatory pathways. Hypermetabolism due to autonomic dysfunction or from increased muscular activity (e.g. with dystonia) may also increase thermogenesis. Neurogenic hyperthermia is essentially a diagnosis of exclusion, as sepsis is very common after significant trauma. However, it should be appreciated that any significant elevation of body temperature is generally regarded to be harmful through its effects on metabolic rate, glutamate release and inflammatory activity.

Initial assessment and stabilization of head-injured patients

Modern initial trauma management follows the standard teaching of a rapid primary assessment to identify and correct catastrophic haemorrhage, life-threatening airway, breathing and circulatory problems ('<C>ABCDE'). The presence of a potential TBI is a highly significant finding. Cerebral oxygen delivery is dependent on adequate oxygenation and CBF, either of which may be disturbed after trauma. Secondary brain damage begins and continues to occur from the moment of injury and for every moment that the patient is hypoxic or hypotensive. Arterial oxygenation saturation <90% and systolic blood pressure <90 mmHg have repeatedly been shown to be predictors of poor outcome. Consequently, it is imperative that cardiorespiratory physiology is quickly restored and optimized. This is the aim of the initial resuscitation phase in head injury.

Pre-hospital assessment and resuscitation

Hypotension and hypoxia are common early pre-hospital findings after traumatic injury. While is generally accepted that long times at the injury scene are associated with increased mortality, airway obstruction (due to reduced consciousness or direct trauma), significant pneumothorax and external haemorrhage can often be quickly remedied. This suggests a therapeutic window of opportunity, and it is the aim of pre-hospital care to identify significant injuries and, where possible, intervene promptly in order to minimize secondary brain injury. Such interventions must be balanced against a need to expedite the rapid evacuation of the patient to hospital for more definitive assessment and management without unnecessary delay.

The scene of an incident may be hazardous, with noise and other environmental factors making it a far from ideal environment for patient assessment. Trauma patients are often young, and as such may initially exhibit a high degree of physiological compensation even after quite major injury. A quick evaluation of the mechanism of injury can be invaluable in predicting the likelihood of otherwise occult injury, so that subsequent decompensation can be anticipated. An assessment of the likely energy transfer should be made: this will be high after rapid decelerations such as with high-speed impacts with rigid objects, intrusion into a vehicle or ejection. The at-scene death of other vehicle occupants should alert the clinician and the receiving team to a significant mechanism of injury. Entrapment is clinically significant after road traffic collisions. Larger forces are typically involved and treatment options for a trapped patient may be significantly limited or unavoidably delayed if access to the casualty is hampered. Both the on-scene and receiving clinician must be wary of insidious hypovolaemia and hypothermia.

The GCS provides a robust starting point in assessing the severity of TBI and any subsequent improvement or deterioration. Hypoxia, hypotension, hypoglycaemia and alcohol or drug intoxication may potentially coexist with TBI and also depress the level of consciousness. This can lead to diagnostic confusion, and the GCS should be regularly reassessed as the patient is resuscitated and once any reversible factors have been corrected. Other gross neurological disability (e.g. pupil size, symmetry and reactivity; limb movement) should similarly be recorded regularly.

Initial resuscitation

Airway obstruction is common immediately after severe traumatic injury and initiates a vicious cycle of hypoxaemia and consequent secondary brain injury. A patent airway must be obtained immediately using simple manoeuvres in the first instance if possible. It will be impossible to clinically rule out spinal injury in any patient with depressed consciousness, and the cervical spine should generally be immobilized in any patient in whom TBI is suspected, as coexisting cervical spine injury is relatively common.

Tracheal intubation remains the gold standard for airway management. Indications for intubation include the following:

- Inability to maintain or protect airway through depressed level of consciousness (typically, but not exclusively, GCS <9).
- Airway obstruction (e.g. through bleeding, maxillofacial trauma).
- Hypoxaemia, not correctable with supplemental oxygen alone.
- Ventilatory failure.
- Patients who are medically unmanageable as a result of a combative state.

The timing, risks and benefits of tracheal intubation must be carefully weighed. It must be remembered that clinical assessment of sedated and mechanically ventilated patients is rendered more difficult. In some cases, the level of consciousness may improve spontaneously or after resuscitation.

Survival of patients with injuries severe enough to allow intubation without drugs is dismal. Pre-hospital endotracheal intubation using rapid sequence induction (RSI) is increasingly available in the UK. The conduct of anaesthesia is essentially the same as that in hospital and is discussed below. However, out-of-hospital induction of anaesthesia, tracheal intubation and positive pressure ventilation of potentially hypovolaemic patients with in-line spinal immobilization is hazardous, and suboptimal performance may explain why a mortality or morbidity benefit is difficult to demonstrate conclusively. A particular difficulty is presented by combative mild/moderate TBI patients in whom simple sedation is clearly hazardous, and the risks and benefits of intubation must be evaluated very carefully.

Irrespective of the setting, anaesthesia and tracheal intubation of the head-injured patient is potentially difficult. Pre-oxygenation is mandatory but may be difficult if the patient is combative, or less effective in the presence of concurrent lung injury. A full stomach must be assumed, and RSI using a titrated low dose of induction agent followed by a rapid-acting muscle relaxant is usual. Manual in-line cervical spine immobilization must be maintained, although this makes laryngoscopy more difficult. Temporary removal of the anterior portion of the hard collar improves mouth opening and laryngoscopy grade. Maxillofacial injury and airway trauma or bleeding result may further complicate airway management, and a difficult airway must always be anticipated. Alternative airway devices (such as the laryngeal mask), or novel airway equipment (such as the Airtraq), may be useful adjuncts in selected patients. Alternative means of oxygenation and ventilation must be immediately available for when laryngoscopy and tracheal intubation is difficult or impossible. If orotracheal intubation is impossible, the airway should instead be secured by cricothyrotomy. Indeed, a primary surgical airway may be safer if the upper airway anatomy is severely distorted, although this is rare. Nasal intubation is hazardous in the presence of a base of skull fracture, may cause bleeding and has a high risk of sinus infection and is therefore best avoided.

As direct laryngoscopy may be difficult and auscultation is unreliable, use of expired gas carbon dioxide monitoring is essential to confirm initial endotracheal tube placement. Capnography also provides a continuous estimate of $PaCO_2$ as well as an early warning of changes in cardiac output.

The choice of anaesthetic agents should allow rapid control of a potentially difficult airway while also conferring haemodynamic stability. Thiopentone and propofol are commonly used as induction agents, but this choice is of less importance than the way the drug is administered. Head-injured patients have low anaesthetic requirements and severe hypotension may occur with induction agent overdose, particularly in the presence of hypovolaemia. Etomidate has a reasonably stable cardiovascular profile but may cause significant adrenal suppression even after a single dose; this may be particularly undesirable, as adrenal insufficiency is already common after TBI. Induction doses of ketamine are regarded by some clinicians as contraindicated after TBI due to concerns regarding its dose-dependent effect on CBV and ICP, although the clinical significance of this may be doubtful.

Laryngoscopy and tracheal intubation are highly stimulating procedures and fentanyl 1–2 µg kg^{-1} IV or lidocaine 1 mg kg^{-1} IV may be a useful adjunct in attenuating the cerebrovascular response. Multiple or prolonged attempts at laryngoscopy are to be avoided if at all possible. Suxamethonium 1–1.5 mg kg^{-1} is commonly used as a muscle relaxant as it reliably and rapidly produces excellent intubating conditions. Suxamethonium may result in a transient rise in ICP from increased carbon dioxide production and cerebral stimulation via afferent muscle activity. However, this is probably not clinically significant in practice, whereas the potential risks of hypoxaemia and hypercapnia from failure to secure the airway are more tangible. The increase in serum potassium associated with the use of suxamethonium in the critically ill or after spinal injury may be an important consideration at later stages but not in the acute setting (<48 h after the initial injury).

Once the airway has been secured, the lungs are mechanically ventilated to maintain adequate arterial oxygen saturation and arterial carbon dioxide tension at the lower end of normality (end-tidal carbon dioxide (EtCO$_2$) between 4.5 and 5.0 kPa). Hypercapnia, leading to vasodilation and potentially a rise in ICP, is clearly undesirable. Hypocapnia (PaCO$_2$ <4.5 kPa), however, must also be avoided (except as a temporary treatment for acute refractory cerebral herniation), as the resultant vasoconstriction may lead to significant ischaemia and may worsen outcome. Oxygenation and ventilation should be verified regularly by arterial blood gas analysis. Capnography should be used to provide a continuous surrogate for PaCO$_2$. However, it must be appreciated that, in the presence of lung injuries, the presence of ventilation–perfusion mismatch may lead to an appreciable arterial–alveolar carbon dioxide gradient. Under these circumstances, EtCO$_2$ may be much lower than PaCO$_2$. Ongoing sedation and muscle relaxation will be required to optimize physiology, reduce CMRO$_2$ and prevent the patient from coughing or straining on the endotracheal tube.

Blood pressure disturbances are common after TBI. Hypertension may be observed as a compensatory response to maintain cerebral perfusion in the face of rising ICP. Therefore, moderate levels of hypertension should generally be tolerated. However, blood pressures above the upper limit of autoregulation (MAP >130 mmHg) should be actively treated, as they will increase CBV and ICP and may worsen any intracranial haemorrhage. Hypotension, on the other hand, must be treated aggressively if CBF is to be maintained. Although uncommon after isolated TBI, hypotension

may occur as a result of other injuries and/or iatrogenically as a result of positive pressure ventilation, sedative drugs or after mannitol-induced diuresis. In the healthy brain, CBF is maintained in the presence of moderate hypotension through autoregulation mediated by reflex vasodilation. In the injured brain, however, systemic hypotension rapidly causes cerebral ischaemia. This may occur either through impaired autoregulation or because vasodilation in the presence of intracranial hypertension increases ICP further, reducing CPP and therefore CBF ('vasodilatory cascade'). In either case, it is essential to avoid systemic hypotension: an analysis by the American National Traumatic Coma Data Bank has demonstrated that systolic blood pressure <90 mmHg is a significant independent factor contributing to poor outcome (Fig. 21.5).

Normotension should be targeted in the first instance until the nature of any cerebral lesion and ICP have been quantified. Hypotension must prompt an immediate and thorough investigation for blood loss with laparotomy and/or thoracotomy if the patient is unstable. Significant hypovolaemia may be masked in the young or by systemic hypertension secondary to intense sympathetic stimulation after TBI. Eventual decompensation with ongoing blood loss, however, is likely to be sudden and potentially catastrophic.

The presence of a head injury has important implications for the resuscitation of the polytrauma patient. A large proportion of trauma-related deaths occur through uncontrollable bleeding. Early haemostasis (<C>ABCDE) is important if a self-perpetuating triad of acidosis, hypothermia and coagulopathy is to be avoided. Although there is increasing interest in permissive hypotensive after major extracranial trauma, this is contraindicated after TBI, and hypovolaemia must be treated sufficiently to maintain adequate CBF.

It is imperative that the source of any haemorrhage be identified as quickly as possible. External bleeding must either be excluded or controlled. Scalp lacerations are common after head injury and may cause hypovolaemia sufficient to precipitate hypotension even in adults, particularly once anaesthetized and mechanically ventilated. Suspicion of significant abdominal or intrathoracic bleeding must prompt immediate imaging and surgical intervention. Clinical examination of the pelvis is often unhelpful and may be dangerous. If there is any reasonable possibility of a pelvic fracture, an external pelvic splint/binder should be applied and the pelvis subsequently 'cleared' radiographically. Blood loss from femoral

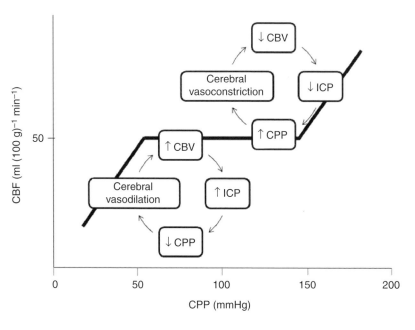

Fig. 21.5. Cerebrovascular autoregulation and vasodilator/vasoconstrictor cascades. At low cerebral perfusion pressure (CPP), the vasodilatory response leads to increased cerebral blood volume (CBV) and therefore intracranial pressure (ICP), further reducing CPP and leading to a vicious cycle of intracranial hypertension. Conversely, CPP elevation not only improves cerebral perfusion but also leads to autoregulatory vasoconstriction, reducing CBV and therefore ICP.

fractures, particularly when bilateral, may be significant and mid-shaft fractures should have traction splints applied.

Either crystalloids or colloids may be used for initial volume expansion. While the use of hypertonic fluids for volume expansion in severely head-injured patients is conceptually attractive, clear clinical benefit has not been shown. However, hypotonic fluids must be avoided, as these may worsen cerebral oedema. Haemodilution will occur with volume expansion, and thromboelastography has demonstrated that a measurable coagulopathy may develop extremely quickly, even when conventional laboratory tests of coagulation remain relatively unchanged. Thus, in the face of significant haemorrhage, blood products should be employed early in the resuscitation phase. Increasing evidence from military trauma suggests that packed red cells and fresh frozen plasma should be transfused in a ratio approaching 1:1 from the outset along with early fibrinogen and platelet replacement. The benefit of such an approach in civilian trauma remains unproven. A haemoglobin concentration of around 10 g dl^{-1} should be maintained to promote oxygen delivery and optimal blood rheology. While rapid or excessive warming is undesirable after neurological injury, deep hypothermia (<33°C) will lead to cardiovascular compromise and coagulopathy, and should be avoided. External haemorrhage must be controlled immediately. Where surgery is required, it should be focused on achieving physiological stability ('damage control' surgery) in the first instance.

The use of glucose-containing solutions should be avoided (except for the treatment of hypoglycaemia), as they are ineffective plasma expanders and may cause hyponatraemia, and because they produce hyperglycaemia, which has been correlated with poor outcome after head injury. Hyperglycaemia should be actively treated and blood glucose levels controlled with an intravenous infusion of rapid-acting insulin. Because many head-injured patients receive mannitol, an adequate urine output is often a poor indicator of volume status in these patients. Central venous pressure monitoring may be helpful in guiding intravascular resuscitation but should be combined with the use of cardiac output monitoring such as pulmonary artery catheterization or pulse contour analysis in the elderly, patients with heart disease and in those patients who require significant or escalating levels of inotropic support.

Cerebral venous drainage should be optimized as far as possible. Compression of the internal jugular vessels may occur with excessively tight endotracheal tube ties or cervical collars. A slight head-up position should be adopted unless contraindicated (e.g. by suspected spinal injuries).

Dilated or unreactive pupil(s), anisocoria, extensor posturing or a sudden deterioration in GCS may signify cerebral herniation. Osmotherapy with mannitol or hypertonic saline should be considered. Under such circumstances, hyperventilation to an EtCO$_2$ of 4.0 (or lower) may be a helpful temporizing measure and this will be discussed in more detail below.

Emergency imaging

Emergency department imaging is aimed at rapidly identifying life-threatening occult injuries. Plain radiographs of the chest and pelvis are useful and usually performed in conjunction with focused ultrasonographic examination ('FAST scan') to rapidly assess the perihepatic, perirenal, pericardial, perisplenic, pelvic and possibly intrapleural spaces for free fluid. Alternatively, whole-body CT imaging may confer a survival benefit after major polytrauma, provided the patient is sufficiently stable to undergo this.

High-resolution head CT is the initial radiological investigation of choice for head-injured patients in the emergency department (Table 21.3). Modern multislice scanners are extremely fast and can assess the extent of both cerebral and bony injuries, even in selected agitated or unstable patients. The images can be viewed online or transmitted electronically to the local neurosurgical unit for specialist neuroradiological or surgical opinion. Facilities for three-dimensional reconstruction may be helpful in characterizing and planning treatment of complex fractures and spinal injuries. Additional acute imaging may subsequently be required, for example angiography to exclude traumatic vascular injury after basal skull fracture or penetrating injury. Neuroimaging is discussed in more detail in Chapter 10.

There is significant morbidity associated with prolonged spinal immobilization. The cervical and thoracolumbar spine should be definitively investigated for unstable fractures by 48–72 h after immobilization. Unfortunately, it will be impossible to clinically rule out spinal injury in obtunded or anaesthetized patients. Anteroposterior and lateral neck plain radiographs alone lack the sensitivity to exclude cervical spine injury even when otherwise technically adequate. Ideally, high-resolution helical CT imaging (and three-dimensional reconstruction) of the entire spine from the craniocervical junction to the T4/T5 disc space should be carried out. The probability of failing to detect an unstable fracture with this investigation is probably <0.5%, although plain films may still be better for detecting ligamentous disruption. If helical CT of the rest of the chest and abdomen has

Table 21.3 Indications for CT head imaging in adults

Immediate CT head imaging (within 1 h):
- GCS <13 on initial assessment in the emergency department.
- GCS <15 at 2 h after the injury.
- Suspected open or depressed skull fracture.
- Any sign of basal skull fracture (haemotympanum, 'panda' eyes, cerebrospinal fluid leakage from the ear or nose, Battle's sign).
- More than one episode of vomiting.
- Post-traumatic seizure.
- Focal neurological deficit.
- Coagulopathy (history of bleeding, clotting disorder, current treatment with warfarin) if there has been some loss of consciousness or amnesia following the injury.

Urgent CT head imaging (within 8 h):
- Amnesia for events >30 min before impact.
- If there has been some loss of consciousness or amnesia following the injury and;
  - Patient ≥65 years.
  - Dangerous mechanism of injury (e.g. pedestrian struck by a motor vehicle, occupant ejected from a motor vehicle or a fall from a height of >1 m or five stairs).

Data from NICE (2007).

not been performed, plain anteroposterior and lateral thoracolumbar radiographs will additionally be required. Urgent MRI of the spine should be considered in patients with neurological deficits if the clinical condition of the patient permits this. Once the spine has been 'cleared', this must be unambiguously documented in the notes.

Secondary transfer of the head-injured patient

Patients with significant head injuries should be discussed with the local neurosurgical service in order to determine whether the patient will benefit or may later benefit from neurosurgical intervention or specialist neurocritical care. Typical referral criteria are given in Table 21.4, although some details may be defined locally. The initial imaging will need to be transferred electronically for review by the specialist centre if this is at a different site.

Once the patient has been stabilized, a decision can be made regarding transfer to a neurosciences unit for further treatment. A secondary transfer will be required if neurosurgical or neurocritical care facilities

Table 21.4 Typical indications for neurosurgical referral of head-injured patients

For discussion of 'surgically significant' findings on head CT imaging.
Persistent Glasgow Coma Scale (GCS) score of ≤8 after resuscitation.
Deteriorating GCS (motor response in particular) or progressive focal neurological signs.
Unexplained confusion persisting for >4 h.
Seizure without full recovery.
Open injury (suspected or confirmed), depressed skull fracture or cerebrospinal fluid leak.

Adapted from NICE (2007).

are not available locally. It is important to plan ahead and prevent avoidable delay due to logistical difficulties such as note gathering and transferring imaging to the receiving centre, particularly if the injury-to-surgery timescale is tight. On the other hand, it is important that preparations for transfer are conducted methodically and not rushed. Interhospital transfer of the head-injured patient is a potentially hazardous procedure and constitutes a significant physiological insult, the risks and benefits of which must be carefully weighed up. It is of paramount importance to discuss the patient with the neurosurgical centre at an early stage, so that treatment priorities can be decided upon and the receiving team is prepared for the arrival of the patient. In any case, the patient must be stabilized as far as possible before transfer is undertaken and then must be accompanied by a suitably qualified and experienced doctor. As the main causes of secondary brain damage are hypoxia and cardiovascular instability, it is of vital importance to avoid either of these during transfer, as resuscitation options are limited while the patient is in transit. A successful and safe transfer involves:

- Adequate resuscitation and stabilization of the patient prior to transfer.
- Adequate monitoring during transfer with appropriate resuscitation equipment and drugs.
- Back-up equipment in the event of pump or ventilator failure, and adequate provision of oxygen and other critical drugs to cover the eventuality of patient deterioration or vehicle breakdown.
- Good communication between the referring and receiving centres and an effective handover to the receiving team.

The fundamental requirement during transfer is to ensure ongoing adequate tissue oxygen delivery and to maintain stable perfusion. The TBI patient is at risk of cardiorespiratory compromise, and this risk is increased during transfer. Any patient with a significantly altered conscious level must be sedated, intubated and mechanically ventilated prior to transfer, as this would be difficult to achieve safely *en route* in the event of clinical deterioration. There is no place for transferring unstable patients to neurosurgical units. Persistent hypotension after resuscitation must be investigated thoroughly and the cause identified and treated prior to transfer. The transferring team must ensure that all lines and equipment are secured before transfer, that they have a sufficient supply of drugs and portable gases, and that there is enough power in battery-operated monitoring equipment for the duration of the journey. Sufficient spare capacity should be provided to allow for unexpected deterioration of the patient, equipment failure or delays due to vehicle breakdown. The mode and urgency of the transfer should be carefully considered. Helicopter or fixed-wing aircraft transfer may be appropriate for longer distances but requires specialist expertise.

Clinical assessment of patients during transfer is difficult, so it is vital that monitoring should be of a standard appropriate to a patient in intensive care. This should include ECG, pulse oximetry, invasive arterial blood pressure monitoring and the use of capnography. Gravity-driven pumps are unreliable in moving vehicles; syringe drivers should be used instead. The transferring team must have appropriate experience in the transfer of patients with head injuries, and should be familiar with the pathophysiology and management of such a patient and with the drugs and equipment they may need to use.

Intraoperative anaesthetic management

Head-injured patients may require anaesthesia for treatment of the primary neurological pathology or for the treatment of a non-neurological injury, including damage control surgery. The optimal timing of such operations will vary, and the decision to operate must be made only after thorough consideration by trauma, neurosurgical and neurocritical care teams. For any operation on the head-injured patient, management priorities remain the avoidance of cerebral ischaemia, optimization of CPP and prevention of intracranial hypertension.

Intraoperative care of the head-injured patient should be a direct continuation of the resuscitation and stabilization process in the neurointensive care unit or the emergency department. Transfer of the patient to and from the operating table must be achieved without subjecting the patient to hypotension or hypoxaemia. The usual considerations for anaesthesia apply. If the patient's head is to be inaccessible during the operation, the anaesthetist must ensure from the outset that the endotracheal tube is secured and ventilation is adequate for maintaining good gas exchange. Cerebral venous drainage must not be obstructed through excessive neck rotation or endotracheal tube ties, and may be aided by gentle head-up positioning where possible.

Because of the dangers of even short periods of cerebral hypoperfusion or hypoxia, it is essential that the patient be continuously and adequately monitored throughout the operation and throughout the transfer to and from the operating environment. Monitoring should include ECG, temperature, urine output, pulse oximetry and invasive arterial blood pressure measurement. Central venous access facilitates the use of vasoactive drugs and may be helpful in guiding fluid therapy. Special emphasis should be placed on $EtCO_2$ monitoring as a means of continuously assessing the level of hyperventilation, and a comparison with $PaCO_2$ is advisable. Cardiac output monitoring, particularly in the elderly and in those with cardiac disease, will allow a more rational approach to fluid replacement, particularly in those patients requiring significant doses of inotropes or vasopressors to maintain an adequate CPP. In patients with neurological injury who require non-neurological surgical intervention, ICP monitoring is recommended, especially if large intraoperative fluid shifts are possible. Intracranial pressure, cerebral venous oxygen saturation (SjO_2) monitoring and the use of TCD are discussed in detail in the respective chapters.

Head-injured patients may have normal anaesthetic requirements: inadequate anaesthesia will allow the surgical stimulus to increase $CMRO_2$, CBF and ICP. The choice of anaesthetic agent and technique will depend on the patient's pre-operative neurological status, his pre-operative medical conditions and the presence of associated injuries. There is little direct evidence for one technique over another; however, the following should be taken into consideration:

- Smooth induction and ongoing haemodynamic stability without sudden or pronounced changes in blood pressure.
- Maintenance of adequate CPP.
- Prevention of a rise in $CMRO_2$, CBF and ICP.
- Rapid post-operative emergence (if the patient is to be woken up immediately after the procedure).

While volatile anaesthetics reduce $CMRO_2$, higher concentrations lead to cerebral vasodilation and increased CBF, which is undesirable. In addition, the inhalational agents impair carbon dioxide reactivity. Sevoflurane appears to be the least problematic agent in both these respects. Nitrous oxide is best avoided, as it stimulates cerebral metabolism, resulting in vasodilation and increased CBF. The epileptogenic properties of enflurane prohibit its use in neuroanaesthesia.

A total intravenous anaesthetic technique using propofol and remifentanil infusions would seem to be ideal. Propofol reduces $CMRO_2$, CBF and ICP up to doses sufficient to cause EEG suppression. Cerebral autoregulation is preserved when combined with remifentanil, which also gives profound analgesia leading to a very stable EEG in the face of a noxious stimulus.

The patient's lungs are ventilated with an oxygen/air mixture to maintain $EtCO_2$ at approximately 4.5–5.0 kPa. Neuromuscular blockade should be maintained intraoperatively in all head-injured patients to prevent coughing or straining, and the extent of neuromuscular block monitored with a neuromuscular stimulator.

Emergence and recovery

Patients with severe TBI who require surgery will need continuing post-operative care in the neurointensive care unit and many will need to remain sedated and mechanically ventilated at the end of the procedure. However, in patients in whom the surgery deals with an isolated lesion responsible for a low GCS (classically an extradural haematoma), it is appropriate to stop sedation at the end of surgery and allow neurological assessment. Similar considerations apply to patients with mild to moderate head injury undergoing, for example, uncomplicated evacuation of an extradural or acute subdural haematoma. A rapid return to consciousness permits early clinical assessment and the detection of any unexpected neurological deficit. This emphasis on rapid emergence makes the maintenance of haemodynamic stability difficult. Care must be taken to avoid excessive coughing and straining, which may cause not only a transient increase in ICP but, more importantly, an increased risk of venous bleeding. Uncontrolled hypertension on emergence may be responsible for intracerebral haemorrhage following neurosurgical procedures. Remifentanil may be useful during emergence to suppress coughing without too much effect on ventilation at low infusion rates. Rises in blood pressure can be controlled with β_1-adrenoreceptor antagonists. Finally, it is important to make sure that the patient is awake, can protect his or her airway, is able to maintain oxygenation and is normocapnic before extubation, in order to avoid increases in ICP.

Neurointensive care management

None of the monitoring techniques and interventions that are widely used by specialist centres in severe head injury has ever been subjected to prospective randomized control trials. Indeed, some procedures such as ICP monitoring are now so widely accepted as being central to the management of patients with severe head injury that it would be ethically impossible to conduct a randomized trial addressing their efficacy. However, the large body of clinical evidence that supports the use of many of these interventions provides a relatively strong basis for their recommendation as treatment guidelines.

Defining therapeutic targets: a rational approach to selecting monitoring modalities

Basic physiology suggests the benefit of maintaining CBF and oxygenation, and these assumptions are confirmed by data from the Traumatic Coma Data Bank (TCDB) and from other sources, which demonstrate the detrimental effects of hypotension (systolic blood pressure <90 mmHg) and hypoxia (PaO_2 levels < 60 mmHg (8 kPa)) in the early and later phases of head injury on outcome. Several studies that have addressed break points for cerebral autoregulation in patients with head injury have suggested preserved cerebrovascular autoregulation with maintenance of CBF at CPP >60–70 mmHg. Ischaemia is a consistent finding in fatal head injury, and retrospective studies from several groups have suggested that outcome is improved in patients who have fewer episodes of CPP or MAP reduction, aggressive CPP management or retained autoregulation. There is, however, some emerging concern that relatively high perfusion pressures may contribute to oedema formation after head injury, and

at least one group has targeted relatively low CPPs in order to minimize oedema formation.

These findings make several points. Firstly, they suggest that autoregulation may be impaired in these patients, as the CPP thresholds for loss of pressure autoregulation are higher than in healthy subjects. Secondly, they emphasize the importance of maintenance of CPP, rather than isolated attention to ICP as a therapeutic target. There are, however, data that show that ICP is primarily an independent determinant of survival rather than quality of outcome in severe head injury.

Monitoring systemic physiology

The need to maintain cerebral oxygenation and CPP requires the continuous measurement of both arterial blood pressure and ICP. The need to rationally manipulate systemic blood pressure also requires the placement of a central venous catheter (or pulmonary artery catheter, if appropriate). Continuous pulse oximetry, regular arterial blood gas analysis, core temperature monitoring and regular measurement of blood sugar are also essential in order to optimize physiology in these patients.

Indications for intracerebral pressure monitoring

The manipulation and optimization of CPP is predicated on the measurement of ICP. Clinical signs of intracranial hypertension are late, inconsistent and non-specific. Furthermore, episodic rises in ICP may occur even in patients with a normal CT scan. A number of technologies are available for ICP measurement, with intraparenchymal micromanometers or fibre-optic probes increasingly being used in preference to ventriculostomy. The insertion of all these devices is not without risk, and ideally should be limited to patients where ICP is likely to be raised (i.e. in whom management may be changed). Unfortunately, this is not always possible to predict with certainty. Severely head-injured patient (post-resuscitation GCS <9) are the most likely to develop intracranial hypertension, and ICP monitoring should be instigated in these patients if the head CT is abnormal (i.e. showing haematomas, contusions, swelling, herniation or compression of the basal cisterns) and they are otherwise potentially salvageable. Intracranial pressure monitoring may also be appropriate in comatose patients with a normal head CT if they have at least two of the following risk factors:

age >40 years, unilateral or bilateral motor posturing, or systolic blood pressure <90 mmHg. Patients with mild to moderate head injury (GCS ≥9) are less likely to develop intracranial hypertension and may be monitored clinically unless they deteriorate.

Intracranial pressure is naturally expected to fluctuate with stimulation (e.g. suctioning), but significant rises should be treated promptly and investigated if sustained. Intracranial pressure thresholds have not been directly subjected to large randomized controlled trials, but there is indirect evidence to suggest an upper limit of 20–25 mmHg above which treatment should be initiated. In addition to static ICP elevations, patients with head injury may develop phasic increases in ICP, often triggered by cerebral vasodilation in response to a fall in CPP. 'A waves' tend to occur on a high baseline pressure and elevate ICP to 50 mmHg or more for several minutes, usually terminated by a marked increase in MAP consequent to a Cushing response, which results in catecholamine secretion. Shorter-lived fluctuations lasting about a minute are referred to as 'B waves'. The frequency of both A and B waves may be decreased by increasing MAP, thus preventing the reflex cerebral vasodilatory cascade that initiates CBV increases and ICP elevation.

Global central nervous system monitoring modalities

While the monitoring described above may help to ensure the maintenance of optimal systemic physiology, detection of local changes in central nervous system (CNS) physiology will require other tools. Commonly used bedside monitoring techniques include TCD ultrasound for non-invasive estimation of CBF, and monitoring of jugular venous saturation (SjO_2) and brain electrical activity. These techniques seek to estimate CBF in the presence of an adequate CPP, estimate the adequacy of oxygen delivery to the brain, and document the consequences of possible oxygen deficit or drug therapy on brain function, respectively.

Transcranial Doppler ultrasonography

Reductions in middle cerebral artery flow velocity provide a useful marker of reduced cerebral perfusion in the setting of intracranial hypertension, but episodic rises in ICP may also be caused by hyperaemia, which may be diagnosed by increases in TCD flow velocity. Transcranial Doppler ultrasonography can also be used as a non-invasive monitor of CPP. As the ICP increases and CPP correspondingly decreases, a characteristic highly pulsatile flow velocity pattern is seen. Continuing increases in ICP result first in a reduction and then loss of diastolic flow, progressing to an isolated systolic spike of flow in the TCD waveform, and eventually to an oscillating flow pattern signifying the onset of intracranial circulatory arrest. The pulsatility index (PI) is one way of mathematically describing the waveform pattern, and correlates with CPP rather than with ICP. This form of monitoring may become particularly useful in patients in whom invasive ICP monitoring is unavailable or may not be clearly indicated (e.g. mild closed head injury). Cerebral vasospasm results in increases in TCD flow velocity, as blood is pushed through narrow arterial segments into a widely dilated microvascular bed.

Jugular venous oximetry

Classically, right jugular venous oximetry has been used to assess the adequacy of CBF in head injury, but a case can be made for targeting the side of the dominant jugular vein for catheterization or for using bilateral catheterization. Reductions in SjO_2 or increases in arteriojugular differences in oxygen content ($AVDO_2$) to >9 ml dl^{-1} provide useful markers of inadequate CBF and can guide therapy, and SjO_2 values below 50% have been shown to be associated with a worse outcome in head injury. Conversely, marked elevations in SjO_2 may provide evidence of cerebral hyperaemia. While SjO_2 monitoring has been widely used in head injury, it is technically difficult. The use of continuous SjO_2 monitoring with a fibre-optic catheter will detect episodes of cerebral desaturation associated with intracranial hypertension, hypocapnia, systemic hypotension and cerebral vasospasm, but as many as half of the episodes identified as cerebral desaturation (SjO_2 <50%) may be false positives. Jugular venous oximetry is discussed in more detail in Chapter 6.

Newer techniques for brain oximetry

The major deficiencies of jugular venous oximetry are its invasiveness and the poor reliability of signal obtained. Other techniques that have been employed investigationally in acute head injury include near-infra red spectroscopy (NIRS), direct tissue oximetry and cerebral microdialysis. These techniques are discussed in Chapters 6 and 7.

Cerebral blood flow measurement

Despite the neuropathological evidence of ischaemia in fatal head injury, antemortem evidence of ischaemia from CBF studies was unconvincing in early studies. Reductions in CBF were generally modest in the first few days following injury. Furthermore, most patients exhibited cerebral $AVDO_2$ in the normal range, implying that the CBF reductions were appropriately coupled to decreases in $CMRO_2$. Two different approaches have provided explanations for these observations. Ultra-early (<12 h) CBF measurements after head injury, in a study by Bouma *et al.* (1991), provided clear evidence that >30% of patients exhibit global CBF reductions below commonly accepted ischaemic thresholds (<18 m $(100 g)^{-1}$ min^{-1}). Later measurements in this study showed elevation of CBF to non-ischaemic levels by 24–48 h post-injury (Fig 21.5). These findings have been generally confirmed by other studies. However, even at early time points, cerebral $AVDO_2$ remained relatively low despite a markedly low CBF (Fig 21.5), with few patients demonstrating increases >9 ml $(100 ml)^{-1}$.

One explanation for the conflict between these clinical findings and the neuropathological evidence of ischaemia may be found in the physiological heterogeneity in the injured brain. Both conventional monitoring methods and newer techniques are limited by the fact that they detect either globally averaged or highly localized abnormalities in cerebral physiology, and may be unable to detect regional abnormalities in the metabolically heterogeneous injured brain. More recently, local CBF has been measured continuously and invasively by thermal clearance. Briefly, an electrically heated tissue probe is introduced. Heat is not only dissipated by passive conduction but is also transported by the flowing blood. The power required to maintain a probe temperature just above brain temperature is therefore a function of local CBF. Such equipment is now commercially available and its clinical role is being evaluated.

Imaging physiology and metabolism in head injury

The need to detect changes in regional physiology and the insensitivity of conventional structural imaging to early, reversible pathology have lead to the conclusion that there is a need to image physiology and metabolism in such patients.

Marked heterogeneity in perfusion patterns and carbon dioxide reactivity in the injured brain have been demonstrated, particularly in the vicinity of contusions. Positron emission tomography (PET) using ^{15}O tracers and ^{18}F-deoxyglucose has been used to image oxygen extraction, CBF, $CMRO_2$ and cerebral glucose metabolism. While such studies have directly demonstrated the presence of a perilesional ischaemic penumbra within the first 24 h of injury, they have also shown that regions of ischaemia and hyperaemia can coexist. Furthermore, metabolic derangements are heterogeneous, and a switch to non-oxidative glucose metabolism may not always be due to classical ischaemia but may be the consequence of microvascular ischaemia, mitochondrial dysfunction or obligate anaerobic metabolism in inflammatory cells. The mechanism of energy failure after TBI is thus highly complex. As bedside techniques exist only for the measurement of either global (hemispheric) or very localized cerebral oxygenation, it is likely that such complexity is not routinely appreciated.

Multimodality monitoring

While individual monitoring techniques provide information regarding specific aspects of cerebral function, the correlation of data from several modalities has several advantages in head injury management. Integration of monitored variables allows cross-validation and artefact rejection, a better understanding of pathophysiology and the potential to target therapy.

Therapy

Achieving target cerebral perfusion pressure values

Most centres agree on the need to maintain a minimum safe CPP of 60–70 mmHg, as cerebral oxygenation falls at lower pressures even if autoregulation is intact.

Cerebral perfusion pressure may be increased either by increasing the MAP or by decreasing ICP (if it is elevated, >25 mmHg). Rosner *et al.* (1995) have been the most enthusiastic proponents of the use of hypertension to increase MAP and induce secondary reductions in ICP. Mean arterial pressure may variously be manipulated by volume expansion, inotropes and vasopressors. The relative efficiency of each of these interventions in maintaining CPP has not been investigated. Indeed, there are no data on the safety of high doses of vasoactive agents in the presence of BBB disruption. However, maintaining MAP may reduce the incidence of jugular venous desaturation.

Intracranial pressure may be reduced by hyperosmolar therapy (using mannitol or hypertonic saline), hyperventilation, the use of CNS depressants (typically barbiturates), drainage of CSF or surgical decompression. Each of these strategies has individual limitations. The advent of intraparenchymal micromanometers and fibre-optic devices for measuring ICP has reduced infection risk but removed the possibility of routine access to ICP drainage in many patients.

It is important to remember that regions of reduced perfusion may still exist, even with an apparently adequate CPP. Still higher thresholds for CPP have not been shown conclusively to improve outcome and, in patients with defective autoregulation, the resultant increase in global CBF may worsen cerebral oedema and paradoxically increase ICP. Furthermore, induced hypertension, hyperventilation and CSF drainage have potential systemic and/or cerebral side effects, and their extent of use will be limited by a risk/benefit ratio. It is likely that several different pathophysiological mechanisms coexist in individual patients, and all approaches are likely to have a role if applied appropriately. Finally, it important to remember that optimization of CPP does not guarantee the absence of regional perfusion defects.

The Lund protocol

In contrast to the discussions above, publications from one centre (Asgeirsson, *et al.*, 1994; Eker *et al.*, 1998) have described the use of a protocol that focuses primarily on the prevention and reduction of cerebral oedema rather than maximizing cerebral perfusion. This protocol accepts CPP values as low as 50 mmHg in adults, with a reduction of MAP using a combination of clonidine and metoprolol and a reduction of CBV with dihydroergotamine and low-dose thiopentone (for sedation). Plasma oncotic pressure was increased by transfusing albumin or plasma to maintain normal albumin levels. These authors reported excellent results (8% overall mortality and 79% good outcome), which compared well with centres using conventional CPP-guided therapy. However, historical controls were used and there is some doubt as to whether the data are truly comparable to those obtained from other centres. In any case, their impressive outcome figures demand further investigation, and it may well be that optimal CPP levels may vary widely both between patients and at different stages after head injury in the same patient.

Hypocapnia for intracranial pressure reduction

Hyperventilation, once the mainstay of ICP reduction in severe head injury, is now the subject of debate. The aim of hyperventilation is to reduce CBV and hence ICP, but this is accompanied by a reduction in global CBF, which may drop below ischaemic thresholds. Although conclusive data are not available, it is likely that these consequences worsen outcome, especially when hyperventilation is prolonged or profound.

In principle, therapeutic hyperventilation may be guided by jugular bulb oximetry, but there is still a risk of inducing regional hypoperfusion secondary to cerebral vasoconstriction. Metabolic imaging with PET has revealed that even moderate reductions in $PaCO_2$ may lead to focal reductions in blood flow to levels that threaten normal oxidative metabolism, and that such induced ischaemia may exist in a significant volume of tissue even when SjO_2 remains normal (Fig. 21.6). It may be that hyperoxia offsets these effects to some extent where brief hyperventilation is contemplated as a rescue manoeuvre.

In addition to concerns regarding ischaemia, the effect of hyperventilation in decreasing ICP may be only short lived due to compensatory reductions in cerebral extracellular fluid (ECF) bicarbonate levels, which rapidly restore ECF pH in normal subjects. Although these compensatory changes may be delayed after TBI, it is still likely that they will, over time, attenuate the effect of low $PaCO_2$ levels on vascular tone, and result in rebound increases in CBV and ICP when $PaCO_2$ is subsequently normalized. It has been suggested that the use of the diffusible hydrogen ion acceptor tetrahydroaminomethane (THAM) may restore ECF base levels and restore cerebrovascular carbon dioxide reactivity. While such an approach has been shown to reduce ICP and the need for intensification of ICP therapy after head injury, it does not alter outcome.

Fluid therapy and feeding

Accurate fluid management may be complicated by continuing or concealed haemorrhage from associated extracranial trauma, but every effort must be made to restore normovolaemia and prevent hypotension. Fluid replacement should be guided by clinical and laboratory assessment of volume status and by invasive haemodynamic monitoring but generally involves the administration of 30–40 ml of maintenance fluid kg^{-1} day^{-1}. The choice of hydration fluid is largely based on inconclusive results from animal data. Fluid flux across

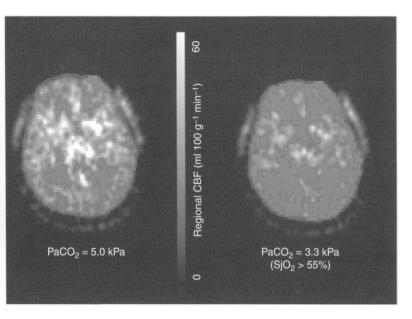

Fig. 21.6. Positron emission tomography imaging showing the effect of hyperventilation in the first 24 h following TBI on regional CBF. Even with an acceptable SjO_2, hyperventilation results in a marked increase in the volume of brain tissue (highlighted areas) below an ischaemic threshold (20 ml $(100 g)^{-1} min^{-1}$) due to vasoconstriction from hypocapnia. See colour plate section.

the normal BBB is governed by osmolality rather than oncotic pressure. Consequently, hypotonic fluids are best avoided and serum osmolality should be maintained at high normal levels (290–300 mOsm l^{-1} in our practice) to minimize fluid flux into the injured brain. Dextrose-containing solutions in particular are avoided because the residual free water after dextrose metabolism can worsen cerebral oedema, and because the associated elevations in blood sugar may worsen outcome. Some clinical data are now available to support these practices.

Increases in plasma oncotic pressure might be expected to provide a distinct advantage in situations where BBB disruption results in a leak of sodium into the brain ECF. Maintenance of oncotic pressure with albumin supplements is one of the cornerstones of the Lund protocol, and the potential advantages of colloid over crystalloid in this setting has been the subject of some debate. Both albumin and gelatins have been used, but the haemostatic disturbances produced by hetastarch may potentiate intracranial haemorrhage. The subgroup analysis from the SAFE Study in 2007 in patients with TBI has raised concerns regarding the safety of albumin solutions in TBI. Certain colloids (such as pentastarch) may be effective in reducing the cerebral oedema associated with cerebral ischaemic and reperfusion injury. Agents that 'plug leaks' by acting as oxygen free-radical scavengers and/or by inhibiting neutrophil adhesion may be the resuscitation fluids of the future.

Head-injured patients have high nutritional requirements and feeding should be instituted early (within 24 h), aiming to replace 140% of resting metabolic expenditure (with 15% of calories supplied as protein) by day 7 post-trauma. Enteral feeding is associated with a lower incidence of hyperglycaemia and may have a protective effect against gastric ulceration, the incidence of which may be increased in these patients. Impaired gastric emptying is common after head injury and can be treated with prokinetic agents such as metoclopramide, erythromycin or cisapride. In those who cannot be fed enterally, parenteral nutrition should be considered together with some form of prophylaxis against gastric ulceration (H_2-receptor antagonists, proton pump inhibitors or sucralfate) and rigorous blood sugar control.

Oxygenation and ventilation

A particular difficulty is faced when mechanically ventilated TBI patients also have respiratory failure secondary to traumatic lung injuries or pneumonia. Such patients may be difficult to ventilate. Cerebral perfusion considerations mandate normocapnia and stringent avoidance of hypoxia. On the other hand, it is well known that, in the absence of TBI, lung-protective ventilation strategies lead to improved survival in patients with acute respiratory distress syndrome (ARDS). Unfortunately, low-volume ventilation may lead to rather higher $PaCO_2$ and lower PaO_2 levels than can be tolerated after TBI. Furthermore, while hypoxia is particularly dangerous after TBI, application of high levels of positive end-expiratory pressure raises jugular venous pressure reducing cerebral venous drainage, which may also be deleterious. Prone positioning may similarly impair venous circulation. Clearly, it is undesirable to adopting a ventilatory strategy that is directly harmful to the brain. However, in some cases, cerebral monitoring may allow the neurointensivist to, at least in part, cautiously adopt some of these strategies provided that ICP, CPP and cerebral oxygenation are not compromised. Furthermore, ICP measurement also allows CPP to be targeted directly. Avoidance of supranormal levels of CPP keeps inotrope and vasoconstrictor requirements to a minimum, which helps to reduce the incidence of ARDS. In many ways, therefore, neuromonitoring techniques allow strategies for the management of extracranial pathology to be individualized to the needs of the individual TBI patient.

Hyperosmolar therapy

Hyperosmolar therapy is traditionally said to reduce ICP by osmotic withdrawal of cerebral water (through an intact BBB) by artificially raising plasma osmolarity. Mannitol is currently the most commonly used agent, although hypertonic saline (HS) solutions are increasingly popular. More recently, it has been realized that these agents also improve microvascular rheology variously by reducing erythrocyte and endothelial cell size, improving erythrocyte deformability and through effects on the nitric oxide pathway and leucocyte adhesion. Experimentally, the time course of ICP reduction after mannitol administration follows the rheological changes even before brain water is measurably affected. This suggests that improved microvascular flow may be a primary mechanism of action. A corollary of this is that CBF may be observed to improve, even if ICP responds only poorly. Typically, these agents are given as boluses to treat relatively acute rises in ICP; their role in the long-term maintenance of ICP is less clear.

Mannitol is a sugar alcohol that has traditionally been used ($0.25–1\,g\,kg^{-1}$, usually as a 20% solution) to elevate plasma osmolarity and reduce brain oedema in the setting of intracranial hypertension. While it is reported to possess antioxidant activity, this is unlikely to be clinically important. Side effects include secondary increases in ICP when the BBB is disrupted and fluid overload from initial intravascular volume expansion. Renal toxicity can be a problem with excessive use, particularly in the face of other nephrotoxic insults. These can be minimized if its use is discontinued when it no longer produces significant ICP reduction, if volume status is monitored and if plasma osmolality is not allowed to rise $>320\,mOsm\,l^{-1}$. It is important to remember that the diuretic effect of mannitol may cause intravascular depletion and arterial hypotension, which must be controlled.

Originally investigated for small volume resuscitation, HS solutions were found to improve outcome in comatose patients suffering from multiple trauma. A number of concentrations are available, and a consensus on the optimal method of administration has not been reached. A dose of $2\,ml\,kg^{-1}$ of 5% saline would be typical, repeated if the serum sodium and plasma osmolarity remain below $155\,mmol\,l^{-1}$ and $320\,mOsm\,l^{-1}$, respectively.

Although HS is generally safe, it may cause central pontine myelinolysis if given to patients with pre-existing chronic hyponatraemia, although this does not appear to be a problem otherwise. Although the dose-response characteristics of hyperosmolar agents are poorly characterized, HS may improves CPP to a greater extent than mannitol and may also improve brain tissue oxygen levels ($PbrO_2$) although further study is warranted. The direct diuretic effect seen with mannitol is not present with HS.

Disordered sodium homeostasis

Abnormalities of sodium homeostasis are relatively common after TBI. Hyponatraemia may worsen cerebral oedema, depress consciousness and lower the threshold for seizures. It is usually considered to occur in the context of either SIADH or CSWS; in practice, the distinction may be less than clear cut and has been questioned. With SIADH, ADH levels are inappropriately high for the plasma osmolarity. The resulting excessive free water retention results in intravascular volume expansion with both urinary sodium and osmolarity being high. In contrast, CSWS is characterized by excessive renal sodium loss mediated by increased plasma natriuretic peptides and inappropriately normal or low aldosterone levels. Urinary sodium and osmolarity are typically less perturbed than in SIADH, and the patients are clinically hypovolaemic. Differentiation between SIADH and CSWS is on the basis of volume status, which can be difficult to assess clinically. Severe and/or symptomatic hyponatraemia may mandate cautious treatment with HS infusion (taking care not to raise serum sodium by $>0.5\,mmol\,h^{-1}$), irrespective of the underlying diagnosis. While fluid restriction can be hazardous in the early stages after TBI, it may be an appropriate first-line treatment for less severe SIADH-related hyponatraemia. Demeclocycline, which antagonizes the renal effect of ADH, may also be effective. In contrast, CSWS may respond to fludrocortisone administration – fluid restriction is ineffective and, indeed, undesirable given the underlying hypovolaemia.

Hypernatraemia in neurocritical care is commonly an iatrogenic effect of repeated hyperosmolar therapy. It may also be seen where damage to the hypothalamic/pituitary axis causes impaired ADH secretion resulting in neurogenic diabetes insipidus. Diabetes insipidus occurs in roughly 1% of head-injured patients and can result in hypernatraemia due to the loss of large volumes of dilute urine (up to 20 l day^{-1}). Mildly raised serum sodium on the neurosciences critical care unit may be tolerated without intervention, or treated with enteral water supplementation. The more severe hypernatraemia and polyuria of diabetes insipidus is treated with the administration of 1-deamino-8-D-arginine vasopressin (DDAVP) and volume replacement with 5% dextrose in water with careful monitoring of blood sugar levels.

Sedation and neuromuscular blockade

Sedation on the neurointensive care unit is usually achieved with a balanced combination of intravenous anaesthetic such as propofol and an infusion of an opioid such as fentanyl for pain control, to minimize ICP elevations and to promote endotracheal tube tolerance. Propofol has a putative cerebral protective effect – pressure autoregulation and the cerebrovascular response to carbon dioxide are maintained, even at doses sufficient to abolish cortical activity, and it decreases CBF, cerebral metabolism and ICP. While the reduction in flow and CBV are secondary to a reduction in metabolism, flow–metabolism coupling is not perfect, and the decrease in CBF may exceed the corresponding decrease in CMRO$_2$, with a widening of the cerebral arteriovenous oxygen content difference. Such uncoupled CBF reductions may be at least partially due to changes in systemic haemodynamics.

Propofol can induce hypotension and decrease CPP, particularly in hypovolaemic patients. The lipid load imposed by a 20 ml h^{-1} continuous infusion of propofol must be taken into account in the calculation of daily caloric intake. In our hands, the use of propofol at 200 µg kg^{-1} min^{-1} to produce burst suppression for long periods has often resulted in unacceptable levels of plasma lipids. These problems with lipid loading have been substantially ameliorated by the introduction of a 2% formulation of propofol. Concerns have emerged over propofol infusion syndrome (PRIS), a rare but potentially fatal clinical entity consisting of lipaemia, hyperkalaemia, hepatomegaly, metabolic acidosis, rhabdomyolysis, renal failure and myocardial dysfunction with refractory bradycardia. The risk of PRIS is increased at high doses of propofol (>4–5 mg kg^{-1} h^{-1}) or after prolonged administration (>48 h), particularly in young patients and in states of tissue hypoperfusion.

Benzodiazepines are often used as an adjunct or alternative to propofol for longer periods of sedation, but even the relatively short-acting agents such as midazolam will tend to accumulate. Midazolam reduces CMRO$_2$, CBF and CBV with both cerebral autoregulation and vasoreactivity to carbon dioxide remaining intact. However, these effects are inconsistent and transient, and even large doses of midazolam will not produce burst suppression or an isoelectric EEG. Opioids generally have minimal effects on CBF and CMRO$_2$. However, the newer synthetic opioids fentanyl, sufentanil and alfentanil can increase ICP in patients with tumours and head trauma due to changes in PaCO$_2$ (in spontaneously breathing subjects) and reflex cerebral vasodilation secondary to systemic hypotension. These changes can be avoided, however, if blood pressure and ventilation are controlled.

Barbiturates are not indicated for routine sedation, as significant accumulation occurs as a result of their zero-order pharmacokinetic terminal elimination characteristics. They may, however, be indicated as a treatment for refractory intracranial hypertension (see below).

Neuromuscular blockade in the head-injured patient receiving intensive care is the subject of some debate. Neuromuscular blockers can play an important role in the head-injured patient by preventing rises in ICP produced by coughing and straining. However, use of these agents is not associated with better outcomes, perhaps because of increased respiratory complications. Profound neuromuscular blockade may mask clinical seizures and destabilize spinal fractures. Furthermore, long-term use of neuromuscular blockade has been associated with continued paralysis after drug discontinuation and acute myopathy, especially with the steroid-based medium-to-long-acting agents. Atracurium, on the other hand, is non-cumulative, is less likely to be associated with myopathy, and theoretical concerns about the accumulation of laudanosine, a cerebral excitatory metabolite of atracurium, in head-injured patients have not been shown to be clinically validated. Nevertheless, because of the risks, neuromuscular blockade should be discontinued as soon as it is safe to do so.

Anti-epileptic therapy

Seizures occur both early (<7 days) and late (>7 days) after head injury, with a reported incidence of 4–25% and 9–42%, respectively. Seizure prophylaxis with phenytoin or carbamazepine can reduce the incidence of early post-traumatic epilepsy but has little impact on late seizures, neurological outcome or mortality. The incidence of post-traumatic seizures is greatest in patients with a GCS <10, and in the presence of an intracranial haematoma, contusion, penetrating injury or depressed skull fractures. As it is important to balance the possible benefit from seizure reduction against the side effects of anti-epileptic drugs, such patients may form the most appropriate subgroup for acute (days to weeks) seizure prophylaxis following head injury. There is increasing interest in the monitoring and treatment of subclinical seizures following TBI – this is discussed in detail in Chapter 27.

Cerebral metabolic suppressants

In higher doses (given as a loading dose followed by an infusion), intravenous barbiturates such as thiopentone can be used to treat otherwise refractory intracranial hypertension by reducing $CMRO_2$. Barbiturates result in cardiovascular depression, increased intensive care stay and an increase in pulmonary infections. However, they may have a significant role to play in selected patients whose problem is intractable intracranial hypertension that is responsive to intravenous anaesthetics. Thiopentone is administered as an intravenous infusion, titrated to produce EEG burst suppression, as this is sufficient to realize near-maximal cerebral metabolic depression. One major disadvantage of barbiturates is prolonged recovery. This might suggest a role for other intravenous anaesthetics (for example, etomidate or propofol) with more desirable pharmacokinetic profiles. However, the efficacy of these agents remains unproven, and they have their own drawbacks. The adrenocortical suppression produced by etomidate infusion has been well documented, and the high doses of propofol required to achieve burst suppression (up to $200\,\mu g\ kg^{-1}\ min^{-1}$), increase the risk of propofol infusion syndrome and necessitate the delivery of high lipid loads with resultant abnormalities in plasma lipid status.

Autoregulation monitoring

Conceptually, an understanding of cerebral autoregulation is central to CPP-guided therapy. The loss of cerebral pressure autoregulation and vasoreactivity to carbon dioxide are indicators of poor prognosis after head injury.

As has been described, autoregulatory behaviour after TBI may be substantially deranged. In principle, determination of the CPP/CBF relationship should allow the clinician to individualize the choice of MAP and therefore optimize CPP. Autoregulation may be assessed by measuring the TCD responses to induced changes in MAP. Direct measurements of the whole autoregulatory curve are, however, not a continuous measure and may require exposing the patient to dangerously high and/or low perfusion states. A number of techniques have been developed to overcome this problem.

One approach is to measure the variability in middle carotid artery flow velocity as measured by TCD due to slow random fluctuations in CPP. Transcranial Doppler flow velocity and CPP are negatively correlated when autoregulation is intact. Thus, the continuous, time-averaged correlation index (mean flow index, Mx) provides a measure of autoregulatory status. An alternative approach is to measure the pressure correlation coefficient (PRx) between MAP and the resultant changes in ICP. With intact cerebrovascular reactivity, a change in MAP should lead to an inverse vasoreactive change in CBV and hence ICP. Under such circumstances, PRx is negative. With disturbed autoregulation, PRx is expected to become increasingly positive. This approach has the advantage that it does not rely on TCD measurement and is easier to apply continuously.

Both Mx and PRx are typically observed to exhibit a U-shaped behaviour with CPP. This defines an 'optimal CPP' where autoregulation is strongest. In practice, if Mx or PRx are time averaged, the random variations of CPP that occur allow the optimal CPP to be mapped out. There is evidence that autoregulation measurements are correlated with outcome, and it may be that Mx or PRx, along with more sophisticated ICP waveform analysis parameters, will be seen to play an increasing role in defining autoregulation-oriented haemodynamic targets in neurocritical care after TBI.

Neurotherapeutics

A large number of complex and interacting cellular and biochemical pathways underpin the pathophysiology of delayed neuronal loss after TBI. These cascades act over a clinically amenable time window and it would seem reasonable to speculate on the existence of neuroprotective therapeutic targets that may prevent the progression of the primary injury. Indeed, a number of theoretically attractive approaches have shown early promise in experimental models of TBI. Unfortunately, such encouraging pre-clinical results have, thus far, failed to translate into successful phase III clinical trials:

- *Corticosteroids.* Glucocorticoids are known to reduce vasogenic oedema associated with inflammatory and neoplastic conditions. However, numerous studies and meta-analyses have found steroids to be ineffective or harmful. Thus, glucocorticoid therapy is not recommended as a routine treatment for TBI, although it should be remembered that adrenal insufficiency is common in this patient group, and steroids may improve haemodynamic responsiveness.

- *Excitatory amino acid antagonists.* High concentrations of glutamate have been demonstrated after TBI. While glutamate is important for normal brain function, high levels may initiate a number of processes resulting in increased calcium influx and cell death. A number of pre- and post-synaptic glutamate antagonists at NMDA and non-NMDA receptors have been investigated as putative neuroprotective agents, as has the novel synthetic cannabinoid dexanabinol, with pluripotent anti-excitotoxic, anti-inflammatory and free-radical scavenging properties. Despite experimental promise, none of these has been proved to be effective in outcome trials. Magnesium has been experimentally demonstrated to have beneficial effects, presumably through several mechanisms including pre-synaptic inhibition of glutamate release, blocking of NMDA receptors and inhibition of calcium influx, but this has failed to translate into a clinical beneficial therapy.

- *Erythropoietin.* Central nervous system erythropoietin and erythropoietin-receptor expression is known to increase after hypoxic insult and may have anti-inflammatory neuroprotective properties experimentally. Clinical benefit has not yet been demonstrated after TBI.

- *Calcium-channel blockers.* Successful clinical trials of nimodipine in SAH prompted trials of this agent in head injury. Trends towards improved outcome have not convincingly reached clinical significance, except possibly in a subgroup of head-injured patients who have traumatic SAH, although this remains controversial and difficult to replicate.

- *Cyclosporin A.* This short peptide has been demonstrated experimentally to have neuroprotective effects that are believed to result from improved cerebral metabolic function through reduced mitochondrial membrane permeability. Phase III data are awaited.

- *Hormones.* Progesterone and oestrogen are both believed to have neuroprotective and neurotrophic effects by multiple mechanisms. Further work is needed to see whether this translates into a useful clinical benefit.

- *Antioxidants.* Animal studies have suggested a prominent role for free radicals in head injury and have demonstrated protection by antioxidants. A number of potential antioxidants have been studied, but no benefits have yet been demonstrated by phase III trials.

- *Statins.* In addition to their effects on lipid metabolism, statins have been shown to have pleiotropic actions that include beneficial effects on the cerebral microvasculature through improved nitric oxide bioavailability, and reduced thrombosis as well as antioxidant, immunomodulatory and anti-excitotoxic properties. Improved neurogenesis, synaptogenesis and angiogenesis have been demonstrated after experimental stroke, and similar effects may occur with TBI. Further studies are required to see whether these finding translate into improvements in outcome.

The above list is not exhaustive but does illustrate the disappointing failure of neurotherapeutic strategies investigated to date. This is perhaps less surprising when one considers the complex and heterogeneous nature of TBI, which is not captured by experimental models. It is, at present at least, unclear which pathophysiological processes are important at a particular time within an individual patient. Some pathways may have both adverse and protective effects, which may additionally be temporally distinct. Furthermore, although it seems natural to concentrate efforts on severe TBI because these patients have worse outcomes, it may be that gains are to be made in mild or moderate TBI where neuronal tissue may be more salvageable. Indeed, even the classification of TBI on the basis of the GCS is undoubtedly a blunt tool, concealing the wide variation in underlying pathology.

Hypothermia

Mild to moderate hypothermia (33–36°C) is proposed to reduce ischaemic tissue damage by lowering cellular energy expenditure, reducing excitotoxicity and attenuating cytokine/chemokine inflammatory cascades. Biochemical evidence for these effects and for outcome improvements is available from animal models. On this basis, induced hypothermia has been widely employed therapeutically for many years and has been the subject of numerous studies. Disappointingly, larger studies such as that by Clifton *et al.* (2001) and several meta-analyses (e.g. Sydenham *et al.*, 2009; Brain Trauma Foundation, 2007) have generally failed to find a convincing outcome benefit. However, the studies to date are methodologically heterogeneous and there is still much we do not know. In contrast to animal models, therapeutic hypothermia is typically achieved hours after the initial insult, and it may be that the intervening period of normothermia is detrimental. Animal data suggests that the inflammatory response is exaggerated in juveniles, and it may be that the effects of hypothermia are age dependent. The effect of different rewarming strategies has not been investigated in detail. The effect of hypothermia may be confounded by other treatments such as barbiturate therapy. Subgroup analysis has demonstrated a trend to improving survival with increasing duration of hypothermia beyond 48 h, and therefore it is possible that negative findings were the result of insufficient duration (or inappropriate timing) of treatment. Perhaps the most important consideration is that induced hypothermia is not a risk-free intervention, and that its benefits may only be realized if it is used in patients who have the greatest likely benefit, and in settings where its known side effects can be carefully monitored, prevented and treated. Clearly, further study is warranted and several trials are currently underway. In the meantime, therapeutic hypothermia should be viewed with caution. It is not without risks, notably increased systemic vascular resistance, myocardial depression and potential coagulation abnormalities. Circulatory depression must be carefully compensated by judicious fluid loading if CPP is to be maintained. Inotrope/vasoconstrictor requirements are generally higher. The pharmacokinetics of commonly used drugs, such as propofol, may be

slowed. At present, therapeutic hypothermia cannot be recommended as a first-line treatment in head-injured patients but is commonly used in refractory intracranial hypertension. On the other hand, hyperthermia has been shown to adversely affect outcome and must be aggressively treated.

Sequential escalation versus targeted therapy for the intensive care of head injury

It is clear that a diverse range of pathophysiological processes operate in acute head injury and that, although a wide range of therapeutic options exist, few of them have proven efficacy. One of two approaches may be used in the choice of therapy in such a setting. The first of these is to use a standard protocol in all patients, and to introduce more intensive therapies in a sequence that is based either on intensity of intervention or on local experience and availability. While such a scheme is simple, it does not provide for individualization of therapy in a given patient.

Alternatively, individual therapies can be targeted at individual pathophysiological processes. Examples are the use of hyperventilation in the presence of hyperaemia, mannitol for vasogenic cerebral oedema and the use of blood pressure elevation in the presence of B-waves. This intellectually appealing approach is hindered by the fact that pathophysiology is usually mixed, and global monitors of CNS physiology may miss critical focal abnormalities. Furthermore, some interventions (e.g. therapeutic hypothermia) are proposed to work via multiple mechanisms and do not easily find a place in a strictly targeted therapy plan.

In practice, many established head injury protocols represent a hybrid approach. Initial baseline monitoring and therapy are applied to all patients, and refractory problems are dealt with by therapy escalation, with the choice of intervention determined by clinical presentation and physiological monitoring. Often, interventions that are more difficult to implement or that present significant risks (e.g. barbiturate coma) are used as a last resort. Figure 21.7 shows the ICP/CPP management protocol used in the Neurosciences Critical Care Unit at Addenbrooke's Hospital, UK.

Prognosis after traumatic brain injury

Outcome after TBI ranges from full recovery through severe disability to vegetative states and death. Prognostication is important not only in determining

Addenbrooke's NCCU: ICP/CPP management algorithm

Fig. 21.7. Addenbrooke's Hospital's Neurosciences Critical Care Unit ICP/CPP management algorithm.

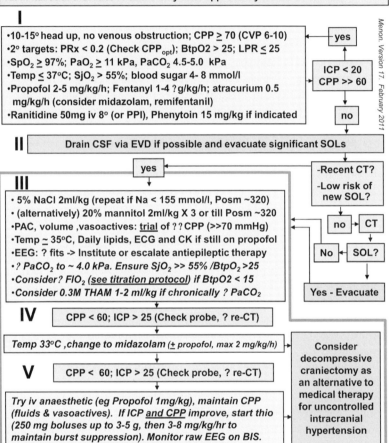

All patients with or at risk of intracranial hypertension *must* have invasive arterial monitoring, CVP line, ICP monitor and Rt SjvO₂ catheter at admission to NCCU.

- Algorithm to be used in conjunction with full protocols; stage III interventions depend on clinical picture & multimodality monitoring (to be established within six hours of admission).
- Early MRI in WBIC if no contraindications, clinical PET for selected patients.
- CPP 70 mmHg set as initial target, but <u>CPP>> 60 mmHg is acceptable in most patients</u>.
- Autoregulation, brain chemistry to individualise targets and titrate hyperoxia as a therapy

Evacuate significant SOLs & drain CSF before escalating medical Rx.
Rx in italics and Grades IV and V only after approval by NCCU Consultant.

I

- 10-15° head up, no venous obstruction; CPP ≥ 70 (CVP 6-10)
- 2° targets: PRx < 0.2 (Check CPP$_{opt}$); BtpO2 > 25; LPR ≤ 25
- SpO₂ ≥ 97%; PaO₂ ≥ 11 kPa, PaCO₂ 4.5-5.0 kPa
- Temp ≤ 37°C; SjO₂ > 55%; blood sugar 4- 8 mmol/l
- Propofol 2-5 mg/kg/h; Fentanyl 1-4 ?g/kg/h; atracurium 0.5 mg/kg/h (consider midazolam, remifentanil)
- Ranitidine 50mg iv 8° (or PPI), Phenytoin 15 mg/kg if indicated

Menon, Version 17, February 2011

yes → ICP < 20 / CPP >> 60

no

II Drain CSF via EVD if possible and evacuate significant SOLs

yes ← -Recent CT? -Low risk of new SOL?

III

- 5% NaCl 2ml/kg (repeat if Na < 155 mmol/l, Posm ~320)
- (alternatively) 20% mannitol 2ml/kg X 3 or till Posm ~320
- PAC, volume ,vasoactives: <u>trial</u> of ??CPP (>>70 mmHg)
- Temp ~ 35°C, Daily lipids, ECG and CK if still on propofol
- EEG: ? fits -> Institute or escalate antiepileptic therapy
- *? PaCO₂ to ~ 4.0 kPa. Ensure SjO₂ >> 55% /BtpO₂ >25*
- *Consider? FIO₂ (see titration protocol) if BtpO2 < 15*
- *Consider 0.3M THAM 1-2 ml/kg if chronically ? PaCO₂*

no → CT

No → SOL?

Yes - Evacuate

IV CPP < 60; ICP > 25 (Check probe, ? re-CT)

Temp 33°C ,change to midazolam (± propofol, max 2 mg/kg/h)

V CPP < 60; ICP > 25 (Check probe, ? re-CT)

Try iv anaesthetic (eg Propofol 1mg/kg), maintain CPP (fluids & vasoactives). If ICP <u>and</u> CPP improve, start thio (250 mg boluses up to 3-5 g, then 3-8 mg/kg/hr to maintain burst suppression). Monitor raw EEG on BIS.

Consider decompressive craniectomy as an alternative to medical therapy for uncontrolled intracranial hypertension

---

the most appropriate treatments but also for informing the patient (where this is possible), and those close to the patient, of what the future is likely to hold. An ideal outcome model would not only be an accurate predictor of ultimate functional outcome in the individual, no matter what the injury, but should also be applicable as early as possible after the primary insult so that the initiation of ultimately inappropriate treatments can be avoided. Unfortunately, the demographics, circumstances, severity and pathology of TBI are so heterogeneous that this is impossible to achieve in practice. Other factors in the resuscitation phase may

contribute to the apparent neurological condition but yet be reversible, so that attempting very early prognostication is inadvisable. Nevertheless, a number of variables have been repeatedly demonstrated to have independent predictive value in regression analyses. Of particular note are initial neurological findings, age, pupil size and reactivity, hypotension and CT findings.

The GCS is a powerful tool for initial/early assessment of injury severity and provides some prognostic information. A significant inverse relationship between initial GCS and survival or favourable outcome has been demonstrated repeatedly. It has several advantages: it is easy to assess, has good reproducibility and is well validated. An accurate initial GCS of 3 predicts a 20% survival (<10% with GCS of 4 or 5). It is important to appreciate that the GCS immediately after injury may be depressed by other factors such as hypoxia, hypotension or intoxicants, the presence of which may not be directly related to the severity of the brain injury. This highlights the importance of assessing the GCS *after* resuscitation. Unfortunately, early sedation and endotracheal intubation will then prevent a full assessment from being made in a substantial proportion of cases. As a result, a low initial GCS alone is typically an overpessimistic predictor of outcome. The long-term accuracy of GCS in predicting good outcome improves when assessed later during the course of treatment, but the optimal timing has not been determined.

Advancing age (approximately >60 years) has been demonstrated to be an independent predictor of mortality and poor outcome. Clearly, pre-existing comorbidity is more prevalent with this age group. However, this is not sufficient to account for the excess mortality. Indeed, TBI in the older age group is aetiologically different, with a greater proportion of falls and less multisystem trauma, suggesting it is primarily the brain injury that determines ultimate outcome. Intracranial haematomas are more common and tend to be larger in older patients, and this itself correlates with poor outcome.

Pupillary size and light reflex involve the pre-tectal and Edinger–Westphal nuclei and therefore, in the absence of afferent damage and direct orbital trauma, test the function of the midbrain and efferent pupilloconstrictor pathway. Direct brainstem compression generally causes bilateral fixed and dilated pupils, whereas temporal lobe herniation typically results in unilateral pupillary signs through compression of the ipsilateral oculomotor nerve. As the brainstem is responsible for numerous essential functions, it is not surprising that the post-resuscitation pupillary dilation (>4 mm) and absence of the pupillary light reflex are predictive of poor outcome, particularly when present bilaterally.

Systemic hypotension (defined as systolic blood pressure <90 mmHg) is well known to be a strong predictor of poor outcome after TBI. The presence of a single hypotensive episode doubles mortality and causes a significant increase in morbidity. Furthermore, hypotension retains statistical significance, even when the presence of extracranial injuries (resulting in hypovolaemia) is controlled, indicating the importance of secondary brain injury on functional survival. Unlike other prognostic variables, hypotension is amenable to intervention. The presence of early hypotension appears to increase the frequency and magnitude of subsequent intracranial hypertension, underlining the need for prompt restoration of cerebral perfusion. Late hypotension, including iatrogenic and intraoperative causes, also correlates with poor outcome.

While correlated with outcome, level of consciousness, age, pupil response and the presence of hypotension do not directly reflect the underlying intracranial pathology. CT imaging allows rapid, early differentiation between focal and diffuse brain injury and assessment of mass effect and brain swelling. A normal CT scan suggests a better prognosis overall. The significance of radiographic abnormalities depends on their nature. While it is not possible to directly measure ICP with imaging, compressed basal cisterns are suggestive of intracranial hypertension and correlate strongly with outcome, with the mortality being at least doubled. A finding of midline shift is also a strong predictor of raised ICP and has prognostic significance particularly for patients with a GCS of 5–7. The degree of shift relates inversely to survival and favourable outcome, particularly in younger patients where baseline prognosis is better. The presence of traumatic SAH also increases mortality and ultimate morbidity depending on its location and extent, with blood in the basal cisterns being of particular significance. Additionally, extensive traumatic SAH is predictive of subsequent secondary ischaemia due to vasospasm. Extracerebral haematomas are easily detected and are prognostically significant in a volume-dependent way, with both mortality and outcome being higher with acute subdural haematomas when compared with extradural haematomas. Intraparenchymal lesions are more difficult to define structurally, but multiple, bilateral or high-density lesions confer a worse outcome.

While CT neuroimaging is crucial in understanding the severity of the underlying pathology of individual TBI, it is a snapshot in time, and repeated scanning is required to appreciate the acute evolution of the injury. Exactly how best to incorporate this into outcome prediction is unclear at present. Furthermore, while CT has good sensitivity for larger regions of haemorrhage and structural changes from space-occupying lesions and mass effects, it is relatively insensitive to more subtle tissue injury. In particular, CT has poor sensitivity for diffuse axonal injury, which is characterized by more microscopic cytoskeletal disruption. Diffuse axonal injury is common after TBI with a GCS of

<9, but carries with it an extremely poor prognosis if severe. Finally, the posterior fossa is relatively poorly visualized with CT and yet lesions within the midbrain and brainstem may have particularly profound sequelae. Other imaging techniques and in particular MRI are becoming more commonplace. While MRI is technically more cumbersome and difficult to perform in acutely ill patients, it gives structural and even functional or metabolic data that cannot be obtained by CT, and it may be that this becomes increasingly important in understanding the functional significance of the underlying injuries.

These multiple factors that affect TBI outcome have been integrated into risk-adjustment schemes that attempt to predict outcome. Two notable prediction models are based on the Medical Research Council CRASH Trial database (2008) and the IMPACT collaboration reported by Steyerberg *et al.* (2008). While these approaches are useful in predicting expected outcomes in groups of patients, their applicability to outcome prediction in individual patients remains unproven.

Further reading

Asgeirsson, B., Grände, P. and Nordström, C. (1994). A new therapy of post-trauma edema based on haemodynamic principles for brain volume regulation. *Intensive Care Med* **20**, 260–4.

Bernard, F., Outtrim, J., Menon, D. and Matta, B. (2006). Incidence of adrenal insufficiency after severe traumatic brain injury varies according to definition used: clinical implications. *Br J Anaesth* **96**, 72–6.

Bouma, G., Muizelaar, J., Choi, S., Newlon, P. and Young, H. (1991). Cerebral circulation and metabolism after severe traumatic brain injury: the elusive role of ischaemia. *J Neurosurg* **75**, 685–93.

Brain Trauma Foundation (2007). Guidelines for the management of severe traumatic brain injury, 3rd edn. *J Neurotrauma* **24**, S1–106.

Brain Trauma Foundation, American Association of Neurological Surgeons, Joint Section on Neurotrauma and Critical Care (2000). Guidelines for the management of severe traumatic brain injury. Intracranial pressure treatment threshold. *J Neurotrauma* **17**, 493–5.

Bullock, R. (1997). Injury and cell function. In P. Reilly and R. Bullock, eds., *Head Injury*. London: Chapman & Hall, pp. 121–41.

Bullock, R. and Povilshock, J. (1996). The role of anti-seizure prophylaxis following head injury. *J Neurotrauma* **13**, 788–93.

Chesnut, R. (1997). Hyperventilation in traumatic brain injury: friend or foe? *Crit Care Med* **25**, 1275–8.

Chesnut, R., Marshall, S., Piek, J. *et al.* (1993). Early and late systemic hypotension as a frequent and fundamental source of cerebral ischaemia following severe brain injury in the Traumatic Coma Data Bank. *Acta Neurochi Suppl* **59**, 121–5.

Clifton, G., Miller, E., Choi, S. *et al.* (2001). Lack of effect of induction of hypothermia after acute brain injury. *N Engl J Med* **344**, 556–63.

Coles, J. (2007). Imaging after brain injury. *Br J Anaesth* **99**, 49–60.

Coles, J., Fryer, T., Smielewski, P. *et al.* (2004). Incidence and mechanisms of cerebral ischaemia in early clinical head injury. *J Cereb Blood Flow Metab* **24**, 202–11.

Coles, J., Fryer, T., Coleman, M. *et al.* (2007). Hyperventilation following head injury: effect on ischaemic burden and cerebral oxidative metabolism. *Crit Care Med* **35**, 568–78.

Cruz, J., Miner, M., Allen, S., Alves, W. and Gennarelli, T. (1991). Continuous monitoring of cerebral oxygenation in acute brain injury: assessment of cerebral haemodynamic reserve. *Neurosurgery* **29**, 743–9.

Czosnyka, M., Smielewski, P., Kirkpatrick, P. *et al.* (1997). Continuous assessment of the cerebral vasomotor reactivity in head injury. *Neurosurgery* **41**, 11–19.

Czosnyka, M., Matta, B., Smielewski, P., Kirkpatrick, P. and Pickard, J. (1998). Cerebral perfusion pressure in head-injured patients: a noninvasive assessment using transcranial Doppler ultrasonography. *J Neurosurg* **88**, 802–8.

Czosnyka, M., Brady, K., Reinhard, M., Smielewski, P. and Steiner, L. (2009). Monitoring of cerebrovascular autoregulation: facts, myths and missing links. *Neurocrit Care* **10**, 373–86.

Edwards, P., Arango, M., Balica, L. *et al.* (2005). Final results of MRC CRASH, a randomised placebo-controlled trial of intravenous corticosteroid in adults with head injury – outcomes at 6 months. *Lancet* **365**, 1957–9.

Eker, C., Asgeirsson, B., Grände, P., Schalén, W. and Nordström, C. (1998). Improved outcome after severe head injury with a new therapy based on principles for brain volume regulation and preserved microcirculation. *Crit Care Med* **26**, 1881–6.

Enevoldsen, E. and Jensen, F. (1978). Autoregulation and CO_2 responses of cerebral blood flow in patients with acute severe head injury. *J Neurosurg* **48**, 689–703.

Fodale, V., Schifilliti, D., Praticò, C. and Santamaria, L. (2008). Remifentanil and the brain. *Acta Anaesthesiol Scand* **52**, 319–26.

Huber-Wagner, S., Lefering, R., Qvick, L.-M. *et al.* (2009). Effect of whole-body CT during trauma resuscitation on survival: a retrospective, multicentre study. *Lancet* **373**, 1455–61.

Jansen, J., Thomas, R., Loudon, M. and Brooks, A. (2009). Damage control resuscitation for patients with major trauma. *BMJ* **338**, 1436–40.

Langlois, J., Rutland-Brown, W. and Wald, M. (2006). The epidemiology and impact of traumatic brain injury: a brief overview. *J Head Trauma Rehabil* **21**, 375–8.

Lobato, R., Rivas, J., Gomez, P. *et al.* (1991). Head injured patients who talk and deteriorate into coma. Analysis of 211 cases studied with computerised tomography. *J Neurosurg* **75**, 256–61.

Maas, A., Stocchetti, N. and Bullock, R. (2008). Moderate and severe traumatic brain injury in adults. *Lancet Neurol* **7**, 728–41.

Martin, N. A., Patwardhan, R.V., Alexander, M. J. *et al.* (1997). Characterization of cerebral hemodynamic phases following severe head trauma: hypoperfusion, hyperaemia and vasospasm. *J Neurosurg* **87**, 9–19.

Matta, B., Lam, A., Strebel, S. and Mayberg, T. (1995). Cerebral pressure autoregulation and CO2-reactivity during propofol-induced EEG suppression. *Br J Anaesth* **4**, 159–63.

Menon, D. K. (1999). Cerebral protection in severe brain injury: physiological determinants of outcome and their optimisation. *Br Med Bull* **55**, 226–58.

Menon, D. K. and Zahed, C. (2009) Prediction of outcome in severe traumatic brain injury. *Cur Opin Crit Care*, **15**, 437–41.

Morris, C., Perris, A., Klein, J. and Mahoney, P. (2009). Anaesthesia in haemodynamically compromised emergency patients: does ketamine represent the best choice of induction agent? *Anaesthesia* **64**, 532–9.

MRC CRASH Trial Collaborators, Perel, P., Arango, M. *et al.* (2008) Predicting outcome after traumatic brain injury: practical prognostic models based on large cohort of international patients. *BMJ* **336**, 425–9.

NICE (2007). *Triage, Assessment, Investigation and Early Management of Head Injury in Infants, Children and Adults.* National Institute for Health and Clinical Excellence.

Polderman, K. H. (2009) Mechanisms of action, physiological effects, and complications of hypothermia. *Crit Care Med* **37** (Suppl.), S186–202.

Reilly, P. L., Graham, D. I., Adams, J. H. and Jennett, B. (1997). Patients with head injury who talk and die. *Lancet* **306**, 375–7.

Robertson, C. S., Valadka, A. B., Hannay, H. J., *et al.* (1999) Prevention of secondary insults after severe head injury. *Crit Care Med* **27**, 2086–95.

Rosner, M., Rosner, S. and Johnson, A. (1995). Cerebral perfusion pressure: management protocol and clinical results. *J Neurosurg* **83**, 949–62.

SAFE Study Investigators, Australian and New Zealand Intensive Care Society Clinical Trials Group, Australian Red Cross Blood Service *et al.* (2007) Saline or albumin for fluid resuscitation in patients with traumatic brain injury. *N Engl J Med*, **357**, 874–84.

Shaz, B., Dente, C., Harris, R., MacLeod, J. and Hillyer, C. (2009). Transfusion management of trauma patients. *Anesth Analg* **108**, 1760–8.

Sheinberg, M., Kanter, M., Robertson, C. *et al.* (1992). Continuous monitoring of jugular venous oxygen saturation in head-injured patients. *J Neurosurg* **76**, 212–17.

Sprenger, K., Farrell, D. and Servadei, F. (2000). Nimodipine in head injury: results of the HIT IV study. In *5th International Neurotrauma Symposium*. Garmisch-Partenjirchen, Germany.

Steyerberg, E. W., Mushkudiani, N., Perel, P. *et al.* (2008) Predicting outcome after traumatic brain injury: development and international validation of prognostic scores based on admission characteristics. *PLoS Med* **5**, e165.

Sydenham, E., Roberts, I. and Alderson, P. (2009). Hypothermia for traumatic head injury. *Cochrane Database Syst Rev* (2), CD001048.

Vespa, P. (2008). Cerebral salt wasting after traumatic brain injury: an important critical care treatment issue. *Surg Neurol* **69**, 230–2.

Vink, R. and Nimmo, A. (2009). Multifunctional drugs for head injury. *Neurotherapeutics* **6**, 28–42.

von Elm, E., Schoettker, P., Henzi, I., Osterwalder, J. and Walder, B. (2009). Pre-hospital tracheal intubation in patients with traumatic brain injury: systematic review of current evidence. *Br J Anaesth* **103**, 371–86.

Zehtabchi, S., Soghoian, S., Liu, Y. *et al.* (2008). The association of coagulopathy and traumatic brain injury in patients with isolated head injury. *Resuscitation* **76**, 52–6.

Chapter

22

Management of aneurysmal subarachnoid haemorrhage in the neurointensive care unit

Frank Rasulo and Basil F. Matta

Introduction

Aneurysmal subarachnoid haemorrhage (aSAH) is a type of haemorrhagic stroke attributable to rupture of an intracranial aneurysm and accounts for 85% of cases of non-traumatic aSAH. Its incidence ranges within the general population from 5 to 25 per 100,000. Aneurysmal SAH occurs more frequently in women than in men, with a ratio of 3:2, but it tends to predominate in men >40 years. The greatest risk of rupture occurs between the ages of 50 and 60 years. At least 15% of people with SAH die before reaching the hospital. Of the 85% of patients who survive the initial SAH, about one-third develop further brain injury due to ischaemia and are at risk of developing delayed ischaemic neurological deficits (DIND), rebleeding and/or hydrocephalus. DIND accounts for most morbidity and 50% of subsequent mortality. Risk factors for aSAH are cigarette smoking, excessive alcohol consumption, hypertension and the presence of a history of aSAH within first-degree relatives. A thorough understanding of the pathophysiology and natural history of aSAH is necessary in order to provide optimal intensive care treatment for these patients. Timely diagnosis and treatment of aSAH-related intra- and extracranial complications may reduce mortality and morbidity.

Pathophysiology

Aneurysms usually occur at the branching sites on the large cerebral arteries of the circle of Willis (Fig. 22.1a). The early precursors of aneurysms are small outpouchings through defects in the media of the arteries. These defects are thought to expand as a result of hydrostatic pressure from pulsatile blood flow and blood turbulence, which is greatest at the arterial bifurcations. A mature aneurysm has a paucity of media, replaced by

connective tissue, and has diminished or absent elastic lamina. The probability of rupture is related to the tension on the aneurysm wall. La Place's Law states that tension is determined by the radius of the aneurysm and the pressure gradient across the wall of the aneurysm. Thus, the rate of rupture is directly related to the size of the aneurysm. Aneurysms with a diameter of ≤5 mm have a 2% risk of rupture, whereas 40% of those 6–10 mm in diameter have already ruptured upon diagnosis. The vessels mostly involved with aneurysm rupture are at the origin of the posterior communicating artery from the internal carotid artery (41%), anterior communicating artery/anterior cerebral artery (34%) and middle cerebral artery (MCA) (20%) (Fig. 22.1b). Both congenital and environmental factors are considered important in aneurysm development. There seems to be an association with inheritable disorders such as fibromuscular dysplasia, Marfan's syndrome, pseudoxanthomaelasticum, Ehlers–Danlos syndrome, polycystic kidney disease and coarctation of the aorta. Multivariate models have found hypertension, smoking and heavy alcohol use to be independent risk factors for aSAH in many industrialized countries. Sympathomimetic drugs, including cocaine and amphetamines, have been implicated as a cause of aSAH, especially in younger patients where cocaine-related SAH has an outcome similar to that in other aSAH patients.

When an aneurysm ruptures, blood extravasates under arterial pressure into the subarachnoid space and quickly spreads through the cerebrospinal fluid (CSF) around the brain and spinal cord and meningeal irritation occurs (Fig. 22.1c). Blood released under high pressure may cause damage directly to local tissues. Blood extravasation causes a global increase in intracranial pressure (ICP).

Core Topics in Neuroanaesthesia and Neurointensive Care, eds. Basil F. Matta, David K. Menon and Martin Smith. Published by Cambridge University Press. © Cambridge University Press 2011.

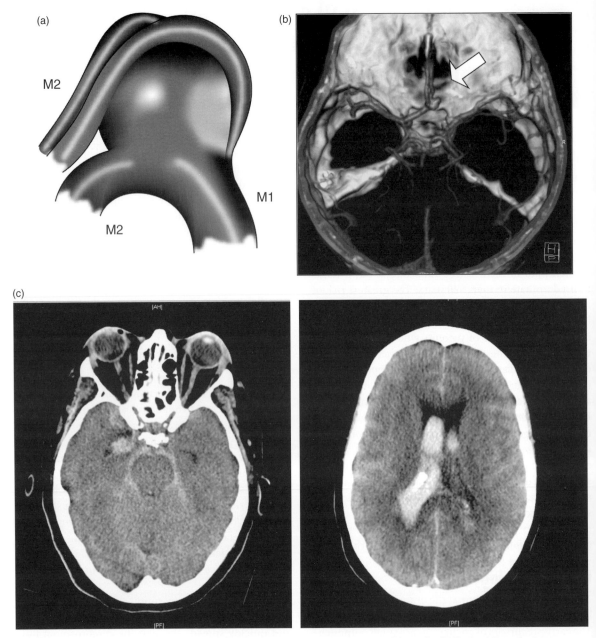

Fig. 22.1. (a) Aneurysms usually occur at the branching sites on the large cerebral arteries of the circle of Willis (middle cerebral artery M1 and M2). The early precursors of aneurysms are small outpouchings through defects in the media of the arteries. (b) CT angiogram demonstrating a lobular aneurysm arising from the anterior communicating artery (arrow). See colour plate section. (c) CT scan showing extensive intraventricular blood, which extends from the lateral to the third and the fourth ventricles. This is more extensive on the right side where there is a cast of acute blood in the mildly dilated right lateral ventricle. There is subarachnoid blood in both Sylvian fissures, more so on the right, and in the basal cisterns and prepontine cisterns.

Early effects of subarachnoid haemorrhage on cerebral blood flow

Pathological findings consistent with an ischaemic injury have been found in the brains of patients dying shortly after aSAH, suggesting that an immediate reduction in cerebral blood flow (CBF) during this early phase. Laboratory studies have established that an increase in ICP, especially within the first minutes after an aneurysm rupture, is a significant factor leading to cerebral perfusion pressure (CPP)-dependent reduction in CBF followed by global ischaemia. Factors that may also be involved in increasing ICP following aSAH may be CSF obstruction due to the presence of blood clots, vasoparalysis and distal cerebral arteriolar vasodilation. However, the reduction in CBF may also be caused by vasospasm of the microvessels and therefore not necessarily be linked to reductions in CPP. This early vasospasm is characterized by a prolonged stage of hypoperfusion, which may last several hours and is associated with decreased CBF, larger haemorrhage, persistent elevations of extracellular glutamate and ultimately poor outcome. This finding is further supported by a recent clinical study observing early vasospasm angiographically in up to 10% of patients. Another mechanism attributed to the early reduction of CBF following aSAH is the depression of cerebral metabolism. In humans, a decrease in the cerebral oxygen consumption and changes in the levels of metabolites related to the cellular oxidative energy are common after SAH. Experimental studies have also shown a reduction in cerebral metabolic requirements for oxygen ($CMRO_2$) and an increase in lactate, free fatty acids and glutamate levels, coupled with reductions in phosphocreatine and hexokinase levels immediately following aSAH. Subarachnoid haemorrhage can cause low cerebral oxygen consumption in the absence of ischaemia and signs of mitochondrial dysfunction during the first minutes after the bleeding, supporting the idea that a decreased metabolism may be an important mechanism reducing brain perfusion acutely after aSAH.

Late effects of aneurysmal subarachnoid haemorrhage on cerebral blood flow (vasospasm)

Cerebral vasospasm is a potentially incapacitating or lethal complication in patients with aSAH. Peak incidence occurs between days 6 and 8, and there is gradual resolution over 2–4 weeks. A consequence of cerebral vasospasm may be DIND, caused by a reduction of CBF below the lower threshold of ischaemia. Besides the thickness of the clot in the basal cisterns, which correlates with the risk of developing vasospasm, microvascular dysfunction due to inflammation, in situ thrombosis or embolism may also contribute to the development and severity of DIND. Subarachnoid haemorrhage is often accompanied by disturbed cerebrovascular autoregulation and, in the presence of vasospasm, CBF becomes directly dependent on CPP, which increases the risk of developing ischaemic brain damage.

Acute management

The emergency setting

The type of hospital and intensive care unit (ICU) to which the patient is admitted influences the outcome of patients with aSAH. Authors have demonstrated that admission of aSAH patients to centres treating greater numbers of patients with this pathology is associated with reduced mortality and is cost-effective. In the emergency setting, a thorough medical history should be obtained and a complete clinical examination should be performed that incorporates at least one established grading system. Clinical grading systems include the Glasgow Coma Scale, Hunt and Hess Stroke Scale and the World Federation of Neurological Surgeons grading scale.

Serial assessments are required because patients may deteriorate in the first few hours after presentation. The initial goals are to stabilize the patient's airway, breathing and circulation. Endotracheal intubation with a rapid-sequence intubation protocol should be performed in those with an inability to protect their airway or with respiratory failure and those who have an important change in the level of consciousness. Consideration should be given to elective intubation of agitated patients to facilitate performing safe and rapid brain imaging. A non-contrast CT scan performed in the first 12 h after SAH has a sensitivity of almost 100%, declining to 95% at 24 h. Blood appears as a high-density signal in the cisterns surrounding the brainstem and the basal cisterns. A CT scan may be falsely negative if the volume of blood is very small, if the haemorrhage occurred several days previously or if the haematocrit is extremely low. The amount of subarachnoid blood is graded according to the Fisher CT scale and represents an important predictor of vasospasm risk. If the CT scan is normal and suspicion of SAH remains strong, a lumbar puncture should be performed. Key factors for the examination of CSF include an understanding of the timing of lumbar puncture in relation to SAH, red and white blood cell counts, the presence of xanthochromia and detection of bilirubin. The presence of xanthochromia may be helpful in distinguishing a traumatic lumbar puncture from a true SAH, especially if it is detected by spectrophotometry.

Conventional catheter four-vessel digital subtraction angiography (DSA) remains the gold standard for detection of intracranial aneurysms and should be performed as soon as possible in order to facilitate early repair of the ruptured aneurysm (Fig. 22.2a). Repeat angiography should be performed within a few days to weeks. Patients with a high-quality complete angiogram that does not identify a source of bleeding have a very low incidence of rebleeding, especially if the blood is limited to the perimesencephalic and ambient cisterns. However, DSA fails to demonstrate the cause of non-traumatic SAH in 15–20% of cases. CT angiography (CTA) is a valid alternative to DSA (Fig. 22.2b). It is more rapid, readily available and less invasive and is characterized by a lower complication rate when compared with DSA. The sensitivity and specificity of CTA for aneurysm detection depend on aneurysm location and size, radiologist experience, image acquisition and the presentation of the images. For aneurysms >5 mm, CTA has sensitivity between 95 and 100%, and between 64 and 83% when aneurysms are <5 mm. Vessel tortuosity decreases the specificity of CTA, leading to misinterpretation as an intracranial aneurysm. CT angiography seems to be becoming the preferred diagnostic mode, especially in North America where it is used more frequently than in Europe (Fig. 22.3).

Magnetic resonance angiography (MRA) has improved the diagnosis of acute SAH. The advantage of MRA is the possibility of obtaining more information regarding the brain and of searching for other causes of SAH. In the presence of negative catheter angiography, a negative CT scan and equivocal lumbar puncture results, MRA is an alternative to evaluate patients with SAH. Although MRA in SAH has evolved over the past decade, it has not replaced catheter-based angiography as the initial test for aneurysm identification and localization. With aneurysms >5 mm, the sensitivity of MRA is of 85–100%, whereas the sensitivity of MRA for detecting aneurysms <5 mm drops to 56%. There are also some limitations for the use of MRA in the emergency setting for acute SAH such as the difficulty in scanning acutely ill patients and longer examination times.

In the first 24 h following SAH, seizures may occur in up to 20% of patients after SAH and must be treated promptly. They are most common when associated with intracerebral haemorrhage, hypertension and middle cerebral and anterior communicating artery aneurysms.

After the initial bleed following a ruptured aneurysm, rebleeding is considered a major cause of death and morbidity in SAH patients. Despite the diffuse use of blood pressure control in an attempt to reduce the risk of rebleeding, there is very little information regarding which is the most efficient antihypertensive strategy. Furthermore, the relationship between blood pressure and acute rebleeding risk has yet to be established with clinical trials. Blood pressure is often elevated following SAH because of pain and anxiety and generalized sympathetic activation, and should be monitored and controlled to balance the risk of stroke and hypertension-related rebleeding, and in order to maintain adequate CPP. Analgesics alone may be effective; otherwise, short-acting continuous-infusion intravenous antihypertensive agents with a reliable dose–response relationship and a favourable safety profile are desirable. The preferred agents include β-blockers, hydralazine and nicardipine. It is reasonable to avoid systemic infusion of sodium nitroprusside in many neurological emergencies because of its tendency to raise ICP and cause toxicity with prolonged infusion. A notable exception to vigorous treatment of hypertension is when hydrocephalus is present. In this situation, blood pressure should be addressed after the hydrocephalus is treated in order to maintain adequate CPP.

Recent evidence suggests that early treatment with a short course of antifibrinolytic agents may be reasonable. These agents may reduce rebleeding, but this is offset by a higher rate of cerebral ischaemia and poor outcome. Antifibrinolytic therapy to prevent rebleeding may be considered in certain clinical situations, as in patients with a low risk of vasospasm and/or when it is necessary to delay surgery.

Cardiac abnormalities are common in the first 48 h after SAH. ECG changes including tall peaked T-waves or cerebral T-waves, ST-segment depression and prolonged QT segments are frequent. Medical management is based on the detection and treatment of cerebral and extracerebral complications of aSAH.

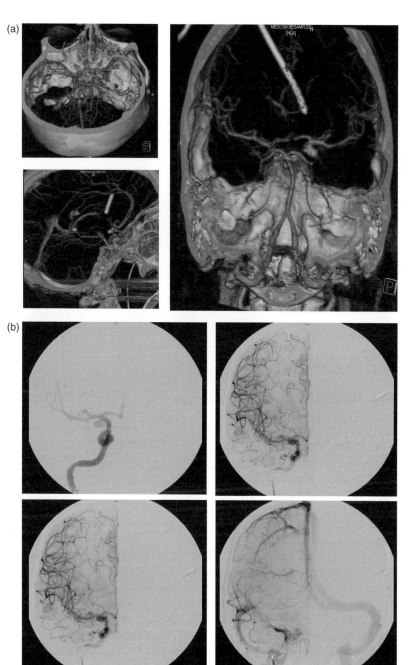

Fig. 22.2. Digital subtraction angiography (a) (see colour plate section) and CT angiography results (b) showing an irregular and elongated (9 mm) aneurysm at the origin of the right posterior communicating artery. The aneurysm is directed posterolaterally, with a small lobule directed medially.

Endovascular coiling versus surgical clipping

A progressive increase in aSAH survival over the past three decades has been reported in several studies. However, evidence of a direct relationship between aSAH outcomes and a specific strategy or intervention is limited. Data regarding management are lacking or equivocal in nature, generating uncertainty and controversy among clinicians. Previous studies showed that overall outcome was not different for early versus delayed treatment after SAH. However, despite a slight increase in frequency of cerebral infarction associated with early treatment, early repair is still beneficial, as the higher risk of cerebral infarction is offset by a lower risk of aneurysm rebleeding.

345

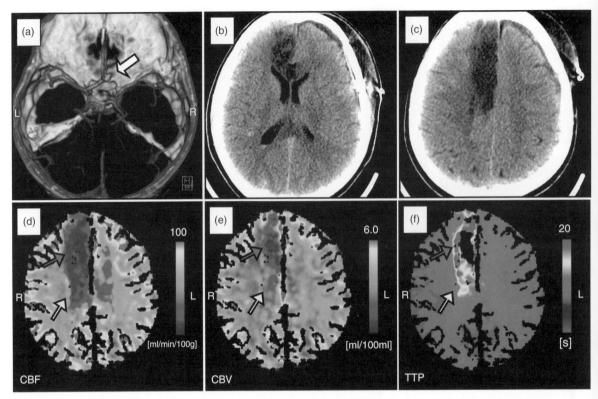

Fig. 22.3. Subarachnoid haemorrhage and ischaemic changes with time. (a) Day of bleed. CT angiogram demonstrating a lobular aneurysm arising from the anterior communicating artery (arrow). Both anterior cerebral arteries originate from the left side with hypoplasia of the right A1. (b, c) Day 10 post-bleed. Plain CT head showing extensive infarction of the right anterior cerebral artery territory involving the genu of the corpus callosum. (d–f) Day 11 post-bleed. CT perfusion showing an established infarct in the right anterior cerebral artery territory (reduced cerebral blood flow (CBF) and cerebral blood volume (CBV), grossly delayed time to peak; red arrows). There is a large, hypoperfused salvageable area extending into the left anterior cerebral artery territory (reduced CBF with maintained CBV and moderately delayed time to peak; yellow arrows). See colour plate section.

The two main and most common therapeutic treatments for cerebral aneurysms are direct clipping of the aneurysm and endovascular coiling. Endovascular coiling emerged as an alternative to surgery in patients with intracranial aneurysms who were deemed poor surgical candidates due to significant neurological injury, the presence of severe medical comorbidities or difficult surgical access to the aneurysm. In recent years, the indication for also treating good-grade SAH patients has increased, and in many centres endovascular coiling of ruptured and unruptured aneurysms has either equalled or surpassed surgical clipping. In order to evaluate the efficacy in terms of outcome between patients treated with surgical clipping or with endovascular coiling, a trial called the International Subarachnoid Aneurysm Trial (ISAT), a multiple-centre, randomized study of endovascular coiling versus surgical clipping conducted in 2143 patients with aSAH who were deemed suitable for either therapy, was performed. At 1 year, endovascular coiling was associated with dependency or death in 23.5% of patients compared with 30.9% in the surgical group, a relative risk reduction of 22.6% ($P = 0.001$). However, non-procedural rebleeding within 1 year was higher in patients randomized to endovascular treatment (40 recurrent aSAHs, with 22 deaths) compared with patients allocated to neurosurgical treatment (33 patients with aSAHs, 30-day mortality in 21 patients). Although regarded as a landmark trial, ISAT has been criticized with regard to biases in patient selection, low rates of randomization of eligible patients, the definition of clinical equipoise, expertise of the neurosurgeons and interventionists, the failure to use an operative microscope, the higher-than-expected morbidity in the surgically treated group, the absence of angiographic data after the initial treatment and the lack of long-term follow-up. A recent report from the ISAT group provided further crucial information regarding long-term outcomes. With a mean follow-up of 4 years, the risk of recurrent aSAH was higher in patients randomized to coiling compared with clipping, but mortality related to recurrent aSAH was equal in both groups. A higher risk for seizures and poor cognitive outcomes was seen in the surgical group, and cumulative 7-year mortality curves showed more deaths in the surgical group compared with coiling. The increased risk of rebleeding in the coiling group did not seem to reverse the early benefit seen with this modality. An important question concerns the influence of surgical or endovascular treatment on the prevalence of cerebral ischaemic complications. In several non-randomized comparisons of surgery and endovascular therapy of ruptured aneurysms, the rate of symptomatic vasospasm was either not significantly different or slightly higher among surgically treated patients. An early non-randomized study of 156 patients had suggested a higher rate of cerebral infarction in patients receiving endovascular versus surgical therapy; however, the proportion of patients with poor initial neurological presentation was higher in the endovascular group. Despite its limitations, the ISAT data indicate that, in patients with good neurological grade aSAH who undergo treatment for aneurysms in the anterior circulation, 1-year outcomes are clearly superior after endovascular coiling when compared with surgical clipping. Long-term (>1 year) clinical trends in patients enrolled in ISAT do seem to suggest that endovascular coiling is likely to retain its advantage over clipping as a superior procedure, and further follow-up of these patients is likely to add insight to this debate.

Cerebral vasospasms

Diagnosis

Vasospasm is traditionally defined as arterial narrowing 3–14 days after SAH. Cerebral ischaemia from vasospasm accounts for up to 30% of the morbidity and mortality that occurs after SAH. A timely diagnosis of delayed cerebral ischaemia may prevent the occurrence of tissue infarction. Almost all patients with SAH, regardless of clinical and radiographic grade, should be monitored intensively for the occurrence of DIND, which presents insidiously with focal neurological abnormalities. A concomitant rise in blood pressure is frequently observed and may be a heralding sign. This rise in blood pressure should not be blunted pharmacologically, as it may serve to maintain adequate CBF.

Serial neurological examinations help to detect DIND and to assess the response to treatment. However, DIND may occur without overt clinical manifestations, especially in comatose patients. Additional diagnostic means are therefore required.

There is a clear relationship between the amount of blood seen in the basal cisterns on initial CT scan and the development of clinically symptomatic vasospasm. Angiographic vasospasm is at its maximal narrowing at 5–14 days after SAH, followed by a gradual resolution up to 4 weeks. Angiographic evidence of arterial narrowing is present in approximately 70% of patients after SAH; however, only 20–30% of these patients will develop DIND. Four-vessel cerebral DSA is the gold standard for diagnosing vasospasm, but given the inherent risks and allocation of time and resources required for this procedure, alternative and complementary diagnostic tools have been proposed. These include transcranial Doppler (TCD), CTA, MRI, radionuclide imaging, cerebral microdialysis, brain tissue oxygenation, near-infrared spectroscopy (NIRS), laser Doppler flowmetry and EEG. Transcranial Doppler ultrasonography is widely used to diagnose vasospasm of the larger arteries. The results can be obtained daily or every other day in patients after SAH. The validity of TCD in diagnosing angiographic vasospasm was summarized in a recent systematic review by Lysakowski and coworkers (2001). For the MCA, the sensitivity of TCD was 67% and specificity was 99%, with a positive predictive value of 97% and negative predictive value of 78%. The accuracy of TCD was considerably less for detecting spasm in vessels other than the MCA. There is debate about the correlation between increased TCD flow velocities and angiographic vasospasm and clinically significant or 'symptomatic' vasospasm. Although mean MCA CBF velocities of $200 \, cm \, s^{-1}$ accurately predict angiographic vasospasm, velocities in the $120–200 \, cm \, s^{-1}$ range have a far lower predictive value. Moreover, it has been observed that TCD is not as reliable in estimating distal MCA vasospasm compared with the more proximal portions of the MCA. Generally, an increase of $50 \, cm \, s^{-1}$ in 24 h was closely associated with angiographic and clinical vasospasm. To overcome the numerical dependence of flow velocities in the measurement of CBF, the Lindegaard index was developed, which normalizes flow velocity in the MCA to that in the ipsilateral extracranial internal carotid artery (an index of 3 is strongly predictive of angiographic vasospasm). However, the ability of TCD to predict which patients will develop neurological symptoms from cerebral vasospasm is poor. Some investigators have proposed that the diagnostic capability of TCD may be enhanced by transcranial colour-coded sonography (TCCD), an ultrasound-based neuroimaging technique that allows real-time visualization of intracranial vascular structures in addition to measurement of CBF velocities. In a prospective study comparing TCCD and conventional TCD in the prediction of angiographic spasm, the sensitivity and specificity of TCCD for MCA and internal carotid artery vasospasm were higher than those for TCD.

Non-invasive angiography (CT and MRI) may have utility in some patients but is less sensitive for vasospasm than conventional angiography. CT angiography is non-invasive, quick and may be performed at the bedside with a portable CT scanner, and is associated with a high positive predictive value for angiographic vasospasm. It is less useful for detecting mild to moderate vasospasm. Combining CTA with a CT perfusion study might increase the diagnostic yield. MR angiography presents some major limits as a useful vasospasm detection method. It takes longer to perform, is subject to more artefacts from aneurysm clips and coils and from metallic intracranial monitoring devices, and has a lower sensitivity for vasospasm than conventional angiography and CTA. As non-invasive angiographic techniques evolve, they may be used more often; presently, neither CTA nor MRA replaces conventional angiography for vasospasm detection.

Recent studies have shifted away from the characterization of vessel lumen diameter to the detection of changes in CBF and of cerebral ischaemia. Perfusion CT, diffusion- and perfusion-weighted MRI, radionuclide-based perfusion studies, cerebral microdialysis and EEG hold promise as techniques that might expand the therapeutic window for treating ischaemia in patients with aSAH.

Monitoring of neurochemical markers of ischaemia with cerebral microdialysis has been proposed as a technique for detecting vasospasm and delayed cerebral ischaemia. In a study of 97 patients with aSAH, neurochemical changes indicative of ischaemia were observed before the onset of symptoms in 83% of patients with DIND. In another report, an ischaemic pattern of cerebral metabolites preceded the occurrence of DIND by a mean interval of 11 h. Although these results are encouraging, several inherent limitations of cerebral microdialysis have been recognized, including the difficulty of extrapolating from measurements made in a very restricted volume of tissue, the development of reactive gliosis around the catheter tip decreasing the accuracy of measurements and the tissue trauma after probe implantation.

Cerebral ischaemia may cause a decrease in the partial pressure of oxygen in the interstitial space of the brain. Direct measurement of brain tissue oxygenation ($PbrO_2$) in individual patients with SAH in the ICU have shown that important decreases in $PbrO_2$ are associated with poor neurological outcome. A Clarke-type electrode may be placed into brain tissue to monitor regional $PbrO_2$ continuously. The LICOX brain tissue oxygen system is a triple-lumen catheter inserted through an intracranial bolt that measures brain tissue temperature and ICP. The critical threshold with this system for impending cerebral hypoxia is brain oxygen < 20 mmHg, where as cerebral ischaemia is present when brain oxygen is < 15 mmHg. A $PbrO_2$ of > 50 mmHg is the threshold indicating a 'luxury perfusion' state. In general, the goal in management is to maintain a $PbrO_2$ > 20–25 mmHg. Practitioners must be mindful of these critical thresholds and have an understanding as to how occurrences of cerebral hypoxia may affect their patients' outcome.

Continuous EEG (cEEG) is emerging as a promising means of detecting cerebral ischaemia. Ischaemia causes characteristic changes in brain electrical activity, and computer algorithms that provide real-time analysis of EEG waveforms have made cEEG a feasible bedside ischaemia detector. Continuous EEG is non-invasive and provides continuous regional and global functional information. It should detect ischaemia regardless of cause and provides additional information about seizures, depth of sedation and prognosis. Computer software displays the location and degree of ischaemia in a real-time bedside graphic display that may alert nurses and physicians to potentially worrisome trends. Continuous EEG may detect ischaemic changes due to vasospasm almost 3 days before changes in the clinical examination and TCD become manifest. Further studies are needed to define the sensitivity and specificity of cEEG for ischaemia detection and its impact on outcome after SAH. Other technologies exist for ischaemia detection, and although none are yet in widespread use, they warrant mention.

Xenon CT and single-photon emission CT (SPECT) provide quantitative CBF information. The former uses inhaled xenon gas and may be performed at the bedside with a portable CT scanner.

Regarding the direct assessment of CBF in aSAH, three diagnostic modalities are used clinically: SPECT, xenon-enhanced CT (sXe-CT) and positron emission tomography (PET) CT. All three methods have been demonstrated to assess CBF directly and to confirm symptomatic vasospasm. However, these methods are characterized by significant clinical drawbacks. Firstly, regional CBF (rCBF) status as determined by these methods cannot be performed at the bedside and requires patient transfer, which often carries a high risk of secondary insults in severely brain-injured patients. Secondly, all of these techniques provide a 'snapshot' impression of the rCBF status only and do not allow continuous monitoring. Lastly, all of these techniques require the use of radioactive or expensive tracers, making them impractical procedures for daily use in intensive care patients.

An innovative technique that uses a thermal diffusion measurement of CBF and which has shown promising results in experimental models is currently being studied in clinical research. The Hemedex® thermal diffusion flowmetry (TDF) represents an effective method for direct and bedside monitoring of CBF. It is performed by inserting a probe into the brain parenchyma through either a burr hole or tunnelization. Cerebral blood flow values obtained by TDF are in agreement with rCBF values obtained in sXe-CT studies. Using this approach, the reliable detection of vasospasm-induced cerebral hypoperfusion has been demonstrated with a sensitivity of 90% and specificity of 75%. Consequently, the rCBF measurements enable the early identification of patients at risk of developing DIND. Nevertheless, as for PbrO$_2$, TDF monitoring provides information regarding blood flow values only in the small area surrounding the implanted microprobe. This modality shows promise and warrants further study to establish its utility as a tool for the detection of DIND.

Management of cerebral vasospasm

The most feared complication following aSAH due to aneurysm rupture is vasospasm, which is correlated to cerebral infarction. A variety of strategies are used to reduce the risk of vasospasm and cerebral infarction and to improve clinical outcome. Due to the delayed onset of vasospasm, both prophylactic and therapeutic strategies are often adopted. While prophylactic modalities aim to prevent, or at least limit, the onset of vasospasm, therapeutic modalities aim to reverse vasospasm and protect the brain from ischaemia and infarction.

Calcium antagonists

Nimodipine, a calcium-channel blocker, is commonly used in the treatment of aSAH patients to reduce their risk of vasospasm and protect their brain from the deleterious effects of secondary ischaemia. Other calcium-channel blockers may also be effective cerebral vasodilators but have not been investigated in randomized clinical trials. Nimodipine is more lipid soluble than the other calcium-channel blockers. Its lipid solubility enables nimodipine to penetrate the blood–brain barrier providing it with a preferential effect on the cerebral vasculature. The ability of nimodipine to reduce cerebral vasospasm comes from some of the earliest experiments in SAH animal models. In a prospective randomized double-blinded study in 70 aSAH patients, the presence of angiographic vasospasm was not significantly lower in those receiving nimodipine compared with the control group, but the severity of clinical vasospasm was less pronounced. The largest randomized controlled trial, carried out by Pickard and colleagues in 1989, included 554 aSAH patients. Follow-up at 3 months showed that 21 days of nimodipine treatment was effective in reducing the incidence of cerebral infarction by one-third (22% with nimodipine compared with 33% with placebo). Nimodipine did not prevent cerebral vasospasm in high-risk patients but did significantly attenuate its severity, reduce the incidence of delayed neurological deficits and improve functional neurological outcome. A meta-analysis concluded that the effectiveness of nimodipine had been well demonstrated and supported routine prophylactic nimodipine administration. In a prospective trial consisting of 204 patients with aSAH, 113 were treated with nimodipine while the others were in the control group. The incidence of post-operative cerebral vasospasm was 16% higher in the nimodipine group than in the control group, but the long-term mortality, morbidity, cognitive benefits and neurological outcome were all better in the nimodipine group. These data suggest that nimodipine may have secondary neuroprotective effects against cerebral ischaemia during vasospasm, leaving the direct effects of nimodipine on vasospasm questionable. Based on the findings in the literature, 60 mg of nimodipine should be administered every 4 h for 21 days after aSAH. An intravenous form of nimodipine for the treatment of cerebral vasospasm is being used in Europe, making it easier to administer to the sedated or comatose patients when oral feeding through nasogastric tubes is not possible. There is no evidence to support the use of other calcium antagonists such as nicardipine.

Hypertension, hypervolaemia and haemodilution

After the aneurysm has been secured, measures are taken to optimize cerebral perfusion. Intracranial hypertension is treated aggressively and blood pressure parameters are liberalized, allowing the patient to mount a hypertensive response. Because intravascular volume depletion is associated with symptomatic vasospasm after aSAH, volume status should be monitored carefully and patients should be kept euvolaemic. When signs of ischaemia are present, management focuses on preventing cerebral infarction, primarily by augmenting CBF. Intravenous fluids and vasopressors are used to induce hypertension. Blood pressure should be raised until signs of ischaemia resolve or until a maximum safely tolerated blood pressure is achieved. There are few data to guide the choice of vasopressor; however, phenylephrine and norepinephrine are reasonable choices. The use of so-called triple-H therapy (hypervolaemia, hypertension and haemodilution) stems from numerous clinical observations noting improvement in patients' clinical symptoms of vasospasm following induced hypertension and volume expansion. Prophylactic volume expansion with triple-H therapy has not been widely supported in literature where it has not shown any benefits. Despite this, a recent survey demonstrated that 39% of survey respondents favoured prophylactic triple-H therapy, and it was more frequent in low-SAH-volume centres and in Europe. Moreover, although there are no clinical trials supporting the use of triple-H therapy, 52% favoured this practice. However, hypotension and hypovolaemia should be avoided in all patients at risk of developing DIND. In future years, functional imaging modalities and invasive cerebral tissue monitoring may lead to refinements in the optimization of cerebral perfusion augmentation therapy. Monitoring of clinical condition, central venous pressure, arterial blood pressure and serial TCD measurements are strongly suggested when adopting this form of therapy, as it is associated with significant complications including pulmonary oedema, myocardial ischaemia and electrolyte abnormalities. Regarding hypertension, by measuring $PbrO_2$ during triple-H therapy, authors were able to demonstrate that vasopressor-induced elevation of mean arterial pressure caused a significant increase of regional CBF and $PbrO_2$ in all patients with SAH. Volume expansion, however, resulted in only a slight effect on regional CBF but reversed the effect on brain tissue oxygenation.

Haemodilution is used to improve blood viscosity in order to augment cerebral perfusion. A recently published prospective study showed that a haemoglobin concentration $<9\,g\,dl^{-1}$ is associated with an increased incidence of brain hypoxia and cell energy dysfunction in patients with poor-grade SAH. Others have also correlated lower haemoglobin levels to adverse outcome following SAH. However, active transfusion of red blood cells was also linked to delayed cerebral ischaemia and poor outcome. These findings warrant further investigation.

Endovascular therapies

Criteria to determine the applicability of endovascular techniques for treating vasospasm following aSAH include the absence of an established infarct on CT scanning, the persistence of neurological deficits despite medical management and angiographic evidence of vasospasm in a distribution consistent with the neurological deficit. Endovascular techniques employed in the therapy of vasospasm include mechanical dilation of major cerebral arteries using transluminal balloon angioplasty (TBA) and local injection of vasodilator agents. Transluminal balloon angioplasty increases CBF, reverses angiographic vasospasm and reduces clinical deficits, although it has not been shown to improve long-term outcome. Complications of TBA include vessel rupture, which has been reported at a rate of 4%, vessel occlusion, thrombus formation and dislodgment of aneurysm clips. Transluminal balloon angioplasty may be used along with pharmacological therapies singularly or in combination. Although the effects of balloon angioplasty are thought to be more durable than those of pharmacological vasodilation, many radiologists still consider any beneficial effects of TBA to be short-lived. Selective endovascular administration of vasodilators may be infused into proximal vessels or, with the use of super-selective micro-catheterization techniques, into distal segments that are not amenable to balloon angioplasty. Intra-arterial carotid injections of nimodipine reduce the systemic side effects of this drug by selectively delivering it at higher concentration to a focused area of the cerebral vasculature. Intrathecal infusion of nimodipine has shown to be promising in the experimental setting;

however, clinical evidence needs to be investigated further. Intravenous administration of papaverine has not been favourable for the treatment of cerebral vasospasm because of its vasodilatory effects on the peripheral vasculature, therefore increasing ICP. For this reason, when using vasodilators it is advisable to monitor ICP.

Novel treatments

Magnesium sulfate

Hypomagnesaemia is associated with vasospasm and with poor outcome. Hence, it should be corrected promptly. Magnesium sulfate was first used in pre-eclamptic pregnant women to reduce uterine smooth muscle contractions and is thought to prevent cerebral vasospasm by a similar mechanism on the smooth muscle of the cerebral vasculature. Its use for cerebral vasospasm has had conflicting outcomes due to various dosing techniques used to administer magnesium sulfate (bolus versus continuous infusion), and different goals for serum and CSF magnesium levels when measured in these studies. An ongoing randomized, placebo-controlled, double-blinded, multicentre trial, the Intravenous Magnesium sulfate in Aneurysmal Subarachnoid Haemorrhage (IMASH) trial, will evaluate the effect of magnesium sulfate infusion on the clinical outcome of patients with aSAH. Preliminary results showed that a 14-day infusion of magnesium sulfate may reduce the incidence of symptomatic vasospasm and justifies the continuation of the study to try and establish a clinically useful prophylactic treatment. This will be the first study to provide level 1 evidence for the effectiveness of magnesium sulfate on the treatment of cerebral vasospasm. Magnesium sulfate levels most suggested in the literature in order to prevent vasospasm range from 2.0 to 3.0 mEq dl^{-1}.

Statins

Statins, 3-hydroxy-3-methylglutaryl coenzyme A (HMG-CoA) reductase inhibitors, are a type of cholesterol-lowering medication that increases endothelial nitric oxide synthase (eNOS) expression and improves its intrinsic function. Nitric oxide relaxes smooth muscle cells in the cerebral arteries, thereby attenuating cerebral vasospasm. In a retrospective study consisting of 115 SAH patients at a single institution, patients who were on statin therapy for at least 1 month before admission were identified and found to have an 11-fold

reduction in the risk of developing cerebral vasospasm compared with those who were not on statin therapy. This led to further studies, which demonstrated that prophylactic therapy with statins improves neurological outcomes and reduces the incidence of cerebral infarction. Statin therapy as a treatment rather than a prophylactic measure has also been demonstrated in a phase II randomized controlled trial where SAH patients were treated with primvistatin within 72 h of the aSAH. The incidences of radiographic and symptomatic vasospasm were reduced by 32 and 42%, respectively, and neurological outcomes were also better when compared with the placebo group. This same team subsequently demonstrated that statin therapy also improved CBF autoregulation. A multicentre randomized controlled phase 3 trial, Simvastatin in Aneurysmal Subarachnoid Haemorrhage (STASH), looking at the potential benefit of simvastatin (40 mg for 21 days) in aSAH is underway and will evaluate the effect of simvastatin on clinical outcome.

Erythropoeitin

Erythropoietin has been suggested to have neuroprotective effects in the central nervous system (CNS) through activation of eNOS; however, a double-blind randomized trial of erythropoietin versus placebo in 73 patients failed to show any beneficial effect on cerebral vasospasm.

Pharmacological implants

Some authors have studied the effect of placing prolonged-release nicardipine implants in the basal cisterns after aneurysm clipping. Results seem promising for the proximal vessels, but the effect has be found to be less prominent on the distal cerebral circulation.

Enoxaparin

There is a significant incidence of deep venous thrombosis in patients who have suffered a SAH. The use of prophylactic enoxaparin, a low-molecular-weight heparin, was found to be safe in randomized trials. However, enoxaparin use has also been shown to reduce the incidence of ischaemic complications from cerebral vasospasm, possibly through a reduction in thrombogenicity. In a prospectively randomized placebo-controlled trial consisting of 120 Hunt–Hess grade 1–3 SAH patients enoxaparin (20 mg SC daily) significantly reduced the incidence of DIND (8.8%), cerebral infarction (3.5%) secondary to cerebral vasospasm and shunt-dependence (1.8%) after 1 year compared with the placebo control group.

Endothelin receptor antagonists

Endothelin, a potent vasoconstrictor, increases after SAH, and stimulation of endothelin receptors induces contraction of vascular smooth muscle cells resulting in vasospasm. Blocking the endothelin receptors through the use of a competitive endothelin-1 receptor antagonist (clazosentan) may decrease the incidence and severity of cerebral vasospasm by inducing arterial relaxation. A phase II multicentre, double-blinded, prospective clinical trial, which evaluated the effects of intravenous clazosentan on preventing cerebral vasospasm in 32 Hunt–Hess grade 3 and 4 SAH patients, demonstrated a reduction in the incidence of cerebral vasospasm (40 vs. 88% in the control group) and new infarctions (15 vs. 44%) without any important side effects. A phase 1 clinical trial reproducing these effects is awaited.

Oestrogen

Laboratory experiments have shown that oestrogen promotes vasodilation by attenuating the upregulation of endothelin-1 receptors after SAH and also by inducing the upregulation of L-type smooth muscle cell calcium ion channels. Tamoxifen, an oestrogen receptor agonist capable of crossing the blood–brain barrier, seems to have neuroprotective properties through at least three mechanisms: inhibition of glutamate cytotoxicity, inhibition of neuronal nitric oxide synthase activity and free radical formation, and antioxidant properties that scavenge oxygen and nitrogen free radicals. Its neuroprotective effects have been proven in experimental animal models by various authors, and future clinical studies are warranted.

Adenosine receptor agonists

Aneurysmal SAH increases inducible nitric oxide synthase (iNOS, vasospastic properties) and reduces eNOS (vasodilatory properties) production after SAH. It has been hypothesized that the adenosine-2A receptor may counteract the effects of SAH on eNOS and iNOS production. Further investigational research is encouraged.

Antifibrinolytics

During the era of late aneurysm surgery, the antifibrinolytic agent ε-aminocaproic acid, a competitive inhibitor of plasminogen activator, has been shown by various authors to reduce rebleeding rates after cerebral aneurysm rupture. Despite the reduced use of ε-aminocaproic acid due to the event of early surgery, and the associated side effects (e.g. deep venous thrombosis, pulmonary emboli, cortical renal necrosis, myopathies and arteriopathic complications) this drug continues to find a place in many centres to reduce rebleeding rates in patients with SAH due to aneurysm rupture. Although antifibrinolytic medications may be beneficial in selected patients, they should not be used routinely. Further study is needed to determine whether certain patient characteristics, other treatment strategies, or timing and dose of drug administration might mitigate the risks associated with antifibrinolytic drugs.

Hypertonic saline

Hypertonic saline is currently used as a therapeutic measure to reduce high ICP following head trauma. In one study, systemic administration of 23.5% hypertonic saline was given in patients with poor-grade spontaneous SAH with enhancement of CBF. Recently, it was also demonstrated that the increment of change in CBF correlated with changes in autoregulation, and it was concluded that bolus systemic hypertonic saline therapy may be used for reversal of cerebral ischaemia to normal perfusion in patients with poor-grade SAH.

Management of complications following subarachnoid haemorrhage

The rupture of an intracranial aneurysm may be associated with an array of severe intracranial and systemic complications, which, if not diagnosed and treated in time, can present a unique challenge for the physician. Cerebral complications of aSAH include recurrent intracranial haemorrhage (especially in the pre-treatment phase), vasospasm (discussed previously in this chapter), cerebral infarction, hydrocephalus, and intracranial hypertension and seizures. Systemic complications include derangements of water and electrolyte homeostasis, myocardial dysfunction, neurogenic pulmonary oedema, sepsis and thromboembolism. Although many of these complications are life-threatening, they are often transient and reversible; hence, early intensive care management improves outcome in the majority of these patients.

Management of intracranial complications

Rebleeding

High blood pressure after aSAH is related to ultra-early rebleeding. Following the initial aneurysm rupture, the risk of rebleeding in untreated aneurysms may be quite significant. It is highest within the first 24 h after the initial rupture. Rebleeding occurs in 20% of patients with an unclipped aneurysm during the first 2 weeks after the initial bleed, in 40% within 6 months, and in 3% for each year following. Approximately 50% of the patients die immediately, whereas another 30% die from further complications after the rebleed. Therefore, it seems prudent to institute medical measures to reduce the risk of rebleeding until definitive treatment is performed. Although blood pressure control has not been definitively shown to affect the risk of rebleeding, significantly elevated blood pressures should be treated with short-acting intravenous medications that have a reliable dose–response relationship. Commonly used medications include nicardipine, labetalol and esmolol. Sodium nitroprusside is avoided because of the risks of elevated ICP and toxicity. It is important to avoid overaggressive lowering of blood pressure, especially in patients with baseline arterial hypertension and in patients with intracranial hypertension, because this may worsen CPP and precipitate cerebral ischaemia. Rebleeding may be related to aneurysmal expansion, which is largely dictated by transmural pressure. For the same reason, lowering pressure outside the aneurysm, in the subarachnoid space, may also predispose to rupture. Therefore, when a ventriculostomy is in place, CSF should not be drained rapidly or aggressively. It is reasonable to keep the drain open and to maintain the collection chamber at 20 cm above the external auditory canal. Ancillary measures to prevent rebleeding include bedrest and adequate treatment of pain and anxiety. Antifibrinolytic agents, such as tranexamic acid and ε-aminocaproic acid, reduce the risk of rebleeding, but, as mentioned previously in this chapter, their benefit is offset by an increased risk of complications, including cerebral infarction. It should be investigated whether immediate administration of tranexamic acid, followed by early aneurysm treatment, discontinuation of antifibrinolytic therapy and aggressive treatment of vasospasm, reduces mortality and the incidence of rebleeding without increasing the incidence of DIND.

Cerebral infarction

The Australian pathologist E. G. Robertson was one of the first to discover the presence of cerebral infarction in 40% of patients with SAH. The presence of both midline shift and angiographically demonstrated vasospasm increases the likelihood of cerebral infarction. Since these early studies, other authors have demonstrated the correlation between vasospasm and cerebral ischaemia. In the pathogenesis of cerebral infarction following SAH, besides the narrowing of cerebral vessels, other factors may be involved, but causality is difficult to prove in critically ill patients. Multiple microthrombi composed of platelet aggregates mixed with multinucleated leucocytes may play an important role. Risk factors for cerebral infarction in good-grade patients include: the amount of blood on the primary brain CT scan, post-operative angiographic vasospasm, early surgery and a history of hypertension. Acute cerebral infarction may present in the first few days following SAH and may be due to the acute effects of haemorrhage and the spike in ICP, but there are few objectively defined risk factors. A recent retrospective study sought to identify patients with cerebral infarction associated with SAH in whom the cerebral infarction was unlikely to be due to vasospasm. The authors found that cerebral infarction occurred in 28% of 103 patients with SAH. Eighteen patients had cerebral infarction that was unlikely to be due to vasospasm because it was visible on a CT scan by day 2 (33%) or because angiography showed no vasospasm in a referable artery (39%), or both (28%). More abnormal acute physiology may indicate a greater risk of cerebral infarction during aneurysm obliteration and greater physiological derangement from the cardiovascular effects of haemorrhage. Alternative mechanisms for cerebral infarction include arterial embolism, hypotension and focal neuronal toxicity due to metabolic derangements (hyperglycaemia, acidosis and hypoxia). Cerebral ischaemia may also be present in asymptomatic SAH patients with vasospasm. In fact, cerebral infarct in the presence of asymptomatic delayed cerebral ischaemia is particularly common in comatose patients and is associated with a poor outcome.

Hydrocephalus

Acute hydrocephalus affects 15–25% of patients with SAH and is associated with poor clinical and radiographic grade. Delayed hydrocephalus can develop anytime from 3 to 21 days post-SAH. Intraventricular blood forming after the bleed frequently leads to a non-communicating form of hydrocephalus; communicating hydrocephalus may also occur. The consequential increase in ventricular size, ventriculomegaly, may be asymptomatic (especially in normal pressure hydrocephalus) or may be accompanied by signs and symptoms of increased ICP, such as headache, sixth-nerve palsy and impaired upgaze, up to a decreased level of arousal. In the last case, a ventriculostomy should be placed, which is often associated with immediate clinical improvement. Complications include ventriculitis (in approximately 15% of patients), bleeding along the catheter tract and cerebral infarction. In symptomatic patients with chronic hydrocephalus, temporary or permanent CSF diversion is recommended after SAH.

Intracranial hypertension

Intracranial hypertension is frequently present in patients with aSAH. Factors that may be involved in increasing ICP may be CSF obstruction due to the presence of blood clots, vasoparalysis and distal cerebral arteriolar vasodilation. Increased ICP may also be caused by cytotoxic oedema due to cerebral ischaemia. Conventional medical strategies may be ineffective, leading to the introduction of therapeutic measures such as hypothermia or decompressive craniectomy. Although there is presently insufficient evidence to support the clinical use of therapeutic hypothermia or decompressive craniectomy for aSAH, many small clinical studies have been published with promising results.

Seizures

The incidence of seizures after SAH varies considerably, and their impact on outcome is still undefined. Most early seizures usually occur prior to medical presentation. Shaking movements are frequently present at the time of the ictus; however, how many of these movements are due to true seizures and not posturing is unknown. Non-convulsive seizures may be under-recognized, occurring in up to 20% of comatose patients following an average of 18 days after the SAH. Data regarding the utility of prophylactic anticonvulsant medications are conflicting. There is some suggestion that cumulative exposure to phenytoin is associated with worse long-term cognitive outcome. Decisions regarding the use of antiepileptic agents should therefore attempt to weigh medication-related risks with seizure-related risks. Early seizure prophylaxis may

be justified during the acute phase, prior to treatment of the aneurysm, where a seizure-related surge in blood pressure may increase the risk of rebleeding. After the aneurysm is secured, the benefit of anticonvulsant medications becomes less clear. Anti-epileptic agents are suggested by some authors to be continued for patients with a pre-morbid history of seizures, for patients who had a seizure around the time of the SAH and for those otherwise deemed to be at high risk for seizures (MCA aneurysm, intraparenchymal haemorrhage, infarction and a history of hypertension). However, the efficacy and harm of this practice have not been evaluated in a randomized trial. The recent American Heart Association guideline recommends that protracted anticonvulsants should be considered only for patients with risk factors such as prior seizure, intraparenchymal haematoma, infarct or MCA aneurysms.

Management of systemic complications

Hyponatraemia and intravascular volume depletion

Following SAH, electrolyte disturbances may be frequent. Hyponatraemia occurs in up to 30% of patients and is independently associated with poor outcome. Risk factors include poor clinical grade, anterior communicating artery aneurysms and hydrocephalus. A potential cause of hyponatraemia after SAH is cerebral salt-wasting syndrome (CSWS), which recently has stimulated frequent debate regarding its true definition. It is due to a renal loss of sodium and is characterized by reduced extracellular volume (hypovolaemic hyponatraemia). The syndrome of inappropriate antidiuretic hormone secretion (SIADH), if untreated, may lead to euvolaemic or hypervolaemic hyponatraemia, and may occasionally coexist with CSWS, therefore requiring the physician to promptly diagnose the electrolytic disturbance in order to change the therapeutic strategy. The key to distinguishing CSWS from SIADH hinges upon determination of volume status, which is frequently difficult and imprecise. However, CSWS may potentially be more harmful, as volume depletion may cause further alterations in CPP. Regardless of the cause of hyponatraemia, salt administration is an appropriate treatment. Most cases of hypovolaemic hyponatraemia are mild and may be treated with isotonic crystalloid – to restore intravascular volume – and with oral or enteral sodium chloride. When hyponatraemia is severe, is acutely symptomatic or occurs in a patient with intracranial hypertension, intravenous hypertonic saline may be required. Two randomized, controlled trials have been performed to evaluate the ability of fludrocortisone to correct hyponatraemia and fluid balance. One found that it helped to correct the negative sodium balance but not volume contraction or hyponatraemia, and the other reported a reduced need for fluids and improved sodium levels with fludrocortisone. One retrospective study has suggested that 3% saline is effective in correcting hyponatraemia. Additional reports suggest that 5% albumin may also be effective. Fludrocortisone has mineralocorticoid properties and may be useful adjunctively to correct hyponatraemia and restore extracellular volume. Mild euvolaemic or hypervolaemic hyponatraemia (SIADH) may be treated with conivaptan, a vasopressin-receptor antagonist. Fluid restriction after SAH is associated with DIND and should be used with extreme caution or not at all.

Cardiac dysfunction

Cardiac enzymes are often mildly elevated and arrhythmias are frequent after SAH, occurring in almost 100% of patients. Troponin levels are frequently elevated and are variably associated with echocardiographic abnormalities. The condition is surprisingly transient and is completely reversed in a few days. In patients with known coronary artery disease, the pattern of echocardiographic changes is often helpful in determining the aetiology. The most important predictors of cardiac dysfunction are those that reflect the severity of the haemorrhage. Following SAH, a variety of ventricular and supraventricular bradyarrhythmias and tachyarrhythmias may occur. The frequency and severity of arrhythmias is greatest in the first 48 h after SAH. Although arrhythmias are usually benign, in rare cases the cardiac abnormities are much more severe. About 5% of arrhythmias are life-threatening, most of them being polymorphic ventricular tachycardia and torsades de pointes. The latter correlates with QT prolongation on ECG. Arrhythmias are treated with standard advanced cardiac life-support protocols. Medications that prolong the QT interval should be used judiciously. Myocardial contractility may be markedly impaired immediately after SAH, leading to a fall in cardiac output and blood pressure. This condition has been referred to as 'stunned myocardium'

and may also include an element of neurogenic pulmonary oedema. Neurogenic stunned myocardium, a reversible cardiomyopathy, occurs in 10–28% of SAH patients and is thought to be related to excessive catecholamine release from the sympathetic nerve terminals innervating the myocardium. A variety of wall motion patterns may be observed, none of which respect an epicardial coronary arterial distribution. Reported risk factors include female sex, younger age, smaller body surface area, higher clinical SAH grade, anterior aneurysm location and prior history of cocaine or amphetamine use. Presenting signs of neurogenic stunned myocardium range from sinus tachycardia to mild to moderate congestive heart failure and pulmonary oedema. Severe cases are accompanied by hypotension or cardiogenic shock. The cardiomyopathy may be accompanied by changes on ECG. ST-segment elevation, mimicking an ST-elevation myocardial infarction, is most common. Non-specific T-wave changes and a new bundle branch block may also be observed. There is a modest elevation in troponin I that correlates with the degree of neurological injury. Cardiac enzyme elevation is typically disproportionally low for the degree of wall motion abnormality compared with myocardial infarction. Brain natriuretic peptide is invariably elevated and correlates with left ventricular end-diastolic pressure. Echocardiography and ventriculography may demonstrate hypokinesis or akinesis of the apical segment of the left ventricle and sparing of the base ('apical ballooning' or 'Takotsubo' pattern). More common after SAH is hypokinesis or akinesis of the mid-segment ('apical sparing' pattern) or hypokinesis or akinesis of the base with preserved apical systolic function ('inverted Takotsubo' pattern). The right ventricle may be involved in some patients and is associated with more severe congestive heart failure. Treatment of neurogenic stunned myocardium is largely supportive. If symptoms are mild, intravenous fluids and phenylephrine may be used to increase afterload and left ventricular cavity size. β-Blockers are of theoretical benefit and may be used as tolerated. If moderate to severe congestive heart failure is present, inotropic medications are used. In theory, a non-catecholamine inotrope such as milrinone should be the drug of choice. Worsening of cardiac function is occasionally observed with catecholamine vasopressors and inotropes. Dynamic left ventricular outflow tract obstruction should be excluded with echocardiography prior to using inotropic medications. Extreme caution should be used with diuretics, given the association between intravascular volume depletion and poor outcome after SAH. When cardiogenic shock is present, standard therapies are used, including vasopressors, inotropes and intra-aortic balloon pump counterpulsation as appropriate. Rare complications of neurogenic stunned myocardium include left ventricular free-wall rupture, formation of intracardiac thrombus and arrhythmias. Prompt management and restoration of a good cardiac output may be beneficial in maintaining an efficient CPP and has been associated with an improvement in neurological outcome.

Neurogenic pulmonary oedema

Neurogenic pulmonary oedema (NPO) is a potentially life-threatening complication in patients with aSAH and is represented by an increase in interstitial and alveolar lung fluid that occurs as a direct consequence of acute or subacute CNS injury. Neurogenic pulmonary oedema is often seen in conjunction with an increase in ICP leading to a reactive increase in the systemic blood pressure, due to α-adrenergic stimulation, and possibly is a result of concomitant increases in left atrial and pulmonary capillary pressures. This is in accordance with the 'blast theory' of Theodore and Robin, where they suggest that a severe transient rise in pulmonary capillary pressure increases pulmonary vascular permeability, leading to an interstitial and alveolar pulmonary oedema.

Haemodynamic changes per se do not explain all of the experimental and clinical data. For example, many clinical studies and animal models of NPO have demonstrated protein-rich oedema fluid and altered pulmonary capillary permeability. It is possible that catecholamines released after brain injury and increased ICP could directly injure pulmonary vessels or cause increases in vessel permeability. In a recent study, elevated ICP values were found in 67% of the patients with NPO, and at time of admission, 33% of the patients showed pupillary disturbances as a sign of severely elevated ICP with start of herniation. Therefore, it can be suggested that elevated ICP during the acute phase is a risk factor for developing NPO. The authors showed that the incidence of NPO was significantly higher in patients with ruptured aneurysm in the posterior circulation, possibly causing compression of the medulla oblongata, essential for a reactive sympathetic reaction.

Symptoms associated with NPO usually present within minutes to hours of a severe CNS insult, although a delayed form of NPO developing more slowly over 12 h to several days has also been described. They include an altered level of consciousness, dyspnea, cyanosis, crackles, hypoxaemia and diffuse pulmonary infiltrates. These clinical features can be mistaken for other causes of pulmonary oedema and may lead to confusion in the diagnosis and therapeutic approach of hypoxaemic respiratory failure in the setting of CNS injury. Chest X-rays typically show a normal heart size with evidence of bilateral diffuse alveolar filling, but they may also appear similar to congestive heart failure with vascular redistribution.

Treatment consists of respiratory support and should focus on the underlying neurological disorder. With general supportive measures including supplemental oxygen, airway protection and mechanical ventilation when necessary, most cases of hypoxaemic respiratory failure are reversible and within 48–72 h. Maintenance of low cardiac filling pressures with diuretics or vasodilators may decrease the formation of oedema but must be done so as not to compromise cardiac output and cerebral perfusion; a pulmonary artery catheter may be helpful in this regard. β-Adrenergic antagonists can reduce histamine-induced augmentation of pulmonary vascular permeability. Dobutamine may increase cardiac output and therefore help decrease pulmonary artery balloon occlusion pressure and promote diuresis.

Rehabilitation

The aim of rehabilitation is to return the patient to the maximum level of independence possible by reducing the effects of disease or injury in daily life. In other words, rehabilitation is the process of re-enabling the patient to live as normally and as independently as possible. Therefore, many believe that rehabilitation begins by preventing secondary neuronal injury. Those patients with minimal deficit require little rehabilitation. However, in patients with major deficits, initial efforts are focused on preventing the development of medical, musculoskeletal, bowel and bladder problems. After this, rehabilitation is aimed at providing optimum medical, social and environmental conditions that will maximize recovery. Coping techniques and compensatory strategies will be taught to allow the patient to become as independent as possible.

Patients who survive aSAH will have a wide spectrum of cognitive and neurological deficits. While many survivors function independently with few or no significant motor or sensory deficits, many suffer from unrecognized subtle cognitive and emotional effects. These include confusion, amnesia, impaired judgement and emotional lability. Medical and nursing staff, family members, therapists, psychologists and social services are all involved in the re-enablement process.

Conclusions

While there has been an improvement in mortality rates for patients presenting with SAH, the final outcome continues to depend on coordinated and aggressive treatment. Early detection of probable complications and prompt treatment will result in the best possible neurological outcome. Future developments focused on improving our understanding of the pathophysiological mechanisms behind secondary neuronal injury will allow the development of novel mechanism-specific targeted therapies, which are likely to improve outcome further.

Further reading

Anon. (2000). Epidemiology of aneurysmal subarachnoid hemorrhage in Australia and New Zealand: incidence and case fatality from the Australasian Cooperative Research on Subarachnoid Hemorrhage Study (ACROSS). *Stroke* **31**, 1843–50.

Baldwin, M. E., Macdonald, R. L. and Huo, D. (2004). Early vasospasm on admission angiography in patients with aneurysmal subarachnoid hemorrhage is a predictor for in-hospital complications and poor outcome. *Stroke* **35**, 2506–11.

Barker, F. G. II and Ogilvy, C. S. (1996). Efficacy of prophylactic nimodipine for delayed ischemic deficit after subarachnoid hemorrhage: a metaanalysis. *J Neurosurg* **84**, 405–14.

Charpentier, C., Audibert, G., Guillemin, F. et al. (1999). Multivariate analysis of predictors of cerebral vasospasm occurrence after aneurismal subarachnoid hemorrhage. *Stroke* **30**, 1402–8.

Crompton, M. R. (1964). The pathogenisis of cerebral infarction following the rupture of cerebral aneurysms. *Brain* **87**, 491–510.

Cross, D. T. III, Tirschwell, D. L., Clark, M. A. et al. (2003). Mortality rates after subarachnoid hemorrhage: variations according to hospital case volume in 18 states. *J Neurosurg* **99**, 810–17.

Dennis, L. J., Claassen, J., Hirsch, L. J. et al. (2002). Nonconvulsive status epilepticus after subarachnoid hemorrhage. *Neurosurgery* **51**, 1136–43.

Ghali, J. K., Koren, M. J., Taylor, J. R. et al. (2006). Efficacy and safety of oral conivaptan: a V1A/V2 vasopressin receptor antagonist, assessed in a randomized, placebo-controlled trial in patients with euvolemic or hypervolemic hyponatremia. *J Clin Endocrinol Metab* **91**, 2145–52.

Groden, C., Kremer, C., Regelsberger, J. et al. (2001). Comparison of operative and endovascular treatment of anterior circulation aneurysms in patients in poor grades. *Neuroradiology* **43**, 778–83.

Gruber, A., Ungersbock, K., Reinprecht, A. et al. (1998). Evaluation of cerebral vasospasm after early surgical and endovascular treatment of ruptured intracranial aneurysms. *Neurosurgery* **42**, 258–67.

Knuckey, N. W. and Stokes, B. A. (1982). Medical management of patients following a ruptured cerebral aneurysm, with epsilon-aminocaproic acid, kanamycin, and reserpine. *Surg Neurol* **17**, 181–5.

Kostron, H., Twerdy, K. and Grunert, V. (1988). The calcium entry blocker nimodipine improves the quality of life of patients operated on for cerebral aneurysms. A 5-year follow-up analysis. *Neurochirurgia* **31**, 150–3.

Kramer, A. H., Gurka, M. J., Nathan, B. et al. (2008). Complications associated with anemia and blood transfusion in patients with aneurysmal subarachnoid hemorrhage. *Crit Care Med* **36**, 2070–5.

Lin, C. L., Shih, H. C., Lieu, A. S. et al. (2007). Attenuation of experimental subarachnoid hemorrhage-induced cerebral vasospasm by the adenosine A2A receptor agonist CGS 21680. *J Neurosurg*; **106**, 436–41.

Lysakowski, C., Walder, B., Costanza, M. C. et al. (2001). Transcranial Doppler versus angiography in patients with vasospasm due to a ruptured cerebral aneurysm: a systematic review. *Stroke* **32**, 2292–8.

Manno, E. M., Gress, D. R., Schwamm, L. H. et al. (1998). Effects of induced hypertension on transcranial Doppler ultrasound velocities in patients after subarachnoid hemorrhage. *Stroke* **29**, 422–8.

McGirt, M. J., Pradilla, G., Legnani, F. G. et al. (2006). Systemic administration of simvastatin after the onset of experimental subarachnoid hemorrhage attenuates cerebral vasospasm. *Neurosurgery* **58**, 945–95.

Molyneux, A., Kerr, R., Ly-Mee, Y. et al. (2005). International Subarachnoid Aneurysm Trial (ISAT) of neurosurgical clipping versus endovascular coiling in 2143 patients with ruptured intracranial aneurysms: a randomized comparison of effects on survival, dependency, seizures, rebleeding, subgroups, and aneurysm occlusion. *Lancet* **366**, 809–17.

Naidech, A. M., Drescher, J., Tamul, P. et al. (2006). Acute physiological derangement is associated with early radiographic cerebral infarction after SAH. *J Neurol Neurosurg Psychiatry*; **77**, 1340–4.

Oddo, M., Milby, A. and Chen, I. (2009). Hemoglobin concentration and cerebral metabolism in patients with aneurysmal subarachnoid hemorrhage *Stroke*. **40**, 75–1281.

Philippon, J., Grob, R., Dagreou, F. *et al.* (1986). Prevention of vasospasm in subarachnoid haemorrhage. A controlled study with nimodipine. *Acta Neurochir* **82**, 110–14.

Pickard, J. D., Murray, G. D., Illingworth, R. *et al.* (1989). Effect of oral nimodipine on cerebral infarction and outcome after subarachnoid haemorrhage: British aneurysm nimodipine trial. *BMJ* **298**, 636–42.

Proust, F., Callonec, F., Clavier, E. *et al.* (1999). Usefulness of transcranial color-coded sonography in the diagnosis of cerebral vasospasm. *Stroke* **30**, 1091–8.

Sarrafzadeh, A. S., Sakowitz, O. W., Kiening, K. L. *et al.* (2002). Bedside microdialysis: a tool to monitor cerebral metabolism in subarachnoid hemorrhage patients? *Crit Care Med* **30**, 1062–70.

Siironen, J., Juvela, S., Varis, J. *et al.* (2003). No effect of enoxaparin on outcome of aneurismal subarachnoid hemorrhage: a randomized, double-blind, placebo-controlled clinical trial. *J Neurosurg* **99**, 953–9.

Skjoth-Rasmussen, J., Schulz, M., Kristensen, S. R. *et al.* (2004). Delayed neurological deficits detected by an ischemic pattern in the extracellular cerebral metabolites in patients with aneurysmal subarachnoid hemorrhage. *J Neurosurg* **100**, 8–15.

Springborg, J. B., Moller, C., Gideon, P. *et al.* (2007). Erythropoietin in patients with aneurysmal subarachnoid haemorrhage: a double blind randomised clinical trial. *Acta Neurochir Wein* **149**, 1089–101.

Treggiari, M. M., Walder, B., Suter, P. M. *et al.* (2003). Systematic review of the prevention of delayed ischemic neurological deficits with hypertension, hypervolemia, and hemodilution therapy following subarachnoid hemorrhage. *J Neurosurg* **98**, 978–84.

Tseng, M. Y., Al-Rawi, P. G., Pickard, J. D. *et al.* (2003). Effect of hypertonic saline on cerebral blood flow in poor-grade patients with subarachnoid hemorrhage. *Stroke* **34**, 1389–96.

Tseng, M. Y., Czosnyka, M., Richards, H. *et al.* (2005). Effects of acute treatment with pravastatin on cerebral vasospasm, autoregulation, and delayed ischemic deficits after aneurysmal subarachnoid hemorrhage: a phase II randomized placebo-controlled trial. *Stroke* **36**, 1627–32.

Vajkoczy, P., Horn, P. and Thome, C. (2003). Regional cerebral blood flow monitoring in the diagnosis of delayed ischemia following aneurysmal subarachnoid hemorrhage. *J Neurosurg* **98**, 1227–34.

Vatter, H., Zimmermann, M., Tesanovic, V. *et al.* (2005). Cerebrovascular characterization of clazosentan, the first nonpeptide endothelin receptor antagonist shown to be clinically effective for the treatment of cerebral vasospasm. Part II: Effect on endothelin(B) receptor-mediated relaxation. *J Neurosurg* **102**, 1108–14.

Wong, G. K., Chan, M. T., Poon, W. S. *et al.* (2006). Magnesium therapy within 48 hours of an aneurysmal subarachnoid hemorrhage: neuro-panacea. *Neurol Res* **28**, 431–5.

Zhang, Y., Milatovic, D., Aschner, M. *et al.* (2007). Neuroprotection by tamoxifen in focal cerebral ischemia is not mediated by an agonist action at estrogen receptors but is associated with antioxidant activity. *Exp Neurol* **204**, 819–27.

Chapter 23

Intracerebral haemorrhage

Fred Rincon and Stephan A. Mayer

Introduction

Spontaneous intracerebral haemorrhage (ICH) is the most devastating type of stroke, and is a leading cause of disability among adults. Primary ICH originates from the spontaneous rupture of small arterioles damaged by chronic hypertension or cerebral amyloid angiopathy (CAA). Secondary ICH is the result of bleeding from vascular malformations, haemorrhagic transformation of an ischaemic stroke, tumours, abnormal coagulation or vasculitis.

Pathophysiology

Spontaneous ICH begins with rupture of a small, chronically damaged and fragmented artery or arteriole. Rapid extravasation of blood into the parenchyma leads to the formation of a space-occupying haematoma, which in turn results in oedema and swelling of the surrounding brain tissue. Chronic hypertension leads to pathological changes within the tunica media of small- and medium-sized arterioles of 100–600 µm in diameter. This vasculopathy is characterized by: (i) degeneration of medial smooth muscle cells; (ii) small miliary aneurysms associated with thrombosis and microhaemorrhages; (iii) accumulation of non-fatty deposits between the intima and media; and (iv) fibrinoid necrosis and hyalinization of the intima, preferentially at bifurcation points and distal portions of the vessel. Primary affected structures include the thalamus, basal ganglia, deep periventricular grey matter, pons and cerebellum. Cerebral amyloid angiopathy leads to spontaneous ICH in elderly people and results from amyloid protein being deposited within the media and adventitia of small- to medium-sized vessels. Cerebral amyloid angiopathy has a predilection for leptomeningeal and penetrating vessels of the cortex, which may undergo fibrinoid necrosis as

seen in chronic hypertension. The apolipoprotein E gene is polymorphic, and apolipoprotein Eε2 (ApoE2) and apolipoprotein Eε4 (ApoE4) genotypes (cognate proteins shown in parentheses) are risk factors for CAA-associated ICH.

Expansion of the haematoma

Following abrupt arterial rupture, rapid accumulation of blood within the brain parenchyma increases local tissue pressure. A degree of physical destruction is inevitable and may be explained by shearing forces of the expanding haematoma. In addition to the relative mass effect, the haematoma itself induces three early pathophysiological changes in the surrounding brain tissue: (i) neuronal and glial cell death due to apoptosis and inflammation; (ii) breakdown of the brain–blood barrier (BBB); and (iii) vasogenic oedema.

Haematoma expansion is an important cause of early neurological deterioration, and the volume of the haematoma is a powerful predictor of outcome after primary ICH. The prevailing theory has been that an expanding haematoma results from persistent bleeding or rebleeding from a single arteriolar rupture. More recent evidence suggests that ICH growth may result from multifocal bleeding into congested and hypoperfused brain tissue surrounding the haematoma. Positron emission tomography (PET) and multisequence MRI protocols, including diffusion-weighted imaging (DWI), indicate that hypoperfused tissue in the periphery of the haematoma is more likely the result of reduced metabolic demand, rather than flow-limiting ischaemia.

Neurotoxic and inflammatory responses

As ischaemia may not be the primary cause of cellular injury after ICH, neurotoxic and inflammatory

Core Topics in Neuroanaesthesia and Neurointensive Care, eds. Basil F. Matta, David K. Menon and Martin Smith. Published by Cambridge University Press. © Cambridge University Press 2011.

mechanisms have been implicated in the pathogenesis of perihaemorrhagic tissue damage. It is feasible that local and systemic inflammatory mediators enhance tissue damage either directly or indirectly by the activation of leucocytes and the generation of prostaglandins and leukotrienes. Several investigators have demonstrated that the upregulation of interleukin-6 (IL-6) and IL-1, and high plasma concentrations of pro-inflammatory molecules such as tumour necrosis factor alpha (TNF-α) and intercellular adhesion molecule 1 (ICAM-1) are correlated with the magnitude of subsequent perihaematoma oedema. This supports the findings of previous experiments in which administration of IL-1 and TNF-α induced opening of the BBB, leading to vasogenic oedema.

Further activation of the complement cascade leads to cell membrane destruction and glutamate excretion. Transient accumulation of high levels of glutamate and other amino acids has been observed within the perihaematoma region of rat brains in experimental models of ICH. Interruption of the inflammatory cascade by complement-complex inhibitors has been shown to reduce brain swelling in experimental ICH models. Additional animal and human studies have also shown evidence of an overwhelming haematoma-induced inflammatory response by the upregulation of matrix metalloproteinases (MMPs), a family of proteases involved in several neuropathological conditions and primarily responsible for extracellular matrix remodelling, chemotaxis and proteolytic cleavage of precursor molecules seen in ICH. The harmful effects of MMPs are manifested by triggering apoptotic cellular responses, which result from cell detachment and loss of integrin signalling. These effects are reduced by treatment with an endogenous inhibitor of MMPs, the tissue inhibitor of metalloproteinase (TIMP).

Effect of extravasated blood products

Extravasated blood is in part directly responsible for the formation of local oedema after ICH. Studies in pigs have proved the deleterious effects of experimental injection of blood and its degradation products into the brain parenchyma. When whole blood was infused into the cerebral lobes of anaesthetized animals, perihaematoma oedema developed within 1 h. Conversely, when only red blood cells (RBCs) were injected, oedema developed after 72 h. Further studies have shown that elements of the coagulation cascade, such as thrombin and fibrin, potentiate brain oedema formation and that

the use of heparinized blood has a protective effect. The inhibition of thrombin by argatroban proved effective in reducing the amount of perihaematomal oedema in rats. Also of potential importance is the platelet-induced activation and release of vascular endothelial growth factor (VEGF) after ICH, which increases vascular permeability and vasodilation via nitric oxide induction, and may trigger free-radical generation, an important mediator of cell membrane damage. Finally, metabolism of haemoglobin by haeme oxygenase (HO) after RBC lysis results in the release of iron, carbon monoxide and biliverdin. The inhibition of HO is associated with attenuation of brain oedema after ICH. These observations suggest that hyperacute oedema (<24 h) is caused by plasma extravasation, leading to oncotically driven water accumulation. Subsequent oedema (24–72 h) may initially be cytotoxic in nature, the result of thrombin release and complement activation. Late oedema (>72 h) may be driven primarily by release of blood degradation products and VEGF activation, leading to breakdown of the BBB and vasogenic oedema.

Diagnostic studies

Non-enhancing CT of the brain is the method of choice to evaluate the presence of ICH (Fig. 23.1). CT scans evaluate the size and location of the haematoma, extension into the ventricular system, degree of surrounding oedema and anatomical disruption. Haematoma volume may easily be calculated from CT images using the (A × B × C)/2 method, a formula derived from that used to calculate the volume of a sphere (Fig. 23.2). CT angiography (CTA) is not performed routinely in most centres but may prove helpful in predicting haematoma expansion and outcomes. MRI techniques such as gradient-echo (GRE, T2*) and susceptibility weighted imaging are highly sensitive for the diagnosis of ICH and may identify distant microhaemorrhages that suggest CAA as the cause of ICH. Conventional diagnostic cerebral angiography should be reserved for patients in whom secondary causes of ICH are suspected, such as aneurysms, arteriovenous malformations, cortical vein or dural sinus thrombosis, or vasculitis. Findings on CT scan or MRI that should prompt angiographic study include the presence of subarachnoid haemorrhage (SAH), primary intraventricular haemorrhage (IVH), vascular structures suggestive of an arteriovenous malformation, ICH at sites typical of aneurysmal haemorrhage or lobar haemorrhage in non-hypertensive younger patients.

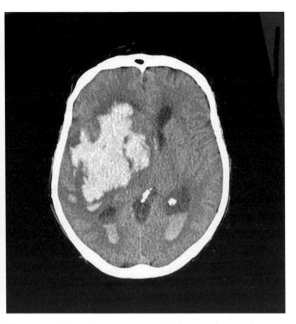

Fig. 23.1. CT scan showing intracerebral haemorrhage with intraventricular extension.

Table 23.1 The ICH score

Component	Score	Points
GCS score	3–4	2
	5–12	1
	13–15	0
ICH volume (ml)	> 30	1
	< 30	0
IVH	Present	1
	Absent	0
Infratentorial ICH	Yes	1
	No	0
Age (years)	> 80	1
	< 80	0

Total Points	30-day mortality (%)
5+	100
4	97
3	72
2	26
1	13
0	0

GCS, Glasgow Coma Scale; ICH, intracranial haemorrhage; IVH, intraventricular haemorrhage.
Data from Hemphill *et al.* (2001).

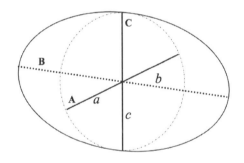

$$V = \frac{\pi \times 4 \times a \times b \times c}{3} = \frac{4 \times \frac{A}{2} \times \frac{B}{2} \times \frac{C}{2}}{} = \frac{A \times B \times C}{2}$$

Fig. 23.2. Calculation of the volume of the haematoma based on the volumetric formula for an ellipse. In this figure *a*, *b*, and *c* are the radius of the sphere; *A*, *B* and *C* are the diameters of the sphere; and π = 3.14.

Prognosis

The mortality after ICH is 30–40% at 30 days and 50% at 1 year. Independent predictors for 30-day and 1-year mortality include: Glasgow Coma Scale (GCS) and/or depressed level of consciousness, age, ICH volume, presence of IVH and infratentorial origin. A simple validated clinical grading scale, the ICH Score, permits rapid calculation of mortality at the bedside. The mortality rates for scores of 0, 1, 2, 3, 4, 5 are 0, 13, 26, 72, 97 and 100%, respectively (Table 23.1). Additional factors associated with high mortality after ICH include arterial hypertension and a widened arterial pulse pressure, hyperglycaemia, and hyperthermia.

Medical management

As the risk of neurological deterioration is highest during the first 24 h after ICH, and because the majority of patients with a depressed level of consciousness require ventilatory support, observation in an intensive care unit (ICU) or a similar setting is strongly recommended. Standard measurements in the ICU indicated for the optimal monitoring of ICH patients include invasive arterial blood pressure and ventricular drainage or placement of an intracranial pressure (ICP) monitor for comatose patients (GCS ≤8). Selected patients may also benefit from central venous pressure, cardiac output, EEG or brain tissue oxygen monitoring.

Blood pressure control

Extreme hypertension often occurs after ICH. Although there is still controversy about the optimal

Table 23.2 Parenteral agents for treating hypertension in acute intracerebral haemorrhage

Drug	Mechanism	Dose	Cautions
Labetalol	α_1-, β_1-, β_2-Receptor antagonist	20–80 mg bolus every 10 min, up to 300 mg; 0.5–2.0 mg min^{-1} infusion	Bradycardia, aggravation of congestive heart failure, bronchospasm
Esmolol	β_1-Receptor antagonist	0.5 mg kg^{-1} bolus; 50–300 µg kg^{-1} min^{-1}	Bradycardia, aggravation of congestive heart failure, bronchospasm
Nicardipine	Calcium-channel blocker	5–15 mg h^{-1} infusion	Use with caution in severe aortic stenosis
Clevidipine	Calcium-channel blocker	Start at 2 mg h^{-1}, increase dose 2–4 mg h^{-1} every 90 s, to a maximum of 16 mg h^{-1}	Lipid vehicle can promote bacterial contamination, therefore tubing requires replacement every 4 h
Enalaprilat	ACE inhibitor	0.625 mg bolus; 1.25–5 mg every 6 h	Variable response, precipitous fall in blood pressure with high-renin states
Fenoldopam	Dopamine-1 receptor agonist	0.1–0.3 µg kg^{-1} min^{-1}	Tachycardia, headache, nausea, flushing, glaucoma, portal hypertension
Hydralazine	Arterial vasodilator	25–75 mg every 8 h	Variable response, headache
Nitroprusside[a]	Nitrovasodilator (arterial and venous)	0.25–10 µg kg^{-1} min^{-1}	Increased intracranial pressure, variable response, myocardial ischaemia, thiocyanate and cyanide toxicity with prolonged use

[a] Nitroprusside is not recommended for use in acute intracerebral haemorrhage because of its tendency to increase intracranial pressure.
Reproduced with permission from Mayer and Rincon (2005).

range for blood pressure control, the American Heart Association (AHA) guidelines indicate that systolic blood pressures >180 mmHg or mean arterial pressure (MAP) >130 mmHg should be managed with continuous infusion of antihypertensive agents such as labetalol, esmolol or nicardipine (Table 23.2). Sodium nitroprusside has serious drawbacks in this setting, since it can lead to vasodilation of the brain vasculature and exacerbation of cerebral oedema and ICP. In the setting of impaired blood flow and autoregulation, excessive blood pressure reduction may exacerbate ischaemia in the area surrounding the haematoma and worsen perihaematomal brain injury. In general, no matter how high the blood pressure is, the MAP should not be reduced beyond 25% over the first 24 h, or below the patient's known baseline blood pressure. Continuous monitoring of the partial pressure of brain tissue oxygen (PbrO$_2$) is a promising method for detecting the 'safe' lower limit of autoregulation when blood pressure is reduced after ICH. Although no prospective study has addressed the timing of conversion from intravenous to oral antihypertensive management, this process can generally be started between 24 and 72 h, as long as the patient's condition has stabilized.

Haemostatic therapy

Baseline ICH volume is an important determinant of mortality, and early haematoma growth causes an incremental increase in the risk of poor outcome. Haemostatic therapy aimed at limiting haematoma growth is a promising but as yet unproven approach for improving survival and outcome after ICH.

Recombinant factor VII (rFVIIa, NovoSeven®; Novo Nordisk) is a powerful initiator of haemostasis that is currently approved for the treatment of bleeding in patients with haemophilia who are resistant to factor VIII replacement therapy. Considerable evidence exists suggesting that rFVIIa may also enhance haemostasis in patients with normal coagulation systems. In 2005, in a randomized, double-blinded, placebo-controlled phase 2B study, 399 patients with spontaneous ICH received treatment with rFVIIa at doses of 40, 80 or 160 µg kg^{-1} within 4 h after ICH

Table 23.3 Emergency management of the coagulopathic intracerebral haemorrhage patient

Scenario	Agent	Dose	Comments	Level of evidence[a]
Warfarin	Fresh frozen plasma (FFP) *or*	15 ml kg^{-1}	Usually 4–6 units (200 ml) each are given	B
	prothrombin-complex concentrate *and*	15–30 U kg^{-1}	Works faster than FFP, but carries risk of DIC	B
	vitamin K IV	10 mg	Can take up to 24 h to normalize INR	B
Warfarin and emergency neurosurgical intervention	*Above, plus* Recombinant factor VIIa	20–80 µg kg^{-1}	Contraindicated in acute thromboembolic disease	C
Unfractionated or low-molecular-weight heparin[b]	Protamine sulfate	1 mg per 100 units of heparin, or 1 mg of enoxaparin	Can cause flushing, bradycardia or hypotension, and anticoagulation	C
Platelet dysfunction or thrombocytopaenia	Platelet transfusion *and/or*	6 units	Range 4–8 units based on size; transfuse to >100,000	C
	Desmopressin (DDAVP)	0.3 µg kg^{-1}	Single dose required	C

[a] Level A, based on multiple high-quality randomized controlled trials; level B, based on single randomized trial or non-randomized studies; level C, case reports and series, expert opinion (2000).
[b] Protamine has minimal efficacy against danaparoid or fondaparinux.
DIC, disseminated intravascular coagulation; FFP, fresh frozen plasma; INR, international normalized ratio.
Reproduced with permission from Mayer and Rincon (2005).

onset. All three doses were shown to limit haematoma growth in a dose-dependent fashion. Regardless of the dose administered, rFVIIa was associated with a 38% reduction in mortality and significantly improved functional outcomes at 90 days, despite a 5% increase in the frequency of arterial thromboembolic adverse events.

With much fanfare in light of the promising results of the phase 2B study, the results of the phase III FAST trial were announced in May of 2007. This study compared doses of 80 and 20 µg kg^{-1} of rFVIIa with placebo in an overall trial population of 841 patients. Despite an even more robust haemostatic effect, no significant difference was found in the main outcome measure, which was the proportion of patients with death or severe disability according to the modified Rankin scale at 90 days (score of 5 or 6). On the basis of these results, routine use of rFVIIa as a haemostatic therapy for non-coagulopathic patients with ICH within a 4-h time window cannot be recommended.

Reversal of anticoagulation

Anticoagulation with warfarin increases the risk of ICH by five- to tenfold in the general population, and approximately 15% of ICH cases overall are associated with its use. Among ICH patients, warfarin increases the risk of progressive bleeding and clinical deterioration, and doubles the risk of mortality. Failure to rapidly normalize the international normalized ratio (INR) to below 1.4 further increases these risks.

Patients with ICH on warfarin therapy should be reversed immediately with fresh frozen plasma (FFP) or prothrombin-complex concentrate (PCC), and intravenous vitamin K (Table 23.3). Treatment should never be delayed in order to check coagulation tests. Unfortunately, normalization of the INR with this approach usually takes many hours, and clinical results are often poor. The associated volume load with FFP may also cause congestive heart failure in the setting of cardiac or renal disease. Prothrombin-complex concentrate contains vitamin K-dependent coagulation factors

363

II, VII, IX and X, normalizes the INR more rapidly than FFP and can be given in smaller volumes but carries the risk of disseminated intravascular coagulation.

Recent reports have described the off-label use of rFVIIa to speed up the reversal of warfarin anticoagulation in ICH patients. A single intravenous dose of rFVIIa can normalize the INR within minutes, with larger doses producing a longer duration of effect. Doses of rFVIIa ranging from 10 to 90 $\mu g \, kg^{-1}$ have been used to reverse the effects of warfarin in acute ICH in order to expedite emergency neurosurgical interventions with good clinical results. When this approach is used, rFVIIa should be used as an adjunct to coagulation factor replacement and vitamin K, as its effect only lasts for several hours. Patients with ICH who have been anticoagulated with unfractionated or low-molecular-weight heparin should be reversed with protamine sulfate, and patients with thrombocytopaenia or platelet dysfunction can be treated with a single dose of 1-deamino-8-D-arginine vasopressin (desmopressin or DDAVP), platelet transfusions or both. Restarting anticoagulation in patients with a strong indication, such as a mechanical heart valve or atrial fibrillation with a history of cardioembolic stroke, can be safely implemented after 10 days.

Management of elevated intracranial pressure

A large-volume ICH leads to a proportionately large amount of cerebral oedema and high ICP. Intraventricular haemorrhage further increases the risk of intracranial hypertension by creating obstructive hydrocephalus and alterations of normal cerebrospinal fluid flow dynamics. All comatose patients with a large-volume ICH or IVH felt to merit aggressive care should be managed with a ventricular drain or parenchymal ICP monitoring device, although this intervention has not been tested in randomized controlled trials. A stepwise approach for treating elevated ICP is shown in Table 23.4.

Basic measures for ICP control include head elevation to 30°, the strict avoidance of free water, seizure prophylaxis and fever control. The first step to definitively control elevated ICP is always neurosurgical intervention, in the form of ventriculostomy, craniotomy or hemicraniectomy. As medical therapy is escalated, the option always remains to 'pull the trigger' on surgical decompression of the intracranial vault. The second line of therapy in ventilated patients with high ICP is

Table 23.4 Stepwise treatment protocol for elevated ICP[a] in a monitored patient

Step	Procedure
1	*Surgical decompression.* Consider repeat CT scanning and definitive surgical intervention or ventricular drainage
2	*Sedation.* Intravenous sedation to attain a motionless, quiet state
3	*CPP optimization.* Pressor infusion if cerebral perfusion pressure (CPP) <70 mmHg, or reduction of blood pressure if CPP > 110 mmHg (preferred agents are phenylephrine, vasopressin and levophed)
4	*Osmotherapy.* Mannitol 0.25–1.5 g kg^{-1} IV or 0.5–2.0 ml kg^{-1} 23.4% hypertonic saline (repeat every 1–6 h as needed)
5	*Hyperventilation.* Target pCO$_2$ levels of 26–30 mmHg
6	*Hypothermia.* Cool core body temperature to 32–33°C
7	*High-dose pentobarbital therapy.* Load with 5–20 mg kg^{-1}, infuse 1–4 mg kg^{-1} h^{-1}

[a] ICP >20 cmH$_2$O.
Adapted from Mayer and Chong (2002).

sedation to produce a quiet, motionless state. Reduction of intrathoracic, jugular venous and arterial pressures is often enough to control surges in ICP. Failing that, cerebral perfusion pressure (CPP) optimization can help to normalize ICP. Extreme hypertension can overwhelm the cerebral circulation and cause vascular engorgement and increased cerebral blood volume. Relative hypotension can alternatively lead to reflex vasodilation in brain regions that have retained the capacity to autoregulate, leading to the creation of a 'plateau wave', which can be terminated by a surge in MAP and CPP.

After sedation and CPP optimization, osmotherapy and hyperventilation usually go hand in hand to attain control of elevated ICP. Mannitol and hypertonic saline have the greatest impact on ICP when they are administered in bolus doses. Central venous pressure monitoring is generally required to avoid volume depletion and overload, respectively. Hyperventilation is generally used sparingly in the ICU because its effect on ICP tends to last only for a few hours. Good long-term outcomes can occur when the combination of osmotherapy and hyperventilation are successfully used to reverse transtentorial herniation.

For intracranial hypertension that is refractory to the above measures, options include hemicraniectomy or other forms of surgical intracranial decompression, paralysis with a neuromuscular blocking agent, barbiturate infusion and mild hypothermia (33–36°C). These techniques generally require advanced expertise in neurocritical care.

Prevention of seizures

Active seizures should be treated with intravenous lorazepam (0.1 mg kg^{-1}), followed by a loading dose of phenytoin or fosphenytoin (20 mg kg^{-1}). Selected high-risk patients with ICH may benefit from prophylactic anti-epileptic therapy, but no randomized trial has addressed the efficacy of this approach. The AHA guidelines have cited anti-epileptic medication for up to 1 month as a treatment option, after which therapy should be discontinued in the absence of seizures. This recommendation is supported by the results of a recent study that showed that the risk of early seizures was reduced by prophylactic anti-epileptic therapy. The 30-day risk for convulsive seizures after ICH is approximately 10%, and the risk of status epilepticus is 1–2%. Lobar location increases this risk. The argument for prophylactic anticonvulsant therapy in stuporous or comatose ICH patients is bolstered by the fact that continuous EEG monitoring demonstrates electrographic seizure activity in approximately 18–28% of these patients, despite prophylactic treatment. The risk of late seizures or epilepsy among survivors of ICH is 5–25%.

Temperature control

Fever after ICH is a common development, particularly with IVH, and should be treated aggressively. Sustained fever after ICH has been shown to be independently associated with poor outcome. A large body of experimental evidence indicates that even small degrees of hyperthermia can exacerbate ischaemic brain injury. Brain temperature elevations have also been associated with hyperaemia, exacerbation of cerebral oedema and elevated ICP.

As a general standard, paracetamol and cooling blankets are recommended for all patients with sustained fever in excess of 38.3°C (101°F), despite the lack of prospective randomized controlled trials supporting this approach. Newer surface and endovascular cooling systems have been shown to be more effective for maintaining normothermia than conventional cooling blankets; however, it remains to be seen whether these measures can improve clinical outcome.

Hyperglycaemia

Hyperglycaemia may play a role in the physiopathology of oedema formation as an osmotic force driving water into the extracellular space. Hyperglycaemia is a potent predictor of 30-day mortality in observational studies of ICH, but it is unclear whether this association reflects a non-specific stress response or whether hyperglycaemia plays a causative role in producing poor outcomes. Strict glycaemic control has been linked to reductions in ICP, duration of mechanical ventilation and seizures in critically ill neurological patients. On the other hand, preliminary microdialysis data suggest that tight glycaemic control can result in critical brain tissue hypoglycaemia in comatose patients. Based on the current evidence, 'loose' intensive insulin therapy directed at maintaining serum glucose levels between 6 and 10 mmol l^{-1} seems reasonable.

Surgical management

Craniotomy and clot evacuation

Craniotomy is the most-studied intervention for ICH. Two earlier smaller trials showed benefit for patients presenting with moderate alterations in the state of consciousness, but a meta-analysis of all pre-2005 trials of surgical intervention for supratentorial ICH showed no significant benefit from this intervention. A pilot study of ultra-early craniotomy performed within 6 h of ICH onset was stopped due to problems with haemostasis in the surgical bed.

The landmark Surgical Treatment for Ischemic Heart Failure (STICH) trial randomized over 1000 ICH patients to emergent surgical haematoma evacuation within 72 h of onset or initial medical management and salvage surgical intervention, if needed. There was no benefit with early surgery. However, it should be kept in mind that certain patients with larger haemorrhages and early worsening from symptomatic mass effect were probably under-represented in this trial because they failed to meet the inclusion criteria of clinical equipoise. In a post-hoc analysis, there was a non-significant trend showing that patients with superficial haematomas and no IVH had better outcomes in the surgical arm. This observation provided support for the STICH-II trial, which is currently enrolling patients.

In contrast to supratentorial ICH, there is much better evidence that cerebellar haemorrhages exceeding 3 cm in diameter benefit from emergent surgical evacuation. Abrupt and dramatic deterioration to coma can occur within the first 24 h of onset in these patients. For this reason, it is generally unwise to defer surgery in these patients until further clinical deterioration occurs.

Minimally invasive surgery

The potential advantages of minimally invasive surgery over conventional craniotomy include reduced surgical trauma, shorter operative time and the possibility of performance under local anaesthesia. Endoscopic aspiration of supratentorial ICH was studied in a small single-centre randomized controlled trial, which showed that this technique was associated with a reduction in mortality at 6 months in the surgical group, particularly in younger patients with superficial haematomas. More recently, pilot studies have demonstrated the safety and feasibility of stereotactic clot aspiration within 72 h of onset. A multicentre randomized trial that examined the utility of stereotactic urokinase infusion administered within 72 h showed a significant reduction in haematoma size and lower mortality rate compared with placebo, at the expense of more rebleeding, but no significant differences in overall outcome.

Thrombolysis for intraventricular haemorrhage

Intraventricular haemorrhage is an independent predictor of mortality after ICH. Administration of thrombolytics via a ventricular drain can accelerate the clearance of an intraventricular clot and may improve outcome by reducing the duration and extent of haemorrhage-related neurotoxicity. Several small studies have reported on the successful use of urokinase or tissue plasminogen activator (tPA) for the treatment of IVH, with the goal of demonstrating safety and accelerated clot lysis. A safety study of 3 mg of rtPA administered via a ventricular drain every 12 h was associated with secondary bleeding in 22% of the patients; subsequent studies showed similar lytic effects and a better safety profile with total daily tPA doses ranging from 0.3 to 3.0 mg. When used off-label, a dose of 1 mg of rtPA every 8 h (followed by clamping of the external ventricular drain for 1 h) is reasonable until clearance of blood from the third ventricle has been achieved. The ongoing Clot Lysis Evaluating Accelerated Resolution (CLEAR) III Intraventricular Thrombolysis Trial is an ongoing phase III trial addressing this issue (http://biosgroup-johnshopkinsmedicine.health.officelive.com).

Hemicraniectomy

Hemicraniectomy with duraplasty has been proposed as a life-saving intervention for catastrophic mass effect from malignant MCA infarction or traumatic brain injury (Fig. 23.3). No randomized controlled trial has been conducted in patients with ICH but in a recent report of 12 consecutive patients with hypertensive ICH treated with hemicraniectomy, 92% survived to discharge and 55% had a good functional outcome. This preliminary data supports the need for better-controlled studies addressing the role of this surgical technique in ICH patients.

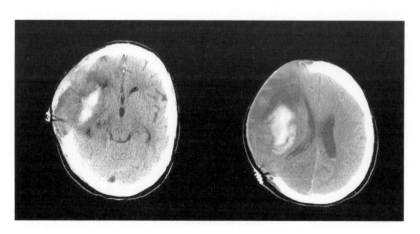

Fig. 23.3. Life-saving hemicraniectomy in a patient with hypertensive lobar intracerebral haemorrhage considered otherwise lethal.

Further reading

Adams, R. E. and Diringer, M. N. (1998). Response to external ventricular drainage in spontaneous intracerebral hemorrhage with hydrocephalus. *Neurology* **50**, 519–23.

Auer, L. M., Deinsberger, W., Niederkorn, K. *et al.* (1989). Endoscopic surgery versus medical treatment for spontaneous intracerebral hematoma: a randomized study. *J Neurosurg* **70**, 530–5.

Bhattathiri, P. S., Gregson, B., Prasad, K. S., Mendelow, A. D. and STICH Investigators (2006). Intraventricular hemorrhage and hydrocephalus after spontaneous intracerebral hemorrhage: results from the STICH trial. *Acta Neurochir Suppl* **96**, 65–8.

Broderick, J., Connolly, S., Feldmann, E., *et al.* (2007). Guidelines for the management of spontaneous intracerebral hemorrhage in adults: 2007 update: a guideline from the American Heart Association/ American Stroke Association Stroke Council, High Blood Pressure Research Council, and the Quality of Care and Outcomes in Research Interdisciplinary Working Group. *Stroke* **38**, 2001–23.

Brott, T., Broderick, J., Kothari, R. *et al.* (1997). Early hemorrhage growth in patients with intracerebral hemorrhage. *Stroke* **28**, 1–5.

Claassen, J. (2007). *Predictors and Significance of Electrographic Seizures and Periodic Discharges after Intracerebral Hemorrhage*. New York: Columbia University Medical Center.

Coplin, W. M. Vinas, F. C., Agris, J. M. *et al.* (1998). A cohort study of the safety and feasibility of intraventricular urokinase for nonaneurysmal spontaneous intraventricular hemorrhage. *Stroke* **29**, 1573–9.

Fernandes, H. M., Siddique, S., Banister, K. *et al.* (2000b). Continuous monitoring of ICP and CPP following ICH and its relationship to clinical, radiological and surgical parameters. *Acta Neurochir Suppl* **76**, 463–6.

Freeman, W. D., Brott, T. G., Barrett, K. M. *et al.* (2004). Recombinant factor VIIa for rapid reversal of warfarin anticoagulation in acute intracranial hemorrhage. *Mayo Clin Proc* **79**, 1495–500.

Gebel, J. M. Jr, Jauch, E. C., Brott, T. G. *et al.* (2002). Relative edema volume is a predictor of outcome in patients with hyperacute spontaneous intracerebral hemorrhage. *Stroke* **33**, 2636–41.

Hemphill, J. C. III, Bonovich, D. C., Besmertis, L., Manley, G. T., Johnston, S. C. (2001). The ICH score: a simple, reliable grading scale for intracerebral hemorrhage. *Stroke* **32**, 891–7.

Juvela, S., Heiskanen, O., Poranen, A. *et al.* (1989). The treatment of spontaneous intracerebral hemorrhage.

A prospective randomized trial of surgical and conservative treatment. *J Neurosurg* **70**, 755–8.

Kothari, R. U., Brott, T., Broderick, J. P. *et al.* (1996). The ABCs of measuring intracerebral hemorrhage volumes. *Stroke* **27**, 1304–5.

Liliang, P. C., Liang, C. L., Lu, C. H. *et al.* (2001). Hypertensive caudate hemorrhage prognostic predictor, outcome, and role of external ventricular drainage. *Stroke* **32**, 1195–200.

Mayer, S. A. and Chong, J. (2002) Critical care management of increased intracranial pressure. *J Int Care Med* **17**, 55–67.

Mayer, S. A. and Rincon, F. (2005). Treatment of intracerebral hemorrhage. *Lancet Neurol* **4**, 662–72.

Mayer, S. A., Lignelli, A., Fink, M. E. *et al.* (1998). Perilesional blood flow and edema formation in acute intracerebral hemorrhage: a SPECT study. *Stroke* **29**, 1791–8.

Mayer, S., Commichau, C., Scarmeas, N. *et al.* (2001). Clinical trial of an air-circulating cooling blanket for fever control in critically ill neurologic patients. *Neurology* **56**, 292–8.

Mayer, S. A., Kowalski, R. G., Presciutti, M. *et al.* (2004). Clinical trial of a novel surface cooling system for fever control in neurocritical care patients. *Crit Care Med* **32**, 2508–15.

Mayer, S. A., Brun, N. C., Begtrup, K. *et al.* (2005). Recombinant activated factor VII for acute intracerebral hemorrhage. *N Engl J Med* **352**, 777–85.

Mayer, S. A., Brun, N. C., Begtrup, K. *et al.* (2008). Efficacy and safety of recombinant activated factor VII for acute intracerebral hemorrhage. *N Engl J Med* **358**, 2127–37.

Mendelow, A. D., Gregson, B. A., Fernandes, H. M. *et al.* (2005). Early surgery versus initial conservative treatment in patients with spontaneous supratentorial intracerebral haematomas in the International Surgical Trial in Intracerebral Haemorrhage (STICH): a randomised trial. *Lancet* **365**, 387–97.

Misra, U. K., Kalita, J., Ranjan, P. and Mandal, S. K. (2005). Mannitol in intracerebral hemorrhage: a randomized controlled study. *J Neurol Sci* **234**, 41–5.

Murthy, J. M., Chowdary, G. V., Murthy, T. V., Bhasha, P. S. and Naryanan, T. J. (2005). Decompressive craniectomy with clot evacuation in large hemispheric hypertensive intracerebral hemorrhage. *Neurocrit Care* **2**, 258–62.

Naff, N. J., Carhuapoma, J. R., Williams, M. A. *et al.* (2000). Treatment of intraventricular hemorrhage with urokinase: effects on 30-day survival. *Stroke* **31**, 841–7.

Nyquist, P. and Hanley, D. F. (2007). The use of intraventricular thrombolytics in intraventricular hemorrhage. *J Neurol Sci* **261**, 84–8.

Ott, K. H., Kase, C. S., Ojemann, R. G. and Mohr, J. P. (1974). Cerebellar hemorrhage: diagnosis and treatment. A review of 56 cases. *Arch Neurol* **31**, 160–7.

Passero, S., Rocchi, R., Rossi, S., Ulivelli, M. and Vatti, G. (2002). Seizures after spontaneous supratentorial intracerebral hemorrhage. *Epilepsia* **43**, 1175–80.

Poungvarin, N., Bhoopat, W., Viriyavejakul, A. *et al.* (1987). Effects of dexamethasone in primary supratentorial intracerebral hemorrhage. *N Engl J Med* **316**, 1229–33.

Qureshi, A. I. and Suarez, J. I. (2000). Use of hypertonic saline solutions in treatment of cerebral edema and intracranial hypertension. *Crit Care Med* **28**, 3301–13.

Qureshi, A. I., Geocadin, R. G., Suarez, J. I. and Ulatowski, J. A. (2000). Long-term outcome after medical reversal of transtentorial herniation in patients with supratentorial mass lesions. *Crit Care Med* **28**, 1556–64.

Rohde, V., Rohde, I., Thiex, R. *et al.* (2002). Fibrinolysis therapy achieved with tissue plasminogen activator and aspiration of the liquefied clot after experimental intracerebral hemorrhage: rapid reduction in hematoma volume but intensification of delayed edema formation. *J Neurosurg* **97**, 954–62.

Rosand, J., Eskey, C., Chang, Y. *et al.* (2002). Dynamic single-section CT demonstrates reduced cerebral blood flow in acute intracerebral hemorrhage. *Cerebrovasc Dis* **14**, 214–20.

Siddique, M. S., Fernandes, H. M., Wooldridge, T. D. *et al.* (2002). Reversible ischemia around intracerebral hemorrhage: a single-photon emission computerized tomography study. *J Neurosurg* **96**, 736–41.

Teernstra, O. P., Evers, S. M., Lodder, J. *et al.* (2003). Stereotactic treatment of intracerebral hematoma by means of a plasminogen activator: a multicenter randomized controlled trial (SICHPA). *Stroke* **34**, 968–74.

Tuhrim, S., Horowitz, D. R., Sacher, M. and Godbold, J. H. (1999). Volume of ventricular blood is an important determinant of outcome in supratentorial intracerebral hemorrhage. *Crit Care Med* **27**, 617–21.

Zazulia, A. R., Diringer, M. N., Videen, T. O. *et al.* (2001). Hypoperfusion without ischemia surrounding acute intracerebral hemorrhage. *J Cereb Blood Flow Metab* **21**, 804–10.

Chapter 24

Spinal cord injury

Rik Fox

Introduction

The consequences of spinal cord injury (SCI) are as sudden as they are devastating. Traumatic injuries tend to occur in young, previously fit individuals who are unprepared for a life of disability. Spinal cord injury also places an enormous burden on patients' relatives and friends and on society in terms of lost opportunities, required resources and healthcare costs.

Demographics and aetiology

Data collection on SCI in the UK is poor compared with that in the USA where the National Spinal Cord Injury Statistics Centre has been in operation since 1973. In the UK, around 1000 people survive SCI each year, with an estimated 40,000 individuals living with chronic SCI. Around 80% of cord injuries in the UK and USA are traumatic, with motor vehicle accidents accounting for 40%. In the UK, falls account for another 40% of cases of traumatic injury, compared with 27% in the USA where acts of violence (mainly gunshot injuries) are responsible for a further 15%. Sports injuries account for around 10% of spinal injuries in the UK, with diving, rugby and horse riding being the main contributors. Various factors can result in non-traumatic cord injury including infection, tumours and ischaemia. The most common infections leading to SCI are *Staphylococcus* or tuberculous abscesses and transverse myelitis. Both primary and secondary (breast, lung, prostate and renal) tumours are associated with SCI, and cord ischaemia may occur during aortic surgery.

Spinal cord injury occurs most commonly in the 18–30-year age group, with a male-to-female ratio of around 4:1. Cervical injuries are most common (50%), with the remainder being spread equally between thoracic, thoracolumbar and lumbosacral regions. Survival

after SCI is related to age at injury and degree of neurological deficit (Table 24.1).

Anatomy

The spinal column comprises the bony elements from C1 to the coccyx. The vertebral canal lies in its centre, with the posterior longitudinal ligament anteriorly and the ligamentum flavum posteriorly. Within the vertebral canal, the spinal cord is surrounded by cerebrospinal fluid, dura and the epidural space, a loose collection of fat and venous plexi. This anatomical arrangement provides a flexible, protective system for the spinal cord within a semi-rigid frame. Under normal circumstances, it is a particularly effective arrangement that allows movement of the spine without putting undue force on the cord and spinal nerves. However, in the presence of a localized space-occupying lesion within the spinal canal, such as an abscess, haematoma or tumour, the rigidity of the bony elements causes compression and ischaemia of the neural tissue.

The main blood supply to the spinal cord is from the anterior spinal artery, which is a branch of the vertebral artery. This is reinforced by numerous small branches entering the vertebral foramina in the cervical and lumbar regions. Usually, there is one major contribution from an intersegmental branch of the descending aorta in the lower thoracic or lumbar area – the arteria radicularis magna or artery of Adamkiewicz – which can contribute the major part of the blood supply to the lower two-thirds of the cord. The two posterior spinal arteries arise from either the vertebral or the inferior cerebellar arteries and are reinforced by radicular arteries along the length of the spine. They supply only the posterior one-third of the cord, with the anterior spinal artery supplying the remainder. There is no overlap in

---

Core Topics in Neuroanaesthesia and Neurointensive Care, eds. Basil F. Matta, David K. Menon and Martin Smith. Published by Cambridge University Press. © Cambridge University Press 2011.

Table 24.1 Life expectancy (years) post-spinal cord injury by severity of injury and age at injury

(a) For persons who survive the first 24 h

Age at injury	Motor function at any level	Paraplegia	Low tetraplegia (C5–C8)	High tetraplegia (C1–C4)	Ventilator dependent at any level
20	52.6	44.8	39.8	35.3	18.1
40	34.1	27.3	23.1	19.6	8.0
60	17.7	12.7	9.8	7.6	1.8

(b) For persons surviving at least 1 year post-injury

Age at injury	Motor function at any level	Paraplegia	Low tetraplegia (C5–C8)	High tetraplegia (C1–C4)	Ventilator dependent at any level
20	53.0	45.5	40.8	36.9	25.1
40	34.5	27.9	23.9	20.8	12.2
60	18.1	13.1	10.3	8.4	3.6

the territories supplied, and the spinal cord is therefore prone to ischaemic insults.

Pathophysiology

Trauma to the spinal cord results in primary and secondary injury. Primary injury occurs because of axonal and cell body disruption due to direct mechanical forces (shear, distraction and compression) and haemorrhage into and around the spinal cord. Within minutes, the primary injury triggers release of inflammatory and other mediators that lead to secondary injury and spinal cord oedema. A variety of complex changes are involved in the secondary injury process and include hypoxia/ischaemia, ionic shifts, free-radical production, lipid peroxidation, excitotoxicty, prostaglandin production and apoptosis. Hypoxia/ischaemia occurs rapidly, particularly in the grey matter, and may be aggravated by failure of autoregulation. Abnormalities in venous drainage may also be associated with worsening ischaemia. Neurological transmission ceases below the level of the injury and this affects most spinal cord function, including reflex activity. Patients therefore present with sensorimotor deficits, areflexic limbs and autonomic imbalance.

It is important to recognize that secondary injury worsens neurological status and the injury level may ascend at some point within the first 48 h after injury. Although numerous mediators have been implicated in secondary SCI, no pharmacological protective agents have had any impact in attenuating the secondary injury response in humans (see below).

Eventually the inflammatory and other injurious processes subside, leaving glial scar tissue around a central cavity that is the major obstacle to neural tissue regeneration and repair. Spinal cord injury results in varying degrees of neurological dysfunction below the level of injury, and ultimate outcome is related to the severity of both the primary and the secondary injury. Clinically, the neurological outcome may not be apparent for up to a year post-injury, although improvement by one somatic level is usual. The worse the initial neurological status, the less likely it is that significant recovery will occur.

The American Spinal Injury Association (ASIA) classification of SCI has been adopted worldwide. As the terms 'complete' and 'incomplete' can be ambiguous when referring to a cord injury level, the injury is now defined as the highest neurological level with normal function. A lesion is 'complete' if there is no sensory or motor function in the S4–S5 (perineal, specifically anal sensation) region and 'incomplete' if there is function in this area. The ASIA scores (Fig. 24.1) allow progress to be documented and should be completed as soon as possible after injury by someone familiar with the scoring system.

Patterns of spinal cord injury

Complete injury now accounts for around 45% of spinal cord injuries, compared with over 60% in previous decades. Cervical and lumbar spine injury accounts for most incomplete cord injury.

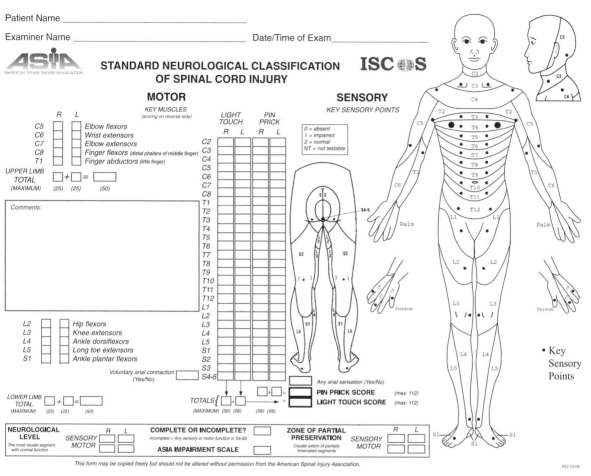

Fig. 24.1. The American Spinal Injury Association (ASIA) neurological classification of spinal cord injury (reproduced with permission from the American Spinal Injury Association. *International Standards for Neurological Classification of Spinal Cord Injury*, revised 2000; Atlanta, GA. Reprinted 2008.)

There are some particular patterns of cord injury that are recognized as distinct entities:

1. *Central cord syndrome* results from some cervical injuries. It occurs because of a diffuse ischaemic insult to the spinal cord in the cervical expansion where the volume of neurological tissue relating to upper limb activity is greater than that of neurons passing through to the lower limbs. Thus, central cord syndrome presents with worse neurological function in upper compared with lower limbs. It is more common in older patients following hyperextension injury and comprises up to 10% of total cervical cord injuries. Respiratory impairment may occur if the C3–C5 segments are involved.

2. *Anterior cord syndrome* is relatively rare and follows ischaemic insults to the anterior spinal artery, often following abdominal or arch aortic surgery. It presents as loss of motor function, pain and temperature sensation below the level of injury.

3. *Posterior cord syndrome* is rare and occurs following interruption of blood supply from the posterior spinal artery. It presents as loss of proprioception and vibration sense with preservation of other sensory and motor functions.

4. *Brown–Séquard syndrome* is characterized by motor, touch and vibration loss ipsilateral to the lesion, with contralateral pain and temperature loss. It is well known among neurologists but particularly rare following trauma. It may occur after traumatic penetrating hemisection of the cord or in association with a space-occupying lesion in the lateral vertebral canal.

5. *Spinal cord injury without radiological abnormality* (SCIWORA) is not a neurological syndrome but a description of cord injury in the absence of radiological bony or ligamentous injury. Cord damage is confirmed by MRI. It is most common in young children with cervical trauma, where ligamentous laxity is greater than cord flexibility. It has been associated with transient neurological symptoms at the time of injury, often with early recovery followed by worsening up to 48 h later.

6. *Cauda equina syndrome* results from damage to the lumbar spinal nerves rather than the spinal cord itself and occurs with spinal column injuries/abnormalities below L2–L3. It normally occurs because of a compressive lesion in the lumbar canal, commonly a prolapsed intervertebral disc. Clinical features include low back pain, bladder and bowel dysfunction and pain, parasthesia, sensory loss and motor dysfunction in the areas supplied by the affected nerve root(s).

Traditionally, the effects of SCI are described as two phases – an acute areflexic flaccid phase, and a chronic hyper-reflexic stage. In practice, the two merge seamlessly from one to the other at some point between 6 days and 6 weeks after injury, with the onset of spasticity marking the transition.

Acute spinal cord injury

Management of acute SCI involves prevention of complications from the sensorimotor deficit, monitoring and management of cardiorespiratory disturbances, spinal immobilization and consideration of surgical intervention, and management of systemic organ dysfunction.

The early management of spinal trauma is focused on the management of life-threatening injuries in accordance with advanced trauma life support protocols. In polytrauma, hypovolaemic shock from chest or abdominal injuries, and associated severe head injury, are common. A spinal injury must be assumed in all polytrauma patients until proven otherwise and spinal precautions should be maintained throughout the resuscitation stage. Once a SCI has been confirmed, the most important aspects of acute management include maintenance of oxygenation, blood pressure support and immobilization. Non-operative care remains the cornerstone of early management, and spinal immobilization is best achieved through meticulous attention

during patient movement, as it is not guaranteed by any type of external stabilization or restraint.

Imaging and surgery

Plain radiographs of the spinal column have largely been replaced by images and reconstructions obtained from spiral CT. However, a well-imaged lateral cervical spine radiograph can often provide sufficient information to allow ongoing management in an emergency situation. MRI is the most sensitive imaging modality for evaluation of soft tissue injury and spinal cord damage.

The timing of surgery after traumatic SCI remains controversial. Although there is no level 1 evidence to support early surgery, most spinal surgeons agree that emergency decompression is indicated in patients with acute and progressive neurological deterioration in the presence of spinal cord compression. There is increasing enthusiasm for emergency surgery, even in patients who present with complete SCI. In terms of fixation of an unstable spine, several studies suggest that early surgery has significant benefit in terms of decreased intensive care unit length of stay, more rapid transfer to rehabilitation and overall decreased hospital costs. However, most studies are not prospective, randomized or controlled. The Surgical Treatment of Acute Spinal Cord Injury Study (STASCIS) is currently underway and aims to identify the optimal timing of surgery. The details of surgery for SCI are discussed in Chapter 15.

Cardiovascular system

Spinal cord injury may be complicated by concomitant haemodynamic alterations that can arise within hours to months after the injury. Neurogenic shock, symptomatic bradycardia, autonomic dysreflexia and orthostatic hypotension are common, and early recognition and management may minimize secondary cord injury and prevent systemic organ system complications.

Autonomic effects

The sympathetic chains form from pre-ganglionic fibres arising from T1 to L2–L3 and are affected by any SCI above L2. Animal studies confirm that at the time of injury there is a mass sympathetic discharge that leads to a short-lived rise in systemic and pulmonary artery pressures. This can be severe enough to disrupt pulmonary capillary endothelium and cause neurogenic pulmonary oedema.

Following the initial generalized sympathetic discharge, SCI results in varying degrees of sympathoparesis depending on the level of injury. In an attempt to maintain blood pressure, vasodilation below the level of injury is counterbalanced by vasoconstriction above. However, this response is limited in the presence of hypovolaemia, so haemodynamic instability is common. With injuries above T6, there is loss of cardiac sympathetic innervation as well as failure of normally innervated vasculature to counteract the loss of peripheral resistance below the injury. This results in bradycardia from loss of cardio-accelerator tone and unopposed parasympathetic activity, and reduction of myocardial contractility and stroke volume. Cord injuries above T6 may therefore present with bradycardia and profound hypotension.

Parasympathetic supply arises mainly from the vagus nerve, which innervates all organs down to the colon. Pelvic organs are supplied by the sacral parasympathetic nerves arising from S2–S4. Unopposed vagal activity frequently results in additional cardiovascular disturbance, particularly severe bradycardia or asystole during vagal stimulation from tracheal suctioning, position changes or intra-abdominal distension. Vascular denervation hypersensitivity to α-agonists can also occur, and this might partly account for the dramatic rises in blood pressure during autonomic dysreflexia and contribute to the propensity to develop pressure sores.

Cardiovascular monitoring

Invasive blood pressure and central venous pressure monitoring are required as a minimum in any patient with haemodynamic instability. Cardiac output and flow monitoring may also be indicated in some patients, but, apart from studies involving Swann–Ganz catheters, none has been evaluated fully in acute SCI.

Management

The acute management of SCI includes maintenance of oxygenation and blood pressure to support spinal cord and systemic organ perfusion.

Blood pressure

Optimization of spinal cord perfusion by maintenance of mean arterial pressure >85–90 mmHg has been associated with improved neurological outcome and reduced morbidity after SCI. Hypotension should initially be treated with volume replacement, bearing in mind that, because of the low systemic vascular resistance, there may be a relatively poor response to filling. Considerable fluid volumes are often required for effective circulatory resuscitation and, in the face of a limited response to filling, vasopressor/inotropic support should be initiated. The choice of agent depends on individual clinical circumstances and no single vasopressor has been shown to be superior to another. Although 5–7 days of blood pressure support is often recommended after SCI, this duration of treatment is not supported by high-level evidence.

Patients with high injuries often suffer from orthostatic hypotension because of a lack of sympathetic tone and reflex activity. This usually becomes apparent during mobilization or changes in position. In the absence of the need for concurrent inotropic support, oral ephedrine, fludrocortisone or midodrine, an oral α-agonist, are the treatments of choice.

Bradycardia

Bradycardia should be treated if associated with low cardiac output. More commonly, it is necessary to pre-treat patients with atropine or glycopyrrolate to prevent vagally induced reductions in heart rate. In the presence of persistent bradycardia, isoprenaline or cardiac pacing should be considered. Bradycardia and exaggerated vagal responses tend to be temporary phenomena that usually improve over a few weeks, so a permanent pacemaker should be avoided if possible, as it will interfere with subsequent MRI scanning.

Autonomic dysreflexia occurs during the chronic phase of a SCI and will be discussed in the next section.

Respiratory system

Loss of respiratory muscle function has a profound effect on morbidity and mortality in both the acute and chronic phases of SCI. Respiratory-related deaths account for the majority of mortality following SCI.

Respiratory muscle function

The diaphragm is the main muscle of respiration. It is innervated via the phrenic nerve from C3–C5, although a contribution from C6 via the accessory phrenic nerve is a well-reported variant. The periphery of the diaphragm also has some sensory innervation from the lower intercostal nerves. The intercostal musculature is innervated from T1 to T11. It exhibits phasic activity during quiet breathing and provides tone to the chest wall, becoming more active during periods of higher ventilation. The extrathoracic insertions of the scalene muscles (innervated by C3–C8) allow them to add to inspiratory activity by their action on the upper rib-cage. The sternomastoid and trapezius muscles have dual innervation from C1–C4 and the accessory (XI) nerve, and can also be useful in very high cervical cord injury by fixing the neck and acting on the clavicle and sternum to lift the upper thorax.

The importance of coughing as a key physiological process is often underestimated. The traditional physiology of a voluntary cough involves an inspiratory phase utilizing the diaphragm, intercostals and possibly accessory muscles, a compressive phase utilizing the abdominal muscles (rectus abdominis (T6–T12), internal and external obliques (T6–L1) and transversus abdominis (T2–L1)) against a closed glottis for 0.2 s, followed by an expulsive phase. As expiratory muscle function is impaired by mid- to low thoracic injuries to a greater degree than inspiratory muscle function, there is a resultant inability to cough. This leads to significant respiratory morbidity.

Respiratory dysfunction

Respiratory function varies with the level of cord injury and also with the time since injury. It is not uncommon for respiratory function to worsen over the first few days, and close monitoring is imperative during this period to avoid a respiratory catastrophe (see below). Conversely, respiratory function usually improves during the first year such that some patients who were ventilator dependent are able to be weaned from support.

It is important for the clinician to understand the effect of the level of cord injury on respiratory function:

1. Lumbar injuries may reduce cough flow and limit the ability to clear secretions. Rarely, this can lead to respiratory failure, usually in those with pre-existing lung disease.
2. Thoracic cord injuries result in loss of intercostal activity below the level of injury, as well as loss of function of all expiratory muscles. In this situation, the affected lower portion of the chest wall has increased compliance and will in-draw during diaphragmatic contraction, leading to a reduction in vital capacity (VC) of 30–50% of predicted. This often leads to atelectasis, particularly in bed-bound patients, and respiratory failure will occur if lung compliance is reduced further. Traumatic thoracic cord injuries

are frequently complicated by rib fractures, pulmonary contusion and haemothorax, all of which compromise respiratory mechanics and increase the risk of respiratory failure.

3. Cervical cord injuries below C5 result in loss of all intercostal activity as well as expiratory muscle activity. Vital capacity can drop to 20% of predicted, and respiratory failure requiring invasive support is required in up to 80% of patients. Patients with cervical cord injuries above C5 may retain some diaphragmatic function but apart from their accessory muscles will have little other respiratory muscle function. Vital capacity can be as low as 5–10% of predicted, and up to 90% of patients require intubation, mechanical ventilation and tracheostomy. Injuries at C2 and above result in instantaneous respiratory paralysis, and patients only survive if respiratory support is provided rapidly at the scene of the injury.

Respiratory function tends to worsen over the first few hours and days after injury because of pulmonary and neurological changes. Pulmonary compliance may worsen because of atelectasis and increased work of breathing, which, in association with respiratory muscle weakness, leads to fatigue and respiratory failure. Loss of cough results in secretion retention and the likelihood of superadded infection. Opioids given for pain reduce respiratory rate and the ventilatory response to raised arterial carbon dioxide tension ($PaCO_2$) and further inhibit the cough reflex. As secondary cord injury develops, cranial extension of the neurological deficit leads to further loss of respiratory muscle function. With mid-cervical injuries, this can mean the difference between the presence of diaphragm function with the ability to self-ventilate and ventilator dependency.

Autonomic dysfunction also adversely affects the respiratory system because of the tendency to bronchoconstriction and increased mucus production from loss of sympathetic tone. Other risk factors for respiratory failure after SCI include age, obesity and previous or current lung disease.

Respiratory monitoring

Repeated VC measurements are the most useful monitor of respiratory function. They are simple to perform, reproducible and correlate well with overall restrictive respiratory dysfunction in SCI. A VC of ≥50% of predicted is compatible with an uneventful respiratory course, whereas a VC between 20 and 30% of predicted requires close monitoring and prophylactic intervention as required. A VC of <20% is an indication for immediate mechanical respiratory support. Other bedside lung function tests that are of value after SCI include maximal inspiratory pressure and cough peak flow.

In the presence of normal lung parenchyma and added inspired oxygen, hypercapnia can be associated with normal arterial oxygen saturation. Pulse oximetry in isolation is therefore an inadequate measure of respiratory reserve after SCI and should be used alongside measurement of $PaCO_2$, using transcutaneous or arterial blood gas analysis. Chest radiography should be performed if clinically indicated to identify areas of pulmonary collapse, consolidation or infection.

Management

The primary aims of respiratory management are to ensure adequate oxygenation to avoid worsening of spinal cord ischaemia and preserve other organ function, maintain lung volumes to minimize the risk of atelectasis and respiratory failure, and enhance secretion clearance. Pneumonia is a common complication in all patients with respiratory muscle dysfunction and is a major cause of morbidity and mortality after SCI. Standard preventative measures are required as well as targeted antimicrobial treatment when signs of respiratory sepsis are identified. The incidence of respiratory complications, pulmonary-related mortality and requirement for tracheostomy are significantly reduced when a ventilator care bundle, or similar respiratory protocol, is used.

Physiotherapy-guided deep-breathing exercises and incentive spirometry may be the only respiratory management required for patients with thoracic and lumbar injuries. In higher-level injury, patient effort will not be adequate to allow appropriate chest expansion, and the intermittent use of non-invasive positive-pressure breathing devices has become standard, despite little evidence to support their use. Non-invasive positive pressure breathing can be facilitated with a mask/mouthpiece and self-inflating resuscitation bag, or with the Bird inspiratory positive pressure or or CoughAssist devices. Non-invasive continuous positive airway pressure (CPAP) can be useful in some patients as it reduces the work of breathing. Non-invasive bilevel positive airway pressure (BIPAP) is indicated if VC is falling or if there are other signs of respiratory failure, such as a rising $PaCO_2$. However, neither technique is suitable for respiratory failure due to retained secretions.

Tracheobronchial secretions must be kept loose in order to facilitate their clearance. Nebulized bronchodilators are often used (even in the absence of bronchospasm) and humidified air/oxygen is essential. Mucolytics such oral carbocysteine or nebulized acetylcysteine are useful in some patients, but bronchoscopic secretion clearance may be required in cases unresponsive to other interventions.

Imminent respiratory failure is indicated by falling VC, hypercarbia or refractory hypoxaemia in association with clinical signs of respiratory distress. Intubation and mechanical ventilation should be undertaken before the patient is *in extremis*. The particular problems associated with endotracheal intubation in patients with an unstable cervical spine have been covered in Chapter 15.

If respiratory failure is due primarily to respiratory muscle weakness, mechanical ventilation is straightforward and gas exchange will normalize with relatively low airway pressures. The mode of ventilation is unimportant, but pressure support ventilation is frequently used. It has been suggested that ventilation using high tidal volumes of $\geq 20\,ml\,kg^{-1}$ might lead to faster weaning after SCI, but this approach potentially risks ventilator-induced pulmonary complications.

Other considerations

Acute SCI has multiple effects on all organ systems, and targeted interventions are associated with reductions in morbidity and mortality.

Gastrointestinal

The autonomic imbalance after acute SCI frequently leads to development of an ileus. This is exacerbated by the effects of opioid analgesia, sedation and coexisting post-traumatic intra-abdominal pathology. The ileus can be prolonged, particularly after cervical cord injury, and may not respond to the usual prokinetic drug regimes. Large bowel function is also compromised, and stimulant laxatives and digital stimulation are required to induce bowel movement. A high-fibre enteral intake may help, but osmotic laxatives can cause excessive gas formation.

Patients with a tracheostomy will not be able to eat normally for some time. Enteral feeding is the optimal route after SCI and should initially be provided via a fine-bore nasogastric feeding tube. This should be converted to a percutaneous endoscopic gastrostomy as soon as practical and safe. Stress ulceration is common after SCI, and patients should be commenced on proton-pump inhibitors until full enteral feeding has been established.

The nutritional requirements following SCI are not fully elucidated, although the effects of trauma, sepsis and multisystem organ failure should be taken into account when determining nutritional support. The acute phase of SCI is characterized by a reduction in metabolic activity and a negative nitrogen balance that cannot be corrected even with aggressive nutritional support. This may last for several weeks, and metabolic demands should be monitored to prevent overfeeding. In the chronic stage, adequate protein and calorie intake minimizes the risk of pressure sores.

Urinary tract

Urinary retention and an atonic bladder are normal during the acute phase of SCI. Catheterization will be required until other urinary management strategies are instituted during the chronic phase of management. Urinary tract infections are a common source of sepsis over the lifetime of the patient.

Temperature control

Temperature control is compromised after SCI for several reasons. Heat is lost rapidly from vasodilated skin, muscles are atonic and cannot contribute to thermogenesis, and afferent temperature input may be absent. After high cervical injury, patients may have no temperature sense at all. Care must be taken to avoid prolonged exposure and heat loss, and consideration given to active warming. Infection may not reliably produce a fever after SCI and, conversely, recurrent fevers can occur in the absence of infection.

Pain

The majority of patients will experience pain, either from a vertebral fracture or as a result of neurological damage. Many will continue to have chronic neuropathic pain around the level of injury, which can be disabling and resistant to treatment.

Thromboembolic disease

Deep vein thrombosis (DVT) and pulmonary emboli are common after SCI because of poor peripheral venous blood flow and immobility. Incidences are varyingly reported from 5 to 67%, with a 1% rate of

pulmonary embolism. Diagnosis of DVT is as difficult as in other clinical scenarios and is frequently made retrospectively following venous thromboembolism (VTE). Clinical presentation of submassive VTE varies depending on the level of spinal injury, but persistent tachycardia and recurrent fever in the absence of sepsis are common features. In tetraplegic patients, chest pain, tachypnoea and dyspnoea may be absent because of loss of afferent pathways. Investigations include CT pulmonary angiography and Doppler ultrasound of lower limb vessels. Venous thromboembolism prophylaxis consists of graduated compression stockings and pneumatic calf or foot compression applied immediately after admission. Care should be taken with compression devices to ensure that skin integrity is not compromised, and regular checks must be made to avoid pressure sores. Pharmacological methods of prophylaxis, currently low-molecular-weight heparin, can usually be administered within 72 h of injury or as soon as considered safe, taking into account any other trauma, coagulopathic states or impending surgery. Prophylaxis should be continued for at least 12 weeks.

Consequences of the sensorimotor deficit

The sensorimotor deficit that accompanies SCI is associated with multiple complications that require careful management.

Pain

Pain is an important sign in any pathological process and SCI is no exception. However, the disruption of sensory pathways can mask injuries and lead to delayed diagnosis and excess morbidity and mortality. Of particular note is the delayed diagnosis of intra-abdominal pathology in patients with SCI. This often presents as ill -defined, vagally mediated pain that is not localized. There is neither guarding nor tenderness to palpation if the cord injury is above the mid-thoracic region. Intra-abdominal blood loss may also be masked by the lack of normal homeostatic cardiovascular reflexes with injuries above T6.

Pressure sores

Pressure sores are a major complication of paralysis and sensory loss, and can develop within minutes. Insensate pressure areas, immobility, reduced muscle tone and alterations in cutaneous blood flow and autoregulation put areas of skin at substantial risk of ischaemia and subsequent necrosis. Areas prone to pressure sores include the heels, sacrum and ischia.

There is also a significant incidence of pressure sore development on the occiput associated with poorly fitting cervical collars. Cervical spine 'clearance' should be undertaken as a priority, and collars and spinal boards removed as soon as practically possible. Particular care and attention is needed during the first few hours after admission to hospital when there will be numerous patient interventions, movements and manipulations. Pressure-relieving procedures must be used every 2 h unless contraindicated by physiological instability. Although pressure-relief mattresses and turning beds assist with the prevention of pressure sores, they are no substitute for carers monitoring areas at risk.

Pressure sores in SCI patients are slow to heal, become colonized or infected, and are associated with severe sepsis and even mortality. The development of a pressure sore also delays rehabilitation and brings additional healthcare costs because of increased length of hospitalization.

Depolarizing muscle relaxants

Suxamethonium is now rarely indicated as superior rapidly acting neuromuscular blocking agents are available. However, it is well worth reiterating its potential complications after SCI. The upper motor neuron-like lesion of an acute SCI results in upregulation of cholinergic receptors on myocyte membranes. When exposed to depolarizing muscle relaxants, these receptors release enough potassium to raise plasma levels substantially, occasionally to levels high enough to cause cardiac arrest. As it takes time for the receptor population to increase, it is generally safe to use suxamethonium during the first 24–72 h after injury. Logically, it should also be safe when spasticity is well established, as the muscles will have reinnervated and the receptor population decreased. However, even at this stage, there can still be areas of continued denervation, so suxamethonium may not be safe in some patients even after the highly quoted 9-month limit.

Neuroprotection and regeneration

While there are many basic science studies that provide optimism for the future of neuroprotection and regeneration after SCI, there are currently no strategies that have proven benefit in the clinical setting.

Steroids

Methylprednisolone is a glucocorticoid that has multiple potential benefits that might ameliorate secondary SCI. These include reduction of the neurotoxic effects of excitatory amino acids and post-traumatic ion shifts, and inhibition of lipid peroxidation and the inflammatory response to trauma. In a post-hoc analysis, the National Acute Spinal Cord Injury Study (NASCIS) II demonstrated that patients treated with methylprednisolone over a 24 h period showed a statistically significant improvement in motor and sensory scores at 6 months. This effect only persisted for motor scores at 1 year, and there were twice as many wound infections and pulmonary emboli in the steroid group compared with controls. NASCIS III compared 24 and 48 h infusions of methylprednisolone started within 8 h of injury and post-hoc analysis revealed improved functional outcome at 6 weeks and 6 months when treatment was initiated 3–8 h after injury and continued for 48 h. However, this potential benefit was also associated with significant rates of pneumonia, sepsis and death.

Following the publication of the NASCIS II data in 1990, methylprednisolone was widely promoted as a standard of care in acute SCI. However, there has been enormous criticism of the interpretation of the NASCIS trials, particularly of their statistical analysis. Current US guidance notes that methylprednisolone for either 24 or 48 h is an option after SCI but cautions that this should only be undertaken in the knowledge that the evidence of harmful side effects is more consistent than any suggestion of clinical benefit. Treatment of acute SCI with steroids is now an individual clinical decision, although current consensus in UK SCI units recommends that high-dose steroids should not be used.

Other neuroprotective agents

There has been interest in the use of GM1 ganglioside for neuroprotection after SCI. An early small study demonstrated a significant improvement in the ASIA motor score at 48 h following GM1 administration, although a subsequent study showed no significant effect on the motor score despite improved bowel and bladder function. GM1 has not been approved for use in the setting of SCI and no further clinical trials are currently in progress.

Other potential neuroprotective agents that have been studied after SCI include tirilazad, thyrotrophin-releasing hormone, naloxone, minocycline and erythopoietin but none has been shown to be of benefit. More recently, pre-clinical research has identified activated macrophages and metalloproteinase inhibition as potential treatment options, and clinical trials of these interventions are awaited. Currently, however, there is no effective pharmacological intervention to ameliorate secondary SCI. Although animal studies have demonstrated a benefit from moderate hypothermia following SCI, the evidence is not compelling and there are currently no high-quality studies that demonstrate efficacy in the clinical situation.

Stem-cell transplantation

Several potential advancements, including transplantation of stem cells into the injured spinal cord, are now at the forefront of SCI research. Phase I studies have been conducted and 1-year follow-up suggests improvements in motor and sensory scores. However, these interventions are not without risk, particularly of uncontrolled regeneration producing pain and tumours. While stem-cell transplantation and tissue engineering hold promise for spinal cord regeneration, these remain research techniques that are some way from clinical application.

Ongoing ventilation and tracheostomy management

As the respiratory muscles remain weak for some time, it is unlikely that rapid weaning from the ventilator will be feasible, despite the presence of adequate gas exchange and ventilator triggering. Artificial ventilation itself worsens respiratory muscle function, but, despite this, the majority of patients who survive a high cervical injury can eventually be weaned from the ventilator.

Tracheostomy

Tracheostomy should be considered early and usually before attempts at ventilator weaning are considered. The only exceptions from this rule are patients with good pre-intubation respiratory function and rapidly reversible lung pathology. The relative merits of surgical and percutaneous tracheostomy placement have not been investigated, but many believe that percutaneous tracheostomy is contraindicated in the presence of an unstable cervical spine. There is no evidence that wound infection rate is affected by tracheostomy placement in patients who have undergone anterior cervical surgery.

The choice and size of tracheostomy tube should be considered carefully as the patient is likely to be partially or wholly ventilator dependent for some time and vocalization will be necessary. The tube diameter should therefore not be so large as to obstruct supraglottic air

flow when the cuff is deflated, nor too small to produce excessive resistance to air flow during spontaneous respiration. Tubes with inner cannulae are easier to clean and are associated with reduced sputum obstruction and accretion. There is little evidence for the benefit of fenestrated tracheostomy tubes but considerable evidence for their potential harm. Tubes with subglottic aspiration ports should be considered in patients with high levels of saliva production.

It is important that patients become accustomed to being ventilated or breathing through their tracheostomy with the cuff deflated. Thus, as soon as pulmonary function has improved and high ventilation pressures are no longer required, intermittent cuff deflation should be attempted. Supraglottic air flow allows speech, which is vitally important for rehabilitation, improves pharyngeal and laryngeal reflexes to allow eating, and reduces the risk of aspiration. When tolerated by the patient, the use of one-way valves or speaking valves is essential.

Weaning from ventilation

Weaning patients from mechanical ventilation with cervical SCI is simple but may take a long time. Physiological changes occurring over the first few weeks after injury make weaning possible in a large proportion of cases. Lung pathology present at the time of (or responsible for) respiratory failure should have improved and spinal cord oedema will have regressed, usually allowing one somatic level of improvement from the original neurological level. This can result in reinnervation to previously non-functioning respiratory muscles. Spasticity and increased muscle tone, which marks the change from the acute to the chronic phase of cord injury, affects the intercostal muscles and improves chest-wall stability. The weaning process itself will also improve function in the remaining respiratory muscles and retrain accessory muscles.

The prerequisites for weaning are similar to those for any critical care patient, that is, adequate oxygenation with the fraction of inspired oxygen (FiO_2) <0.4, positive end-expiratory pressure (PEEP) <8 cmH$_2$O, a stable cardiovascular and metabolic state, manageable tracheobronchial secretions, and an alert and cooperative patient. There should also be some evidence of spontaneous respiratory activity that has been quantified by measurement of VC and/or maximal inspiratory pressure off ventilatory support. Different methods have been used to wean patients with SCI, but the most reliable is the ventilator-free breathing technique. As the name suggests, this involves intermittently removing the patient from ventilatory support for short periods of time, guided by their VC:

- VC <250 ml – start with 5 min periods of spontaneous respiration.
- VC <500 ml – start with 15 min periods of spontaneous respiration.
- VC >750 ml – start with 30 min periods of spontaneous respiration.
- VC >1000 ml – start with 60 min periods of spontaneous respiration.

The periods of ventilator-free breathing should be repeated frequently during the day, with the patient rested on pressure support ventilation at night. It is important that fatigue should not occur, and the VC should be measured at the start and end of each ventilator-free breathing episode. If at the end it is <70% of the initial measurement, the rest time between episodes should be lengthened or the episode duration shortened.

Tetraplegic patients experience a drop in VC of up to 15% when moving from a supine to an upright position because their diaphragms are drawn down to a less mechanically efficient curvature by the abdominal contents, which are not supported because of the lack of abdominal wall tone. It is therefore recommended that weaning episodes are performed supine and that weaned patients wear an abdominal binder when upright. In order to reduce the reduction in functional residual capacity associated with breathing through a tracheostomy tube, it is also advisable to provide a small amount of CPAP or to use a speaking valve when the tube cuff is deflated.

The intermediate weaning aim is to have the patient ventilator-free by day and rested with minimal ventilatory support at night. Patients with respiratory muscle weakness often hypoventilate when sleeping, especially during rapid eye movement (REM) sleep. Therefore, those who are weaned during the day with a VC of <30% of predicted should have oxygen saturation (SpO_2) and transcutaneous carbon dioxide monitoring during periods of ventilator-free sleep.

Decannulation

The tracheostomy tube is no longer needed when the patient is free from ventilatory support and has adequate secretion clearance. Prior to decannulation, the tracheostomy tube should be downsized so as not to interfere with tracheal air flow when it is capped. The duration of capping will depend on the perceived need for continued emergency airway access. Secretion removal depends on air flow through the trachea and glottis, and it has been suggested that decannulation should be considered when the cough peak flow is >160 l min^{-1}. It is of note that the tracheostomy tube itself may be a cause of sputum production and decannulation can itself result in reduced secretion volume.

Ineffectual coughs can be augmented by an assisted cough technique, where a carer, in synchrony with the patient's own cough attempt, provides a vigorous abdominal thrust to increase intrathoracic pressure and improve tracheal air flow. This is a particularly effective technique when performed correctly and has few reported side effects. The technique can be improved by providing the patient with a maximal inspiratory capacity breath using a bag and mask/mouthpiece prior to the cough, or by using glossopharyngeal breathing (see Long-term ventilation below). A similar effect can be achieved with a positive-pressure breathing device. A mechanical device (CoughAssist by Phillips Respironics) is available that provides high airway pressure breaths followed by high negative expiratory air flows, mimicking the high tracheal air flow produced by a cough. It requires cooperation and coordination by the patient but is highly effective. Inspiratory muscle training using a variable resistance device is also of assistance to some patients.

Chronic spinal cord injury

In the chronic phase of SCI, lack of descending, mainly inhibitory, control causes changes in spinal cord physiology that render sensorimotor reflex arcs more sensitive to minor stimuli. Thus, the muscle response is more exaggerated and many patients develop spasms. Reflex activity may affect contralateral muscle groups or even ascend to include all muscles up to the level of the cord injury. Reflex activity also appears in the sympathetic nervous system and, if the injury is above T6, may manifest as autonomic dysreflexia. Resting muscle tone below the injury may increase, causing spasticity. The development of the features of chronic SCI varies considerably, and may occur from 6 days to never in a few patients. However, on average, these symptoms and signs occur at around 6 weeks after injury.

The majority of chronic SCI patients prefer to be managed for ongoing medical needs in a spinal injury unit and are therefore infrequently seen outside a small number of hospitals. Common causes for readmission to hospital include pneumonia, sepsis from the renal tract or pressure sores, autonomic dysreflexia and perioperative care. Rarer causes include ventilatory failure, peripartum care and because of complications of intrathecal baclofen treatment (see below).

Spasticity

Spasms and increased muscle tone often start innocuously but can become dramatic and painful and may seriously interfere with a patient's life. The advent of reflex spasms is often misinterpreted by relatives as the beginning of recovery. A degree of spasticity is to be welcomed, as muscle activity maintains muscle bulk and helps protect against pressure sores. Treatment should therefore be started only if the spasms are interfering with some other aspect of management.

Pharmacological treatment

Baclofen, a γ-aminobutyric acid B ($GABA_B$) agonist that acts on inhibitory interneurons in the spinal cord, is the first-line pharmacological treatment of spasticity. Low initial doses should be increased every few days until spasms become manageable. Baclofen is generally well tolerated, but large doses can cause drowsiness. Abrupt withdrawal of high-dose baclofen should be avoided. Tizanidine is a centrally acting $α_2$-agonist that can be used in conjunction with baclofen if spasticity remains uncontrolled, or alone if there is intolerance to baclofen. Clonidine, another $α_2$-agonist, is available as a transdermal patch and is used in some patients as an adjunct to other medication. Dantrolene, which alters excitation–contraction coupling in skeletal muscle, is rarely used because it causes global muscle weakness. Diazepam is often used for hypersensitivity spasms and clonazepam to control night-time spasticity. The use of medical-grade cannabinoids has been inconclusive in studies of spasticity, but there are undoubtedly some individuals who benefit. Non-prescribed cannabis is widely used and is usually commended by patients.

Intrathecal baclofen

When spasms are uncontrolled with high doses of medication, or if side effects interfere with normal life, consideration should be given to administration of intrathecal baclofen. A test dose of 10–50 μg is administered intrathecally and, if the response is good, consideration should be given to insertion of an indwelling intrathecal catheter and associated pump implantation. Subsequent management is usually uneventful, but there are two situations in which complications can become medical emergencies. Rebound hyperspasticity is a rare condition seen with sudden pump failure or extrathecal catheter fracture. Patients present with uncontrolled continuous spasms, hyperthermia, autonomic dysreflexia and respiratory failure. This can progress to rhabdomyolysis and renal failure, and there have been several fatalities from multisystem organ failure related to this condition. The mainstay of treatment is control of the muscle contractions, either by modulation of the reflex cord activity or the muscle itself, followed by rapid reintroduction of oral or intrathecal baclofen. Benzodiazepenes are helpful, but dantrolene is not. In extreme circumstances, propofol infusion, with or without neuromuscular blockade, should be considered. The second emergency situation arises from accidental overdose of baclofen due to pump malfunction or programming error, or following an accidental bolus while investigating catheter placement. Cranial diffusion of baclofen leads to progressive ascending weakness and an acutely atonic patient, nausea, vomiting, respiratory muscle weakness, confusion and coma. Respiratory and cardiovascular support may be needed for up to 48 h following the overdose.

Autonomic dysreflexia

Autonomic dysreflexia occurs as a result of mass sympathetic discharge consequent on an autonomic stimulus in patients with cord injuries above T6. It is more common in those with complete cord injury and generally occurs during the chronic phase of injury and only very rarely in the acute phase.

Loss of supraspinal control of sympathetic preganglionic neurons in association with denervation hypersensitivity of vascular smooth muscle leads to abnormal cardiovascular control. Sympathetic discharge below the level of injury causes central and peripheral vascular contraction and a rapid rise in blood pressure. The intact baroreceptor reflex, innervated by cranial nerves IX and X, leads to intense bradycardia. The remaining functioning sympathetic system attempts to counteract the rise in blood pressure by dilation of the remaining controlled vasculature, resulting in cutaneous flushing, sweating and intracerebral vasodilation. The rise in blood pressure can be mild, around 20–30 mmHg from baseline. In the context of the low resting blood pressure in many patients, this brings blood pressure within a normal range and the condition may be unnoticed by an inexperienced observer. However, blood pressure rises to >200 mmHg systolic and >100 mmHg diastolic are common, and systolic blood pressure >300 mmHg has been reported. Immediate morbidity and mortality are usually related to hypertension-related myocardial ischaemia, intra-cerebral haemorrhage or seizures. Detached retina and other visual disturbances may also occur. The long-term consequences of autonomic dysreflexia are unknown.

Common stimuli for the precipitation of autonomic dysreflexia are bladder and colonic distension from blocked urinary catheters or faecal loading. Symptoms include headaches, nausea and sweating, but their severity is unrelated to the degree of blood pressure elevation, and some patients may be asymptomatic. The duration of an episode of autonomic dysreflexia is short if the cause is found and treated, although continuous relapsing dysreflexic episodes can sometimes last for several days.

The management of autonomic dysreflexia consists primarily of removal of the causative stimulus and manoeuvres to lower blood pressure. Patients in the community use physical adjuncts, such as sitting or standing, to garner any orthostatic assistance in lowering blood pressure. This is often all that is required. A number of pharmacological agents, usually rapid-onset and short-acting vasodilators, are recommended if simple manoeuvres fail. Drugs used in the community include sublingual nifedipine or glyceryl trinitrate, but in hospital practice almost every vasodilator has been used, with the choice determined by individual circumstances. Novel treatments such as sildenafil, prostaglandins and phenoxybenzamine have also been reported, as has magnesium in the critical care setting. Prophylactic treatment with conventional antihypertensive medication is not recommended, as many patients are normally hypotensive because of the underlying sympathoparesis.

Autonomic dysreflexia can also occur during intra-abdominal and pelvic surgery and is seen in >60% of tetraplegic women in labour, when it is usually timed with contractions. Epidural anaesthesia is well documented as being effective in controlling blood pressure in these circumstances, as it blocks both stimulus input and efferent output from the sympathetic chain.

Long-term ventilation

Patients are considered to be ventilator dependent if they are unable to maintain spontaneous respiration indefinitely. This definition encompasses those who are dependent on ventilator support 24 h a day, as well as those who require nocturnal support to improve respiratory function during the day. It does not, however, include patients who require CPAP or BIPAP at night for obstructive or central sleep apnoea.

Overall, 1–2% of all patients with SCI become ventilator dependent each year and, in the UK, this means that there are 200–250 ventilator-dependent SCI patients at any one time. Ventilator dependency has a major effect on prognosis after SCI and is associated with a 30–40% 1-year survival (Table 24.1). Thereafter, survival rates are also considerably worse than similar, non-ventilated patients with SCI.

Predicting ventilator dependence

Predicting whether a patient will be ventilator dependent is not straightforward. Changes to spinal cord physiology and respiratory mechanics over time mean that those with absent respiratory function initially may regain sufficient function to allow weaning from mechanical ventilation up to 1 year post-injury. The level of cord injury at presentation correlates approximately with ventilator dependence, but, because the level of injury between C0 and C4 is determined mainly by sensory testing, any motor function is ill-defined. A significant proportion of patients with injuries above C4 can be weaned from ventilation, but, conversely, some with injuries below C4 cannot. A proportion of patients with injuries at C2 and above have no respiratory muscle activity at all, whereas others have sufficient activity to support ventilator-free breathing for a few minutes per hour, providing a safety window in the event of ventilator failure.

Assessment of respiratory function requires off-ventilator spirometry to allow determination of forced vital capacity and maximum inspiratory pressure. These measurements should be repeated every few weeks to monitor progress. Diaphragmatic activity can be confirmed by fluoroscopy but has little predictive value in terms of determining the future likelihood of weaning. However, inspiratory force diaphragm needle electromyography (EMG) is a useful predictor of the ability to wean.

Ventilators for long-term use

Small discreet ventilators suitable for long-term use are manufactured by a number of companies in Europe and the USA, and new models appear regularly. The majority offer volume or pressure ventilation in support or control modes and the ability to adjust most ventilatory parameters. Newer features such as average volume assured pressure support are now being included. Most devices incorporate single limb circuits with pneumatic exhalation valves, or fixed leak exhalation ports situated close to the patient, although some can also run dual limb circuits. All have pressure and/or volume monitoring for alarm purposes and built-in batteries. To allow them to be classified as life support systems, the ventilators should run on batteries from 2 to 6 h and be licensed for invasive use. However, the important issues from a patient's point of view are a quiet, reliable device with good battery life that will sit inconspicuously on the back of a wheelchair.

The ideal aim of the patient–ventilator interface is the ability to speak through an uncuffed tracheostomy during ventilation to near-normal arterial blood gasses, without the need to change ventilator settings from day to day. The patient should be able to swallow safely while being ventilated and should ideally be adequately ventilated at night with the same ventilator settings as during the day.

Speech is facilitated by large tidal volumes, with some inspired gas being used for speech. Patients become able to control the partition of flow such that they are often mildly hypocapnic. In-line, one-way valves are available that augment speech by diverting the whole tidal volume through the larynx. Swallowing takes some time to learn as coordination with ventilation is essential. Sleep ventilation may require adjustment to ventilator settings as laryngeal relaxation during REM sleep can lead to hypoventilation. In extreme cases, a cuffed tracheostomy tube may be required, with the cuff partially inflated at night.

Spontaneous breathing techniques

Patients with sternomastoid or scalene innervation can train these muscles to lift the upper chest wall and generate small tidal volume respiration that can occasionally be sufficient to allow several minutes of ventilator-free breathing. This manoeuvre is extremely reassuring for patients, as it gives them the reassurance that death is not inevitable if their ventilator fails.

Glossopharyngeal breathing is another technique that has been in use for decades. A mouthful of air is passed into the lungs and held by glottic closure while another mouthful is taken in. It is a difficult technique to master and obviously not possible with an open

tracheostomy. However, experienced patients can 'swallow' a tidal volume in five mouthfuls, taking a few seconds to do so.

Phrenic nerve pacing

Patients with injuries above C4 and intact phrenic nerves may be suitable for phrenic nerve pacing. Phrenic nerve integrity depends on the anterior horn cells of C4 (and C3 and C5) being unaffected by the cord injury.

Testing for phrenic nerve activity is performed some time after injury when cord oedema has completely resolved. Transcutaneous electrical stimulation is applied in the neck at the anterior border of sternomastoid and magnetic stimulation over C2 at the back of the neck. The resultant diaphragmatic EMG is detected by cutaneous electrodes placed over the anterior insertion of the diaphragm or by needle electrodes inserted percutaneously into the diaphragm. An intact nerve produces a characteristic waveform with a latency of 5–10 ms. Additional functional measures, such as inspiratory pressure and volume measurement using fluoroscopic diaphragm imaging, are also recommended.

Currently, there are three devices available for phrenic nerve pacing. Two are fully implantable (produced by Atrotech and Avery Labs) and use external electromagnetic energy transfer coils to power and control the pacers. Electrodes are implanted around the phrenic nerve in the neck or mediastinum, and the pacing characteristics simulate normal phrenic nerve neurophysiology. Patients can become ventilator-free indefinitely after a period of retraining, although many choose to use the pacers only during the day. The third device developed at the Neurological Institute, University Hospitals Case Medical Center, Ohio, USA, uses laparoscopically implanted wire electrodes in the motor points of each hemi-diaphragm and an external pacing device attached via a percutaneous connection. The physiological and psychological benefits of phrenic nerve pacing over invasive ventilation are proven. There is also evidence that there is a lower incidence of respiratory tract infection in patients using phrenic nerve pacers and the cost of the equipment (£30,000–£40,000 in 2010) may well be offset by a reduction in the number of respiratory-related admissions to hospitals.

Long-term care

The main aim of the rehabilitation of patients with SCI is their reintegration into the community to live as independently as possible. This applies as much to tetraplegic ventilator-assisted individuals as to those with less severe injuries. Independence in this scenario also means verbal independence, as patients must be able to express their needs and instructions to their carers. Ideally, patients should also understand their ventilator and other apparatus so that they can instruct carers how to trouble-shoot and manage all aspects of their respiratory care. Tetraplegic patients require so many aids to allow independent living that their respiratory management is a relatively small part of their overall care package. However, for social or logistical reasons, some patients can never be discharged to their own homes, and there are limited numbers of care homes in the UK with the resources to manage such complex patients.

Further reading

Ackland, G. L. and Fox, R. (2005) Low-dose propofol infusion for controlling acute hyerspasticity after withdrawal of intrathecal baclofen therapy. *Anesthesiology* **103**, 663–5.

Adams, M. M. and Hicks, A. L. (2005) Spasticity after SCI. *Spinal Cord* **43**, 577–86.

Bach, J. R. and Saporito, L. R. (1996). Criteria for extubation and tracheostomy tube removal for patients with ventilatory failure. *Chest* **110**, 1566–71.

Berney, S., Bragge, P., Granger, C., Opdam, H. and Denehy, L. (2010). The acute respiratory management of cervical spine cord injury in the first 6 weeks after injury: a systematic review. *Spinal Cord* **49**, 17–29.

Bracken, M. B., Shepard, M. J., Collins, W. F. *et al.* (1990). A randomized controlled trial of methylprednisolone or naloxone in the treatment of acute SCI. *New Engl J Med* **322**, 1405–11.

Bravo, G., Guízar-Sahagún, G., Ibarra, A., Centurión, D. and Villalón, C. M. (2004). Cardiovascular alterations after spinal cord injury: an overview. *Curr Med Chem Cardiovasc Hematol Agents* **2**, 133–48.

Chiodo, A. E., Scelza, W. and Forchheimer, M. (2007) Predictors of ventilator weaning in individuals with high cervical spinal cord injury. *J Spinal Cord Med* **31**, 72–7.

Coffey, R. J., Edgar, T. S., Francisco, G. E. *et al.* (2002). Abrupt withdrawal from intrathecal baclofen: recognition and management of a potentially life-threatening syndrome. *Arch Phys Med Rehabil* **83**, 735–41.

Como, J. J., Sutton, E. R., McCunn, M. *et al.* (2005). Characterising the need for mechanical ventilation following cervical spinal cord injury with neurological deficit. *J Trauma* **59**, 912–16.

Gelis, A., Dupeyron, A., Legros, P. *et al.* (2009). Pressure ulcer risk factors in persons with spinal cord injury: part I: acute and rehabilitation stages. *Spinal Cord* **47**, 99–107.

Gore, R. M., Mintzer, R. A. and Calenoff, L. (1981) Gastrointestinal complications of spinal cord injury. *Spine* **6**, 538–44.

Green, D., Hartwig, D., Chen, D., Soltysik, R. C. and Yarnold, P. R. (2003). Spinal cord injury risk assessment for thromboembolism (SPIRATE Study). *Am J Phys Med Rehabil* **12**, 950–6.

Gupta, R., Bathen, M. E., Smith, J. S. *et al.* (2010). Advances in the management of spinal cord injury. *J Am Acad Orthop Surg* **18**, 210–22.

Guterrez, C. J., Harrow, J. and Haines, F. (2003). Using an evidence-based protocol to guide rehabilitation and weaning of ventilator-dependent cervical spinal cord injury patients. *J Rehabil Res Dev*, **40**, 99–110.

Hurlbert, R. J. (2006). Strategies of medical intervention in the management of acute spinal cord injury. *Spine* **31**, S16–21.

Khan, S., Plummer, M., Martinez-Arizala, A. and Banovac, K. (2007). Hypothermia in patients with chronic spinal cord injury. *J Spinal Cord Med*, **30**, 27–30.

Krassioukov, A., Warburton, D. E., Teasell, R. *et al.* (2009). A systemic review of the management of autonomic dysreflexia after spinal cord injury. *Arch Phys Med Rehab* **90**, 682–95.

Lynch, A. C., Palmer, C., Lynch, A. C. *et al.* (2002). Nutritional and immune status following spinal cord injury: a case controlled study. *Spinal Cord* **40**, 627–30.

Mansel, J. K. and Norman, J. R. (1990). Respiratory complications and management of spinal cord injuries *Chest* **97**, 1446–52.

National Spinal Cord Injury Statistical Center (2009). Spinal cord injury facts and figures at a glance. Available at: https://www.nscisc.uab.edu/.

Onose, G., Anghelescu, A., Muresanu, D. F. *et al.* (2009). A review of published reports on neuroprotection in spinal cord injury. *Spinal Cord* **47**, 716–26.

Peterson, W. P., Barbalata, L., Brooks, C. A. *et al.* (1999). The effect of tidal volumes on the time to wean persons with high tetraplegias from ventilators. *Spinal Cord* **37**, 284–8.

Ploumis, A., Yadlapalli, N., Fehlings, M. G., Kwon, B. K. and Vaccaro, A. R. (2010). A systematic review of the evidence supporting a role for vasopressor support in acute SCI. *Spinal Cord* **48**, 356–62.

Prigent, H., Roche, N., Laffont, I. *et al.* (2009). Relation between corset use and lung function postural variation in spinal cord injury. *Eur Respir J* **35**, 1126–9.

Schilero, G. J., Spungen, A. M., Bauman, W. A., Radulovic, M. and Lesser, M. (2009). Pulmonary function and spinal cord injury. *Arch Phys Med Rehabil* **166**, 129–41.

Sekhon, L. H. and Fehlings, M. G. (2001). Epidemiology, demographics and pathophysiology of acute spinal cord injury. *Spine* **26**, S2–12.

Short, D. J., El Masry, W. S. and Jones, P. W. (2000). High dose methylprednisolone in the management of acute spinal cord injury – a systematic review from a clinical perspective. *Spinal Cord* **38**, 273–86.

Stiens, S. A., Bergman, S. B. and Goetz, L. L. (1997). Neurogenic bowel dysfunction after spinal cord injury: clinical evaluation and rehabilitative management. *Arch Phys Med Rehabil* **78**, S86–99.

Thibault-Halman, G., Casha, S., Singer, S. and Christie, S. (2010). Acute management of nutritional demands after spinal cord injury. *J Neurotrauma* **27**, 1–11.

Vale, F. L., Burns, J., Jackson, A. B. and Hadley, M. N. (1997). Combined medical and surgical treatment after acute spinal cord injury: results of a prospective pilot study to assess the merits of aggressive medical resuscitation and blood pressure management. *J Neurosurg* **87**, 239–46.

Winslow, C. and Rozovsky, J. (2003). Effect of spinal cord injury on the respiratory system. *Am J Phys Med Rehabil* **82**, 803–14.

Occlusive cerebrovascular disease

Lorenz Breuer, Martin Köhrmann and Stefan Schwab

Ischaemic stroke

Stroke is the third leading cause of death after myocardial infarction and cancer, and the leading cause of permanent disability and of disability-adjusted loss of independent life years in western countries. Aside from the tragic consequences for patients and their families, the socio-economic impact is enormous, as stroke patients with permanent deficits such as hemiparesis and aphasia are frequently unable to live independently or pursue an occupation. The direct and indirect cost estimates of a survived stroke episode vary between US$35,000 and US$50,000 per year. In the face of an ageing population, the incidence and prevalence of stroke is expected to rise, and an effective and widely applicable treatment of this devastating disease is desperately needed.

General management and diagnosis

It is essential to evaluate and stabilize vital signs and other physiological variables before initiating specific stroke therapy. The patient's neurological status should be assessed urgently using standard stroke scales such as the National Institutes of Health Stroke Scale, and the time point of stroke onset identified. Close monitoring of neurological status, heart rate and rhythm, blood pressure, oxygen saturation (SpO_2), body temperature and laboratory variables, such as blood glucose, is crucial. Oxygen should be administered if SpO_2 falls below 95% and serum glucose levels >18.0 mmol l^{-1} (180 mg dl^{-1}) treated with insulin infusion.

Up to 70% of ischaemic stroke patients present with elevated blood pressure, but this usually normalizes within the first hours and days after stroke onset. Normal autoregulation of cerebral blood flow (CBF) can be impaired in the acute phase after stroke, and perfusion of ischaemic brain is likely to depend primarily on systemic blood pressure. As vessel occlusion or stenosis may be (partly) compensated by collaterals and acute elevation of blood pressure, substantial reductions in blood pressure should be avoided early after stroke onset. Guidelines from the American Heart Association and the European Stroke Organisation recommend that blood pressure should be lowered only if systolic blood pressure (SBP) exceeds 220 mmHg and diastolic blood pressure (DBP) exceeds 120 mmHg. Early initiation of co-therapies including speech, physical and occupational therapies minimize complications such as aspiration pneumonia, thrombosis and limb contractures. Secondary prophylaxis with antiplatelet agents, statins and antihypertensives is recommended to avoid early recurrent strokes. Optimal management of vascular risk factors also requires that smoking be discouraged and patients who are overweight managed with regular physical activity and a weight-reducing diet.

Imaging

There are several imaging modalities that can be used to identify patients who may benefit from acute recanalization therapy after ischaemic stroke. Options include non-contrast CT and advanced CT techniques using CT angiography (CTA) and CT perfusion. Multiparametric MRI stroke protocols, including diffusion-weighted imaging (DWI), fluid-attenuated inversion recovery (FLAIR), gradient-recalled echo (GRE) and MR angiography (MRA), provide additional information (Fig. 25.1). A simple non-contrast CT to exclude intracranial haemorrhage is sufficient within the early 3–4.5 h time window, whereas advanced imaging techniques are able to identify patients who are likely to benefit from therapy delivered in extended time windows (see below).

Core Topics in Neuroanaesthesia and Neurointensive Care, eds. Basil F. Matta, David K. Menon and Martin Smith. Published by Cambridge University Press. © Cambridge University Press 2011.

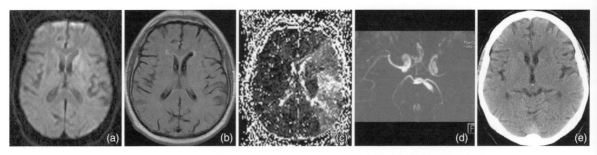

Fig. 25.1. Imaging of a 76-year-old man with occlusion of the proximal left middle cerebral artery (MCA). (a–d) Pre-treatment MRI scans (a, diffusion-weighted imaging (DWI); b, fluid-attenuated inversion recovery; c, perfusion-weighted imaging (PWI); d, magnetic resonance angiography) showing a large PWI/DWI mismatch in the MCA territory. (e) Post-treatment (intravenous thrombolysis) CT scan showing only minor infarction in the left MCA territory.

Acute specific therapy

Intravenous thrombolysis

Occlusion of a brain vessel leads to an immediate reduction in cerebral perfusion and to ischaemic infarction in a central core of irreversible damaged brain tissue within minutes. Surrounding this is an area of hypoperfused but still vital brain tissue (the ischaemic penumbra), which can potentially be salvaged by rapid restoration of blood flow. The underlying rationale for the application of thrombolytic agents is the lysis of occluding thrombus and subsequent re-establishment of tissue reperfusion.

Currently, the only approved reperfusion therapy is CT-guided intravenous recombinant tissue plasminogen activator (rtPA) administered according to recognized inclusion and exclusion criteria within 3 h of stroke onset. The standard regimen is rtPA 0.9 mg (kg body weight)$^{-1}$ (maximum dose 90 mg) with 10% of the dose given as an initial bolus and the remaining dose over the following hour. Findings from the European Cooperative Acute Stroke Study (ECASS) III suggest some benefit of rtPA up to 4.5 h from stroke onset. However, pooled analysis of data from rtPA trials confirms that, even within a 3 h window, earlier treatment results in better outcome.

Several large observational studies as well as smaller randomized trials have successfully utilized MRI sequences to select patients for intravenous thrombolysis (IVT) in time windows extended up to 9 h after stroke onset. MRI-guided treatment appears to be safer than standard CT-guided treatment and is at least as effective. However, such extended time windows for IVT are not yet incorporated into routine clinical practice, and MRI is logistically more difficult to perform than CT in the acute phase.

Intra-arterial thrombolysis and interventional therapy

Another strategy in thrombolytic therapy is an intra-arterial, interventional approach. Compared with IVT, it has the advantage of providing a higher concentration of the thrombolytic agent at the target site, while minimizing systemic concentration and therefore complications. The technique requires cerebral angiography to localize the occluding clot, navigation of a microcatheter to the side of the clot and administration of the lytic agent at the level of, or inside, the clot. The higher technical demands and specialist equipment usually cause a considerable time delay compared with IVT and the limiting factor is often the availability of an interventional neuroradiologist. Intra-arterial thrombolysis (IAT) may be combined with mechanical recanalization devices, such as the Mechanical Embolus Removal in Cerebral Embolism retriever (MERCI retriever) or the Penumbra device, and with remodelling techniques including percutaneous transluminal angioplasty (PTA) and/or stenting. Although the Intra-arterial Prourokinase for Acute Ischemic Stroke (PROACT) II study demonstrated an outcome benefit of IAT in proximal middle cerebral artery (MCA) occlusion with pro-urokinase within 6 h of stroke onset, this was not sufficient for this therapy to be approved by the US Food and Drug Administration. Prourokinase is no longer available and, although there are no randomized controlled data on IAT using other agents, rtPA is often used as an individual treatment option for patients with proximal MCA or acute basilar artery occlusion (see below). Common intra-arterial doses of rtPA should not exceed 40 mg.

Combined intravenous/intra-arterial thrombolysis

The combination of IVT and IAT allows early IVT to 'buy time' until IAT can be undertaken and is often

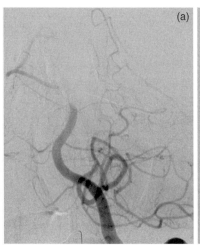
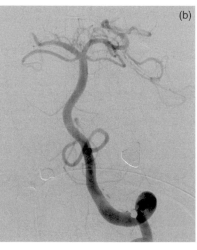

Fig. 25.2. Digital subtraction angiography (DSA) of an 80-year-old male with acute basilar artery occlusion. (a) Pre-treatment DSA showing complete basilar artery occlusion. (b) Post-treatment DSA. After combined intravenous/intra-arterial thrombolysis and mechanical intervention, there is complete recanlization of the basilar artery.

referred to as the 'bridging approach'. As with IAT alone, there is no formal approval for this combination, but it is being used in some centres for patients with proximal MCA or acute basilar occlusion. The Emergency Management of Stroke (EMS) and the Interventional Management of Stroke (IMS) I and II trials suggest that a reduced dose of intravenous rtPA (0.6 mg (kg body weight)$^{-1}$, maximum dose 60 mg) should be administered immediately after exclusion of ICH, with overall and intra-arterial rtPA doses not exceeding 90 and 40 mg, respectively. Bridging lysis may also be combined with mechanical clot removal devices or PTA.

Acute basilar artery occlusion

Although basilar artery occlusion (BAO) is rare, it is the most severe type of ischaemic stroke, with a case fatality rate of up to 90%. In younger patients, it is usually related to embolism from cardiac sources or, less commonly, vertebral artery dissection, whereas local atherothrombosis is more common in the elderly.

Basilar artery occlusion and other ischaemic infarctions in the vertebrobasilar territory are associated with variable symptoms but often present with progressive or hyperacute brainstem symptoms, tetraplegia and alterations in consciousness ranging from somnolence to coma. Typical cerebellar symptoms may occur with or without visual deficits and loss of cranial nerve functions. Specific symptoms depend on the affected vessel and exact localization of the abnormality within the vessel. Different patterns include caudal vertebro-basilar, mid-basilar and top-of-the-basilar thrombosis syndromes, the first being mostly of atherothrombotic

causes and the last of embolic origin. Top-of-the-basilar syndrome is defined by bilateral thalamic, mesencephalic, superior cerebellar artery and posterior cerebral artery infarctions with coma, vertical ocular paresis and skew deviation. Extensive basilar artery thrombosis may result in a 'locked-in' syndrome.

Due to the poor prognosis of untreated acute BAO, diagnostic vessel imaging using either non-invasive methods (CT/CTA or MRI/MRA) or digital subtraction angiography (DSA) should be initiated as early as possible (Fig. 25.2). MRI is superior to CT at identifying ischaemic lesions within the brainstem and will confirm the extent of the infarction. Differential diagnoses of acute BAO range from intoxication to a post-seizure reduction of consciousness. Therefore, other aetiologies should be considered and additional diagnostic procedures, such as lumbar puncture and EEG, may be useful in clarifying the diagnosis.

Treatment of basilar artery occlusion

Patients with persistent BAO face an almost inevitably grim prognosis, and those with suspected BAO need immediate referral to a specialist centre for further imaging and possible rescue therapy. In the case of proven BAO, IVT, IAT or both, in combination with mechanical recanalization, is usually recommended, although the lack of randomized studies means that the optimal treatment remains unclear. However, most national guidelines favour endovascular thrombolysis in combination with mechanical removal of the thrombus. Regardless of the treatment modality, acute recanalization is the single most important predictor of improved outcome. Multiple case series have been published in the last 25 years, but most include small numbers with only a few studies recruiting even 40 or 50 patients. In observational studies, survival rates range from 30 to 73%, although a recent meta-analysis showed that, notwithstanding improved recanalization rates after IAT, survival rates were comparable to IVT. Therefore, in centres without interventional neuroradiologists, IVT is a viable alternative for patients with BAO.

A multicentre observational study demonstrated that the 'bridging approach', using combined treatment with intravenous platelet glycoprotein IIb/IIIa receptor inhibitors and IAT with rtPA, combined with PTA or stenting in cases of severe residual stenosis after IAT, might improve neurological outcome compared with IAT alone. Recently, bridging therapy with intravenous platelet glycoprotein IIb/IIIa inhibitors plus IAT with rt-PA has been shown to be associated with a significant increase in recanalization rates without an increased risk of bleeding complications compared with IAT alone.

Intensive care management of acute ischaemic stroke

Although most ischaemic stroke patients can be treated in high-dependency or dedicated stroke units, some require admission to a (neurological) intensive care unit (ICU). Indications for ICU admission may be related to general medical issues or specific to the acute ischaemic stroke (Table 25.1). The focus of ICU management therefore includes general medical measures, such as airway management, mechanical ventilation and cardiovascular support, as well as disease-specific interventions such as treatment of space-occupying brain oedema and other stroke-related complications.

Prevention and management of general complications

Up to 50% of patients with a hemiplegic stroke are initially dysphagic, and early evaluation of swallowing function is essential to prevent aspiration pneumonia, the most common stroke-related complication on the ICU. The prevalence of dysphagia declines to approximately 15% within 3 months after stroke onset. It is associated with a higher incidence of medical complications and a higher rate of malnutrition, which is itself a predictor of poor functional outcome and increased mortality. Early feeding via a nasogastric tube is

Table 25.1 Indications for ICU admission after acute ischaemic stroke

Stroke related	Large MCA territory stroke
	Brainstem stroke
	Significant brain oedema causing raised ICP and midline shift
	Decreased consciousness
	Dysphagia, pulmonary aspiration
	Respiratory insufficiency, mechanical ventilation
	Severe cardiac arrhythmia
	Circulatory shock
	Recurrent epileptic seizures
	Extended monitoring after:
	• Thrombolysis
	• Neurosurgical intervention (e.g. hemicraniectomy)
	• Neuroradiological interventions
General medical conditions	Pneumonia
	Sepsis, other infections
	(Multi)organ failure
	Pre-existing comorbidities

ICP, intracranial pressure; MCA, middle cerebral artery.

essential, and a percutaneous gastrostomy should be considered in patients in whom dysphagia might be prolonged. Early feeding also prevents bacterial aspiration pneumonia, although diminished cough and immobilization increase its risk.

Another feared complication of stroke is the development of deep vein thrombosis (DVT) and pulmonary embolism (PE). Up to 50% of patients develop DVT, and PE occurs in 3–39%. Pulmonary embolism accounts for around 2% of early deaths after acute stroke. Early rehydration and graduated compression stockings are recommended to reduce the risk of venous thromboembolism (VTE). Several large trials have demonstrated that low-molecular-weight heparin is safe in stroke patients and significantly reduces the incidence of DVT and PE. The PREvention of VTE after Acute Ischemic Stroke with LMWH Enoxaparin (PREVAIL) study showed a 43% relative risk reduction in VTE events in patients receiving enoxaparin compared with unfractionated heparin for the development

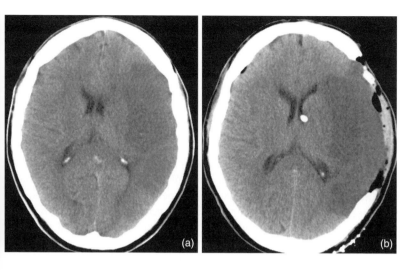

Fig. 25.3. Cranial CT scan of a 58-year-old male with left-sided middle cerebral artery (MCA) infarction. (a) Subtotal left-sided MCA infarction with oedema and early midline shift. (b) Post-treatment scan showing decompressive hemicraniectomy and ventriculostomy.

of symptomatic or asymptomatic DVT and symptomatic and/or fatal PE during the treatment period. Deep vein thrombosis prophylaxis using low-molecular-weight heparin should therefore be administered to all stroke patients showing persisting motor deficits.

Other common complications in stroke patients include urinary tract infection, focal or secondary generalized epileptic seizures, pressure ulcers, gastric ulcers and critical illness polyneuropathy. Treatment of these complications is identical to that in non-stroke patients.

Management of stroke-specific complications

Malignant hemispheric infarctions

Subtotal or complete MCA territory infarctions (Fig. 25.3), with or without additional ischaemia of the anterior or posterior cerebral artery territories, constitute up to 10% of patients with supratentorial infarction. In the majority of patients, a rapid neurological deterioration occurs because of associated oedema formation and critical brain swelling, usually between the second and fifth day after stroke onset. The resulting mass effect leads to increased intracranial pressure (ICP) with damage to formerly healthy brain tissue and the risk of midline shift and transtentorial or uncal herniation. Despite maximal conservative treatment, case fatality rates of up to 80% were observed in early observational studies and this led to the introduction of the term 'malignant' MCA infarction.

Medical treatment of brain oedema and intracranial pressure

Medical therapy in patients with malignant MCA infarction and brain oedema is based mostly on observational data. Basic management includes head-up positioning to 30%, adequate oxygenation, normalization of body temperature, avoidance of noxious stimuli and adequate pain relief. Intravenous mannitol is the first-line medical therapy in the presence of clinical or radiological signs of raised ICP, or measured increases in ICP. Intravenous hypertonic saline solutions are likely to be similarly effective. Severe increases in ICP resistant to other therapies may be treated with intravenous thiopental, but this should only be administered in the presence of ICP and haemodynamic monitoring, as it runs the risk of a significant reduction in blood pressure and cerebral perfusion pressure (CPP). EEG monitoring may also be used to guide therapy.

Decompressive hemicraniectomy

For decades a large, space-occupying infarction was invariably regarded as an untreatable disease with an inevitably fatal outcome. However, the introduction of decompressive hemicraniectomy has fundamentally changed this view (Fig. 25.3). After early observational studies, several randomized trials confirmed the efficacy of craniectomy. In 2007, a pooled analysis of the three major European hemicraniectomy trials – the DEcompressive Surgery for the Treatment of malignant INfarction of the middle cerebral arterY (DESTINY), DEcompressive Craniectomy In MALignant middle cerebral artery infarcts (DECIMAL), and the

Hemicraniectomy After Middle cerebral artery infarction with Life-threatening Edema Trial (HAMLET) trials – was published. Overall, more patients undergoing decompressive surgery within 48 h of stroke onset reached a modified Rankin Scale (mRS) of ≤3 or <4 compared with conservative management, with numbers needed to treat of 2 and 4, respectively. Survival in the surgical group was 78% compared with 29% in the conservative treatment group and surgery did not result in a higher proportion of survivors with an mRS of 5. No difference was observed in the benefit of surgery in relation to predefined subgroups including age (above and below 50 years), the presence or absence of aphasia and time to randomization (within or later than 24 h).

The rationale of decompressive surgery is to remove a part of the cranium to allow expansion of the swollen brain, thus normalizing ICP, avoiding ventricular compression and preventing brain tissue shifts. Furthermore, by reducing ICP, CBF and CPP increase, leading to improved oxygenation of brain tissue at risk of infarction and minimizing final infarct volume. Decompressive surgery consists of a large hemicraniectomy and duraplasty – an ICP monitor can be inserted for post-operative monitoring.

Based on the results of the individual DESTINY, DECIMAL and HAMLET studies, as well as their pooled analysis, early hemicraniectomy before the onset of herniation is recommended. The DECIMAL trial included only patients treated within 48 h and did not show a difference in the benefits of surgery before or after 24 h. Of the individual trials, only HAMLET included delayed surgery (up to 99 h after stroke onset) and found that beyond 48 h there was no evidence for improved functional outcome after surgery.

There is no definitive evidence to identify an upper age limit for decompressive hemicraniectomy in malignant MCA infarction. The upper age limits in the three large European trials were between 55 and 60 years. Several small studies suggest an unfavourable outcome in elderly patients and recommend an upper age limit for intervention of between 50 and 60 years. On the basis of this, an upper age limit of 60 years is often applied in clinical practice, but it is important to take into account the patient's 'biological' as well as chronological age. The decision to perform decompressive surgery should therefore be made on an individual basis. Treatment of patients with malignant infarction of the dominant hemisphere is also controversial, but there

is no evidence that patients do not benefit from treatment. However, more data on post-operative quality-of-life issues are required.

Restorative cranioplasty is generally performed between 3 and 6 months and should never be undertaken earlier than 6 weeks after the initial surgery.

Hypothermia

Elevated body temperature during the first 72 h after stroke onset worsens the extent of ischaemic damage and is an independent predictor of mortality and poor outcome. Spontaneous hypothermia, on the other hand, is associated with reduced mortality and improved outcome. Therapeutic hypothermia is increasingly used during neurocritical intervention for neuroprotection in hypoxic brain injury (see Chapter 29). Presumed mechanisms of action include induction of ischaemic tolerance by reduced brain metabolism and excitatory neurotransmitter release, inhibition of apoptosis and metalloproteinase expression, reduced inflammatory response and inhibition of blood–brain barrier disruption.

Animal studies have demonstrated that the neuroprotective effects of hypothermia after acute stroke are more pronounced when started early and continued for >24 h. High-quality clinical data on cooling after stroke are limited, but moderate hypothermia may reduce mortality in malignant ischaemic brain infarction. Hypothermia is an invasive intervention that should only be delivered by experienced practitioners in an ICU environment, as mechanical ventilation, muscle relaxation and measurement of ICP are required. Hypothermia is also associated with a high rate of complications, including pneumonia, severe bradycardia, cardiovascular compromise, thrombocytopaenia and coagulopathy. During the rewarming phase, patients may develop rebound increases in ICP and severe electrolyte disturbance.

To date, there are insufficient data to guide when or if hypothermia should be initiated after stroke, and for how long it should be continued. Because of the lack of conclusive data from randomized trials, hypothermia is currently restricted to selected patients treated in experienced centres, or for whom hemicraniectomy is not an option. Hypothermia in isolation is less effective than hemicraniectomy, but a combination of the two may be a promising approach. In one small randomized controlled study, mild hypothermia (35°C) in addition to decompressive surgery produced a trend

Table 25.2 Complications of space-occupying cerebellar infarction

Compression of the brainstem
Hydrocephalus due to blockage of the fourth ventricle
Aspiration (bulbar palsy and impaired consciousness)
Respiratory insufficiency
Cardiac arrhythmias
Haemorrhagic transformation
Upward herniation after ventriculostomy

towards a better clinical outcome than decompressive surgery alone.

Space-occupying cerebellar infarction

Space-occupying oedema occurs in 17–54% of patients with cerebellar infarction. It may cause life-threatening deterioration because of obstructive hydrocephalus due to the blockage of the fourth ventricle or from direct compression of the midbrain and pons. Upward herniation of the superior cerebellar vermis through the tentorial notch, or downward herniation of the cerebellar tonsils through the foramen magnum, may also occur. Patients with total or subtotal cerebellar infarction should therefore be monitored closely on an ICU and should undergo repeat imaging if their conscious level is impaired. Complications of space-occupying cerebellar infarction are shown in Table 25.2.

Randomized controlled studies are lacking, but, based on clinical experience and non-randomized trials, surgical treatment including ventriculostomy and decompression of the posterior fossa should be considered early, and certainly before signs of herniation are present. When the procedure is life-saving, prognosis and clinical outcomes can be very good, even in patients who were comatose before surgery.

Carotid endarterectomy

Approximately 20% of all ischaemic strokes are caused by carotid stenosis. The main mechanism for infarction is atherosclerosis secondary to artery-to-artery embolism rather than the haemodynamic effects of the stenosis. The prevalence of asymptomatic stenosis >50% is between 5 and 7% in patients >65 years. The incidence of high-grade carotid stenosis is much higher (20–30%) in patients with previous myocardial infarction and peripheral artery disease. Decisions regarding the use of invasive procedures to treat carotid disease must balance the long-term risk reduction of ipsilateral stroke against the immediate risks of the intervention.

Indications

Carotid endarterectomy (CEA) is the treatment of choice for symptomatic carotid stenosis, with several studies confirming its efficacy in the secondary prevention of ischaemic stroke. In terms of primary prophylaxis of asymptomatic carotid stenosis, the risk reduction of CEA is around 1% overall. Carotid endarterectomy is therefore only recommended for primary prophylaxis in male patients with >80% stenosis and a life expectancy >5 years. Carotid endarterectomy should be performed in high-volume centres where the perioperative morbidity and mortality is <3%. Currently, there is no evidence to support the use of carotid artery angioplasty and stenting (CAS) in the routine management of carotid disease. However, selected patients with severe symptomatic stenosis in whom endarterectomy cannot be performed safely may benefit from endovascular management. Although its equivalence has not been proven in randomized trials for symptomatic patients, CAS has found its way into more routine practice in some centres.

Perioperative complications

Carotid endarterectomy is a high-risk procedure, and patients require close monitoring and management to minimize the risk of perioperative complications. Several factors, including prior ipsilateral hemispheric neurological symptoms (stroke, transient ischaemic attack), severe contralateral stenosis of the carotid artery, stenosis of the distal internal carotid or external carotid arteries, chronic renal failure, smoking, diabetes and hyperlipidaemia, are associated with poor outcome. In addition, CEA patients are at risk of cardiovascular complications, particularly myocardial infarction, because of the relatively high incidence of comorbidities including peripheral vascular and coronary artery disease, heart failure, chronic pulmonary disease, diabetes mellitus and hypertension.

Perioperative ischaemic stroke caused by thromboembolism or temporary local hypoperfusion may result in new neurological symptoms, and restenosis or occlusion of the carotid artery may occur in the early phase after intervention. Untreated hypertension can predispose to cerebral hyperperfusion syndrome (see below) or intracranial haemorrhage. Post-operative airway complications related to airway narrowing because of oedema and wound haematoma occur in 3–8% of patients, and reintubation and emergency wound exploration may be required.

Arterial blood pressure management

Arterial pressure is often labile and difficult to control after CEA, and perioperative haemodynamic instability is associated with increased morbidity and mortality. Particularly in chronically hypertensive patients with carotid stenosis, CBF often depends on collateral circulation, and autoregulation may be impaired. Aggressive antihypertensive therapy in these circumstances can predispose to cerebral ischaemia. The incidence of severe hypertension after CEA is around 66% and, although its aetiology is multifactorial, it can partly be explained by impaired baroreceptor function. The baroreceptors in the carotid sinus can be affected directly by the stenosis, by the surgical intervention and by anaesthesia and concurrent therapies. Furthermore, altered sensitivity of the receptors is not uncommon in patients who have recently suffered an ischaemic stroke or transient ischaemic attack.

Although it is agreed that strict perioperative control of arterial blood pressure is associated with improved neurological and cardiovascular outcomes after CEA, there are few data on which to base guidelines for blood pressure management. In particular, there is no conclusive evidence favouring one antihypertensive agent over another or for specific blood pressure targets. Severe hypertension (SBP >180 mmHg or DBP >115 mmHg) predisposes to perioperative arrhythmias and myocardial ischaemia and, in the absence of definitive data, SBP >160 mmHg is widely used as a threshold for treatment. However, close haemodynamic and neurological monitoring, in association with individualized titration of antihypertensive therapy, are more important than specific targets. First-line drugs include α- or β-adrenergic antagonists such as labetalol, esmolol or metoprolol, but they have the potential to worsen CEA-induced bradycardia. Second- and third-line therapies include hydralazine and glyceryl trinitrate (GTN). Nifedipine and sodium nitroprusside are usually avoided because they can cause brain oedema secondary to cerebral vasodilation in patients with impaired autoregulation.

Late post-operative management

To preserve the long-term benefits of CEA, arterial blood pressure and other cerebrovascular risk factors such as hyperlipidaemia and diabetes mellitus should be monitored and treated as appropriate. Secondary medical prophylaxis with antiplatelet agents, including aspirin, the combination of aspirin with extended-release dipyridamole or clopidogrel, is indicated. Depending on existing comorbidities, oral anticoagulation with warfarin might also be appropriate. Duplex carotid ultrasonography should be performed regularly after CEA to detect restenosis.

Cerebral hyperperfusion syndrome

Cerebral hyperperfusion syndrome (CHS), sometimes called reperfusion syndrome, is a rare but serious complication of carotid revascularization after CEA or CAS. It occurs in approximately 1% of patients after CEA and evolves between 2 and 7 days after surgery. Classic symptoms include ipsilateral severe headache, (transient) neurological deficits and seizures. There is an increase in CBF compared with pre-operative values because of two interlinked mechanisms – impaired cerebral autoregulation and arterial hypertension. High-grade extracranial stenosis very often causes exhaustion of the autoregulatory mechanism leading to maximum dilation of the cerebral arterioles. The effect of post-operative hypertension is likely to be related to impaired baroreceptor function, although CHS can occur in normotensive patients. Before CEA, relatively high blood pressure is required to ensure adequate distal cerebral perfusion and prevent 'watershed' cerebral ischaemia. After CEA, the distal vessels that were previously protected by the stenosis are suddenly exposed to this relatively high pressure, leading to uncontrolled increases in CBF and fluid transudation and vasogenic white-matter oedema.

Generally, CHS has a favourable prognosis but can be fatal if it results in intracerebral haemorrhage (ICH). There are no data from randomized studies clarifying how CHS can be prevented or treated. Close monitoring of blood pressure and CBF (e.g. using transcranial Doppler ultrasonography) and meticulous control of post-operative blood pressure are essential. Seizures should also be treated aggressively. Because CHS symptoms can occur days after intervention, patients should be advised to return to hospital immediately if they develop severe headache or new neurological symptoms.

Cerebral venous thrombosis

Cerebral venous thrombosis (CVT) is a rare cause of cerebral infarction (<1%) but is of importance because it has a relatively high morbidity and mortality and different diagnostic and therapeutic approaches compared with other causes of cerebral infarction. The exact incidence of CVT is uncertain. Previously, it was usually diagnosed at post mortem and was therefore believed to be a rare (3–4 cases per million population) and fatal disease. However, modern imaging techniques and the increasing numbers of examinations performed has led to a reappraisal of the incidence of CVT, which is almost certainly higher than previously believed. With increased diagnosis comes earlier intervention, and this has led also to a reappraisal of the grim outcome prospects. Mortality in untreated cases is likely to lie between 14 and 48%.

Causes and risk factors

Up to 75% of adult patients with CVT are female, with the puerperal period being a particular risk. The peripartum frequency of CVT is 12 per 100,000 births. No racial predilection is identified. There is a uniform age distribution for the presentation of CVT in men, whereas 61% of women with CVT are aged 20–35 years, presumably related to pregnancy or the use of oral contraceptives.

Two distinct entities are recognized – infectious and non-infectious CVT. Infectious CVT occurs secondary to local infections, including sinusitis, otitis media, mastoiditis, dental infections and meningitis, or because of systemic bacterial, viral and parasitic infections. There are multiple causes of non-infectious CVT including coagulation disorders, trauma and malignancies (Table 25.3).

Clinical presentation

Because of the great variability in collaterals of the cerebral venous system, many thromboses are asymptomatic and only around one-third of patients present with symptoms. Headache is the most common and often the first symptom of CVT and occurs in 75–95% of symptomatic patients. The typical description is of a dull, oppressing, slowly worsening pain, although a thunderclap headache as seen in subarachnoid haemorrhage may occur, particularly in patients with venous ICH. About 30–40% of patients develop focal or generalized epileptic seizures. Nausea, vomiting and

impaired vision may also occur and are likely to be related to elevated ICP. Depending on the affected venous vessel, consciousness may vary from fully alert and oriented, through mild confusion to coma. Deep CVT most commonly presents with coma. Focal neurological deficits such as hemiparesis, aphasia, ataxia, dizziness, chorea, hemianopia and cranial nerve syndromes can also occur.

Cerebral venous thrombosis-related cerebral infarction and haemorrhage

Initially, there is intracranial compensation for the venous congestion associated with CVT, but at some point the rising cerebral blood volume causes an increase in ICP. A local reduction in CBF is followed initially by cytotoxic and later by vasogenic oedema, and persistent local tissue hypoxia leads to venous infarction. In 40% of patients, the blocked venous outflow will ultimately result in intracranial, subarachnoid, subdural or intraventricular haemorrhage.

Diagnosis

Modern non-invasive imaging techniques using venous CTA (v-CTA) or MRA (v-MRA) are the first-line diagnostic tools to confirm CVT. These techniques have replaced the use of DSA, which carries its own interventional risks. The absence of flow void in the normal venous channels is diagnostic of CVT. Venous MRA is an excellent method of visualizing larger cerebral veins and dural venous sinuses (Fig. 25.4). Venous CTA is equivalent to v-MRA in identification of dural sinus thrombosis and therefore the investigation of first choice in patients with suspected sinus thrombosis, as it is easier and faster to perform than MRA and produces fewer flow artefacts. Plain CT in association with v-CTA is also used in an emergency situation, as it can detect even very small congestive haemorrhages. However, infarction cannot be identified by CT for up to 48–72 h, whereas MRI is able to confirm an infarct pattern that does not follow the distribution of an expected arterial occlusion much earlier. The 'empty delta sign' is the classic finding of CVT on contrast scans. It is characterized by enhancement of collateral veins in the superior sagittal sinus walls surrounding a non-enhanced thrombus in the sinus, although this sign is frequently absent. The 'dense triangle' sign formed by fresh coagulated blood in the superior sagittal sinus and the 'cord sign' representing

Table 25.3 Risk factors and causes of cerebral venous thrombosis

Infectious causes	
Local infections	Sinusitis
	Otitis media
	Mastoiditis
	Dental infections
	Furuncles of the face
	Subdural empyema
	Bacterial meningitis
Systemic infections	Bacterial, viral, mycotic and parasitic (including subacute bacterial endocarditis)
Non-infectious causes	
Local	Trauma, neurosurgical procedures
	Tumour
	Infusions into the internal jugular vein
	Pregnancy/puerperal
Hormonal	Oral contraception
	Therapy with steroids or androgens
Medication	Chemotherapy
Drug abuse	
Coagulation disorders	Antiphospholipid syndrome
	Protein S and C deficiencies
	Antithrombin III deficiency
	Lupus anticoagulant
	Leiden factor V mutation
	Disseminated intravascular coagulation
	Heparin-induced thrombocytopaenia
Predisposing factors	
Heart disease	Congenital heart disease
	Heart failure
	Cardiac pacemaker
Gastrointestinal diseases	Cirrhosis of the liver
	Crohn's disease, ulcerative colitis
Vasculitis	Systemic lupus erythematosus
	Horton's disease
	Wegener's granulomatosis
Haematological disorders	Polycythaemia
	Sickle-cell disease
	Paroxysmal nocturnal haemoglobinuria
Malignancies	Lymphoma
	Leukaemia
	Carcinoid
	Histiocytosis X
Other	Dehydration
	Diabetes mellitus
	Sarcoidosis
	Nephrotic syndrome

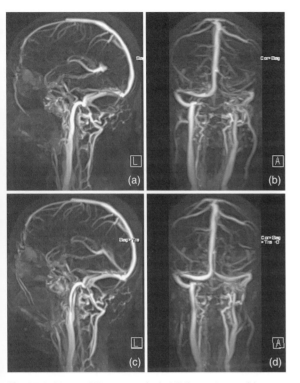

Fig. 25.4. Venous MR angiography (v-MRA) in a 38-year-old female with cerebral venous thrombosis. (a, b) Venous MRA showing thrombosis affecting the straight sinus, confluent sinus and both transverse sinuses. (c, d) Repeat v-MRA at 6 months after oral anticoagulation showing complete recanalization of the sinuses.

a thrombosed cortical vein are rare. CT angiography and MRA are also useful in ruling out other conditions such as neoplasm and in evaluating coexistent lesions such as a subdural empyema.

D-dimers can be of assistance in the diagnosis of CVT. Although they cannot be used as a screening method because of poor specificity, their high sensitivity (up to 97%) and negative predictive value (99%) means that normal D-dimers are unlikely to be found in patients with CVT. Screening for thrombophilia should also be performed to detect underlying systemic disease.

Treatment

Patients with an acute CVT usually receive anticoagulation with intravenous heparin to maintain the partial thromboplastin time at 60–80 s for 10–14 days in order to minimize clot propagation. There are only a few studies of anticoagulation after CVT, but these confirm a tendency towards improved outcome after anticoagulation. One study even showed improvement

in outcome with heparin in the presence of CVT-associated ICH. Subcutaneous low-molecular-weight heparin has also been used to treat CVT. Local thrombolysis is a therapeutic option of last resort if symptoms progress despite adequate systemic anticoagulation. In the case of infection-related CVT, antibiotic therapy should be started early and a possible local focus identified and surgically drained. Seizures should be treated with appropriate anticonvulsants.

Although there are few data to guide the switch from heparin to warfarin oral anticoagulation, many recommend that this should occur sometime between 10 and 14 days after presentation. Warfarin should be continued for at least 3–6 months to maintain the international normalized ratio (INR) at 2.5. The International Study on Cerebral Vein and Dural Sinus Thrombosis (ISCVT) demonstrated a 2.2% recurrence rate of CVT after a mean of 7.7 months of oral anticoagulation. Life-long anticoagulation is therefore only recommended in cases of recurrent CVT or if there is an underlying prothrombotic condition.

Prognosis

Recanalization of the affected vein or sinus is usually seen within the first months after treatment, and the rate of recurrent CVT is low (5%). The prospective ISCVT included 624 patients with CVT treated between 1998 and 2002 and found an 8.3% mortality rate. At 6 months, 57% of patients were symptom free and 13% had unfavourable outcome (mRS ≥3). Age >37 years, male sex, congestive ICH, thrombosis of deep veins, cerebral infection and neoplasm were all associated with a worse outcome.

Further reading

Eames, P., Blake, M., Dawson, S., Panerai, R. and Potter, J. (2002). Dynamic cerebral autoregulation and beat to beat blood pressure control are impaired in acute ischaemic stroke. *J Neurol Neurosurg Psychiatry* **72**, 467–72.

Eckert, B., Koch, C., Thomalla, G. *et al.* (2005). Aggressive therapy with intravenous abciximab and intra-arterial rtPA and additional PTA/stenting improves clinical outcome in acute vertebrobasilar occlusion: combined local fibrinolysis and intravenous abciximab in acute vertebrobasilar stroke treatment (FAST): results of a multicenter study. *Stroke* **36**, 1160–5.

European Stroke Organisation (ESO) Executive Committee and ESO Writing Committee (2008). Guidelines for management of ischaemic stroke and transient ischaemic attack 2008. *Cerebrovasc Dis* **25**, 457–507.

Ferro, J., Canhão, P., Stam, J. *et al.* (2004). Prognosis of cerebral vein and dural sinus thrombosis: results of the International Study on Cerebral Vein and Dural Sinus Thrombosis (ISCVT). *Stroke* **35**, 664–70.

FOOD Trial Collaboration (2003). Poor nutritional status on admission predicts poor outcomes after stroke: observational data from the FOOD trial. *Stroke* **34**, 1450–6.

Gosk-Biersak, I., Wysokinski, W., Brown, R. D. Jr *et al.* (2006). Cerebral venous sinus thrombosis: incidence of venous thrombosis recurrence and survival. *Neurology* **67**, 814–19.

Hacke, W., Schwab, S., Horn, M. *et al.* (1996). 'Malignant' middle cerebral artery territory infarction: clinical course and prognostic signs. *Arch Neurol* **53**, 309–15.

Hacke, W., Donnan, G., Fieschi, C. *et al.* (2004). Association of outcome with early stroke treatment: pooled analysis of ATLANTIS, ECASS, and NINDS rt-PA stroke trials. *Lancet* **363**, 768–74.

Hacke, W., Albers, G., Al-Rawi, Y., *et al.* (2005). The Desmoteplase in Acute Ischemic Stroke Trial (DIAS): a phase II MRI-based 9-hour window acute stroke thrombolysis trial with intravenous desmoteplase. *Stroke* **36**, 66–73.

Hacke, W., Kaste, M., Bluhmki, E. *et al.* (2008). Thrombolysis with alteplase 3 to 4.5 h after acute ischemic stroke. *N Engl J Med* **359**, 1317–29.

Hofmeijer, J., Kappelle, L. J., Algra, A. *et al.* (2009) Surgical decompression for space-occupying cerebral infarction (the Hemicraniectomy After Middle Cerebral Artery infarction with Life-threatening Edema Trial [HAMLET]): a multicentre, open, randomised trial. *Lancet Neurol* **8**, 326–33.

IMS II Trial Investigators (2007). The Interventional Management of Stroke (IMS) II Study. *Stroke* **38**, 2127–35.

Kamphuisen, P., Agnelli, G. and Sebastianelli, M. (2005). Prevention of venous thromboembolism after acute ischemic stroke. *J Thromb Haemost* **3**, 1187–94.

Karapanayiotides, T., Meuli, R., Devuyst, G. *et al.* (2005). Postcarotid endarterectomy hyperperfusion or reperfusion syndrome. *Stroke* **36**, 21–6.

Leonardi-Bee, J., Bath, P. M., Phillips, S. J., Sandercock, P. A. and IST Collaborative Group (2002). Blood pressure and clinical outcomes in the International Stroke Trial. *Stroke* **33**, 1315–20.

Lindsberg, P. and Mattle, H. (2006) Therapy of basilar artery occlusion: a systematic analysis comparing intra-arterial and intravenous thrombolysis. *Stroke* **37**, 922–8.

Mas, J., Chatellier, G., Beyssen, B. *et al.* (2006). Endarterectomy versus stenting in patients with symptomatic severe carotid stenosis. *N Engl J Med* **355**, 1660–71.

Martino, R., Foley, N., Bhogal, S. *et al.* (2005). Dysphagia after stroke: incidence, diagnosis, and pulmonary complications. *Stroke* **36**, 2756–63.

Muir, K. (2008). The PREVAIL trial and low-molecular-weight heparin for prevention of venous thromboembolism. *Stroke* **39**, 2174–6.

Nagel, S., Schellinger, P. D., Hartmann, M. *et al.* (2009) Therapy of acute basilar artery occlusion: intraarterial thrombolysis alone vs bridging therapy. *Stroke* **40**, 140–6.

Posner, S., Boxer, L., Proctor, M. *et al.* (2004). Uncomplicated carotid endarterectomy: factors contributing to blood pressure instability precluding safe early discharge. *Vascular* **12**, 278–84.

Schellinger, P., Fiebach, J. B., Mohr, A. *et al.* (2001). Thrombolytic therapy for ischemic stroke – a review. Part I. Intravenous thrombolysis. *Crit Care Med* **29**, 1812–18.

Schellinger, P., Fiebach, J. B., Mohr, A. *et al.* (2001). Thrombolytic therapy for ischemic stroke – a review. Part II. Intra-arterial thrombolysis, vertebrobasilar stroke, phase IV trials, and stroke imaging. *Crit Care Med* **29**, 1819–25.

Schellinger, P., Thomalla, G., Fiehler, J. *et al.* (2007). MRI-based and CT-based thrombolytic therapy in acute stroke within and beyond established time windows: an analysis of 1210 patients. *Stroke* **38**, 2640–5.

Schwab, S., Georgiadis, D., Berrouschot, J. *et al.* (2001). Feasibility and safety of moderate hypothermia after massive hemispheric infarction. *Stroke* **32**, 2033–5.

SPACE Collaborative Group, Ringleb, P., Allenberg, J. *et al.* (2006). 30 day results from the SPACE trial of stent-protected angioplasty versus carotid endarterectomy in symptomatic patients: a randomised non-inferiority trial. *Lancet* **368**, 1239–47.

Stam, J. (2005). Thrombosis of the cerebral veins and sinuses. *N Engl J Med* **352**, 1791–8.

Vahedia, K., Hofmeijer, J., Juettler, E. *et al.* (2007). Early decompressive surgery in malignant infarction of the middle cerebral artery: a pooled analysis of three randomised controlled trials. *Lancet Neurol* **6**, 215–22.

Chapter

26

Neuromuscular disorders

Nicholas Hirsch and Robin Howard

Introduction

The origin of the intensive care treatment of neuro-muscular disease lies in the development of specialized respiratory units in Scandinavia to treat respiratory failure due to poliomyelitis during the epidemic in 1952. While many patients survived due to acute respiratory intervention, a proportion required long-term respiratory support, and the principles gained from this experience remain in use today.

Although primary neuromuscular disease is a relatively uncommon cause for admission to the general intensive therapy unit (ITU), it is important that intensivists understand the diversity of these conditions and the problems that they pose. Other individuals develop neuromuscular diseases as a consequence of their critical illness. Management of both groups requires close cooperation between many disciplines including intensivists, anaesthetists, neurologists, neurophysiologists, therapists and experts in neurorehabilitation.

This chapter discusses the general medical care of patients with neuromuscular disease and gives an account of the more common conditions seen in the intensive care setting.

General medical care of patients with neuromuscular disease

This section will review the general principles of the complex and challenging management of patients with neuromuscular disease.

Respiratory system

Patients with neuromuscular disease require tracheal intubation and mechanical ventilation either because of acute respiratory insufficiency or because they are unable to protect their airway as a consequence of poor bulbar function. The onset of respiratory failure may be acute (e.g. Guillain–Barré syndrome), acute-on-chronic (e.g. Duchenne muscular dystrophy), slowly progressive (e.g. acid maltase deficiency) or relapsing (e.g. myasthenia gravis). In many neuromuscular diseases, bulbar weakness and respiratory insufficiency coexist, resulting in failure to clear secretions, pulmonary aspiration and bronchopneumonia.

The pathophysiology of respiratory muscle weakness in neuromuscular disease is complex and is condition dependent. For example, respiratory failure in motor neuron disease and acid maltase deficiency occurs primarily because of diaphragmatic failure, whereas in Duchenne and myotonic muscular dystrophies, expiratory muscle dysfunction, resulting in poor cough, predominates. The onset of respiratory failure in chronic neuromuscular disease is often insidious, and symptoms and signs may be subtle (Table 26.1). Generally, ventilation is required if patients exhibit daytime symptoms or if there is sleep study evidence of nocturnal hypoventilation. However, many patients can be managed effectively using domiciliary non-invasive nasal positive-pressure ventilation (NIV) during sleep.

Respiratory muscle strength can be monitored using a variety of techniques, including maximal inspiratory and expiratory mouth pressures and maximal nasal sniff pressure, but the most reproducible is forced vital capacity (FVC). When FVC is performed correctly, serial decreases effectively indicate deteriorating ventilatory function. When FVC falls below 15–20 ml kg^{-1} (normal value 75 ml kg^{-1}), tracheal intubation and mechanical ventilation is indicated, as the patient will be unable to generate a cough that is sufficiently strong to clear their airway. Earlier intubation should be considered if bulbar weakness coexists. Reliance on arterial blood gas analysis can be misleading, even

Core Topics in Neuroanaesthesia and Neurointensive Care, eds. Basil F. Matta, David K. Menon and Martin Smith. Published by Cambridge University Press. © Cambridge University Press 2011.

Table 26.1 Symptoms and signs of chronic neuromuscular respiratory weakness

Symptoms	Signs
Dyspnoea	May be none
Disrupted and restless sleep	Tachypnoea and use of accessory muscles
Witnessed apnoea	Paradoxical inward abdominal movement of the abdomen on inspiration
Excessive daytime sleepiness	> 30% decrease in forced vital capacity on lying from standing position
Morning headache	Hypoxaemia, hypercarbia and increased bicarbonate level on arterial blood gas analysis
Poor concentration and irritability	Oxygen desaturation during sleep
Orthopnoea	
Nocturia	

in acute neuromuscular disease, because hypoxaemia and hypercarbia may occur late and often not until the FVC has fallen below 15 ml kg^{-1}.

In many cases, prolonged ventilation will be required while awaiting recovery from the underlying condition and, as soon as this is obvious, a tracheostomy should be performed. A tracheostomy affords greater patient comfort, allows more efficient tracheal suction, facilitates mechanical ventilation without the need for sedation and provides the potential for eating and speaking as bulbar function allows. However, a tracheostomy does bring a risk of long-term dependence in progressive conditions such as motor neuron disease and Duchenne muscular dystrophy (DMD).

Mechanical ventilation and weaning

In patients with respiratory failure due to acute neuromuscular disease, ventilation is usually initiated with synchronized intermittent mandatory ventilation until recovery of respiratory muscle function occurs. Again, FVC provides the most useful method of monitoring recovery. When FVC has risen to 15–20 ml kg^{-1}, weaning may begin by transferring the patient onto pressure support ventilation. When pressure support has been successfully weaned to 10 cmH$_2$O, short periods of continuous positive airway pressure (CPAP) support, interspersed with pressure support ventilation, can be introduced. It is important initially to restrict these periods to 5–10 min h^{-1} and only increase the time spent on CPAP as respiratory muscle strength increases. Eventually CPAP can be replaced by unsupported spontaneous breathing through the tracheostomy while maintaining adequate humidification either through a 'wet circuit' or a Swedish nose. It is important to understand that patients with

chronic neuromuscular disease may require long-term respiratory support at night (predominantly due to their reduced nocturnal respiratory drive), even when successfully weaned from ventilation during the day.

Cardiovascular system

Cardiovascular monitoring is similar to that in the general ITU population. However, autonomic disturbances resulting in cardiac arrhythmias and labile blood pressure are common manifestations of many neuromuscular diseases, and invasive blood pressure monitoring is mandatory. Severe bradyarrhythmias may occur during suctioning and turning of the patient and may require temporary or permanent cardiac pacing. Cardiac failure secondary to cardiomyopathy is commonly seen in DMD and myotonic dystrophy.

Gastrointestinal system

Protein catabolism is almost inevitable in critically ill patients as a result of an inadequate supply of calories and increased substrate requirement associated with the stress response to injury and sepsis. The resultant generalized muscle loss also affects respiratory muscles, further compounding the poor respiratory reserve in patients with neuromuscular disease. Enteral feeding, initially via a nasogastric tube, should be started as soon as possible to provide protein-sparing calories, to protect against peptic ulceration and decrease the risk of bacterial translocation and nosocomial infection. If early enteral feeding can be established, there is no need for the prophylactic use of H$_2$-receptor antagonists or proton-pump inhibitors, which increase the incidence of ITU-associated infections.

Disorders of gastrointestinal motility are common in neuromuscular disorders. Constipation occurs because of a combination of autonomic dysfunction, immobility, opioid analgesics and a relative lack of fibre in enteral feed. The resulting abdominal distension causes diaphragmatic splinting, which impedes weaning from mechanical ventilation. The majority of patients require regular laxatives such as lactulose and senna. Ileus may occur in the acute phase of a number of neuromuscular diseases including GBS and high cervical cord lesions. It usually resolves within 48 h, although prokinetic agents such as metoclopramide and erythromycin may be required. Total parenteral nutrition is rarely needed.

Nosocomial infection

Although patients with neuromuscular respiratory failure can usually be weaned from mechanical ventilation, this may take many months. Nosocomial infection is the major cause of morbidity and mortality during this period of recovery. Common sites of infection include the urinary tract, respiratory tract (especially ventilator-associated pneumonia) and vascular cannulae (catheter-related sepsis). Infection control requires meticulous staff hygiene (handwashing before and after each patient contact), rigorous aseptic techniques for invasive procedures, early identification and appropriate treatment of infection by routine microbiological screening, the use of disposable equipment and the isolation of infected patients. It is also important to obtain daily input from a medical microbiologist.

Anticoagulation

Thromboembolic disease is an important cause of death in patients with neuromuscular disease nursed for long periods on the ITU. In some patients, this may be a result of a hypercoagulable state due to protein S or C deficiency or resistance, antithrombin III deficiency, malignancy or sepsis. However, in the majority of cases, it is related to long periods of immobility due to neuromuscular paralysis. Prophylaxis against venous thrombosis using low-molecular-weight heparin is essential, and all patients should also wear graduated compression stockings and receive intermittent mechanical calf compression.

Patient comfort

Patients with respiratory failure secondary to neuromuscular disease often require prolonged periods of mechanical ventilation, and it is neither feasible nor desirable to keep them sedated during their ITU stay. Furthermore, continuous sedation does not allow clinical neurological assessment and impairs subsequent weaning from mechanical ventilation. However, sedative and analgesic agents are necessary in the early stages to aid tolerance of the endotracheal tubes and facilitate mechanical ventilation, tracheal suction and physiotherapy. Intravenous propofol and fentanyl is a suitable combination. The former has a short context-sensitive half-time, which allows rapid wakening on discontinuation.

Pain

Pain is a prominent feature of many neurological conditions treated on the ITU and it is important that this is recognized and treated. Combinations of opioid and non-opioid analgesics, including agents directed towards neuropathic pain (e.g. amitriptyline, gabapentin), may be required.

Communication

Even in patients requiring mechanical ventilation, speech is often possible via a tracheostomy. Fibre-optic evaluation of vocal cord function can lead to early speaking trials. These require specialist valves and, more importantly, the expertise of an experienced speech and language therapist. If speech is impossible, other communication aids will be required.

Sleep

Sleep deprivation is almost inevitable in patients nursed in the ITU for long periods. Factors include disruption of day/night cycles, environmental factors such as noise and patient factors such as fear. These result in agitation, confusion and the development of ITU psychosis. Furthermore, sleep deprivation has a direct effect on respiratory muscle function, catabolism and the immune response. It is vital to recognize the problem early and re-establish a normal sleep–wake cycle by the use of hypnotic agents (e.g. benzodiazepines, zopiclone) and sedative antidepressants. Melatonin has proved useful in resistant insomnia.

Primary neuromuscular diseases

Respiratory failure due to neuromuscular disease may be caused by diseases affecting the anterior horn cells, peripheral nerves, neuromuscular junction or the respiratory muscles themselves (Table 26.2).

Table 26.2 Primary neuromuscular causes of ventilatory insufficiency

Anterior horn cell diseases

Motor neuron disease (amyotrophic lateral sclerosis)

Poliomyelitis

Rabies

Polyneuropathies

Guillain–Barré syndromes

- Acute inflammatory demyelinating polyneuropathy (AIDP)

- Acute motor axonal neuropathy (AMAN)

- Acute motor and sensory axonal neuropathy (AMSAN)

- Fisher syndrome

Other polyneuropathies

- Acute porphyria

- Organophosphate poisoning

- Diphtheria

Neuromuscular junction disease

Lambert–Eaton myasthenic syndrome

Botulism

Tetanus

Myasthenia gravis

Animal toxins

Organophosphate poisoning

Primary muscle disease

Muscular dystrophies

- Duchenne muscular dystrophy

- Myotonic dystrophy

Congenital myopathies

- Central core disease

- Nemaline myopathy

Metabolic muscle disease

- Acid maltase disease

- Mitochondrial disease

Periodic paralyses

Anterior horn cell diseases

Motor neuron disease

Motor neuron disease (MND) is a progressive condition characterized by degeneration of motor neurons and cranial nerve nuclei. It has an incidence of 6 per 100,000 of the population, more commonly affects men and has a mean onset age of 63 years; 90% of patients die within 5 years of diagnosis. Approximately 5% of cases of MND are familial.

Amyotrophic lateral sclerosis is the commonest clinical form of MND. It is characterized by upper and lower motor neuron involvement of the bulbar, limb and trunk muscles resulting in muscle wasting, fasciculation, weakness, spasticity and brisk reflexes. Progressive respiratory and bulbar muscle weakness results in respiratory failure and death from bronchopneumonia. Patients with MND may occasionally present to the ITU with acute respiratory failure due to selective diaphragmatic weakness or chest sepsis, and tracheal intubation and mechanical ventilation may be required before the diagnosis of MND becomes apparent. However, in those in whom the diagnosis has already been established, careful discussion about the inevitability of respiratory failure allows the preparation of a patient-specific plan regarding the appropriateness of mechanical ventilation under such circumstances. Early intervention with NIV improves the length of survival and quality of life by ameliorating the daytime symptoms caused by nocturnal hypoventilation. However, this must be balanced against the wishes of the patient, the practicalities of providing support and the distress of prolonging life in the terminal stages of the disease.

Poliomyelitis

Despite widespread (and largely successful) vaccination programmes aimed at eradication, cases of sporadic and vaccine-induced polio still occur. The disease is caused by an enterovirus that gains access via the gastrointestinal tract. After an incubation period of 7–14 days, minor flu-like symptoms are followed by a meningitic phase as the virus reaches the central nervous system (CNS). The onset of spinal polio is characterized by myalgia, severe muscle spasms and an asymmetrical flaccid weakness, which reaches its peak in 48 h. Respiratory muscle involvement can lead to respiratory failure, often requiring prolonged periods of mechanical ventilation. Post-polio syndrome refers to functional deterioration some years after the initial paralytic illness and includes the development of chronic respiratory failure requiring NIV.

Rabies

Although officially eradicated from the UK in 1920, occasional cases of rabies are seen in patients who have contracted the disease abroad, most commonly

Table 26.3 Guillain–Barré syndrome (GBS) variants

Guillain–Barré subtype	Features
Acute inflammatory demyelinating polyradiculopathy (AIDP)	Classical GBS caused by demyelination Accounts for approximately 90% of cases in the UK and USA
Acute motor and sensory axonal neuropathy (AMSAN)	Motor and sensory axons affected
Acute motor axonal neuropathy (AMAN)	Motor axons selectively affected
Fisher syndrome	Triad of ophthalmoplegia, ataxia and areflexia Overlap syndromes occur where the triad is accompanied by neuropathy causing limb and respiratory weakness

in India. In the USA, two to three cases are reported each year. The disease is caused by a neurotropic RNA virus usually transmitted via saliva following the bite of an affected dog or bat. The virus spreads to the CNS by axoplasmic flow. The incubation period is between 30 and 90 days but may extend for years. Prodromal symptoms include itching and pain at the site of inoculation, fever, myalgia, irritability and depression leading to encephalopathy.

Furious rabies is the most common presentation. Early symptoms and signs include cranial nerve lesions, autonomic disturbance, painful laryngospasm and fear of swallowing (hydrophobia). These may progress to generalized extensor spasm and cardiopulmonary arrest. Even with supportive intensive care, death is almost inevitable. In contrast, the rarer paralytic rabies (which usually results from Latin American bat bites) causes a flaccid paralysis resulting in respiratory and bulbar failure. Early treatment of suspected rabies, including thorough wound cleaning and active and passive immunization, can prevent the onset of clinical symptoms. If immunization is delayed or not performed, around 15% of those exposed to the rabies virus will contract the disease, leading to almost inevitable death.

Polyneuropathies

Guillain–Barré syndrome

Guillain–Barré syndrome (GBS) is the collective term for at least four subtypes of acute peripheral neuropathy that have specific clinical features (Table 26.3).

Acute inflammatory demyelinating polyradiculopathy (AIDP) is the most common form of GBS in Europe and North America and has an incidence of approximately one to two cases per 100,000 of the population. In 60% of cases, GBS follows an upper respiratory tract infection or gastroenteritis. Organisms most commonly associated with GBS include *Campylobacter jejuni*, cytomegalovirus, Epstein–Barr virus and *Mycoplasma pneumoniae*. It is likely that antibody to various infective agents cross-reacts with myelin sheath or axonal antigens, thereby damaging the peripheral nerves. This hypothesis is supported by the presence of a number of circulating antibodies to neural gangliosides in some forms of the disease. Guillain–Barré syndrome has also been reported following vaccination and major surgery.

Clinical features and diagnosis of Guillain–Barré syndrome

The classical presentation of AIDP is an ascending distal and proximal weakness accompanied by mild sensory disturbance (usually glove-and-stocking parasthesia) and areflexia. Pain may be a prominent presenting feature, especially in children. Facial, ocular and bulbar weakness occur in 50% of cases. Progression of the weakness is often rapid, with 50% of cases reaching a nadir within 2 weeks and 90% by 4 weeks. If progression continues beyond 4 weeks, a diagnosis of chronic inflammatory demyelinating polyradiculopathy (CIDP) should be considered. Differentiation between GBS and CIDP is essential, as their treatments are fundamentally different. Autonomic involvement is common in severe GBS and manifestations include tachy- and bradyarrhythmias, hypotension, episodic hypertension and ileus.

Although the diagnosis of GBS is based largely on clinical evidence and exclusion of other causes of neuromuscular weakness, it is supported by the demonstration of a raised cerebrospinal fluid (CSF) protein (especially after the first week) and neurophysiological investigations that allow differentiation between the various subtypes of GBS.

Other variants of Guillain–Barré syndrome

Around 50% of cases of GBS in China, Japan and central America are the axonal forms – acute motor and sensory axonal neuropathy (AMSAN) and acute motor axonal neuropathy (AMAN). These are often associated with *Campylobacter* infection and antibodies to GM1 ganglioside are commonly identified. Onset of weakness is characteristically more rapid than in AIDP, and prolonged ventilatory support is often required.

Fisher syndrome consists of ophthalmoplegia, ataxia and areflexia. Although its course is generally relatively benign, overlap syndromes can occur when the triad is accompanied by limb and respiratory muscle weakness. Antibodies to the GQ1b ganglioside are often present.

Treatment of Guillain–Barré syndrome

Plasma exchange (PE) was the first treatment shown to be beneficial in GBS, and it shortens the time to recovery and reduces the need for mechanical ventilation. It is more beneficial when performed within 7 days of the onset of symptoms. Subsequently, intravenous immunoglobulin (IVIg) has been shown to be equally effective, and is now the favoured treatment in non-specialist centres because of its relative ease of administration compared with PE. No benefit has been demonstrated by combining PE and IVIg, and corticosteroids have no role in the treatment of GBS.

Intensive care management of Guillain–Barré syndrome

Guillain–Barré syndrome patients with a low or rapidly declining FVC, poor bulbar function or autonomic instability should be monitored carefully in an ITU setting. Approximately 25% of patients with GBS require mechanical ventilation while awaiting recovery of respiratory muscle function. Suxamethonium must be avoided during tracheal intubation because of the risk of hyperkalaemia and cardiac arrest. Tracheostomy should be performed if respiratory failure lasts longer than 7–10 days.

Other aspects of the critical care management of GBS include treatment of autonomic dysfunction (cardiac pacing may be necessary for severe bradyarrhythmias), early initiation of enteral feeding, thromboembolic prophylaxis and meticulous nursing care. An adequate means of communication should be established as soon as possible. Musculoskeletal and neuropathic pain is almost invariable and often requires treatment with combinations of opioid and non-opioid analgesics, tricyclic antidepressant agents and gabapentin. Passive and active physiotherapy is essential to maximize residual muscle function and prevent tendon shortening. Psychological support with regular patient updates on progress may need to be supplemented by antidepressant therapy.

Recent advances in treatment have reduced the overall mortality rate of GBS to around 6%. Mortality rates are higher in those requiring mechanical ventilation and lower in patients treated in specialist neuroscience centres with experience of GBS. Death usually occurs because of sepsis, thromboembolic events or unrelated conditions. Eventual prognosis is variable and depends on the need for mechanical ventilation and the extent of axonal loss. Worse outcome occurs in the elderly, those with a preceding diarrhoeal illness and those with a poor disability score 2 weeks into the disease.

Acute porphyria

The acute hepatic porphyrias (acute intermittent porphyria, variegate porphyria and hereditary coproporphyria) are a group of autosomal dominant disorders of haem synthesis that affect the central, peripheral and autonomic nervous systems. Each type of porphyria occurs because of a deficiency of a specific enzyme in the haem synthetic pathway, resulting in a lack of haem and accumulation of intermediate metabolites. The most prominent neurological manifestation is a polyneuropathy, which produces acute, severe, generalized weakness. Most attacks are precipitated by drugs including barbiturates, anti-epileptic agents (especially phenytoin), sulfa antibacterial agents and oestrogens. Exacerbations may also occur during menstruation, pregnancy, infection and starvation.

Porphyric crises typically begin with acute abdominal and low back pain, followed by symmetrical limb weakness mainly affecting the proximal muscles. Flaccid tetraparesis and respiratory failure may follow. Autonomic disturbances including pyrexia, gastrointestinal stasis and labile blood pressure are common. Central nervous system involvement includes seizures, confusion and encephalopathy. The major differential diagnoses are GBS, and strychnine and heavy-metal poisoning (particularly lead). The diagnosis of porphyria can be confirmed by the presence of markedly raised levels of porphobilinogen in a spot urine sample. Detailed biochemical analysis of blood, urine and faeces allows subsequent classification of the specific porphyria. In an acute attack, urine turns reddish brown due to polymerization of bilinogen.

The intensive care treatment of acute porphyric crisis includes discontinuation of any precipitating medication, rehydration with glucose-containing fluids (which suppress porphyrin synthesis), correction of electrolyte abnormalities and supportive care. In severe cases, haematin (haem arginate) may be administered to reduce porphyrin levels. Treatment of seizures can be difficult because many anti-epileptic agents exacerbate porphyria. However, clonazepam and sodium valproate have been used successfully.

Diphtheria

Although diphtheria is uncommon in developed countries because of mass immunization, sporadic cases still occur, especially as immunization does not confer life-long immunity. It is caused by infection with *Corynebacterium diphtheriae*, a Gram-positive organism, which causes local mucosal necrosis and the formation of a thick 'pseudomembrane' of fibrin, epithelial cells, bacteria and neutrophils affecting the skin and throat. The incubation period is 1–7 days. Systemic involvement follows dissemination of the toxin and may lead to myocarditis and neurological complications characterized by cranial nerve involvement and peripheral neuropathy. The diagnosis of diptheria is made initially on clinical grounds and confirmed by throat swabs and toxin detection.

Palatal and posterior pharyngeal wall paralysis commonly follows pseudomembrane formation and is associated with progressive cranial neuropathy leading to bulbar weakness manifest as dysarthria, dysphagia and aspiration. Ocular involvement may also occur. A mixed sensorimotor peripheral neuropathy develops later in the course of the disease, often many months after its onset. Proximal weakness, which may extend distally, can result in severe paralysis and areflexia. Diaphragm and respiratory muscle weakness may also develop, requiring tracheal intubation and prolonged periods of mechanical ventilation. Distal sensory impairment affects all modalities, and autonomic involvement, manifest as sinus tachycardia, postural hypotension and urinary retention, is common.

Treatment involves the immediate administration of diphtheria antitoxin to neutralize circulating toxin, antibiotic treatment against *C. diphtheriae* (penicillin or erythromycin) and supportive management of cardiac, respiratory, bulbar and secondary infective complications. As immunity may wane, booster immunization should be offered every 10 years. Contacts are at considerable risk, and throat swabs should routinely be collected from them.

Disorders of the neuromuscular junction

The neuromuscular junction (NMJ) forms the link between myelinated motor nerves and skeletal muscle. In health, it acts as an efficient biological amplifier, converting minute nerve action potentials into muscle contraction. The NMJ consists of pre-synaptic, synaptic and post-synaptic components (Fig. 26.1).

Arrival of an action potential at the nerve terminal leads to membrane depolarization and opening of voltage-gated calcium channels arranged in parallel arrays at the active zones. This leads to a rise in free calcium ions within the terminal, which, through a number of events, leads to mobilization of acetylcholine (ACh) vesicles from their actin matrix, docking at the active zone and release of ACh into the synapse. The ACh diffuses across the synapse within a few microseconds. Approximately 50% of the released ACh reaches the post-synaptic membrane and the remainder is hydrolysed by acetylcholinesterase contained within the basement membrane of the synapse. On arrival at the post-synaptic region, ACh binds to the N-terminal domain of the junctions of the $\alpha\delta$ and $\delta\epsilon$ subunits of the ACh receptor (AChR) causing opening of the pore, influx of sodium ions and depolarization of the muscle membrane, which, following a number of steps, results in muscle contraction. A number of neurological diseases affect the pre-synaptic and post-synaptic components of the NMJ.

Pre-synaptic neuromuscular junction disorders

Lambert–Eaton myasthenic syndrome

Lambert–Eaton myasthenic syndrome (LEMS) is a rare autoimmune disease in which IgG antibodies are raised against the pre-synaptic voltage-gated calcium channels. This results in a decreased influx of calcium ions following depolarization of the nerve ending and leads to reduced ACh release from the pre-synaptic terminal. Although proximal limb muscles are usually affected, respiratory muscle involvement may occasionally

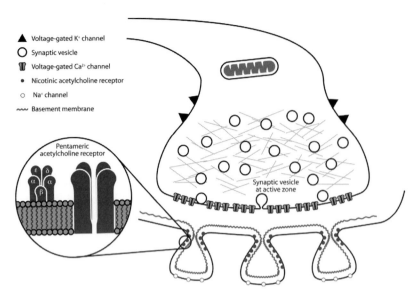

Fig. 26.1. Components of the neuromuscular junction.

Table 26.4 Autoimmune diseases associated with myasthenic syndromes

Hypo/hyperthyroidism
Rheumatoid disease
Systemic lupus erythematosus
Pernicious anaemia
Polymyositis
Diabetes mellitus

result in respiratory failure. Fifty per cent of cases are associated with underlying malignancy, usually small-cell carcinoma of the bronchus. In the remainder, there may be coexisting autoimmune disease. The condition is characterized by ptosis, weakness and prominent autonomic dysfunction. Diagnosis consists of detection of anti-voltage-gated calcium-channel antibodies and characteristic neurophysiological findings including an incremental response to high-frequency repetitive stimulation. Therapy includes treatment of the underlying malignancy, immunosuppression and 3,4-diaminopyridine, which increases pre-synaptic quantal release of ACh by blocking voltage-gated potassium channels and thereby prolonging the duration of the action potential.

Anaesthesia for patients with LEMS poses certain problems. They often have the associated features of malignancy and smoking-related disease and may also have other autoimmune conditions (Table 26.4). Many

will be receiving corticosteroids and require hydrocortisone 'cover' at induction of anaesthesia. Pre-operative PE or IVIg may be necessary if weakness is pronounced. Patients also show extreme sensitivity to depolarizing and non-depolarizing neuromuscular blocking agents and these should be avoided if possible. Other non-anaesthetic drugs may further compromise NMJ transmission (Table 26.5).

Botulism

Botulism is the clinical syndrome caused by neurotoxins produced by the anaerobic Gram-positive organism *Clostridium botulinum*. Neurotoxins A, B and E account for the majority of human cases. The toxins target various proteins at the pre-synaptic junction necessary for release of ACh. Food-borne botulism is the most common and is caused by ingestion of food contaminated with *Clostridium* spores or toxins produced under anaerobic conditions (e.g. home canning). Wound botulism results from contamination of surgical or other wounds. Recent outbreaks have been reported in drug abusers injecting black tar heroin subcutaneously ('skin popping'). Infant botulism occurs in children (usually <1 year old) who produce the toxin within the gastrointestinal tract as a result of ingesting *Clostridium* spores (classically in infected honey).

Clinical features of botulism include nausea, vomiting and abdominal pain (within 36 h of ingesting infected material) and autonomic dysfunction (blurred vision, diplopia, bradycardia and hypotension),

Table 26.5 Drugs to be avoided or used with caution in myasthenic conditions

Drug	Examples
Neuromuscular blocking agents	
Antibacterial agents	Aminoglycosides, polymixins, quinolones, clindamycin, erythromycin
Antiarrhythmics	Quinidine, procainamide
β-Adrenergic receptor antagonists	
Calcium-channel blocking drugs	
Immunosuppressive agents	Corticosteroids, cyclophosphamide
Statins	
Others	Penicillamine, phenytoin, dantrolene

followed by a descending flaccid paralysis. Although mild cases of botulism may not require mechanical ventilation, bulbar and respiratory failure progress rapidly and patients should therefore be monitored in a critical care area. In addition to its effect on the NMJ, botulinum toxin also blocks cholinergic synapses in the autonomic nervous system, resulting in cardiovascular instability and gastrointestinal disturbances.

The diagnosis of botulism depends on detecting botulinum toxin and *C. botulinum* from serum, faeces or wound exudates. The mouse inoculation test remains the most sensitive assay for the toxin, but results may be delayed. A modified ELISA-based detection method may provide a more rapid diagnosis. Although electrophysiological testing may be helpful, the diagnosis relies mainly on clinical suspicion.

Patients with recent-onset food-borne botulism should receive equine trivalent (ABE) antitoxin, which shortens the course of the disease and decreases mortality. Those allergic to the antitoxin and those with infant botulism should receive human botulism immunoglobulin. In addition, patients with wound botulism should undergo thorough wound debridement and treatment with metronidazole.

Tetanus

Tetanus is the clinical syndrome caused by neurotoxins produced by the anaerobic Gram-positive organism *Clostridium tetani*. Inoculation of *C. tetani* spores can occur through often insignificant skin wounds. The spores then germinate under anaerobic conditions and produce the toxin tetanospasmin, which, having bound to peripheral nerve terminals, migrates via retrograde axonal transport to the spinal cord and brainstem. The toxin eventually reaches pre-synaptic terminals where it inhibits the release of the inhibitory neurotransmitters γ-aminobutyric acid (GABA) and glycine. Without their inhibitory influence, unchecked α-motor neuron activity results in muscle rigidity. Preganglionic sympathetic fibres are also affected, resulting in sympathetic 'storms'. Muscle weakness is also seen in tetanus as tetanospasmin inhibits pre-synaptic release of ACh at the NMJ.

Tetanus accounts for approximately 0.5 million deaths worldwide annually but is rare in countries where tetanus immunization is performed routinely. Since 2003, approximately five cases occur in the UK and 45 cases in the USA each year. Tetanus is characterized by an acute onset of painful increased muscle tone and spasms, classically beginning in the masseter muscles and resulting in trismus or 'lockjaw'. This is usually followed by pain and stiffness in the neck, shoulder and back muscles. Respiratory failure may occur because of respiratory muscle spasm or laryngospasm. Autonomic dysfunction is also common and leads to tachyarrhythmias, labile blood pressure, profuse sweating and ileus. Cephalic tetanus is a variant in which only cranial nerve-innervated muscles are affected. Neonatal tetanus affects children born to unimmunized mothers.

Tetanus is a clinical diagnosis that should be suspected in patients with an increased tone in facial, paraspinal and proximal limb muscles. The spatula test has a very high sensitivity and specificity for the diagnosis of tetanus. In tetanus, a wooden spatula placed in contact with the oropharynx results in spasm of the masseter muscles and biting of the spatula. More sophisticated tests, including examination of the CSF and electromyography (EMG), are rarely helpful.

Treatment of tetanus starts with removal of the source of the toxin by thorough debridement of the wound and eradication of any remaining vegetative spores with metronidazole. Control of rigidity and spasms is achieved by nursing the patient in a quiet environment and, if required, the use of benzodiazepines, such as diazepam or midazolam, anticonvulsant agents (including phenobarbital and chlorpromazine) and propofol. The successful use of dantrolene and intrathecal baclofen has also been reported. However, if spasms are not controlled with sedation alone, administration of neuromuscular blocking agents (e.g. atracurium) and mechanical ventilation may be necessary. Autonomic instability often requires the use of β-adrenergic receptor antagonists or clonidine. Magnesium has been used with some success to control both rigidity and autonomic dysfunction in both ventilated and non-ventilated patients with tetanus.

The mortality of tetanus depends on the facilities available for treatment. In developing countries with limited intensive care facilities, mortality approaches 50%, whereas mortality rates of 15% are reported in patients treated in modern ITUs. Death is usually related to sudden cardiac events or the respiratory complications of prolonged mechanical ventilation.

Postsynaptic neuromuscular junction disorders

Myasthenia gravis

Types of myasthenia gravis

There are several types of myasthenia gravis (MG):

1. *Acquired MG* is an archetypical autoimmune disease in which antibodies are raised against the NMJ. In the majority of cases, an IgG antibody is directed at the post-synaptic AChR. Those without AChR antibodies (so-called seronegative MG) often have antibodies directed towards the muscle-specific receptor kinase (MuSK) at the NMJ. This receptor has a role in directing the agrin-dependent clustering of AChRs during their development. Although the precise aetiology of the autoimmune process remains unknown, most patients with seropositive MG have abnormalities of the thymus gland – either hyperplasia or thymoma. This clearly plays a part in the generation of the anti-AChR antibodies, which cause complement-mediated destruction of the AChR and a decreased receptor density at the post-synaptic membrane. This loss of AChRs leads

to the generation of an insufficient threshold of the end-plate potential (EPP), which is necessary to produce effective muscle contraction. Acquired MG is an uncommon disease with a prevalence of approximately 20 per 100,000 of the population and an annual incidence of 2–10 per million. Its incidence has a bimodal distribution, being more common in young women (<40 years) and older men (>50 years).

2. *Neonatal MG* occurs in approximately 10% of babies born to myasthenic mothers and is due to placental transfer of AChR antibodies. Spontaneous recovery tends to occur within 6 months, although a period of mechanical ventilation may be necessary.

3. *Congenital myasthenic syndromes* are a rare group of inherited diseases that can affect the presynaptic, synaptic and post-synaptic elements of the NMJ. The commonest form involves mutations of the α-subunit of the AChR and presents in early adolescence with facial, limb and respiratory muscle weakness. The last may result in respiratory failure.

4. *Drug-induced myasthenia* is usually associated with penicillamine therapy and often resolves on discontinuation of the drug.

Clinical features of acquired MG

Myasthenia gravis is characterized by fatigable weakness of skeletal muscle. Muscle strength may fluctuate from hour to hour and classically improves with rest. Ocular weakness is common and manifests with ptosis and diplopia. In 15% of patients, MG is confined to the eyes (ocular myasthenia), but in the remainder the disease is generalized with bulbar, limb and respiratory muscles affected to varying degrees. Although the course of MG is extremely variable, maximum progression occurs within the first 2 years. Approximately 10% of patients experience spontaneous remission.

Diagnosis of MG

Confirmatory tests for the diagnosis of MG include the edrophonium (Tensilon™) test, electrophysiological testing and detection of anti-AChR antibodies. Edrophonium is a short-acting anti-acetylcholinerase agent that prolongs the presence of ACh at the NMJ and therefore increases the duration and amplitude of the EPP. This results in a transient increase in muscle power in MG. Its diagnostic sensitivity for the diagnosis of MG is about 75%, but its specificity is limited. The mainstay of electrophysiological testing is repetitive nerve stimulation (at 2–5 Hz), which shows a progressive decrease in amplitude of the compound muscle action potential (CMAP), termed decrement or fade. Single-fibre EMG shows 'jitter' and blocking and has a greater sensitivity than conventional EMG if affected muscles are specifically sampled. Anti-AChR antibodies are found in approximately 85% of patients with generalized MG and, in addition, anti-striated muscle antibodies are found in the majority of patients with thymoma. Anti-MuSK antibodies should be measured in those without anti-AChR antibodies. A chest CT or MRI should also be performed to exclude the presence of a thymoma.

Treatment of MG

The first-line treatment of MG consists of oral anticholinesterase agents such as pyridostigmine, usually in a dose of 30–90 mg every 4–6 h. Higher doses can result in cholinergic symptoms and may worsen muscle weakness. Although patients with mild MG may be managed using these agents alone, most also require immunosuppression with corticosteroids, azathioprine, cyclosporin or mycophenolate, either alone or in combination. Exacerbations of MG require short-term immunomodulation with either PE, which temporarily reduces autoantibody levels, or IVIg, which appears to interfere with antibody binding. The indications for thymectomy remain unclear, although most authorities suggest that it should be considered in patients under the age of 60 with generalized seropositive MG and in those with thymoma, regardless of age.

Anaesthesia and MG

The anaesthetic management of a patient with MG requires careful pre-operative assessment and optimization in order to minimize post-operative complications. A consistently reduced FVC and poor bulbar function are strong indicators of the need for prolonged post-operative mechanical ventilation. Pre-operative physiotherapy and rationalization of MG treatment are necessary in all cases and, if indicated, pre-operative PE or IVIg should be offered. Associated autoimmune conditions (Table 26.4) may also influence the course and management of anaesthesia.

Pre-medication is normally avoided in those with decreased pulmonary reserve. Anticholinesterase therapy is traditionally withheld on the morning of surgery, as it interferes with the metabolism of both depolarizing and non-depolarizing neuromuscular blocking agents. Patients taking corticosteroids require hydrocortisone cover on induction of anaesthesia. Due to the decreased number of AChRs, patients with MG show a relative resistance to the action of suxamethonium, and adult patients often require twice the normal dose. In addition, a phase II block readily occurs. In contrast, there is undue sensitivity to non-depolarizing neuromuscular blocking agents, which have a faster onset and a more prolonged action than normal. Atracurium (at 40–60% of the normal dose) is the drug of choice because of its rapid, spontaneous metabolism. Tracheal intubation can usually be performed without the use of muscle relaxants, but. if they are used, neuromuscular function should be monitored. The neuromuscular blocking properties of the volatile anaesthetic agents are exaggerated in MG, and this is useful in providing adequate muscular relaxation without resorting to neuromuscular blocking agents.

Most patients can have their tracheas safely extubated at the end of the procedure, but those with severe MG may benefit from a period of post-operative ventilation. Anticholinesterase therapy is often restarted in the immediate post-operative period, although requirements may be decreased in the first 48 h.

Myasthenic crisis

Myasthenic crisis is defined as weakness resulting from MG that is severe enough to require tracheal intubation for ventilatory support or airway protection. It occurs in about 15% of patients during the course of their disease and usually within the first 2 years after diagnosis. It is more common in those with pronounced oropharyngeal symptoms. Mortality from myasthenic crisis has decreased considerably with modern intensive care and improved therapies for MG, and now remains steady at about 5%.

Although myasthenic crisis may be the presenting feature of previously undiagnosed MG, most cases occur in those with known disease. In one-third of patients no precipitating cause is found, and in the remainder deterioration is associated with sepsis (typically respiratory tract infections), initiation or changes in corticosteroid therapy, menstruation, pregnancy or surgery (especially post-thymectomy). Acute cholinergic weakness due to overtreatment with anticholinesterase agents is rarely seen in practice, but myasthenic crises may be precipitated or worsened by other medications known to affect the NMJ (Table 26.5).

Recognition of worsening respiratory and bulbar dysfunction in the myasthenic patient requires clinical acumen. Although objective measures of ventilatory reserve (e.g. FVC, sniff pressure, arterial blood gas analysis) may be helpful, clinical signs are more reliable. A breathless patient using their accessory muscles of respiration, unable to swallow their saliva, talking in short sentences and looking exhausted always requires tracheal intubation and ventilation. Non-invasive nasal positive-pressure ventilation has been used successfully in some patients to manage myasthenic crises without tracheal intubation. Patients in myasthenic crisis also require supportive treatment while the causes of the crisis are treated. Remission of myasthenic weakness is promoted by the use of high-dose corticosteroids, PE and/or IVIg.

Animal toxins

A number of animals, including snakes, ticks, fish and spiders, produce toxins that cause neuromuscular paralysis by interfering with NMJ function. Over 20 species of North American snakes produce neurotoxins that cause rapid neuromuscular failure. Black widow spider venom contains α-latrotoxin, which causes massive release of ACh at the pre-synaptic terminal and blocks its reuptake. Anti-venoms are available for a number of specific animal venoms.

Tick paralysis results from inoculation of a neurotoxin from a tick's salivary gland and typically presents 2–7 days following the bite. Respiratory failure may ensue. Treatment is largely supportive, and symptoms subside rapidly following removal of the embedded tick. Marine toxins are produced by dinoflagellates within the fish or, in the case of the puffer fish, by the animal itself. All affect depolarization by interfering with sodium-channel function. Treatment is supportive while awaiting recovery.

Organophosphate poisoning

Organophosphorus compounds are oxydiaphoretic acetylcholinesterase inhibitors and are commonly found in insecticides but also in some chemical weapons (e.g. sarin). They may be absorbed through the gastrointestinal tract, lungs or skin. They act as a substrate for acetylcholinesterase, and the intermediate complex formed is hydrolysed only slowly, resulting in inhibition of the enzyme for weeks. Recovery requires synthesis of new acetylcholinesterase.

Widespread effects include peripheral enzyme inhibition resulting in both muscarinic (bronchospasm, increased secretions, abdominal cramps, bradycardia) and nicotinic (muscle twitching and weakness, hypertension, tachycardia) effects. Proximal muscle weakness occurs 24–96h after the cholinergic crisis due to post-synaptic inhibition at the NMJ. Effects on the CNS include tremor, confusion, encephalopathy and convulsions. A delayed polyneuropathy may be seen 2–4 weeks after the poisoning. Respiratory failure results from peripheral weakness, CNS depression and increased tracheobronchial secretions.

Diagnosis is based on history, tolerance to atropine therapy, an acetylcholine assay and detection of organophosphorus and metabolites in blood and urine. Treatment is largely supportive, with care taken to avoid contamination of clinical staff. Large doses of atropine may be required to treat bradycardia. Pralidoxime administered within 24–36h of poisoning accelerates the rate of acetylcholinesterase production.

Primary muscle diseases

Although muscular weakness is often acquired as a consequence of critical illness and its treatment (see below), a number of primary muscle diseases may result in respiratory failure. These include the muscular dystrophies, congenital muscle disease, metabolic muscle disease and the periodic paralyses.

Muscular dystrophies

The muscular dystrophies are a large group of inherited diseases caused by genetic defects in muscle proteins. These include defects of sarcolemmal structural proteins (e.g. dystrophin), nuclear envelope proteins and muscle enzymes. Although respiratory failure may be a feature of a number of these conditions, the two most commonly encountered are DMD and myotonic dystrophy.

Duchenne muscular dystrophy

Duchenne muscular dystrophy is an X-linked recessive disease that has a frequency of 1 in 3500 live male births. It occurs because of a genetic defect in dystrophin, a protein that stabilizes the sarcolemma during muscle contraction. Death occurs from respiratory muscle failure that is often exacerbated by an associated scoliosis and dilated cardiomyopathy. With improved supportive care, including NIV, mean survival in DMD is now 25 years. Patients may present to the ITU with worsening respiratory function, often associated with respiratory infection. There are major ethical considerations in the decision to intubate and ventilate a patient with DMD who may never be able to be weaned from mechanical ventilation.

Patients with DMD are particularly vulnerable to the effects of general anaesthesia and sedation. Volatile anaesthetic agents and suxamethonium may result in a malignant hyperthermia-like reaction characterized by rhabdomyolysis, hyperkalaemia and cardiac arrest. There is also a greatly increased need for respiratory support following anaesthesia. If general anaesthesia is necessary, total intravenous techniques should be used, and patients with markedly reduced FVC should receive nasal intermittent positive-pressure ventilation following tracheal extubation. Gastrointestinal pathology may lead to acute gastric dilation resulting in further diaphragmatic dysfunction and an increased risk of aspiration of gastric contents.

Myotonic dystrophy (dystrophia myotonica)

Myotonic dystrophy is an autosomal dominant disease of muscle characterized by myotonia, i.e. persistent contraction of muscle following stimulation. It occurs because of a genetic abnormality of the voltage-gated chloride channels in skeletal muscle. Unlike other congenital myotonias, myotonic dystrophy is a multisystem disease (Table 26.6).

Anaesthesia for patients with myotonic dystrophy requires careful pre-operative assessment and perioperative management. Myotonic dystrophy is associated with extreme sensitivity to the respiratory depressant effects of pre-medication, induction agents and opioids. Suxamethonium may result in generalized myotonia severe enough to make laryngoscopy and ventilation impossible, as well as severe hyperkalaemia. Similarly, anticholinesterase agents, surgical manipulation and shivering may worsen myotonia. The duration of action of the non-depolarizing neuromuscular blocking agents may be prolonged.

Congenital myopathies

The congenital myopathies are a group of rare muscle disorders that are defined on the basis of distinctive morphological muscle features. Central core disease and nemaline myopathy have particular implications for the anaesthetist and intensivist.

Central core disease

Central core disease is an autosomal dominant disorder that may present as neonatal hypotonia or with a later onset. It occurs because of a mutation in the

Table 26.6 Systemic manifestations of myotonic dystrophy

System	Abnormalities
Respiratory	Respiratory muscle weakness with alveolar hypoventilation and poor cough
	Central and obstructive sleep apnoea
	Poor pharyngeal control and tendency to aspiration
Cardiac	Conduction defects, which may result in sudden death
	Cardiomyopathy
	Septal defects
	Valve disease
Gastrointestinal tract	Dysphagia
	Decreased gastric motility
Endocrine	Diabetes mellitus
	Hypothyroidism
Other	Hypersomnolence
	Cataracts

RYR1 gene, which encodes the skeletal muscle ryanodine receptor. Muscle weakness is usually mild and cardiorespiratory involvement rare. Central core disease is associated with an increased risk of malignant hyperthermia, with around 30% of central core disease patients having susceptibility to malignant hyperthermia.

Nemaline myopathy

Nemaline myopathy is an autosomal dominant or recessive myopathy. It may present following birth with severe muscle weakness, respiratory failure and cardiomyopathy or as a milder adult-onset form with the development of proximal weakness between the ages of 20 and 50 years. Respiratory muscle weakness is rare, but, when it does occur, patients often require respiratory support.

Metabolic muscle disease

Acid maltase disease

Acid maltase disease is an autosomal recessive glycogenosis characterized by excessive accumulation of glycogen in lysosomal-derived vacuoles. The severe infantile form (Pompe's disease) leads to death from cardiac failure in the first 2 years of life. The juvenile and adult forms are milder, but respiratory failure due to early diaphragmatic paralysis and scoliosis often requires nocturnal ventilatory support.

Mitochondrial muscle disease

Normal functioning of the mitochondrial respiratory chain is essential for generation of sufficient ATP to support cellular function. Defects in the chain lead to CNS and skeletal muscle dysfunction because of their high energy requirements. Although a large variety of clinical phenotypes exist, proximal myopathy in combination with CNS manifestations is common. These include mitochondrial encephalomyopathy with lactic acidosis and strokes (MELAS) and mitochondrial encephalomyopathy with ragged red fibres (MERRF).

Patients with mitochondrial disease may present to the ITU with respiratory or bulbar failure, metabolic encephalopathy, recurrent lactic acidosis or status epilepticus.

Periodic paralyses

The periodic paralyses are a group of autosomal dominant disorders of skeletal muscle characterized by generalized or focal weakness of variable duration. They are examples of muscle channelopathies and have been classified on the basis of changes in serum potassium levels during the attacks.

Hyperkalaemic periodic paralysis

Hyperkalaemic periodic paralysis causes recurrent attacks of muscle weakness starting in the first decade of life. It occurs because of a point mutation in muscle sodium channels. Attacks vary in severity from mild weakness to total paralysis, and may be precipitated by rest following exercise, cold, potassium ingestion or stress. Recovery usually occurs spontaneously within 2 h, but respiratory support may be required during this period. Acute attacks can be terminated by ingestion of carbohydrate or inhaled salbutamol. Prophylaxis against attacks includes the use of acetazolamide or a thiazide diuretic. Anaesthesia may result in prolonged paralysis, especially if suxamethonium is used. Total intravenous anaesthesia is favoured.

Hypokalaemic periodic paralysis

Hypokalaemic periodic paralysis occurs as a result of a point mutations in skeletal muscle calcium (or less commonly sodium) channels. Weakness may be severe and generalized and is often precipitated by strenuous exercise or a large carbohydrate meal on the preceding day. Other precipitants include infection, menstruation and stress. Attacks may be treated with oral potassium

Table 26.7 Neuromuscular manifestations of critical illness

Critical illness polyneuropathy (or acute motor neuropathy)
Critical illness muscle disease:
• Diffuse non-necrotizing cachectic myopathy
• Critical illness myopathy
• Acute necrotizing myopathy

preparations, and prophylaxis with carbonic anhydrase inhibitors may be effective.

Intensive care unit-acquired neuromuscular weakness

Neuromuscular weakness is common in patients recovering from critical illness. It usually manifests as difficulty with weaning from mechanical ventilation and results in extended periods in the ITU and hospital. Symptoms may persist for long periods following discharge from hospital. If a primary neuromuscular disorder has been excluded, weakness in an intensive care unit (ICU) patient is most likely to be related to one of the neuromuscular manifestations of critical illness (Table 26.7).

Critical illness polyneuropathy

Critical illness polyneuropathy (CIP) is an acute sensorimotor axonal neuropathy (or occasionally a pure motor neuropathy), which is increasingly recognized as a potent cause of failure to wean from mechanical ventilation. It is characterized by severe distal flaccid weakness, reduced or absent reflexes, and marked muscle wasting. Accurate estimates of the incidence of CIP are difficult because of different diagnostic criteria and selection bias in the reported series. However, it is likely to affect around 60% of patients with prolonged ICU admission, rising to 80% in those with a systemic inflammatory response syndrome (SIRS) or multiorgan failure.

Pathophysiology

The precise aetiology of CIP remains unclear, but a number of mechanisms, which may not be mutually exclusive, have been proposed. Although CIP has been described in patients with 'uncomplicated' respiratory failure, its association with SIRS in the majority of cases has led to the suggestion that pro-inflammatory cytokines, including tumour necrosis factor alpha (TNF-α) and interleukin-1, are implicated in its development. Cytokines increase expression of cell-adhesion molecules such as E-selectin, which in turn leads to leucocyte-mediated vascular tissue injury. Immunological factors may also play a role and anti-ganglioside antibodies have been identified in patients with CIP. Finally, cellular metabolic derangement resulting in energy failure in nerve tissue may contribute. Nerve biopsy and autopsy studies have confirmed motor and sensory axonal degeneration without evidence of primary inflammation or demyelination.

A number of other factors may be associated with the development of CIP. These include hypoalbuminaemia, hyperglycaemia and insulin deficiency, corticosteroids (which also to appear to have an important role in critical illness myopathy), non-depolarizing neuromuscular blocking agents, aminoglycosides and vasopressors. However, some of these associations may merely reflect the severity of the underlying critical illness.

Diagnosis

The diagnosis of CIP tends to be considered when the patient fails to wean from mechanical ventilation during the recovery phase of critical illness. Diagnostic clinical signs are difficult to elicit in the uncooperative patient, and confirmation relies on exclusion of other causes of neuromuscular weakness and characteristic neurophysiological findings. These confirm reduction in the amplitude of motor and sensory CMAP, with preservation of normal conduction velocities. Fibrillation potentials and positive sharp waves indicating axonal damage usually appear later. Abnormalities in the acute axonal form of CIP are confined to motor CMAPs.

Prognosis and treatment

Critical illness polyneuropathy is usually self-limiting and the overall prognosis is influenced by the severity of the underlying critical illness, which accounts for the majority of CIP-related mortality. Outcome is associated with the severity of sepsis, the extent and severity of the neuropathy, time spent on the ITU and the presence of hyperglycaemia, hyperosmolality and hypoalbuminaemia. Recovery is relatively rapid and complete when CIP is mild or moderate, but more severe polyneuropathy results in high mortality and limited recovery in survivors. Follow-up studies show that persisting weakness and residual, clinically relevant, motor and sensory deficits are common in survivors of protracted critical illness. These lead to chronic weakness, fatigue and difficulty with mobilization. In some patients, the weakness is still present up to 4 years after discharge from the ICU. Neurophysiological evidence of chronic partial denervation, consistent with previous CIP, is found in >90% of long-stay ICU patients >5 years after discharge.

Critical illness polyneuropathy results in the need for prolonged respiratory support. Apart from rapid and effective management of SIRS, no specific prophylaxis or treatment of CIP exists. High-dose IVIg has failed to show benefit, but excellent glycaemic control might minimize the risk of developing CIP. Patients may also benefit from strict potassium control, including early renal replacement therapy in those with elevated serum potassium secondary to renal failure. As axonal hypoxia appears to be an important aetiological factor for CIP, providing optimal oxygenation and perfusion must be important.

Critical illness muscle disease

Neurophysiological and biopsy studies suggest that critical illness-related myopathy occurs more frequently than previously recognized. Three main types have been identified: critical illness myopathy, diffuse non-necrotizing cachectic myopathy and acute necrotizing myopathy of intensive care.

Critical illness myopathy

Critical illness myopathy (CIM) is an acute primary myopathy causing weakness and paralysis in critically ill patients. It is also called myopathy with selective loss of thick filaments (myosin), acute quadriplegic myopathy, acute illness myopathy, acute myopathy of intensive care and rapidly evolving myopathy with myosin-deficient fibres. It is an under-recognized cause of failure to wean from mechanical ventilation and is more common than critical illness neuropathy with which it often coexists. The term critical illness polyneuromyopathy has been proposed to describe this association.

Pathophysiology

Epidemiological and animal data has established the association of CIM with SIRS and the use of corticosteroid therapy, both of which have been shown to interfere with muscle membrane excitability and sodium-channel function. Other associated factors include prolonged non-depolarizing neuromuscular blockade, nutritional deficiencies, hyperglycaemia, renal and hepatic dysfunction, and metabolic and electrolyte disturbances.

Diagnosis

In common with CIP, CIM usually manifests in difficulty in weaning from mechanical ventilation. Clinical features include predominantly proximal muscle weakness, facial and neck muscle weakness and reduced reflexes. Blood creatine kinase levels are raised in <50% of cases. Although neurophysiological studies may be helpful in cooperative patients, without cooperation they are neither sensitive nor specific. Definitive diagnosis requires muscle biopsy and identification of characteristic pathological changes. These include abnormal variation of muscle fibre size, fibre atrophy, angulated fibres, internalized nuclei, rimmed vacuoles, muscle fibre fatty degeneration and single fibre necrosis without inflammatory changes. There is also selective loss of thick (myosin) myofilaments and preservation of thin (actin) myofilaments and Z discs.

Prognosis

The outcome of CIM is better than CIP, and most patients make a full recovery unless paralysis has been severe and prolonged.

Non-necrotizing cachectic myopathy

Non-necrotizing cachectic myopathy presents with muscle wasting and associated proximal or generalized weakness. It is associated with prolonged ITU admission, sedation or paralysis causing muscle disuse and poor nutrition with protein catabolism. Creatine kinase levels and EMG are normal, and biopsy shows type 2 fibre atrophy and neurogenic atrophy.

Acute necrotizing myopathy of intensive care

This is a rare myopathy, which may be a form of rhabdomyolysis. It is associated with the use of neuromuscular blocking agents with or without corticosteroid therapy, but may also occur after infective or metabolic insults. Serum creatine kinase is usually markedly elevated and myoglobinuria is common. Muscle biopsy reveals patchy or widespread fibre necrosis with vasculitic infarction within the muscle. Recovery of muscle power is often poor.

Conclusion

Neuromuscular disorders are an important cause of respiratory failure or failure to wean from mechanical ventilation. They may have been present before admission to ITU or develop as a consequence of critical illness. A review of the medical history, careful neurological examination and neurophysiological studies usually allow an accurate diagnosis to be made. Although specific treatment is available for some disorders, supportive care is the mainstay of treatment for most.

Further reading

Anderson, K. E., Bloomer, J. R., Bonkovsky, H. L. *et al.* (2005). Recommendations for the diagnosis and treatment of the acute porphyrias. *Ann Intern Med* **142**, 439–50.

Baraka, A (1992). Anaesthesia and myasthenia gravis. *Can J Anaesth* **39**, 476–86.

Bolton, C. F. (2005). Neuromuscular manifestations of critical illness. *Muscle Nerve* **32**, 140–63.

Cook, T. M., Protheroe, R. T. and Handel, J. M. (2001). Tetanus: a review of the literature. *Br J Anaesth* **87**, 477–87.

Farrero, E., Prats, E., Povedano, M. *et al.* (2005). Survival in amyotrophic lateral sclerosis with home mechanical ventilation. *Chest* **127**, 2132–8.

Hirsch, N. P. (2007). Neuromuscular junction in health and disease. *Br J Anaesth* **99**, 132–8.

Howard, R. S., Radcliffe, J. and Hirsch, N. P. (2003). General medical care on the neuromedical intensive care unit. *J Neurol Neurosurg Psychiatry* **74** (Suppl. 3), iii 10–15.

Howard, R. S., Tan, S. V. and Z'Graggen, W. J. (2008). Weakness on the intensive care unit. *Prac Neurol* **8**, 280–95.

Hughes, R. A. and Cornblath, D. R. (2005). Guillain–Barré syndrome. *Lancet* **366**, 1653–6.

Hughes, R. A., Swan, A. V., Raphaël, J. C. *et al.* (2007). Immunotherapy for Guillain–Barré syndrome: a systematic review. *Brain* **130**, 2245–57.

Jani-Acsadi, A. and Lisak, R. P. (2007). Myasthenic crisis: guidelines for the prevention and treatment. *J Neurol Sci* **261**, 127–33.

Karalliedde, L. (1995). Animal toxins. *Br J Anaesth* **74**, 319–27.

Meriggioli, M. N. and Sanders, D. B. (2009). Autoimmune myasthenia gravis: emerging clinical and biological heterogeneity. *Lancet Neurol* **8**, 475–90.

Russell, S. H. and Hirsch, N. P. (1994). Anaesthesia and myotonia. *Br J Anaesth* **72**, 210–16.

Simonds, A. K. (2006). Recent advances in respiratory care for neuromuscular disease. *Chest* **130**, 1879–86.

Chapter 27

Seizures

Brian P. Lemkuil, Andrew W. Michell and David K. Menon

Introduction

Status epilepticus (SE) is a medical emergency that requires rapid and aggressive treatment. The definition of SE varies and has evolved over time. For epidemiological purposes, SE has traditionally been defined as a single clinical seizure lasting >30 min, or repeated seizures over a period of >30 min without intervening recovery of consciousness. Other definitions (primarily of convulsive SE) have utilized a temporal threshold of 20 min, 10 min, and more recently, by Lowenstein (1999), as 'at least 5 minutes of persistent generalized, convulsive seizure activity or two or more discrete seizures between which there is incomplete recovery of consciousness'. This more recent definition provides a practical working definition for clinicians in light of improved understanding of the pathophysiological mechanism and treatment of SE.

Status epilepticus is a dynamic and complex electroclinical syndrome, which is not easily defined by a single clinical, electrophysiological or mechanistic definition. There are multiple classifications of SE, each with unique clinical and electrical characteristics that evolve with continued seizure activity. This chapter will focus primarily on non-convulsive SE (NCSE) as seen in the comatose patient in the intensive care unit (ICU) as well as generalized convulsive SE (GCSE), including its typical clinical evolution into subtle convulsive SE.

Classification and terminology

There are multiple ways to classify SE based on the electrophysiological characteristics and clinical manifestations of seizure activity. Understanding the classification and terminology is important for discussing SE, especially prognosis, as well as for evaluating clinical studies. In some clinical situations, classification may dictate how aggressively seizure activity is treated. It is critical, however, when discussing seizure classification, that one does not fall into thinking of SE as a disease in and of itself but rather as a manifestation of an underlying pathological process.

Focal/partial seizures

Focal seizures involve a discrete region of the cortex at onset and are subcategorized as 'complex' (impaired consciousness) or 'simple' (preserved consciousness). As part of a persistent epilepsy disorder, focal seizures may have a relatively benign symptomatology lacking clinical urgency; however, focal seizures may become secondarily generalized, thus requiring more immediate attention. In the ICU or in the context of an acute cerebral insult, persistent focal complex seizure activity should be treated promptly; however, the aggressiveness of therapy should be dictated by patient factors on a case-by-case basis.

Generalized seizures

Generalized seizures are those with electrical and clinical evidence of global cortical involvement. They are subcategorized as either primary or secondarily generalized, the latter being of focal onset initially. The term 'generalized seizure' is often equated with 'grand mal' or tonic–clonic seizure activity but also includes 'petit mal' or absence seizures. Absence seizures may be brief or quite prolonged (absence SE), typically with relatively benign clinical symptoms. Generalized convulsive SE, on the other hand, is clinically obvious at onset and represents a true medical emergency, frequently requiring ICU admission.

Convulsive and non-convulsive status epilepticus

Classification of SE into either *convulsive* or *non-convulsive* is common and clinically convenient. Convulsive status epilepticus (CSE) typically refers to generalized epileptiform activity, loss of consciousness and recurrent or continuous tonic and/or clonic motor activity. Focal motor seizures may also be convulsive, but they are clinically distinct and carry a very different prognosis and treatment to GCSE, which is universally considered a medical emergency requiring rapid and aggressive medical treatment. Some of these patients will be refractory to medical therapy necessitating transfer to the ICU for infusion of coma-inducing anaesthetics and ventilatory support.

Non-convulsive status epilepticus lacks a formal definition but refers to ongoing focal or generalized electrical seizure activity, often with an altered level of consciousness, with either a complete absence of motor symptoms or very subtle activity that may easily be overlooked. It therefore incorporates the end stage of CSE when there is 'burn out' of the motor component. It is important to form the distinction between the comatose patient with generalized NCSE and the functional outpatient with NCSE. Absence SE is a type of generalized NCSE that occurs in a specific group of epileptic patients with a susceptibility to these types of attacks. They often remain ambulatory, although slightly confused or fidgety. Their symptoms may be overlooked by inexperienced clinicians, and hence the diagnosis may be delayed. However, treatment typically occurs in the outpatient setting with a characteristically excellent clinical response. The clinical setting, aetiology, treatment and prognosis of these patients are distinct from the comatose ICU patient with generalized NCSE and therefore will not be discussed further.

In this chapter, NCSE will refer more broadly to persistent electrical seizure activity, either focal or generalized, without overt motor activity in the comatose ICU patient.

Aetiology-based classification of status epilepticus

Status epilepticus may be categorized into one of three aetiologies:

1. Symptomatic SE: associated with an identifiable cause.

2. Cryptogenic SE: unidentified but probably due to an unidentified cause.

3. Idiopathic SE: most probably due to genetic predisposition.

In the ICU, SE is assumed to be symptomatic until proven otherwise. The aetiology is the most significant prognostic indicator of SE and thus this classification is of particular clinical importance.

Epidemiology

In industrialized countries, the average incidence of SE is reported at 20 per 100,000 person years within Caucasian populations. This number probably represents a gross underestimation of the true incidence for multiple reasons. These estimates come primarily from population-based studies with typical inclusion criteria of 'clinically evident' seizure activity, resulting in significant underestimation of NCSE, particularly within critically ill patients. The recent trend towards a more inclusive definition of SE may result in a higher reported incidence from future studies. The demographics of the population studied will also have a profound effect on the reported incidence owing to a bimodal distribution, with peaks during the first 12 months of life and again in adults over the age of 60 years.

Non-convulsive seizures (NCSZ) and NCSE are frequently detected following various acute brain insults. The reported occurrence of NCSE is quite variable (3–18%) depending on patient selection, screening tools/protocol, diagnostic criteria utilized and the predominant sedation practices. Although discussed further under Monitoring, the increased incidence of NCSE often reported from the USA may result from greater use of continuous EEG (cEEG) screening, opioid-based sedation regimes and more liberal inclusion criteria. In contrast, the lower rates reported in Europe probably reflect increased use of propofol, more stringent diagnostic criteria and less frequent use of cEEG. The reported incidences of NCSZ and NCSE associated with specific cerebral insults using cEEG screening in the ICU are as follows:

- Neurointensive care unit mixed cohort: 18–34% NCSZ, 10% NCSE.
- Traumatic brain injury: 18–33% NCSZ, 8% NCSE.
- Central nervous system (CNS) infections: 33% NCSZ, 17% NCSE.
- Intracerebral haemorrhage: 18–28% NCSZ, 7% NCSE.

- Subarachnoid haemorrhage: 8–18% NCSZ, 13% NCSE.
- Acute ischaemic stroke: 9% NCSZ, 7% NCSE.

Aetiology

Aetiology is recognized as one of the most critical determinants of SE outcome. The most frequently encountered aetiologies depend on the age of the patient population evaluated. For example, the most common aetiology in childhood is febrile seizure or infection with fever, which represents about 50% of all cases. Other significant paediatric aetiologies include remote symptomatic causes (identifiable structural lesion temporally unrelated to SE onset) followed by low anti-epileptic drug (AED) levels in known epileptics. The most common aetiologies in adulthood are markedly distinct from those found in childhood. The major contributors are: (i) acute symptomatic (50–70%), most notably due to low AED levels and cerebral vascular accidents (CVAs); (ii) remote symptomatic, most notably due to previous CVAs; and (iii) metabolic causes. As indicated by population-based data, SE in the neurointensive care unit probably represents symptomatic aetiology (acute or chronic) warranting an immediate and thorough evaluation, as the underlying aetiology may be readily treatable. Thus, in addition to pharmacological treatment, a timely and thorough evaluation of aetiologic triggers is critically important. Figure 27.1 represents common population-based aetiologies of adult SE and their approximate frequency with a more inclusive list of aetiological triggers found in Table 27.1.

Mechanism of status epilepticus

The brain has both neurotransmitters and neuropeptides, which are either excitatory or inhibitory in nature. Typically, a balance between the two prevents excessive and prolonged excitatory neuronal activity, which is known to be harmful to the CNS. During the rare occasions when seizure activity is not prevented, animal and human brains alike employ robust mechanisms aimed at quickly terminating this activity, resulting in the spontaneous termination of the vast majority (90%) of seizures within 1–2 min. Continued seizure activity beyond this interval probably implies failure of these adaptive mechanisms, thus allowing seizures to continue or recur in rapid succession. As such, seizure activity persisting beyond a couple of minutes should

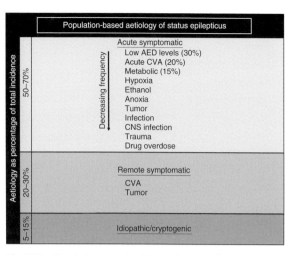

Fig. 27.1. Population-based aetiology of status epilepticus. AED, anti-epileptic drug; CNS, central nervous system; CVA, cerebrovascular accident.

be considered to have a high likelihood of becoming self-sustaining. This represents part of the rationale for defining GCSE as continued seizure activity for >5 min.

A 5 min diagnostic threshold for GCSE is also intended to prevent delay of treatment. Continued SE results in the well-recognized (both clinically and in experimental models) phenomenon of pharmacoresistance whereby AEDs are less frequently effective and require much higher doses as seizure activity continues. Experimental evidence suggests that various biochemical mechanisms probably contribute to this phenomenon. Within minutes of sustained seizure activity, there is a change in neuronal receptor trafficking, primarily γ-aminobutyric acid (GABA) (inhibitory) and glutamate (excitatory), resulting in reduced inhibitory and increased excitatory receptors at the synaptic membrane. Downregulation of $GABA_A$ receptors, the site of benzodiazepine action, explains the clinical experience of early benzodiazepine resistance. As seizure activity continues and neuronal molecular reserves are depleted, changes in gene expression are induced. The result is decreased inhibitory neuropeptides and increased excitatory peptides. This further shifts the balance towards neuronal excitation and failure of inhibitory mechanisms. These pathophysiological mechanisms, along with others not mentioned, help explain the clinical experience of time-dependent pharmacoresistance to nearly all AEDs and provide the rationale for early aggressive treatment of GCSE.

Table 27.1 Under-recognized causes of status epilepticus

Cause	Examples
Systemic infection	Sepsis
Central nervous system infection	Neurosyphilis, prion disease, neurobartonellosis, rabies, viral encephalitis, tuberculosis, non-viral infectious encephalitis, abscess, meningitis
Withdrawal	Alcohol, benzodiazepines, barbiturates, baclofen, opioids
Structural	Occult cortical dysplasias
Vascular	Arteriovenous malformation, central venous thrombosis, antiphospholipid syndrome, primary angiitis of the central nervous system, eclampsia
Metabolic	Hepatic encephalopathy, uraemia, hyponatraemia, pyridoxine deficiency, hypophosphataemia, hypocalcaemia, hypomagnesaemia, hypoglycaemia, non-ketotic hyperglycaemia
Iatrogenic	Tricyclic antidepressants, metronidazole, isoniazid, flumazenil, penicillin G, clozapine, imipenem, lithium, theophyllines, insulin, local anaesthetics, meperidine, cyclosporin, phenytoin, tramadol, cephalosporins, quinolones, radiographic contrast
Illicit drugs	Cocaine, amphetamines, heroin, phencyclidine (PCP), ecstasy
Toxins	Domoic acid and marine toxins, other causes of toxic leukoencephalopathy
Genetic	Mitochondrial disorders, porphyria
Oncological	Paraneoplastic limbic encephalitis
Perfusion	Hypertensive encephalopathy, post-carotid endarterectomy hyperperfusion syndrome, hypotension, eclampsia, posterior reversible encephalopathy syndrome
Autoimmune	Antiphospholipid syndrome, acute disseminated encephalomyelitis, neurosarcoidosis, autoimmune encephalitis/limbic encephalitis, Hashimoto's encephalopathy, multiple sclerosis, systemic lupus erythematosus

Diagnosis and pathogenesis

Generalized convulsive status epilepticus

Both the clinical and EEG features of GCSE evolve over time. The characteristic clinical features of GCSE initially include bilaterally symmetric tonic and/or clonic movements that are continuous but wane over time in an unconscious patient. As seizure activity continues, convulsive movements may become more subtle, lateralized or focal, confined to intermittent facial/ocular twitches, or even undetectable. Likewise, the EEG also changes over time but not always in a well-defined sequence. Initial generalized epileptiform discharges may eventually give way to periods of relative flattening and periodic epileptiform discharges.

Non-convulsive status epilepticus in the intensive care unit

The diagnosis of NCSE in a comatose patient in the ICU can be difficult. The first step is recognition that SE can and does exist with considerable frequency without an obvious motor component. Clinical suspicion is confirmed with EEG; however, the interpretation of EEG findings can be especially difficult in this setting. Particularly troublesome is distinguishing true epileptiform activity from similar patterns reflective of injured brain or medication effects (see Monitoring below).

The clinical significance of NCSE has been debated along with the necessity and urgency of treatment. It seems clear that NCSE may be associated with metabolic deterioration in the injured brain, but it remains unclear whether this is a causal mechanism or simply a marker of severe tissue damage. The impact of NCSE on outcome remains unclear, as does the justification for recommending aggressive treatment of all detected cases.

Systemic manifestations of generalized convulsive status epilepticus

The initial systemic effects of GCSE are primarily those of increased sympathetic discharge. Serum levels of epinephrine and norepinephrine are substantially elevated, resulting in increased systemic and pulmonary artery pressures, heart rate and blood glucose, as well as increased incidence of arrhythmias. Status epilepticus is also associated with a rapid and profound metabolic acidosis that is significantly attenuated by pharmacologically induced muscle paralysis. The degree of acidosis is independent of neuronal damage and typically recovers quickly following seizure cessation. Hyperkalaemia typically is not clinically significant, although it may be profoundly elevated along with creatinine kinase in cases of prolonged convulsive activity and muscle necrosis. Such cases may also experience profound hyperthermia, which is an independent predictor of morbidity and CNS damage. Cerebral blood flow is initially appropriately increased in proportion to cerebral oxygen consumption but begins to drop along with systemic blood pressure in the latter stages (>30 min). Other systemic effects associated with SE are leukocytosis and cerebrospinal fluid (CSF) pleocytosis. Although infection must be excluded as the cause of seizures, systemic leukocytosis and mild CSF pleocytosis themselves are not necessarily indicative of an infectious aetiology. As SE continues beyond 30 min, many of the haemodynamic effects revert back to baseline levels or below. The latter stages may also be associated with respiratory insufficiency due to exhaustion, resulting in respiratory acidosis.

Prognosis

Mortality

The short-term mortality rate following SE has been reported to be near 20% by two US studies and significantly lower (<10%) by two European studies that excluded SE resulting from anoxic brain injury. As these studies demonstrate, mortality and outcome are highly dependent on the underlying aetiology. It is not surprising that those with a more malignant aetiology, such as anoxic brain injury, do far worse than those with an aetiology of alcohol withdrawal or low AED levels. Other key factors associated with a higher mortality include age (>65 years), sex (male > female) and duration of SE (>60 min). Although the mortality of SE is difficult to isolate from the underlying aetiology, there is some evidence to suggest that SE itself carries a 3% mortality rate.

Long-term mortality is also dependent on the underlying aetiology, patient age and duration of SE, as well as the type of SE. The highest long-term mortality is associated with anoxia and hypoxia, followed by other symptomatic (acute or remote) aetiologies. Rather benign acute aetiologies such as alcohol withdrawal or low AED levels are associated with lower long-term mortality. Interestingly, patients without a symptomatic cause (idiopathic or cryptogenic), who survive the first 30 days, have 10-year mortality rates equivalent to the general population.

Central nervous system dysfunction and injury

The association between seizure activity and hippocampal neuronal damage was first reported in the 1800s by Bouchet and Cazauvielh, and later by Sommer.

Since then, whether hippocampal neuronal damage is the cause or the result of seizure activity has been a contentious topic. Multiple experimental animal models have demonstrated that SE induced by a variety of mechanisms does result in damage to specifically vulnerable hippocampal neurons independent of secondary systemic complications. These models suggest that a threshold of 45–60 min of continuous electrographic seizure activity is necessary to induce such damage, which incidentally corresponds to the duration of GCSE associated with worse clinical outcomes.

Quantifying any neuronal dysfunction due to SE alone is extremely difficult, as neuronal injury probably results from a complex interaction between seizure type, duration and the underlying aetiology. In GCSE, there is a duration-dependent risk of neuronal injury (independent of systemic complications) while injury associated with NCSE is less certain. In the outpatient setting, diagnosis and treatment of NCSE (absence SE) is often delayed, yet is associated with an excellent prognosis, although most patients are not formally assessed for mild cognitive or memory impairment. The same is often true of focal complex SE without an acute brain lesion. However, as discussed above, ambulatory patients with NCSE are drastically different from comatose patients in the ICU. In the ICU setting, NCSE may act synergistically with other factors to induce further neuronal injury and cognitive impairment. Therefore, an argument could be made that all sustained seizure activity, even if non-convulsive, should be treated urgently in the neurointensive care unit. However, clinical proof for aggressive treatment of NCSE is lacking. Therefore, the aggressiveness of treatment should be determined on a case-by-case basis with consideration for the patient's age, comorbidities and underlying aetiology, and the potential side effects of therapy.

Epilepsy

Long-term epilepsy is a well-established sequela of SE. Status epilepticus increases the risk of developing long-term epilepsy fourfold compared with a single-seizure episode, while refractory SE – seizure activity not responsive to first- and second-line treatment – may result in even greater risk of developing long-term epilepsy.

Management of convulsive status epilepticus

Convulsive status epilepticus is a medical emergency that warrants aggressive and early treatment using a rationally based protocol that takes into account the

clinical stage of SE. As previously discussed, repetitive seizures without intermittent recovery or a single seizure persisting beyond 5 min probably represents a failure of adaptive mechanisms intended to prevent sustained, excessive neuronal activity. Status epilepticus results in a time-dependent pharmacoresistance to nearly all AEDs. Although the mechanism behind this is incompletely understood, it appears in part to be due to receptor trafficking and altered expression of inhibitory and excitatory neuropeptides. In addition, prolonged GCSE (>60 min) appears to be associated with an increased likelihood of systemic complications, CNS injury and mortality. Thus, limiting the duration of SE and preventing the development of refractory SE may improve clinical outcomes and is the basis for early, aggressive treatment with combination AED therapy at high therapeutic doses. Figure 27.2 summarizes the pharmacological treatment of GCSE.

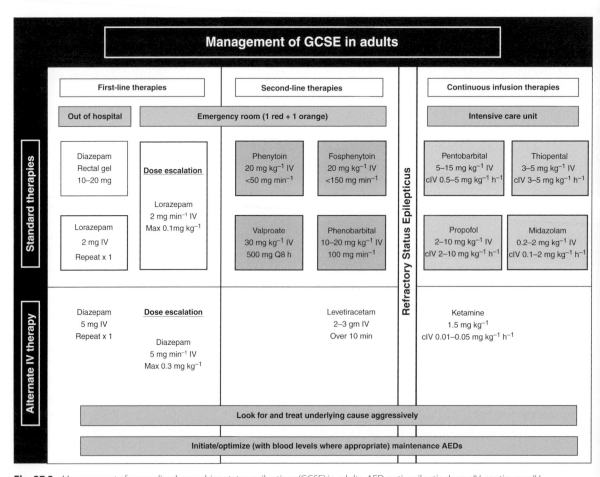

Fig. 27.2. Management of generalized convulsive status epilepticus (GCSE) in adults. AED, anti-epileptic drug; cIV, continuous IV.

Out-of-hospital management

Randomized controlled trials have documented the benefit of initiating therapy outside the hospital with benzodiazepines. Lorazepam (LZP) and diazepam (DZP) are the most studied and utilized members of their class. Multiple studies suggest nearly equivalent efficacy with a trend favouring LZP. The more sustained clinical effect of LZP has made it the preferred agent for initial management of SE. Benzodiazepine therapy reduces the duration and recurrence of SE with a concomitant reduction in systemic complications and short-term mortality compared with placebo. Out-of-hospital therapy may be initiated by family members of patients with a history of epilepsy or SE, who are educated to administer diazepam (10–20 mg rectally) for seizure activity persisting longer than usual. Alternatively, emergency medical personnel may administer LZP (2 mg, repeat ×1) or DZP (5 mg, repeat ×1) intravenously and draw blood for basic toxicology screening, electrolytes analysis and serum glucose evaluation. If there is concern for hypoglycaemia, a glucose bolus along with 100 mg of thiamine should be given without delay. This out-of-hospital treatment is provided simultaneously with basic life-support measures, oxygen supplementation and basic monitoring.

Emergency department management

Emergency department treatment of SE should be a continuation and escalation of therapy initiated out of the hospital. Additional benzodiazepine should be administered by repeated boluses (LZP 2 mg min^{-1}, DZP 5 mg min^{-1}) until seizure cessation or until a cumulative LZP dose equivalent to 0.1 mg kg^{-1} or DZP dose of 0.3 mg kg^{-1} (max. 15–20 mg). As benzodiazepine resistance may develop relatively early, administration of a second agent concomitantly with or immediately following benzodiazepine therapy is recommended. Depending on patient age, comorbidities and drug availability, phenytoin or fosphenytoin administration at a dose of 15–20 mg kg^{-1} IV is often the next therapy. Valproate (30 mg kg^{-1}) is an alternative second-line agent, which, like phenytoin, may be administered rapidly with minimal sedative effects. Phenobarbital, an additional second-line agent, is being utilized less frequently owing to both sedative and respiratory depressant effects, which may necessitate mechanical ventilation. Persistence of seizure activity following rapid administration of maximal therapeutic doses of both a first- and second-line agent is defined as refractory SE (RSE). In cases of RSE, an additional second-tier agent may be considered, although the reported utility of this has been marginal. In any case, plans for initiating continuous-infusion therapy and transfer to the ICU for monitoring and ventilatory support should occur without delay.

Intensive care unit management of refractory status epilepticus

Refractory status epilepticus may occur in up to 35–45% of patients with SE and will typically require transfer to the ICU for more aggressive treatment. Refractory status epilepticus carries a higher mortality rate, which may reflect a combination of a more severe underlying aetiology, side effects associated with therapy and the effects of prolonged seizure activity itself. The ICU treatment of RSE typically involves administration of coma-inducing anaesthetic agents guided by continuous or intermittent EEG monitoring. There are limited prospective clinical trials by which to guide treatment of RSE, and thus recommendations largely reflect case reports and expert opinion.

Traditional therapies used in the ICU setting have been anaesthetics such as midazolam, propofol and barbiturates (pentobarbital/thiopental). These anaesthetics are typically initiated with a loading dose aimed at seizure cessation and maintained by titration of a continuous infusion for a period of 12–48 h before gradual weaning. The end point for continuous anaesthetic infusion has traditionally been EEG burst suppression, although this end point has not been shown to improve outcomes. The level of burst suppression suggested for this purpose has been 10–15 s periods of EEG flattening between electrical bursts. An alternative target, especially if anaesthetic dose requirements are high or associated with limiting side effects (hypotension, risk of propofol infusion syndrome), is suppression of electrographic seizure activity. Regardless of the end point used, it is helpful if clinicians are familiar with the ictal EEG characteristics of the monitored patient.

Following 12–48 h of seizure-free therapy and adequate serum levels of maintenance AEDs (phenytoin level 10–20 µg ml^{-1}, phenobarbital level 35–50 µg ml^{-1}, valproate level 80–120 µg ml^{-1}), the infusion therapy should be slowly titrated off. Typically, this is done by reducing the dose by 25–50% every 8–12 h, followed by a period of observation and EEG evaluation. Seizure

Table 27.2 Comparison of the pharmacokinetic properties of benzodiazepines

Property	Diazepam	Lorazepam	Midazolam
Octanol/H_2O partition coefficient	309	73	34 (pH 3) 475 (pH 7.4)
Distribution half-life (min)	1–49	9–10	2–4
Elimination half-life (h)	20–40	12 (adults)	1–5
Metabolism	CYP2C19/CYP3A4	Glucuronidated	CYP3AS (high first-pass metabolism)
Active metabolites	Desmethyldiazepam	None	α-Hydroxymidazolam
Protein binding (%)	99	91	94–97

breakthrough during treatment or therapy withdrawal requires transition to an alternative anaesthetic infusion and perhaps initiation of additional maintenance AED therapy.

It is important to recognize that the therapeutic ranges for these heavily protein-bound drugs pertain to patients with normal levels of plasma proteins, and it is important to correct plasma levels for low albumin levels in critically ill patients. For phenytoin, it is conventional to use the Sheiner–Tozer equation, which assumes that the normal unbound fraction of phenytoin is 0.1:

Corrected phenytoin concentration = measured total concentration

$$0.9 \ (albumin_{patient}/albumin_{normal}) + 0.1$$

Intensive care unit evaluation

Intensive care management of patients with SE may fall into one of four groups: (i) those responsive to aggressive emergency department treatment with the resultant need for weaning from mechanical ventilation; (ii) those responsive to treatment who require ICU admission primarily to manage the underlying aetiology; (iii) those unresponsive who require coma-inducing infusions of anaesthetic agents to control their seizure activity; and (iv) those who develop SE subsequent to hospital admission.

Each of these groups of patients will have different critical care needs but all require a careful and thorough evaluation to diagnose and possibly treat an underlying aetiology. As indicated in Fig. 27.1, the vast majority of SE (85–95%) has a symptomatic aetiology with an underlying pathological process, which should be identified and treated simultaneously with anticonvulsant therapy. Evaluation will typically involve basic

blood (and sometimes CSF) screening, and either a CT scan or a well-planned MRI evaluation, depending on the clinical situation. In other cases, the aetiology may not be detected easily, and screening for less common aetiologies may be required (Table 27.1).

Antiseizure medications

Benzodiazepines (first-line therapy)

Benzodiazepines, the gold standard first-line therapy for SE, are a family of $GABA_A$ receptor agonists that augment neuronal inhibition. In the out-of-hospital setting, benzodiazepine administration is relatively easy and safe with excellent efficacy; however, higher doses may be associated with hypnosis and respiratory suppression. Multiple routes of administration are possible including intravenous, buccal, rectal, intramuscular and intranasal. The primary routes used for treatment of adult SE are rectal and intravenous. The key pharmacokinetic characteristics of commonly used benzodiazepines are presented in Table 27.2.

Lorazepam

Lorazepam is considered by many to be the preferred benzodiazepine for initial treatment of SE due to a more prolonged therapeutic effect (12 h) compared with DZP and midazolam (MZP). Its clinical efficacy approaches 65% when given alone (0.1 mg kg^{-1} IV) in the early stages of SE. The relatively limited lipid solubility of LZP compared with other family members dictates intravenous administration. It is metabolized hepatically with an intermediate elimination half-life. As a first-line agent, it may be administered by emergency medical personnel as a 2 mg IV bolus (repeated once). In the emergency department, the dose should be escalated to a maximum of 0.1 mg kg^{-1}.

Diazepam

Diazepam, the other commonly used benzodiazepine for initial treatment of SE, may be administered rectally in the out-of-hospital setting with therapeutic concentrations achieved within 10–15 min. It is highly protein bound and has a long half-life of 20–40 h. Intravenous DZP may be equivalent to LZP with regard to initial seizure termination but has a greater rate of seizure recurrence. Its non-sustained clinical effect is a result of redistribution to other body compartments owing to its increased lipid solubility compared with LZP. In the out-of-hospital setting, it may be administered rectally (10–20 mg) or intravenously (5–10 mg). In the emergency department, therapy is escalated with repeated intravenous boluses every minute until seizure cessation or a maximum dose of 0.3 mg kg^{-1}.

Midazolam

In the setting of SE, MDZ is most commonly used as a continuous infusion for seizure suppression in the ICU. For this use, it is favoured over other family members due to its relatively short elimination half-life (1–5 h). However, as a first-line agent, its utility is limited due to its rapid redistribution and short elimination half-life. In children, it may be administered intranasally or buccally as initial therapy before intravenous access is obtained. Midazolam, as commercially prepared (buffered to pH of 3), has an ionized open-ring structure with low lipid solubility and is quickly converted to its lipid-soluble form at physiological pH. Rectal absorption, therefore, is inconsistent due to the low water content of the rectal cavity and subsequent slow conversion to its lipid-soluble form.

Second-tier therapy

Second-tier therapy should be administered concomitant with or immediately following benzodiazepine therapy. There are limited data to support the use of one particular agent over the other. Ideal second-tier agents would have a rapid clinical onset with high efficacy, be safely and quickly administered intravenously, and have very little sedative or ventilatory suppressant effects. The limited data that is available suggests that, regardless of the chosen therapy, it may be reasonable to expect less than a 10% response rate if benzodiazepine treatment has already failed.

Phenytoin

Phenytoin is a commonly used second-tier drug chosen more out of familiarity and cost efficacy than clinical evidence of superiority. Like other AEDs, it is subject to time-dependent pharmacoresistance and thus is prepared and administered immediately following benzodiazepine therapy. Phenytoin works by mechanisms independent of benzodiazepines with a relatively rapid clinical effect. It is hepatically metabolized, a potent inducer of the P450 system, and is highly bound to albumin. The active, unbound fraction varies with the albumin level, which is used to calculate its true therapeutic concentration (goal: 10–20 µg ml^{-1}; which equates to ~35–70 µmol l^{-1}). Favourable characteristics attributed to phenytoin include haemodynamic stability, limited sedative effects and relative ease of oral conversion. Unfortunately, phenytoin is plagued by complicated pharmacokinetics that may be altered in critically ill patients. Phenytoin toxicity may occur from low albumin levels or displacement from albumin by other drugs. Rapid administration of phenytoin carries systemic risks of hypotension and cardiac conduction abnormalities, particularly in older patients with pre-existing conduction defects. Drug administration requires continuous ECG and blood pressure monitoring. Phenytoin administration may also cause local toxicity in the form of phlebitis or purple glove syndrome due to its high alkaline pH (pH 12). The loading dose for SE is 15–20 mg kg^{-1} and should not exceed a rate of 50 mg min^{-1}.

Fosphenytoin

Fosphenytoin, a water-soluble pro-drug of phenytoin, is rapidly and completely converted to phenytoin (conversion half-life = 10–15 min) and has been approved for the treatment of SE since 1996. It has a rapid clinical effect and is hepatically metabolized with an elimination half-life of >12 h. Its neutral pH addresses the local irritant concerns associated with intravenous phenytoin and allows a faster rate of administration (150 mg min^{-1}). However, fosphenytoin still has the potential to cause hypotension or heart block if administered rapidly in sensitive patients and thus requires appropriate cardiovascular monitoring. Cost and availability are the main drawbacks, but it is quickly replacing phenytoin in many institutions.

Valproate

Sodium valproate (VPA) is a hepatically metabolized second-line agent (half-life 12–24 h) with rapid therapeutic efficacy and broad-spectrum anti-seizure activity. Clinical evidence suggests that it may be as effective as, and possibly more effective than, phenytoin. Some recent consensus guidelines have included VPA as an alternative second-tier agent. However, it is often still reserved for patients with phenytoin allergy or cardiac conduction defects. Valproate is highly protein bound (80%) and may induce phenytoin toxicity if the two are co-administered. Rapid VPA administration is considered safe with minimal hypnotic or haemodynamic effects. Unlike phenytoin, it is a P450 inhibitor, which may affect metabolism of concurrently prescribed medications. The typical loading dose is 30 mg kg^{-1} over 10 min with a targeted therapeutic serum concentration of 80–120 µg ml^{-1}. Some guidelines advocate an additional 10–20 mg kg^{-1} if the initial dose is ineffective. Although adverse systemic effects related to acute VPA administration are rare, adverse effects include hyperammonia-induced pancreatitis and encephalitis, hepatic dysfunction and thrombocytopaenia. As such, VPA is contraindicated in patients with pre-existing liver dysfunction, hyperammonaemia or urea cycle disorders, and thrombocytopaenia.

Phenobarbital

Phenobarbital is one of the oldest AEDs with good efficacy and a rapid therapeutic effect but may cause prolonged sedation and respiratory insufficiency (especially at higher doses). In light of these concerns and the presence of newer non-sedating intravenous agents, clinical use of phenobarbital has declined. Like many of the other agents, it is metabolized hepatically and carries a risk of local venous irritation due to polypropylene solvent. Phenobarbital has low protein binding but a prolonged half-life (100 h), resulting in a sustained clinical effect. The typical loading dose in SE is 10–20 mg kg^{-1} at a maximum rate of 100 mg min^{-1} with a targeted serum level of 35–50 µg ml^{-1}.

Levetiracetam

Levetiracetam is a newer intravenous AED with great potential, although it is not yet licensed for the treatment of SE. Its unique mechanism is believed to be mediated by binding the synaptic vesicular protein SV2A, thus providing a potentially useful addition to the treatment of RSE. Rapid administration of levetiracetam appears safe, with minimal hypnotic or haemodynamic risk to the patient. Unlike other AEDs, it has insignificant hepatic metabolism and few drug interactions. Intravenous levetiracetam may also easily be transitioned to the oral formulation for maintenance therapy. Clinical experience of treating SE with levetiracetam is accumulating, confirming both its safety and

efficacy in doses of 2–3 g infused over 15 min. Unlike the other second-tier agents mentioned so far, its clinical effect may be somewhat delayed. Randomized control trials will probably be needed to confirm its efficacy as a second-tier agent before it is included universally in protocols and consensus guidelines. At the moment, its utility is typically reserved for patients with liver dysfunction or an allergic reaction to other second-tier agents or as a maintenance AED initiated during continuous-infusion therapy.

Continuous-infusion therapy for refractory status epilepticus

Third-line therapy typically involves transfer to the ICU for continuous infusion of coma-inducing anaesthetic agents and mechanical ventilation. Limited clinical research suggests an unlikely response (2–3%) to further trials of second-tier agents if both first- and second-line therapies have been ineffective. In light of this, plans should be made to proceed without delay to continuous-infusion therapy. However, in cases where intubation would best be avoided, it may be reasonable to try an additional second-tier agent if readily available.

A few of the most commonly used anaesthetic drugs are highlighted below. All agents are typically loaded until EEG evidence of seizure activity has ceased (clinical manifestations are unreliable due to electromechanical dissociation). A continuous infusion of the anaesthetic is then titrated to either cessation of seizure activity (if this occurs prior to burst suppression) or burst suppression. Typically, infusions are continued for a 12–48 h seizure-free interval before initiating a slow drug withdrawal. Transition to an alternative anaesthetic infusion is recommended for breakthrough or recurrence of seizure activity.

Pentobarbital

Pentobarbital is a common barbiturate used for coma induction in the ICU and treatment of RSE. Although its primary mechanism involves agonism of GABA$_A$ receptors, it may also involve ion-channel (calcium) modulation. The extended half-life (24 h) of pentobarbital, which may be significantly lengthened by prolonged infusions or high doses, may deter clinical use. Although considered a potent seizure inhibitor, it is often associated with significant vasodilation, cardiac depression and hypotension. Pentobarbital is typically loaded by repeated slow boluses of 5 mg kg^{-1} until cessation of neuronal seizure activity (maximum 15 mg kg^{-1}) followed by a maintenance infusion of 0.5–5 mg kg^{-1} h^{-1}. During drug withdrawal, a periodic or paroxysmal EEG pattern may appear. The significance of this pattern is unknown and may resolve spontaneously without further treatment. Definite recurrence of the characteristic ictal EEG pattern should prompt initiation of an alternative drug infusion.

Thiopental

Thiopental is another barbiturate that is favoured by some owing to its shorter elimination half-life (3–9 h) compared with pentobarbital. Its high lipid solubility results in a rapid clinical effect but allows significant redistribution to fatty tissues, which may prolong elimination. It is metabolized by the liver primarily to inactive metabolites that are renally excreted. The typical loading dose required for seizure cessation is 3–5 mg kg^{-1}, which is followed by a continuous infusion of 3–5 mg kg^{-1} h^{-1}. With regard to haemodynamic effects, thiopental is quite similar to pentobarbital.

Propofol

Propofol is an anaesthetic with hypnotic and amnestic properties thought to work through GABA$_A$ agonism but may involve modulation of calcium and sodium channels as well. Propofol is a highly lipid-soluble agent with rapid clinical onset and redistribution, necessitating continuous-infusion administration. Like barbiturates, it also causes significant hypotension from cardiac depression and vasodilation. Propofol may be favoured over other agents due to its short elimination half-life. Even patients on prolonged infusions (>3 days) typically wake up within 4 h of infusion termination. Loading is achieved with repeated boluses of 1–2 mg kg^{-1} (maximum 10 mg kg^{-1}) until cessation of neuronal seizure activity, followed by a maintenance infusion of 2–10 mg kg^{-1} h^{-1}. A maximal infusion of 5 mg kg^{-1} h^{-1} should be used for those maintained on propofol for multiple days to minimize the risk of propofol infusion syndrome. Although first described in children, critically ill adults receiving high-dose propofol for multiple days are also at risk. The typical manifestations of the syndrome include metabolic acidosis, renal failure, development of a Brugada-type ECG pattern, arrhythmias, cardiac failure and rhabdomyolysis. The incidence of the syndrome is related to both peak and cumulative propofol dose, and patients with SE who are on prolonged propofol infusions need to be monitored carefully for its occurrence.

Midazolam

Midazolam, a benzodiazepine with a short half-life, is often chosen for coma induction in this setting because it may have fewer cardiovascular depressant effects than propofol or barbiturates. The anaesthetic effects of midazolam are mediated by GABA$_A$ agonism and primarily result in anterograde amnesia and anxiolysis at typical clinical doses. Although reported to be 1–5 h, the half-life of midazolam may be prolonged with sustained infusions due to accumulation in other compartments. It is metabolized hepatically with renal excretion of an equipotent metabolite. Tachyphylaxis to midazolam may occur within 48 h in patients receiving high-dose infusions. Midazolam is typically initiated with repeated intravenous boluses of 0.2 mg kg^{-1} (max. 2 mg kg^{-1}) followed by an infusion of 0.1–2 mg kg^{-1} h^{-1}.

Ketamine

Ketamine is a dissociative anaesthetic that works primarily through N-methyl-D-aspartate (NMDA) receptor antagonism by binding the phencyclidine (PCP) site inside the channel. Unlike other therapies, ketamine is more efficacious in prolonged SE than in the early stages. As discussed above, this is probably due to SE-induced receptor trafficking resulting in upregulation of NMDA receptors at neuronal synaptic membranes. Haemodynamically, ketamine is unique among most anaesthetics causing increased cardiac output, heart rate and systemic blood pressure. Ketamine may increase cerebral blood flow and should be used with caution if increased intracranial pressure is a concern. Experimental models of SE suggest that ketamine may also possess neuroprotective effects. Case reports of ketamine treatment of SE in humans are relatively few with moderate outcomes. Therapy is initiated as a 1.5–2 mg kg^{-1} loading dose, followed by a 10–50 μg kg^{-1} min^{-1} infusion.

Novel therapies in highly refractory status epilepticus

Failure of continuous-infusion therapy despite adequate serum levels of maintenance AED therapy and a thorough evaluation and treatment of any underlying aetiology carries a poor prognosis. Trials of various novel therapies may be considered. These therapies are based on anecdotal reports and small case series and are not supported by systematic clinical trials.

One emerging cause of highly refractory SE that often responds quite well to alternative therapeutic modalities is acute autoimmune encephalitis. Specific antibodies to various antigens (e.g. NMDA receptors, voltage-gated potassium channels) have been linked with the development of limbic encephalitis, which is occasionally associated with highly refractory seizures or SE. Limbic encephalitis may be of paraneoplastic or non-paraneoplastic origin. The former obviously necessitates treatment of the associated neoplasm and tends to respond poorly to immunotherapy, whereas non-paraneoplastic limbic encephalitis frequently responds to immunotherapy (e.g. plasmapharesis, methylprednisolone, intravenous immunoglobulin).

Surgery

Although surgical treatment of persistent focal epilepsy is well established, it is an uncommon treatment for RSE. Although only a small minority of patients with RSE are likely to have a focal lesion suitable for resection, awareness of this option for specific individuals may be life-saving. The 'ideal candidates' are 'patients with convulsive or non-convulsive RSE who have a high degree of concordance between semiology, imaging, functional imaging with PET [positron emission tomography] or SPECT [single-photon emission CT], and EEG (scalp as well as invasive) indicating a single epileptogenic zone, with focal cortical dysplasia as the underlying pathology', as defined by Lhatoo and Alexopoulos (2007). With very few reports of surgically treated RSE, the optimal timing of surgery is unknown. A 2-week trial of medical management prior to surgery has been advocated previously. However, waiting for an arbitrary 2-week period must be balanced against the risk of CNS injury associated with ongoing seizure activity, as well as the risks inherent in prolonged sedation and mechanical ventilation in the ICU. Certainly, in 'ideal candidates', consideration may be given to more expedient surgical intervention following failure of continuous-infusion therapy, regardless of the duration of therapy.

Miscellaneous therapies

Isoflurane and desflurane are inhalational anaesthetics that work primarily through $GABA_A$ potentiation. Small case series utilizing these agents report good control of seizure activity with mortality rates between 43 and 67%.

Etomidate is another haemodynamically stable anaesthetic with an imprecisely defined mechanism of action that has been used for continuous-infusion therapy in SE. However, prolonged infusions cause reversible cortisol suppression, necessitating replacement therapy.

Lidocaine infusions have also been used in SE with some reported success. Lidocaine is a class Ib anti-arrhythmic known to modulate sodium channels. Reported doses in SE have been as high as $5\,mg\,kg^{-1}$ followed by a continuous infusion of $6\,mg\,kg^{-1}\,h^{-1}$. Such high doses of lidocaine have the potential to cause CNS toxicity themselves by inducing seizure activity.

Verapamil is a calcium-channel blocker and inhibitor of P-glycoprotein, a drug efflux transporter found at the blood–brain barrier. Status epilepticus is known to increase expression of this transporter, which may be responsible for reducing the brain concentration of certain AEDs and thus contributing to pharmacoresistance. Although anecdotal reports of its use for RSE are rare, it is a relatively safe drug for which there is substantial clinical experience.

Similarly, magnesium is another drug for which there is substantial clinical experience (treatment of eclampsia), little of which involves treatment of SE. It, too, is a relatively benign treatment option, assuming toxic serum levels are avoided.

Other treatments with anecdotal reports include a ketogenic diet, electroconvulsive therapy, steroids, plasma exchange, intravenous immunoglobulin, vagal nerve stimulation and therapeutic hypothermia.

Monitoring

Overt seizures: EEG in patients with refractory status epilepticus

A small number of patients are admitted to the ICU for treatment of clinically overt RSE. The incidence of subclinical seizures and NCSE is high in this population following initial treatment due to electromechanical dissociation often characteristic of prolonged CSE. In this setting, EEG not only helps guide infusion therapy but also helps detect ongoing subclinical seizure activity (Fig. 27.3b) that would otherwise pass unnoticed. However, the classical spike and wave abnormalities commonly seen in patients with epilepsy (Fig. 27.3a) are infrequently seen in the ICU setting as a result of the infusion therapy itself or EEG evolution that naturally occurs with sustained seizure activity. The initial goal of infusion therapy is usually EEG burst suppression (Fig. 27.4), as this results

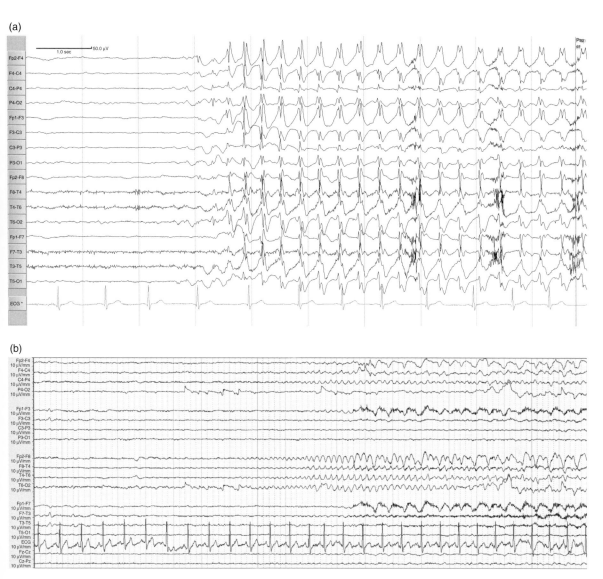

(a)

(b)

Fig. 27.3. (a) Classic high-amplitude spike–wave activity in childhood absence epilepsy. Such clear epileptiform discharges are not commonly seen during seizures in critically ill patients. (b) Evolution of a right temporal seizure. Note that the EEG during a seizure may not contain spikes or sharp waves.

in fewer breakthrough seizures than a goal of seizure suppression alone while minimizing the risks associated with deeper levels of anaesthesia that accompany complete EEG suppression.

Subclinical seizures: incidence in the intensive care unit

Many studies have been published on seizure occurrence in the ICU. Unfortunately, the studies are extremely heterogeneous making them nearly

impossible to compare, while larger studies often contain mixed patient populations.

The sources of heterogeneity in these studies are manifold. Firstly, the underlying disease process affects the likelihood of seizures, with a high incidence following intracerebral infection, cortical pathology or neurosurgical intervention. Secondly, patient age appears to be a significant factor – perhaps unsurprising given that the incidence of epilepsy peaks in both the young and the old. Thirdly, the predominant sedation regimens (propofol vs. opioid) employed by different ICUs

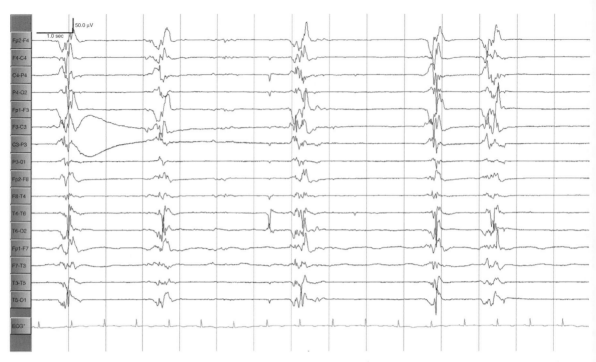

Fig. 27.4. EEG burst suppression. The burst suppression ratio (BSR) is the proportion of time during which the EEG is isoelectric (less than +5 µV). It is common to aim for a BSR of 50–90% during treatment of refractory status epilepticus.

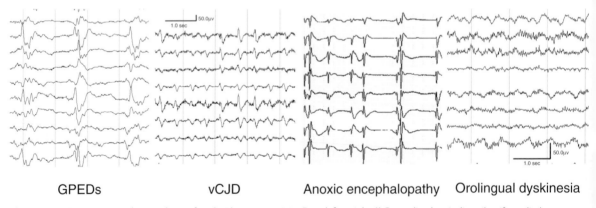

| GPEDs | vCJD | Anoxic encephalopathy | Orolingual dyskinesia |

Fig. 27.5. EEG appearances that may be confused with seizure activity. From left to right: (i) Generalized periodic epileptiform discharges (GPEDs). These may be lateralized and are then referred to as periodic lateralized epileptiform discharges. (ii) Triphasic/periodic discharges in a patient with variant Creutzfeldt–Jakob disease (vCJD). (iii) Cortical discharges in anoxic encephalopathy. These reflect anoxic neuronal injury, rather than ongoing epilepsy-movement artefacts due to orolingual dyskinesia (iv) in a patient with anti-NMDA (N-methyl-D-aspartate) receptor antibody-mediated disease. While the condition can cause seizures, these appearances are due to a non-seizure movement disorder.

may contribute to the frequency of seizure detection. Finally, the screening protocol used, including diagnostic criteria, will significantly affect the rate of seizure activity reported.

The EEG diagnostic criteria utilized, as well as the reliability of interpretation, is particularly problematic and is central to studying the incidence of nonconvulsive seizure and NCSE. In some instances, the distinction between periodic epileptiform discharges, triphasic waveforms and established NCSE can be difficult, especially in sedated patients. Other EEG patterns that may be misinterpreted include stimulus-induced rhythmic activity seen in a proportion of patients in the ICU and the EEG seen after anoxic brain injury (Fig. 27.5). Suggested EEG criteria for NCSE have been published, but in general these have not been widely used, and the EEG criteria for determining a non-convulsive seizure or SE is not overtly stated in many papers. Rather concerning is a recent study suggesting that, even using published criteria, the inter-observer reliability of EEG interpretation of NCSE is relatively poor, albeit in an artificial setting in which only sections of the EEG were shown to participants. In some settings, a benzodiazepine trial may help determine whether a patient is truly in NCSE, but this may not be helpful in heavily sedated ICU patients where an appreciable clinical/EEG response is unlikely.

When to request an EEG and how long to monitor

In a cohort of comatose patients in whom cEEG detected a seizure, 50% of cases had a first seizure detected within 1 h, 80% within 24 h and 87% within 48 h of the initial recording. In this group, the EEG was requested because of suspected NCSE or for titration of continuous-infusion therapy. These findings raise a number of important questions, such as when and how long to monitor, and whether to treat subclinical seizures aggressively.

Many centres do not have cEEG routinely available, and thus it is important to consider when to request a 'routine' EEG to maximize yield when resources are limited. In the ICU, NCSE should be suspected in patients with subtle ocular movement abnormalities (nystagmus, hippus and sustained eye deviation in any direction), particularly in those with risk factors for seizures including a previous stroke, intracerebral tumour, neurosurgery, dementia and meningitis.

Where cEEG is available, the raw data can be inspected visually, but this is time-consuming. Alternatively, this data can be manipulated into a user-friendly bedside cerebral function display, reducing analysis time but at the cost of potentially missing important data or misinterpreting artefacts. There are pros and cons to each approach, but, even if subclinical seizures are detected, it is not yet clear how aggressively they should be treated. On the one hand, it would seem desirable to suppress seizures given the wealth of basic scientific evidence that they are detrimental to neurons. On the other hand, aggressive treatment will prolong ICU admission and potentially increase respiratory and other complications. There is a need for prospective trials in highly selected patient groups with tightly controlled criteria for diagnosing and treating non-convulsive seizures. One of the many problems to be overcome in designing such a trial is that increasingly

severe cerebral injury is more likely to be associated with seizures and also with poor outcome, and so, because of injury severity, the incidence of seizures will tend to be greatest in patients with poorer outcome.

Further reading

Abend, N. S. and Dlugos, D. J. (2008). Treatment of refractory status epilepticus: literature review and a proposed protocol. *Pediatric Neurol* **38**, 377–90.

Abend, N. S., Dlugos, D. J., Hahn, C. D., Hirsch, L. J. and Herman, S. T. (2010). Use of EEG monitoring and management of non-convulsive seizures in critically ill patients: a survey of neurologists. *Neurocrit Care* **12**, 382–9.

Abou Khaled, K. J. and Hirsch, L. J. (2008). Updates in the management of seizures and status epilepticus in critically ill patients. *Neurol Clin* **26**, 385–408, viii.

Alldredge, B. K., Gelb, A. M., Isaacs, S. M. *et al.* (2001). A comparison of lorazepam, diazepam, and placebo for the treatment of out-of-hospital status epilepticus. *N Engl J Med* **345**, 631–7.

Amantini, A., Fossi, S., Grippo, A. *et al.* (2009). Continuous EEG-SEP monitoring in severe brain injury. *Neurophysiol Clin* **39**, 85–93.

Chin, R. F. M., Neville, B. G. R. and Scott, R. C. (2004). A systematic review of the epidemiology of status epilepticus. *Eur J Neurol* **11**, 800–10.

Chin, R. F. M., Neville, B. G. R., Peckham, C. *et al.* (2006). Incidence, cause, and short-term outcome of convulsive status epilepticus in childhood: prospective population-based study. *Lancet* **368**, 222–9.

Claassen, J. (2009). How I treat patients with EEG patterns on the ictal-interictal continuum in the neuro ICU. *Neurocrit Care* **11**, 437–44.

Claassen, J., Hirsch, L. J., Emerson, R. G. *et al.* (2001). Continuous EEG monitoring and midazolam infusion for refractory nonconvulsive status epilepticus. *Neurology* **57**, 1036–42.

Claassen, J., Mayer, S. A., Kowalski, R. G., Emerson, R. G. and Hirsch, L. J. (2004). Detection of electrographic seizures with continuous EEG monitoring in critically ill patients. *Neurology* **62**, 1743–8.

Coeytaux, A., Jallon, P., Galobardes, B. and Morabia, A. (2000). Incidence of status epilepticus in French-speaking Switzerland: (EPISTAR). *Neurology* **55**, 693–7.

Costello, D. J. and Cole, A. J. (2007). Treatment of acute seizures and status epilepticus. *J Intensive Care Med* **22**, 319–47.

DeLorenzo, R. J., Hauser, W. A., Towne, A. R. *et al.* (1996). A prospective, population-based epidemiologic study of status epilepticus in Richmond, Virginia. *Neurology* **46**, 1029–35.

DeLorenzo, R. J., Waterhouse, E. J., Towne, A. R. *et al.* (1998). Persistent nonconvulsive status epilepticus after the control of convulsive status epilepticus. *Epilepsia* **39**, 833–40.

Friedman, D., Claassen, J. and Hirsch, L. J. (2009). Continuous electroencephalogram monitoring in the intensive care unit. *Anesth Analg* **109**, 506–23.

Fujikawa, D. G. (1996). The temporal evolution of neuronal damage from pilocarpine-induced status epilepticus. *Brain Res* **725**, 11–22.

Fujikawa, D. G. (2005). Prolonged seizures and cellular injury: understanding the connection. *Epilepsy Behav* **7** (Suppl. 3), S3–11.

Gilmore, E., Choi, H. A., Hirsch, L. J. and Claassen, J. (2010). Seizures and CNS hemorrhage: spontaneous intracerebral and aneurysmal subarachnoid hemorrhage. *Neurologist* **16**, 165–75.

Hesdorffer, D. C., Logroscino, G., Cascino, G., Annegers, J. F. and Hauser, W. A. (1998). Incidence of status epilepticus in Rochester, Minnesota, 1965–1984. *Neurology* **50**, 735–41.

Hirsch, L. J. (2008). Levitating levetiracetam's status for status epilepticus. *Epilepsy Curr* **8**, 125–6.

Hirsch, L. J., Claassen, J., Mayer, S. A. and Emerson, R. G. (2004). Stimulus-induced rhythmic, periodic, or ictal discharges (SIRPIDs): a common EEG phenomenon in the critically ill. *Epilepsia* **45**, 109–23.

Holtkamp, M., Othman, J., Buchheim, K. and Meierkord, H. (2005). Predictors and prognosis of refractory status epilepticus treated in a neurological intensive care unit. *J Neurol Neurosurg Psychiatry* **76**, 534–9.

Iyer, V. N., Hoel, R. and Rabinstein, A. A. (2009). Propofol infusion syndrome in patients with refractory status epilepticus: an 11-year clinical experience. *Crit Care Med* **37**, 3024–30.

Jordan, K. G. and Hirsch, L. J. (2006). In nonconvulsive status epilepticus (NCSE), treat to burst-suppression: pro and con. *Epilepsia* **47** (Suppl. 1), 41–5.

Kaplan, P. W. (2005). The clinical features, diagnosis, and prognosis of nonconvulsive status epilepticus. *Neurologist* **11**, 348–61.

Kaplan, P. W. (2007). EEG criteria for nonconvulsive status epilepticus. *Epilepsia* **48** (Suppl. 8), 39–41.

Knake, S., Rosenow, F., Vescovi, M. *et al.* (2001). Incidence of status epilepticus in adults in Germany: a prospective, population-based study. *Epilepsia* **42**, 714–8.

Knake, S., Hamer, H. M. and Rosenow, F. (2009). Status epilepticus: a critical review. *Epilepsy Behav* **15**, 10–4.

Kurtz, P., Hanafy, K. A. and Claassen, J. (2009). Continuous EEG monitoring: is it ready for prime time? *Curr Opin Crit Care* **15**, 99–109.

Lhatoo, S. D. and Alexopoulos, A. V. (2007). The surgical treatment of status epilepticus. *Epilepsia* **48** (Suppl. 8), 61–5.

Logroscino, G., Hesdorffer, D. C., Cascino, G. D. *et al.* (2002). Long-term mortality after a first episode of status epilepticus. *Neurology* **58**, 537–41.

Lothman, E. (1990). The biochemical basis and pathophysiology of status epilepticus. *Neurology* **40** (Suppl. 2), 13–23.

Lowenstein, D. H. (1999). Status epilepticus: an overview of the clinical problem. *Epilepsia* **40** (Suppl, 1), S3–8; discussion S21.

Lowenstein, D. H. and Cloyd, J. (2007). Out-of-hospital treatment of status epilepticus and prolonged seizures. *Epilepsia* **48** (Suppl. 8), 96–8.

McDaneld, L. M., Fields, J. D., Bourdette, D. N. and Bhardwaj, A. (2010). Immunomodulatory therapies in neurologic critical care. *Neurocrit Care* **12**, 132–43.

Meierkord, H. and Holtkamp, M. (2007). Non-convulsive status epilepticus in adults: clinical forms and treatment. *Lancet Neurol* **6**, 329–39.

Pandian, J. D., Cascino, G. D., So EL, Manno, E. and Fulgham, J. R. (2004). Digital video-electroencephalographic monitoring in the neurological–neurosurgical intensive care unit: clinical features and outcome. *Arch Neurol* **61**, 1090–4.

Robakis, T. K. and Hirsch, L. J. (2006). Literature review, case report, and expert discussion of prolonged refractory status epilepticus. *Neurocrit Care* **4**, 35–46.

Ronner, H. E., Ponten, S. C., Stam, C. J. and Uitdehaag, B. M. (2009). Inter-observer variability of the EEG diagnosis of seizures in comatose patients. *Seizure* **18**, 257–63.

Rosenow, F., Hamer, H. M. and Knake, S. (2007). The epidemiology of convulsive and nonconvulsive status epilepticus. *Epilepsia* **48** (Suppl. 8), 82–4.

Rossetti, A. O. (2009). Novel anaesthetics and other treatment strategies for refractory status epilepticus. *Epilepsia* **50** (Suppl. 12), 51–3.

Rossetti, A. O., Logroscino, G. and Bromfield, E. B. (2005). Refractory status epilepticus: effect of treatment aggressiveness on prognosis. *Arch Neurol* **62**, 1698–702.

Shneker, B. F. and Fountain, N. B. (2003). Assessment of acute morbidity and mortality in nonconvulsive status epilepticus. *Neurology* **61**, 1066–73.

Shorvon, S. (2007). What is nonconvulsive status epilepticus, and what are its subtypes? *Epilepsia* **48** (Suppl. 8), 35–8.

Simon, R. P. (1985). Physiologic consequences of status epilepticus. *Epilepsia* **26** (Suppl. 1), S58–66.

Theodore, W. H., Porter, R. J., Albert, P. *et al.* (1994). The secondarily generalized tonic–clonic seizure: a videotape analysis. *Neurology* **44**, 1403–7.

Towne, A. R., Pellock, J. M., Ko D and DeLorenzo, R. J. (1994). Determinants of mortality in status epilepticus. *Epilepsia* **35**, 27–34.

Treiman, D. M., Walton, N. Y. and Kendrick, C. (1990). A progressive sequence of electroencephalographic changes during generalized convulsive status epilepticus. *Epilepsy Res* **5**, 49–60.

Treiman, D. M., Meyers, P. D., Walton, N. Y. *et al.* (1998). A comparison of four treatments for generalized convulsive status epilepticus. Veterans Affairs Status Epilepticus Cooperative Study Group. *N Engl J Med* **339**, 792–8.

Vespa, P. M., Miller, C., McArthur, D. *et al.* (2007). Nonconvulsive electrographic seizures after traumatic brain injury result in a delayed, prolonged increase in intracranial pressure and metabolic crisis. *Crit Care Med* **35**, 2830–6.

Wasterlain, C. G. and Chen, J. W. Y. (2008). Mechanistic and pharmacologic aspects of status epilepticus and its treatment with new antiepileptic drugs. *Epilepsia* **49** (Suppl. 9), 63–73.

Young, G. B., Jordan, K. G. and Doig, G. S. (1996). An assessment of nonconvulsive seizures in the intensive care unit using continuous EEG monitoring: an investigation of variables associated with mortality. *Neurology* **47**, 83–9.

Chapter
28

Central nervous system infections and inflammation

Amanda Cox

Central nervous system infections

Infection within the CNS can result in meningitis, encephalitis or the formation of abscesses and empyemas. Infection is often due to spread from a systemic source, but can occur in isolation.

Meningitis

Meningitis is the term used to describe inflammation of the meninges, irrespective of the cause. If bacterial meningitis is suspected, treatment with high-dose broad-spectrum antibiotics should be initiated without delay. Delay in initiating antimicrobial therapy is associated with poor outcome. Bacterial meningitis, particularly meningococcal disease, can kill within 12 h of symptom onset if left untreated.

Clinical presentation

Classically, patients experience fever, headache, photophobia, vomiting and neck stiffness. Seizures are a feature in up to 40% of cases. Infection or inflammation can spread beyond the meninges to cause cerebral dysfunction, drowsiness, delirium and coma. The emergence of focal neurological signs at any point should initiate a hunt for focal pathology. Commonly, complications such as cortical vein or sinus thrombosis, subdural empyemas, abscess formation or the development of hydrocephalus are responsible.

Diagnosis

A detailed history taken from the patient or informant will identify clues as to the aetiology of the infection, such as an unusual travel history, animal encounters and insect bites, intravenous drug use, chronic alcohol misuse, immunosuppression or head and neck trauma. Symptoms of systemic illnesses may lead to the source of infection, or identify a systemic illness associated with aseptic meningitis. A history of neuroleptic use should raise the possibility of neuroleptic malignant syndrome as a non-infective cause of fever, neck stiffness and coma.

Blood cultures, a platelet count and assessment of coagulation should be performed as soon as possible in all patients. In adults, if there is no haemostatic defect, and a CT scan of the head is normal, then a lumbar puncture to confirm the presence and identity of the pathogen is the mainstay of diagnosis. Lumbar puncture is rarely performed in children. The cerebrospinal fluid (CSF) constituents are often helpful in directing empirical treatment prior to confirmation of the pathogen (see Table 28.1). Lumbar puncture is contraindicated in the setting of raised intracranial pressure (ICP), coagulopathy or thrombocytopaenia (particular care needed with meningococcal disease) or severe shock. In the vast majority of cases, but always in the setting of reduced consciousness and focal neurological signs, imaging (usually with CT) should be performed prior to lumbar puncture.

Peripheral blood cultures, skin rash aspirates and posterior pharyngeal swabs can confirm meningococcal disease. Viral studies and investigations to identify systemic infections (e.g. an echocardiogram in bacterial endocarditis) may also be helpful.

Aetiology

Bacterial meningitis

Bacterial meningitis carries a mortality rate of 20%. If suspected, treatment should be initiated without delay. The infective organisms responsible vary according to patient age and immune status (see Table 28.2).

Three important and common pathogens are *Neisseria meningitidis* (meningococcus), *Streptococcus pneumoniae* (serotypes 6, 9, 14, 18 and 23) and,

Core Topics in Neuroanaesthesia and Neurointensive Care, eds. Basil F. Matta, David K. Menon and Martin Smith. Published by Cambridge University Press. © Cambridge University Press 2011.

Table 28.1 Guide to central nervous system infection based on cerebrospinal fluid (CSF) constituent

Cause	CSF pressure	Cells	Protein	Glucose
Acute bacterial	Often ↑	↑ – mainly PMNs (100–5000). NB: *Listeria* can have normal CSF, or a monocytosis (most classical), or lymphocytosis	↑	↓ (<1/3 of serum; <1/4 carries a poor prognosis)
Acute viral	N/↑	↑ – mainly lymphocytes (5–500). NB: in children, enterovirus can cause ↑ PMNs	N/↑	N except in mumps, HSV and CMV
Fungal	↑	↑ (mainly lymphocytes, 30–100)	↑	↓
Acute syphilis	↑	↑ (mainly lymphocytes, 100–800)	↑	N
Tuberculosis	↑	↑ mainly lymphocytes (PMNs early stage) 5–100	↑	↓
Carcinomatosis	N/↑	N/↑ (0 to several hundred mononuclear/ malignant cells)	↑	↓
Neurosarcoidosis	N/↓	N/↑ (<100 lymphocytes)	Slightly ↑	↓ in 50% of cases

CMV, cytomegalovirus; HSV, herpes simplex virus; N, normal; PMN, polymorphonuclear cells.

Table 28.2 Probable pathogen causing meningitis based on age/risk factors of patient

Age/risk factor	Pathogen
<3 months	*Escherichia coli* (Gram-negative bacillus), Group B *Streptococcus*, *Listeria*
3 months–18 years	*Haemophilus influenzae*, *Neisseria meningitidis*, *Streptococcus pneumoniae*
18–50 years	*Neisseria meningitidis*, *Streptococcus pneumoniae*, *Staphylococcus aureus*, (*Listeria*)
>50 years	*Streptococcus pneumoniae*, *Listeria*, Gram-negative bacilli
Immunocompromised	Gram-negative bacilli, *Listeria*
Neurosurgical procedure/head trauma	*Staphylococcus aureus*, Gram-negative bacilli, *Streptococcus pneumoniae*
Diabetes mellitus	*Streptococcus pneumoniae*. *Staphylococcus aureus*, Gram-negative bacilli
Chronic alcoholic	*Streptococcus pneumoniae*
Neutropaenia	*Pseudomonas* spp.

particularly in those <5 years, *Haemophilus influenzae*. A child or adult who appears well can die within hours from meningococcal meningitis. It commonly emerges in the setting of septicaemia and is most common in the under-12s with a prodrome of a throat infection. Later, a petechial or purpuric rash may develop. Its course is frequently complicated by shock and disseminated intravascular coagulation (DIC). *Haemophilus influenzae* generally infects younger children aged <5 years. Its onset is generally slower and it has a tendency to cause subdural collections of pus. It can be associated with the syndrome of inappropriate anti-diuretic hormone (SIADH). Pneumococcal meningitis is often a complication of pulmonary infections but can also occur de novo or following skull fractures and sinus/middle-ear infections. Thick basal exudates often form, which can precipitate complications such as sinus thrombosis, cerebral oedema, SIADH and deafness.

Viral meningitis

Viral meningitis is generally a benign and self-limiting condition that requires no treatment other than symptomatic. The CSF is sterile, with a lymphocytosis, although the pathogenic organism can sometimes be identified by polymerase chain reaction (PCR).

Fungal meningitis

Fungal infections of the CNS are most common in the setting of immunosuppression (human immunodeficiency virus (HIV) infection, chemotherapy/

Table 28.3 Suggested empirical treatment of suspected bacterial meningitis based on patient age and risk factors

Demographic/risk factor	Recommended antibiotics
Pre-hospital/emergency department	Parenteral penicillin or ceftriaxone
Neonates	Ampicillin and a third-generation cephalosporin
Children and adults	Third-generation cephalosporin
Adults >50 years	Ampicillin and a third-generation cephalosporin
Area with high cephalosporin resistance rates	Add vancomycin or rifampicin
Neutropaenia	Meropenem and an aminoglycoside (to cover *Pseudomonas* spp.)
Immunosuppression (lymphopaenic/lymphocyte dysfunction)	Ampicillin (for *Listeria* cover)
Allergy to β-lactam antibiotics	Vancomycin or chloramphenical (with co-trimoxazole if *Listeria* suspected)

malignancy, post-neurosurgery) and tend to present with a more chronic form of the disease over several weeks. They are often complicated by abscess formation and vascular invasion causing stroke and, therefore, focal neurological signs. Common pathogens include *Candida* spp., *Cryptococcus neoformans* and *Aspergillus* spp.

Tuberculous meningitis

Chronic alcoholics, the immunosuppressed and travellers from endemic areas are at risk of tuberculous meningitis. Symptoms tend to be subacute in evolution but can mimic fulminant bacterial meningitis. Infection often localizes to the basal meninges resulting in cranial nerve palsies and spasticity. Microabscess formation can cause further focal neurological signs. The CSF should be interrogated specifically for mycobacteria – a Ziehl–Neelsen stain allows direct visualization of the organism, but often culture or PCR are required to secure the diagnosis. Treatment should be guided by local sensitivities, and accompanied by high-dose steroids for the first 4 weeks.

Other infections

Particularly with the increase in foreign travel, of which a careful history should be taken, the possibility of non-endemic infections should be considered. Rickettsial meningitis, for example, can be contracted worldwide via tick and mite bites, and the symptoms may only emerge when the traveller returns home. Rickettsial infections include Rocky Mountain spotted fever (seen in the Americas), typhus and Q fever (ubiquitous). All these infections present with high fever, skin rash and headache along with meningoencephalitis.

If suspected, the treatment of choice is tetracycline or doxycycline. *Listeria* meningitis may be associated with late development of a rhombencephalitis, which involves the brainstem.

Non-infectious causes of meningitis

An inflammatory reaction in the subarachnoid space can be caused by mechanisms other than infection. Autoimmune diseases such as Behçet's disease and sarcoidosis can cause aseptic meningitis. Neoplastic disease can also cause aseptic meningitis; haematological malignancies such as lymphoma and leukaemia are most commonly involved, although leptomeningeal carcinomatosis can also occur as a consequence of metastatic spread from tumours such as breast, lung and melanoma. Finally, a number of drugs can trigger aseptic meningitis, including non-steroidal anti-inflammatory drugs (NSAIDs), intravenous immunoglobulins, azathioprine, carbamazepine, penicillin and isoniazid.

Treatment

If bacterial meningitis is suspected, treatment should not be delayed by investigations. Broad-spectrum antimicrobial therapy, given intravenously and in high doses, should be commenced; initial empirical treatment is guided by the age of the patient and particular risk factors identified in the history (Table 28.3); this is modified when the causative organism is identified (Table 28.4). In-house treatment protocols, reflecting local bacterial resistance, should be sought.

The release of bacterial cell-wall products into the CSF, in part as a consequence of antimicrobial treatment, results in inflammation. There is evidence for the beneficial effect of corticosteroids in the treatment of

Table 28.4 Guide to treatment of meningitis when the causative pathogen is identified

Pathogen	Recommended antibiotic
Listeria	Ampicillin (co-trimoxazole if allergic)
Meningococcus	Benzylpenicillin
Haemophilus influenzae type b and pneumococcal	Third-generation cephalosporins
Group B *Streptococcus*	Penicillin or ampicillin
Staphylococcus aureus	Flucloxacillin (vancomycin if allergic or organism resistant/hospital acquired)
Coagulase-negative staphylococci (e.g. shunt infections)	Vancomycin ± rifampicin
Gram-negative bacilli	Third-generation cephalosporins *and* meropenem

bacterial meningitis by reducing this inflammation. In adults, dexamethasone 10 mg should be given on suspicion of bacterial meningitis, with or just before the first dose of antibiotics. It should then be continued, if the diagnosis is confirmed, at a dose of 10 mg every 6 h for 4 days. In children, a dose of 0.15 mg kg^{-1} is given every 6 h for 4 days. This improves outcome in most cases but particularly in those with pneumococcal meningitis.

Encephalitis

Encephalitis occurs when there is an inflammatory reaction in the brain parenchyma, either as the primary site of infection (such as in herpes simplex virus (HSV) encephalitis), or secondary to subarachnoid space infection (meningoencephalitis). Presentations range from mild with headache and confusion to more severe with seizures, focal neurological deficits, raised ICP and coma.

The most common causes of encephalitis are viral. Areas of inflammation may be focal or generalized. Treatment is supportive, with the exception of HSV for which intravenous acyclovir should be given without delay. In HSV infection, the diagnosis may be suspected based on imaging demonstrating changes in the temporal lobes (Fig. 28.1), and EEG demonstrating periodic epileptiform activity lateralized to the site of infection. Diagnosis is confirmed by PCR of the CSF.

Members of the arbovirus and enterovirus family also cause encephalitis – treatment is supportive only. Infection of the CNS with varicella-zoster virus (VZV) is normally benign and self-limiting; however in immunocompromised patients, a post-infectious encephalomyelitis occurs, which may be treated with acyclovir. Another important worldwide cause of encephalitis is rabies, which carries a 100% mortality

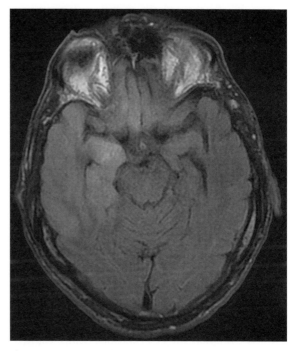

Fig. 28.1. Herpes simplex virus encephalitis. Axial fluid attenuation inversion recovery (FLAIR) image of a 73-year-old man showing increased signal intensity and swelling in the anterior and medial right temporal lobe.

rate. The bite by a rabid dog may precede the CNS infection by months. Along with headache and fever, patients develop paraesthesias and pain at the inoculation site.

The main differentials in the setting of encephalitis are the myriad causes of encephalopathy (disturbance of brain function) due to non-CNS diseases such as systemic infections (e.g. urinary tract infections), metabolic disturbances (e.g. uraemia or hepatic encephalopathy) or drug toxicity.

433

(a) 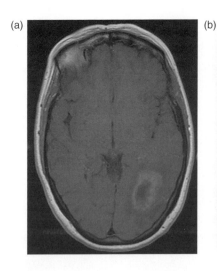 (b)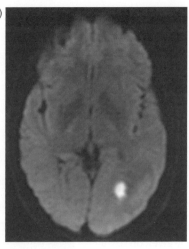

Fig. 28.2. Cerebral abscess. (a) Axial contrast-enhanced T1-weighted image in a 37–year-old woman shows a ring enhancing lesion in the left occipitotemporal white matter with low-signal intensity surrounding vasogenic oedema. (b) Diffusion-weighted imaging showing increased signal intensity in the central part of the abscess.

Cerebral abscesses and subdural empyemas

Cerebral abscesses can be caused by bacterial or fungal infections, and often present with headache, fever, seizures and focal neurological signs. They are more common in young men, and are often due to the haematological spread of infection from a distant source (e.g. bacterial endocarditis, suppurative lung disease), the direct extension of local infections (e.g. purulent sinus infections, dental abscesses) or direct inoculation of pathogens during neurosurgery or trauma. Immunosuppressed patients are more vulnerable to developing brain abscesses, particularly those on high-dose steroids.

The route of infection usually dictates which organism is causative. For example, various streptococcal species may infect the ear, nose and throat and form abscesses through direct extensions. More unusual organisms such as Gram-negative rods, or fungi such as *Aspergillus* and *Candida* spp. are typical in neutropaenic patients. T-cell dysfunction exposes patients to abscess formation by *Listeria*, *Nocardia*, *Mycobacterium tuberculosis* (tuberculosis (TB)), *Toxoplasma gondii* (toxoplasmosis) and *Cryptococcus*.

If a cerebral abscess is suspected, lumbar puncture is contraindicated. Diagnosis is made on the basis of typical imaging findings and identification of the organism through blood cultures or surgical biopsy/drainage (Fig. 28.2). A search should be made, if appropriate, for the source of infection to ensure this is adequately treated.

The management and treatment is determined by the degree of mass effect imposed by the abscess.

Aspiration of the abscess may also be required to confirm the diagnosis and identify the pathogenic organism. If foreign bodies (e.g. bone fragments) are associated with infection, these should be removed. The choice of empirical antibiotics is governed by the likely source of infection; in most cases, a third-generation cephalosporin with metronidazole, and the addition of vancomycin if staphylococcal infection is suspected, is used.

Spinal epidural abscesses may present with acute cord compression (weak legs, and bowel and bladder dysfunction). These require urgent surgical decompression, followed by prolonged antimicrobial treatment. Subdural empyemas can have a more subacute presentation.

Other specific central nervous system infections

Neurocysticercosis

In its acute form, this parasitic infection can cause both arachnoiditis and parenchymal cysts. Arachnoiditis presents with headache and cranial nerve dysfunction, and offers a poor prognosis, despite treatment. Up to 50% of patients develop hydrocephalus, which can deteriorate on initiation of treatment; it is recommended that a shunt is placed prior to commencing drug therapy.

Parenchymal cysts often present with partial/secondary generalized seizures. In the acute phase, oedema and mass effect cause raised ICP. In the inactive phase, cysts become calcified and can present with partial seizures.

Human immunodeficiency virus

Human immunodeficiency virus is a retrovirus and spreads between humans in body fluids to infect cells of the immune system and CNS. Therefore, in addition to direct infection, HIV causes disease in the CNS through immunosuppression. The virus infects CNS tissue early; therefore, CSF abnormalities (raised lymphocyte numbers and protein, with a normal glucose) are seen in up to 20% of untreated HIV-infected individuals in the absence of CNS symptoms and cannot be relied on to diagnose infections alone.

Primary HIV infection can cause aseptic meningitis or meningoencephalitis during seroconversion, often accompanied by lymphadenopathy and a maculopapular rash. At this time, individuals are highly infectious with high viral loads. Diagnosis is confirmed by the identification of free viral RNA in the context of normal serology. The role of antiretroviral therapy in this setting is contentious; it may hasten recovery from what is normally a self-limiting illness; however, early treatment could promote multidrug-resistant strains of HIV.

A later consequence of primary HIV infection is HIV encephalopathy or the 'AIDS dementia complex'. This usually manifests as slow cognitive decline; however, sudden acute deteriorations can occur with confusion and delirium. In this setting, CSF analysis to exclude infection is necessary. MRI often demonstrates atrophy and diffuse white-matter abnormalities.

Human immunodeficiency virus infection renders its host vulnerable to secondary, or opportunistic, infections of the brain. Reactivation of dormant JC virus causes progressive multifocal leukoencephalopathy (PML). This is a white-matter disease; the virus causes demyelination resulting in either uni- or multifocal lesions, with corresponding signs (Fig. 28.3). Diagnosis is confirmed by demonstrating JC virus in the CSF. The condition is usually fatal; however, there may be some improvement with the introduction of highly active antiretroviral therapy (HAART). Focal CNS lesions can also arise secondary to infection with *Toxoplasma* and *Cryptococcus*, when CD4 counts drop below 200 μl⁻¹. In these circumstances, fungal and tuberculous infections are also common.

Toxoplasmosis arises through the reactivation of latent cysts of *Toxoplasma gondii*; their rapid division results in expanding masses of necrotic tissue typically occuring around the basal ganglia. Securing a firm diagnosis may be difficult due to false-positive IgG levels consequent to prior exposure. Ring-enhancing

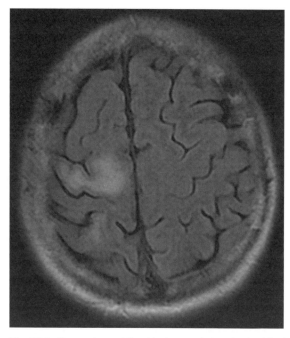

Fig. 28.3. Progressive multifocal leukoencephalopathy. Axial fluid attenuation inversion recovery (FLAIR) image in a 38-year-old man with AIDS showing asymmetrically increased signal intensity in the right frontal and parietal white matter with involvement of the subcortical U-fibres.

lesions on MRI are suggestive of toxoplasmosis, along with the response to treatment. If CSF can be obtained, it may be possible to identify *Toxoplasma* by PCR. Cerebral biopsy is indicated if the diagnosis is not certain, or if there is no response to treatment with pyrimethamine and sulfadiazine within 2–3 weeks.

Cryptococcosis is caused by the encapsulated yeast-like fungus *Cryptococcus neoformans*. It typically causes meningitis, which may be acute or subacute in evolution and often presents as a painful radiculopathy. Abscesses can also form. The diagnosis is made following the identification of cryptococcus in the CSF using an India ink stain, or by detection of the cryptococcal polysaccharide antigen (CrAg) in serum. Initial treatment is with amphotericin B, possibly combined with flucytosine. This is then followed with fluconazole.

The incidence of TB is rising with HIV infection. Tuberculosis can present with focal CNS lesions, or more diffusely with tuberculous meningitis. It is important to consider neoplastic disease, particularly lymphoma, as a differential for focal CNS lesions, to which AIDS patients are prone.

More diffuse CNS infections include HSV, VZV and cytomegalovirus (CMV); it is important to also consider non-opportunistic infections to which patients may be prone. Human immunodeficiency virus vasculitis is a rare complication, which can result in cerebral infarctions.

Human immunodeficiency virus infection is treated using HAART. Patients are usually required to take a complex regime of at least three different drugs, which work by a variety of mechanisms (reverse transcriptase inhibitors, protease inhibitors or inhibitors of HIV fusion with, and entry into, cells). Patients on antiretroviral treatments are at risk of drug-related side effects; rarely, the drugs themselves can cause both encephalopathy and neuropathy.

Spirochaete infections

Spirochaete infections, including syphilis, leptospirosis and Lyme disease, are important to consider if features in the history allude to their possibility.

Tertiary syphilis, caused by *Treponema pallidum*, is increasing in incidence with HIV infection. It can present with a variety of symptoms ranging from apathy to seizures, dementia, myoclonus, tremor and dysarthria. It can cause acute meningitis within 2 years of the primary infection. The diagnosis is confirmed by performing a Venereal Disease Research Laboratory (VDRL) test on CSF, in which a raised protein and lymphocyte count but normal glucose is the typical pattern. Treatment is with high-dose intravenous procaine penicillin for 2–3 weeks (or until CSF clearance is achieved). Corticosteroids should be given for the first 24 h of treatment, as these patients are at risk of Jarisch–Herxheimer reactions.

In the tick-borne infection caused by *Borrelia burgdorferi*, Lyme disease, symptoms are often heralded by erythema chronicum migrans at the bite site. This characteristic rash represents the first stage of the disease, while neurological manifestations occur in the second stage (1–6 months after the initial bite). These include meningitis/meningoencephalitis (which occurs in about 10% of patients), radiculoneuritis, cranial nerve abnormalities and a mononeuritis multiplex. The diagnosis is made on the basis of serological tests. Lyme disease should be treated with intravenous ceftriaxone, or high-dose penicillin, for a minimum of 2 weeks.

Weil's disease is caused by infection with leptospires, usually following contact with rat's urine on river banks or polluted water sources. Therefore, farmers, sewage workers, fishermen and miners, as well as watersports enthusiasts, are at risk of infection. The average incubation period is 1–2 weeks. The severity of symptoms varies from subclinical infection to a fulminant, lethal disease. It commonly presents with fever, headache, gastrointestinal symptoms and myalgia. Typically, patients report muscle pain, especially of the calves, abdomen and back, as a prominent feature. Conjunctivitis is another common manifestation. In 5–10% of cases, the syndrome evolves to a second phase, causing meningitis or meningoencephalitis; severe headache, neck stiffness, seizures and coma can occur. The CSF is sterile with a variable white-cell response, probably as this phase of the disease is driven by the host response to infection. Liver, renal and clotting impairments are common. Diagnosis is made by serological confirmation or isolation of the organism. These tests are not widely available, are expensive and lack sensitivity; therefore, Weil's disease is often a clinical diagnosis. Treatment with high-dose intravenous antibiotics should be initiated on suspicion of infection; Leptospires are sensitive to most antibiotics, but amoxicillin (or oral doxycycline in milder cases) is generally used. As in the treatment of syphilis, patients are at risk of Jarisch–Herxheimer reactions.

Malaria

Cerebral malaria has a mortality rate of up to 50% and can lead to death within 72 h of symptom onset. It manifests as a generalized encephalopathy, caused by cerebral vasculitis and microthrombosis, resulting in diffuse ischaemic damage. Patients may have experienced a non-specific flu-like syndrome prior to the onset of cerebral symptoms, which may be heralded by seizures followed by prolonged coma. Swinging pyrexia (on a 48 h cycle) is classical. Acute tubular necrosis, acute respiratory distress syndrome and disseminated intravascular coagulation commonly co-occur. The clinical picture may be complicated by the presence of persistent hypoglycaemia, worsening seizures and prolonging coma.

The disease is caused by infection with *Plasmodium falciparum* following a bite from an infected mosquito. The infection is endemic in large parts of Asia, sub-Saharan Africa, central and south America and the Middle East. It is important to consider this infection if working in non-endemic areas of the world, particularly in emigrants returning from their native countries whose previous immunity may have waned. Holidaymakers and travellers will also be at risk, and pregnancy increases susceptibility to infection.

Rarely, hitchhiking mosquitoes bite residents local to airports.

The diagnosis of cerebral malaria relies on identification of the parasite on thick and thin blood films – a test that should be repeated every 6–8 h for at least 48 h in order to confirm or exclude malaria infection. If clinical suspicion is high, treatment should be commenced prior to investigation. Quinine is used most widely: an initial dose of 7 mg kg^{-1} is given intravenously over 30 min, followed by 10 mg kg^{-1} over the following 4 h, repeated every 8–12 h thereafter. If the parasite load is high and the patient very ill, exchange transfusions can be considered. If quinine is not available, quinidine or artemisimin derivatives may be used. Care should be taken to consider the possibility of and treat superimposed bacterial infections, particularly Gram-negative septicaemia to which seriously ill patients are vulnerable.

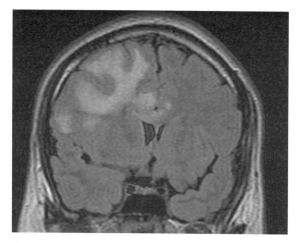

Fig. 28.4. Acute disseminated encephalomyelitis. Coronal fluid attenuation inversion recovery (FLAIR) image in a 25-year-old man showing increased signal intensity and swelling in the right frontal subcortical white matter with mass effect on the adjacent corpus callosum.

Central nervous system inflammation

Many non-infectious conditions result in inflammation in the CNS; these may be post-infectious, paraneoplastic or the consequence of a chronic autoimmune disease. Sudden acute neurological dysfunction can occur, either at the time of disease onset or during relapse of the disease, resulting in focal neurological deficits or coma (encephalopathy). Such patients may require intensive care support in the setting of opportunistic or severe infections due to the combination of chronic disability and the use of long-term immunosuppressive treatments.

Post-infectious central nervous system inflammation

Acute disseminated encephalomyelitis (ADEM) is a monophasic demyelinating autoimmune disease of the CNS that can affect multiple sites in both the brain and spinal cord concurrently. While it can occur spontaneously, this condition often follows (by between 1 and 6 weeks) a febrile illness or, more rarely, vaccination. In the UK, a non-specific respiratory tract infection may be the precipitant, but varicella-zoster virus, mumps virus, rubella virus, measles virus, rabies virus, enterovirus, Epstein–Barr virus, human herpesvirus 6, human T-cell lymphotropic virus type 1, *Chlamydia* and many more infectious agents have been reported to cause the disease. It most commonly affects children and young adults, with a male preponderance. Characteristically, altered consciousness (ranging from irritability to coma), seizures, meningism and focal neurological signs occur. The diagnosis is made on MRI appearances (large ill-defined deep white-matter lesions suggestive of demyelination; Fig. 28.4) and CSF analysis (raised protein and cell count). As no diagnostic tests exist, it is important to exclude other differentials such as HSV encephalitis, *Listeria* meningoencephalitis and TB meningitis, as well as multiple sclerosis, cerebral vasculitis, multiple septic emboli, and multifocal primary and secondary central neoplasms. Multiple sclerosis (MS) is the condition most commonly confused with ADEM; however, it is unusual for MS to present with such a severe, polysymptomatic illness (Table 28.5). Multiple sclerosis is the more likely diagnosis if the history or scan suggests that some of the lesions were acquired prior to the acute clinical presentation, or if new lesions evolve on future scans with or without symptoms.

In a small proportion (around 30%), the peripheral nervous system is also involved, with evidence of demyelination. Acute (necrotizing) haemorrhagic leucoencephalitis is a more fulminant form of ADEM.

The condition is initially treated with high-dose corticosteroids: methylprednisolone 1 g daily for 3–5 days. This is often followed by plasma exchange or intravenous immunoglobulins if the response to steroids is inadequate. In the setting of a large inflammatory load causing cerebral oedema, ICP monitoring and

Table 28.5 Comparison of the clinical features of acute disseminated encephalomyelitis (ADEM) and multiple sclerosis (MS)

Clinical feature	ADEM	MS
Sex	Male preponderance	Female preponderance
Age at onset	Common in children	Common in adults
Level of consciousness	Often ↓	Normal
CSF white cells	↑	Normal
CSF oligoclonal bands	Absent (may be transiently present in 10% cases)	Present
MRI lesions	Large 'fluffy' WM lesions, disappear over time	Well-defined WM 'plaques' that persist
Evidence of PNS involvement	Occurs clinically in 30%	Never occurs

CSF, cerebrospinal fluid; PNS, peripheral nervous system; WM, white matter.

management is required. In these situations, a decompressive craniotomy may be considered. It is important to identify and treat acute, recurrent or superimposed infection, which may be driving or complicating the neurological syndrome.

Most patients recover fully; 20–30% have significant neurological sequelae, which is most common following mumps and measles. In a small percentage, the condition is fatal.

Paraneoplastic disease involving the central nervous system

Paraneoplastic disease can take many forms in the CNS including encephalopathy, seizures and movement disorders. They are associated with, and may be caused by, antibodies produced in response to neoplastic disease. Early recognition and treatment can potentially prevent permanent severe neurological dysfunction.

There are a number of recognizable clinical syndromes (limbic encephalopathy, cerebellar degeneration, stiff-person syndrome, opsoclonus myoclonus), but more commonly the presentation is less specific, with many areas of the nervous system affected, and is better described as a paraneoplastic encephalomyelitis. The onset of symptoms can be rapid and progression fulminant, making infection the initial working diagnosis.

The diagnosis is confirmed by the demonstration of 'anti-neuronal' antibodies (Table 28.6) and the primary neoplasm driving the immune response. A large number of these antibodies are now recognized. Some

antibodies are directly pathogenic; voltage-gated potassium-channel and NMDA receptor antibodies cause neuronal injury or dysfunction in patients with limbic encephalitis. In other situations, the antibodies probably mediate a cellular immune response responsible for the paraneoplastic syndrome, the probable mechanism driving paraneoplastic cerebellar syndromes. Finally, antibodies may be an epiphenomenon. Often, the same antibody can cause a number of different syndromes, and a single syndrome can be caused by a number of different antibodies. It is critical to search hard for the tumour, which may well be small in the setting of a vigorous autoimmune antitumour response.

The autoimmune attack within the CNS may manifest on MRI with signal changes in the relevant areas (especially with multifocal or limbic encephalitis), but imaging may also be normal, even in the setting of marked neurological deficits. Similarly, the CSF may be abnormal, with rises in both mononuclear cell counts and protein and the presence of oligoclonal bands, but it can also be normal. When a paraneoplastic syndrome is suspected, the diagnostic work-up is tailored towards identifying the underlying malignancy. Careful testicular and breast examinations, followed by appropriate imaging, and a chest X-ray are indicated. A transvaginal ultrasound, or pelvic MRI, is recommended in women presenting with encephalitis of paraneoplastic origin, as small ovarian tumours may be missed with other imaging modalities. When initial tests fail to reveal a malignancy, 18-fluorodeoxyglucose positron emission tomography (FDG-PET) may be a useful screening tool.

Table 28.6 A non-exhaustive list of major paraneoplastic syndromes and their associated tumours and antibodies

Paraneoplastic syndrome	Associated tumours	Associated autoantibody
Multifocal encephalomyelitis	SCLC and various carcinomas	Anti-Hu, anti-CV2, anti-Ri, anti-ANNA3, anti-amphiphysin, (anti-Ma1 with testicular tumours)
Stiff-person syndrome	SCLC, breast, others	Anti-amphiphysin, anti-Ri, anti-GAD
Cerebellar degeneration	SCLC, Hodgkin's lymphoma, breast and ovary	Anti-Hu, anti-CV2, PCA-2, ANNA-3, anti-amphiphysin, anti-VGCC, anti-Ri, anti-Zic4, anti-Tr, anti-mGluR1, anti-Yo
Limbic encephalitis	SCLC, ANNA-3	Anti-Hu (ANNA-1)
	Ovarian teratoma, testicular tumours	Anti-NMDA receptor antibodies
	Thymoma, SCLC	VGKCA, anti-CV2
	Testicular tumours, breast and non-SCLC	Anti-Ma1, anti-Ma2
	Breast, SCLC	Anti-amphiphysin
Brainstem encephalitis	SCLC, breast, testicular, others	Anti-Hu, anti-Ri, anti-Ma2

NMDA, N-methyl-D-aspartate; SCLC, small-cell lung cancer; VGKCA, voltage-gated potassium-channel antibodies.

The management of paraneoplastic syndromes requires identification and, where possible, removal or treatment of the causative tumour. This alone can result in a dramatic improvement in the neurological syndrome. Prior to this, suppression of the immune response to the tumour, using steroids, intravenous immunoglobulins or plasma exchange, is often required acutely. Cyclophosphamide, azathioprine and other immunosuppressants have also been used with varying efficacy.

A small number of patients with paraneoplastic CNS syndromes will make a significant recovery with removal of the tumour and treatment. The extent of recovery is influenced by the time to diagnosis and amenability of the tumour to treatment. However, in the majority of cases, these syndromes carry a poor prognosis.

Autoimmune disease

Multiple sclerosis

Multiple sclerosis is an autoimmune disease of the CNS, characterized by episodes of demyelination, with consequent degeneration of axons. Typically, it presents in the third and fourth decades, more commonly in females. In the early stages, patients typically experience relapses during which neurological symptoms evolve subacutely, persist for days to weeks and, in most cases, improve. The nature and severity of the symptoms depend on the location of the autoimmune attack. Common manifestations include optic neuritis,

transverse myelitis, sensory symptoms and brainstem syndromes (diplopia, ataxia, dysarthria, pyramidal signs). Rarely, a relapse affecting the brainstem or high cervical structures results in an inability to swallow and respiratory compromise requiring intensive care support. In contrast to ADEM, encephalopathy is exceedingly rare. Relapse frequency varies enormously, but on average patients experience a relapse once every 2 years.

Diagnosis is made on the basis of a typical history of relapsing and remitting neurological symptoms and the appearance of typical periventricular white-matter lesions or 'plaques' on MRI (Fig. 28.5). When diagnostic uncertainty remains, the presence of oligoclonal bands in otherwise normal CSF, or delay in visual evoked responses, are supportive.

Acute relapses are treated with high-dose pulsed methylprednisolone; this treatment aims to hasten recovery, although it does not influence the long-term outcome. Occasionally, in the setting of severe or life-threatening relapses, plasma exchange is used if no response is achieved with steroids.

In patients with frequent disabling relapses, immunosuppressants are introduced in an attempt to modify the disease course. The β-interferons and glatiramir acetate offer a modest reduction in relapse rate and few side effects. However, if these fail, more powerful immunotherapies are introduced. The recently licensed monoclonal antibody, natalizumab, which blocks the traffic of T lymphocytes into the CNS, is reasonably effective in stopping relapses. However, a small number

439

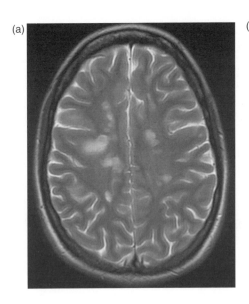

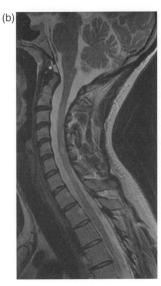

Fig. 28.5. Multiple sclerosis. (a) Axial T2-weighted image in a 29-year-old woman showing multiple ovoid white-matter lesions in the periventricular white matter, orientated perpendicular to the long axes of the lateral ventricles. (b) Sagittal T2-weighted image of the spinal cord in the same patient showing a hyperintense plaque in the spinal cord at C5.

of patients (fewer than 1 in 1000) develop progressive multifocal leukoencephalopathy, a fatal infection due to reactivation of dormant JC virus. Mitoxantrone, a synthetic antineoplastic drug, is also used in severe MS. It has long-term immunosuppressive effects, although its use is limited by cardiac toxicity. Recipients are at increased risk of developing acute leukaemias.

Prognosis is dependent on the rapidity with which individuals accumulate disability, either through axonal transaction during acute severe relapses (resulting in a stepwise worsening in ability) or secondary to early axonal degeneration in areas previously the target of immune attack. Life expectancy is reduced by 10–15 years on average.

Neuromyelitis optica (NMO; Devic's disease) is a demyelinating disease similar to MS. However, in NMO, attacks are restricted to the spinal cord and optic nerves. Relapses tend to be more severe and can render patients blind and/or para-/tetraplegic. The condition is associated with the presence of anti-aquaporin antibody in 50% of cases. Imaging of the cord demonstrates large lesions often spanning several vertebral heights (diagnostically, at least three levels are required). Acute attacks are managed with steroids or plasma exchange. In many, longer-term immunosuppression is required; azathioprine, methotrexate and rituximab are used, with varied reports of success.

Neurosarcoid

Sarcoidosis is a multisystem, non-caseating, granulomatous autoimmune disease. It most commonly affects the lungs, but in 5% it affects the CNS, following either a monophasic, relapsing or chronically progressive course. The estimated prevalence in Caucasians living in the UK is around 10–20 per 10,000 of the population (more common in African-Americans). However, the incidence may be higher, as sarcoidosis is frequently identified incidentally in asymptomatic individuals.

Most patients present with CNS symptoms in their second and third decades and the disease is more common in women. Only one-third of cases are known to have sarcoidosis. Most commonly, patients present with cranial neuropathies. Optic neuritis occurs in around one-third of presentations and is often severe with disc oedema. The optic nerve can also be compressed due to raised ICP (secondary to a large parenchymal lesion or hydrocephalus). Other cranial nerves can also be affected, particularly the facial nerve; neurosarcoidosis is a cause of bilateral facial nerve palsies, which can mimic the early stage of Guillain–Barré syndrome. Spinal cord and brainstem disease involvement are also frequent manifestations. Meningeal infiltration is common, and can extend along the Virchow–Robin spaces to enter the brain parenchyma, particularly around the base of the brain. Symptomatically, this presents with aseptic meningitis with or without cranial neuropathies, or with hydrocephalus due to obstruction of CSF outflow. The structures within the pituitary–hypothalamic axis are vulnerable to granulomatous infiltration, causing, typically, diabetes insipidus (although panhypopituitarism and other endocrine deficits can occur) and changes to circadian rhythm and thermo-dysregulation. Finally, patients may present non-specifically with cognitive decline, neuropsychiatric illness or encephalopathy. Rarely, granulomatous infiltration may occur in blood vessel walls, resulting in spontaneous subarachnoid haemorrhage, intraparenchymal haemorrhage or stroke. The peripheral nervous system may also be affected.

The diagnosis of neurosarcoidosis is definite when histological samples can be taken from the CNS (demonstrating sarcoid-like granulomas). However, when this is not possible, a probable diagnosis can be based on a typical clinical presentation, exclusion of other differentials, demonstration of CNS inflammation and confirmation of the disease in tissue from other organs/lymph nodes. Only approximately one-third of patients will have an abnormal chest X-ray (most commonly with hilar lymphadenopathy). In the CSF, inflammation may be evident as elevation in CSF protein or a pleocytosis (up to 250 cells, usually lymphocytes). Oligoclonal bands may be present in the CSF alone, indicating local synthesis, or may spill over into the CSF from serum. Angiotensin-converting enzyme (ACE) in the CSF can be measured, and when elevated is specific (95%; also elevated with tumours and infection), although sensitivity is low. Serum and urinary calcium may be helpful but are rarely elevated in the setting of neurosarcoidosis. Similarly, a normal erythrocyte sedimentation rate does not exclude the diagnosis. An FDG-PET scan can reveal subclinical neurosarcoid lesions. A gallium-67 scan can demonstrate the presence of sarcoidosis in the salivary and lachrymal glands, spleen and chest. Neuroimaging, using MRI, most commonly demonstrates multiple white-matter lesions, which can also be evident in the spinal cord and brainstem. Meningeal and optic nerve enhancement may also be seen. Transbronchial lung biopsy is the most lucrative site for tissue diagnosis; however, blind conjunctival biopsy offers a negligible complication rate and moderate sensitivity (increased by bilateral procedures) in the absence of ocular symptoms. There is also increasing interest in blind muscle biopsies to provide diagnostic tissue.

The mainstay of treatment (although there are no controlled trials proving efficacy) is with corticosteroids, often delivered initially in the form of pulsed methylprednisolone, followed subsequently by oral prednisolone, tapering if possible. Further immunosuppressants such as cyclophosphamide, azathioprine, hydroxychloroquine and methotrexate may be introduced in the absence of a response to or failure to wean from steroids. There are anecdotal reports of a response to the anti-tumour necrosis factor-alpha (TNF-α) monoclonal antibody infliximab, and to thalidomide. Cerebral irradiation has also been used in the setting of drug-resistant neurosarcoidosis, and rarely surgical decompression of hydrocephalus or large parenchymal lesions is indicated.

Overall, disease presenting in the spinal cord or optic nerve and the presence of epilepsy carries the worst prognosis. Patients are more prone to infections due to defects in swallowing and micturition, poor mobility and the long-term use of immunosuppressive treatments.

Behçet's disease

Behçet's disease is a chronic, relapsing, autoimmune, multisystem disorder. As symptoms often appear asynchronously, the diagnosis can be difficult, delaying the administration of appropriate immunosuppressive treatments. The major diagnostic criteria for Behçet's disease require patients to have experienced at least two of the following symptoms: oral ulcers recurring at least three times per year, genital ulcers or scars, eye disease (such as anterior or posterior uveitis, hypopyon or retinal vasculitis), skin lesions (erythema nodosum, folliculitis, acneiform lesions) or a positive pathergy skin test (development of a sterile pustule at a skin site pricked by a sterile needle) observed by a physician. Minor diagnostic criteria include arthritis or arthralgia, deep venous thromboses, subcutaneous thrombophlebitis, epididymitis, a family history, and gastrointestinal, CNS or vascular involvement.

Neurological manifestations occur in up to 50% of cases, usually during active disease. It is unusual, but not impossible, for neurological manifestations to be the only feature at presentation. Common CNS manifestations include brainstem, diencephalic or corticospinal tract dysfunction, acute confusion, venous sinus thrombosis and meningoencephalitis (although these rarely co-occur). There are no diagnostic tests; the diagnosis is based on clinical findings, alongside the exclusion of other differentials. Cerebrospinal fluid can be normal, but increased pressure, protein, white cells, complement C3 levels, immunoglobulins and oligoclonal bands can be seen in neurological manifestations of Behçet's disease. CT brain imaging can be normal, even in the setting of extensive lesions, and therefore MRI should be undertaken where possible, which will often reveal an extensive lesion load, particularly in the brainstem, basal ganglia or the pontobulbar junction. Brainstem atrophy is seen following chronic disease. Enhancement with gadolinium is seen in the context of acute parenchymal or meningeal involvement. Treatment is with corticosteroids and other immunosuppressants, as described for neurosarcoidosis.

Cerebral vasculitis

Cerebral vasculitis is an inflammatory disease in which structural damage to the walls of arteries and/or veins in the CNS occurs, often accompanied by thrombosis and ischaemic damage to surrounding tissues. When no systemic disease (such as Wegener's granulomatosis) or precipitants such as drugs (amphetamines, cocaine), malignancy (such as lymphoma) or infections (TB, mycoplasma) can be identified, it is considered to be a primary CNS vasculitis.

Primary cerebral vasculitis

Primary cerebral vasculitis is rare; it can present with any symptom or sign depending on which vessels, and consequent tissue, is affected. Headaches and confusion are common, and neurological lesions tend to be multifocal, accumulating over time (days to months). Despite this heterogeneity, disease tends to present in one of three ways: with an acute/subacute encephalopathy (progressive confusion leading to coma), with multifocal lesions similar to those seen in MS (presenting with a relapsing phenotype but with unusual features such as headache and seizures), or with large intracranial mass lesions causing headache, focal signs and raised ICP. Spinal cord lesions may also occur as the first manifestation, presenting with progressive myelopathy and back pain.

Investigation of the patient has two aims: to secure the diagnosis of vasculitis and to exclude secondary causes. Urine and renal function should be scrutinized for evidence of renal involvement suggesting systemic disease. Erythrocyte sedimentation rate may be raised, but in the setting of primary cerebral vasculitis an immunological screen (e.g. for rheumatoid factor, anti-neutrophil cytoplasmic antibody, complement levels or cryoglobulins) will be normal. Two-thirds of patients will have evidence of inflammatory disease in the CSF (helpful in differentiating from MS and other mimics), such as raised protein and mononuclear cells. MRI, particularly T2-weighted and fluid attenuation inversion recovery (FLAIR) sequences, is sensitive but non-specific in vasculitis, although assessing the distribution of discrete lesions can be helpful. Together, a normal MRI and CSF analysis have a high negative predictive value. With modern MRI techniques, angiography is less commonly required. Its findings of beading of the vessels, aneurysms, circumferential or eccentric vessel irregularities and multiple occlusions with sharp cut-offs are non-specific, and its sensitivity is only 60%. The absolute gold standard for diagnosis of primary cerebral vasculitis is brain or meningeal biopsy; however, one-quarter of these will be falsely negative. Yield is increased by sampling both brain and meninges, or by targeting radiographically abnormal areas.

Untreated, this condition is fatal, and severe disability may result from delayed diagnosis. The mainstay of treatment is with immunosuppression. High-dose corticosteroids and cyclophosphamide are usually the initial treatments of choice.

Small-vessel vasculitis

Wegener's granulomatosis (WG), Churg–Strauss syndrome (CSS) and the less well-defined microscopic polyangiitis (MPA) cause systemic disease through small-vessel necrotizing vasculitis. They share many clinical features as well as the presence of the hallmark serological finding of anti-neutrophil cytoplasmic autoantibodies (ANCA) in the majority of patients with active disease. Patients can present in a myriad of ways; some will present with acute, life-threatening disease resulting in admission to the intensive care unit. Again, complications may occur due to chronic disability and immunosuppressive therapies resulting in susceptibility to severe and opportunistic infections.

Wegener's granulomatosis is characterized by the development of necrotizing granulomatosis and vasculitis affecting small- and medium-sized arteries. It tends to present in the fifth decade, most commonly with upper and lower respiratory tract symptoms and renal disease (glomerulonephritis). The extent and severity of the disease varies widely among individuals, and can be life-threatening in some due to respiratory and renal failure. Approximately three-quarters of patients will also experience musculoskeletal symptoms, and there may be eye involvement in 50% of individuals. This can be due to retro-orbital inflammatory mass lesions, or vasculitis resulting in optic nerve infarction. Similarly, there may be local disease of the retinal artery leading to occlusions and ischaemia. Conjunctivitis, uveitis or episcleritis can also occur.

Fifty per cent of patients with WG will have neurological involvement, although in 50% of these, symptoms and disease are restricted to the peripheral nervous system, taking the form of a polyneuropathy or mononeuritis multiplex. Only 10% of patients are likely to encounter disease in the CNS; this can take many forms including cranial neuropathies and headache. Less commonly, diabetes insipidus can occur due to infiltration of the posterior pituitary gland, and rarely WG can result in ischaemic stroke, intracerebral haemorrhage, cerebritis, myelopathy or venous sinus thrombosis.

While the cause of the condition is unknown, there is a clear association with positivity for ANCA, and specifically in WG for ANCA directed against proteinase 3 (PR3), which is present in 90% of cases (in 3% of cases, ANCA directed against myeloperoxidase (MPO) will be identified). Rarely, WG is thought to be induced by medication (e.g. hydralazine or propylthiouracil).

The differential diagnosis includes other vasculitidies such as microscopic polyarteritis (usually MPO positive and lacking granuloma formation on biopsy), and chronic infections such as TB, fungal infections and syphilis.

Prior to the introduction of prednisolone and cyclophosphamide as treatments for WG, this was a fatal condition. Now, 80% survive at least 10 years from diagnosis. Death results not only from the disease directly but also from complications of treatment (e.g. infection, cytopaenia, cyclophosphamide-induced cystitis/bladder carcinoma, lymphoma, myelodysplasia). Prednisolone is used alone in disease localized to the lower respiratory tracts. Methotrexate is considered in the setting of non-life-threatening systemic disease and cyclophosphamide for severe disease. Azathioprine can be used for maintenance therapy, and rituximab has been used in treatment-resistant cases.

It is rare for vasculitis to occur in the CNS as a consequence of CSS, another ANCA-positive small-vessel vasculitis characterized by peripheral eosinophilia and asthma. However, this condition commonly damages the peripheral nervous system causing a peripheral neuropathy or mononeuritis multiplex. However, cranial neuropathies can occur, as can cranial haemorrhage or infarction (likely to be cardioembolic).

As with many of these conditions, the gold standard for diagnosis comes from tissue histology. Serological tests for perinuclear ANCA are positive 50–70% of the time and are generally MPO specific. The condition is treated in a very similar way to WG,

with immunosuppressants being introduced according to disease severity and progression, starting with steroids.

Collagen vascular diseases

This is a group of conditions with diverse phenotypes but a common pathological basis of diffuse inflammatory changes in connective tissue, particularly in the wall of blood vessels. The neurological manifestations, which can be lethal, are dependent on the extent of arteritis. Again, treated with systemic immunosuppression, patients are susceptible to opportunistic infections. There are many variants: systemic lupus erythematosus (SLE), polyarteritis nodosa (PN) and Sjögren's syndrome are common examples that can have CNS involvement.

Systemic lupus erythematosus is a multiorgan vasculitis, which mainly occurs in women (85%) and is characterized on biopsy by fibrinoid degeneration of blood vessel walls. It typically effects small arteries and arterioles but also causes microvascular lesions either directly or as a consequence of coexisting antiphospholipid antibodies. The most common non-CNS organ manifestations involve the skin, kidneys, joints, heart and bone marrow.

The neurological manifestations are varied, and can be bizarre. Seizures and acute episodes of psychosis feature in 30% of cases. It is thought that this is caused by microvascular disease, often undetectable on MRI. Other neurological consequences of the same pathology include chorea, cranial nerve palsies, mononeuritis multiplex, peripheral neuropathy, polymyositis and Guillain–Barré syndrome. There is an increased incidence of cerebrovascular accidents in patients with SLE.

The condition can be drug-induced; however, most commonly it arises spontaneously. It is most commonly treated with immunosuppressive therapies, although it is important to note that, due to bone marrow suppression, patients may already be lymphopaenic or have low complement levels.

Polyarteritis nodosa (PN) is rare but is the most severe of the collagen vascular diseases. It causes a pan-arteritis, with destruction of all layers of the blood vessel wall. Its most common neurological manifestation is with mononeuritis (which may be multiplex), caused by infarction of the nerve roots. When multiple nerve roots are affected, it has a predilection for roots C5–C7 and L2–L4. Cranial nerve palsies and cerebrovascular accidents occur but are uncommon. The most life-threatening complication of the disease is renal arteriolar disease resulting in uncontrollable hypertension. The condition can be drug induced (e.g. sulfonamides, penicillin) but is most commonly idiopathic. Treatment is with immunosuppression, commonly high-dose steroids. Intracranial PN can result in the development of cerebral aneurysms.

Sjögren's syndrome is a collagen vascular disorder with the hallmark features of dry eyes and dry mouth (sicca syndrome). Many of its neurological manifestations involve the peripheral nerves; however, it can cause cerebral and cord lesions that mimic those seen in MS on MRI, and can present with myelopathy or even meningoencephalitis. It is diagnosed based on its autoantibody profile (ANA, SSA/Ro, SSB/La positive) and the presence of sicca syndrome. Again, treatment revolves around the use of immunosuppressant therapy.

Acknowledgements

I thank Dr Alasdair Coles (Consultant Neurologist, Addenbrookes Hospital, Cambridge, UK) and Dr Daniel Scoffings (Consultant Neuro-radiologist, Addenbrookes Hospital, Cambridge, UK) for their help.

Further reading

Baringer, J. R. (2008). Herpes simplex infections of the nervous system. *Neurol Clin* **26**, 657–74, viii.

Be, N. A., Kim, K. S., Bishai, W. R. and Jain, S. K. (2009). Pathogenesis of central nervous system tuberculosis. *Curr Mol Med* **9**, 94–9.

Compston, A. and Coles, A. (2002). Multiple sclerosis. *Lancet* **359**, 1221–31.

de Gans, J. and van de Beek, D. (2002). European Dexamethasone in Adulthood Bacterial Meningitis Study Investigators. Dexamethasone in adults with bacterial meningitis. *N Engl J Med* **347**, 1549–56.

Lennon, V. A., Wingerchuk, D. M., Kryzer, T. J. *et al.* (2004). A serum autoantibody marker of neuromyelitis optica: distinction from multiple sclerosis. *Lancet* **364**, 2106–12.

Price, R. W. and Spudich, S. (2008). Antiretroviral therapy and central nervous system HIV type 1 infection. *J Infect Dis* **197** (Suppl. 3), S294–306.

Sakane, T., Takeno, M., Suzuki, N. and Inaba, G. (1999). Behçet's disease. *N Engl J Med* **341**, 1284–91.

Seki, M., Suzuki, S., Iizuka, T. *et al.* (2008). Neurological response to early removal of ovarian teratoma in anti-NMDAR encephalitis. *J Neurol Neurosurg Psychiatry* **79**, 324–6.

Semple, D., Keogh, J., Forni, L. and Venn, R. (2005). Clinical review: vasculitis on the intensive care unit – part 1: diagnosis. *Crit Care* **9**, 92–7.

Semple, D., Keogh, J., Forni, L. and Venn, R. (2005). Clinical review: vasculitis on the intensive care unit – part 2: treatment and prognosis. *Crit Care* **9**, 193–7.

Van de Beek, D., de Gans, J., Tunkel, AR and Wijdicks, E. F. (2006). Community-acquired bacterial meningitis in adults. *N Engl J Med* **354**, 44–53.

Young, N. P., Weinshenker, B. G. and Lucchinetti, C. F.. (2008). Acute disseminated encephalomyelitis: current understanding and controversies. *Semin Neurol* **28**, 84–94.

Zajicek, J. P. (2000). Neurosarcoidosis. *Curr Opin Neurol* **13**, 323–5.

Chapter 29

Intensive care of cardiac arrest survivors

Andrea Lavinio and Basil F. Matta

Post-resuscitation care: the fifth link of the chain of survival

Prompt recovery of spontaneous circulation (ROSC) is only the first step towards the goal of best achievable outcome following a cardiac arrest. Adequate post-resuscitation care of cardiac arrest survivors – the advocated *fifth link of the chain of survival* – can also dramatically improve outcome (Fig. 29.1). Until recently, the treatment of patients with coma after resuscitation from cardiac arrest was largely supportive. A new era of post-resuscitation care began in 2002 with the publication of two strikingly successful trials of therapeutic hypothermia in comatose cardiac arrest survivors by Bernard and co-workers. The cumulative results of these two studies yielded a formidable number needed to treat of six; this means that only six patients need to be treated with hypothermia to prevent one death or other unfavourable neurological outcome following cardiac arrest. This kind of effectiveness was unheard of in the realm of neurological therapeutics and neurological intensive care.

Therapeutic hypothermia following cardiac arrest is far more successful than many of the treatments that we tout as effective, such as intravenous tissue plasminogen activator for acute stroke, surgery for refractory temporal lobe epilepsy or any available treatment for traumatic neurological injury.

The provision of adequate post-resuscitation care of cardiac arrest survivors confers major public health benefits. Based on a estimated yearly European incidence of 375,000 cardiac arrests, and limiting the potential benefits of hypothermia to the 8% of patients fitting the inclusion criteria of the trial (witnessed out-of-hospital cardiac arrest, ventricular fibrillation or non-perfusing ventricular tachycardia as the initial cardiac rhythm, age of 18–75 years) the Hypothermia after Cardiac Arrest Study Group estimated that hypothermia alone would prevent 1200–7500 unfavourable neurological outcomes in Europe each year. Healthcare institutions have a responsibility to develop, implement and audit evidence-based protocols tailored to local resources. A survey of all intensive care units (ICUs) in the UK showed that, by 2006, only 27% of units had ever used mild hypothermia to treat post-cardiac arrest patients. By 2010, the percentage of ICUs implementing therapeutic hypothermia had increased to 86%.

The complexities of the intensive care management of cardiac arrest survivors are best understood in the framework of the so-called post-cardiac arrest syndrome. From the moment of resumption of spontaneous circulation, a complex set of pathophysiological processes including anoxic–ischaemic brain injury, post-cardiac arrest myocardial dysfunction and systemic ischaemia/reperfusion response jeopardize the patient's chances of recovery. Post-cardiac arrest care bundles that include therapeutic hypothermia, control of blood sugar and early coronary reperfusion strategies – along with state-of-the-art supportive care – can tackle these processes and improve survival and neurological outcome after cardiac arrest. The scope of the present chapter is to provide the reader with a pragmatic approach to ICU admission, acute treatment and prognostication of cardiac arrest survivors.

Indications for intensive care unit admission of cardiac arrest survivors

Patients admitted to the ICU represent only a small proportion of all those treated for cardiac arrest. Most cardiac arrest victims do not survive to get to ICU, and some patients are resuscitated so rapidly that they do not need ICU admission. In the UK, mechanically ventilated survivors of cardiac arrest account for

Core Topics in Neuroanaesthesia and Neurointensive Care, eds. Basil F. Matta, David K. Menon and Martin Smith. Published by Cambridge University Press. © Cambridge University Press 2011.

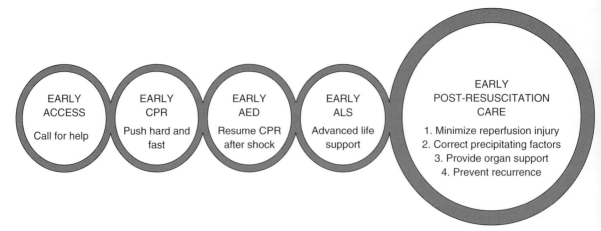

Fig. 29.1. The five links of the chain of survival. CPR, cardiopulmonary resuscitation; AED, automated external defibrillator; ALS, advanced life support.

approximately 6% of all ICU admissions. Of these, approximately 30% survive to hospital discharge. The criteria for ICU admission should be based on the prioritization of patients who are likely to benefit from ICU care. Given the inability to issue an early accurate prognosis and the potential benefits of intensive care, all appropriately resuscitated patients with obtunded cerebral function and/or requiring organ support despite sustained ROSC should be admitted to an ICU.

Patients who are excluded from ICU admission are usually referred to as patients who are 'too well to benefit' or 'too sick to benefit' from critical care services. Survivors of cardiac arrest can be considered 'too well to benefit' from ICU care if they were resuscitated rapidly, if they do not have neurological symptoms, if they do not require organ support and if they have a negligible chance of recurrence of the event. For a minority of patients fitting the above criteria, ICU or high-dependency-unit admission can still be warranted on the basis of monitoring and clinical observation in an appropriately equipped and staffed area, pending adequate diagnostic work-up. The admission of these patients should be prioritized on the basis of local availability of intensive care resources.

The category of patients achieving sustained ROSC that can be considered 'too sick to benefit' from critical care services is, in practice, limited to patients with an incurable primary disease who were resuscitated inappropriately. Optimized post-cardiac arrest care is resource intensive and should not be continued when the effort is clearly futile. However, it must be pointed out that drugs administered during resuscitation

weaken the reliability of early neurological assessments and prognostication. Early neurological prognostication is therefore insufficiently specific to inform withdrawal of care in patients with sustained ROSC in the first hours after arrest only on the basis of presumed anoxic–ischaemic brain injury. Even in the presence of ominous signs such as fixed and dilated pupils, patients have a significant chance of meaningful survival and they should be admitted to an ICU for continued care.

Early investigation of the patient's and the patient's relatives' wishes should be carried out whenever possible to identify potential donors, as transplant outcomes of organs donated by cardiac arrest survivors are similar to those achieved with organs from other brain-dead donors.

Post-cardiac arrest syndrome

The resumption of spontaneous circulation after prolonged, complete ischaemia represents an unnatural pathophysiological state created by successful cardiopulmonary resuscitation. Prolonged whole-body ischaemia causes global tissue and organ injury, and additional damage occurs during and after reperfusion.

The expression 'post-cardiac arrest syndrome' was introduced in 2008 to describe a combination of pathophysiological processes compounding the primary condition that led to cardiac arrest. The concept dates back to the early 1970s. The expression 'post-cardiac arrest syndrome' replaces the previous formulation 'post-resuscitation disease', which somewhat implied that the act of resuscitation ended with ROSC. The pathophysiological processes involved in post-cardiac arrest syndrome are treatable and include: (i) a systemic ischaemia/reperfusion response; (ii) post-cardiac arrest myocardial dysfunction; and (iii) post-cardiac arrest brain injury. The severity of these disorders and their individual contributions to outcome vary in individual patients based on the duration of arrest and severity of the ischaemic insult, the primary cause of cardiac arrest and the patient's comorbidities.

Systemic ischaemia/reperfusion response

The systemic ischaemia/reperfusion response begins with the abrupt cessation of oxygen and metabolic substrates delivery and the accumulation of toxic metabolites in organs and tissues. Inadequate oxygen delivery persists during cardiopulmonary resuscitation (CPR), and even after ROSC due to post-cardiac arrest myocardial dysfunction and ongoing microcirculatory failure. The ischaemia/reperfusion sequence triggers generalized activation of immunological and coagulation pathways, leading to multiple organ failure with mechanisms resembling those described in severe sepsis. As early as 3 h after cardiac arrest, blood concentrations of various cytokines, soluble receptors and endotoxin increase; the magnitude of these changes correlates with outcome. The stress of total-body ischaemia/reperfusion also affects adrenal function. Although an increased plasma cortisol level occurs in many patients after out-of-hospital cardiac arrest, relative adrenal insufficiency, defined as failure to respond to corticotrophin stimulation, is common. Low basal cortisol levels are associated with refractory shock and early death. Other common manifestations of the systemic ischaemia/reperfusion response include intravascular volume depletion, impaired vasoregulation and increased susceptibility to infection. The analogies between the systemic ischaemia/reperfusion response and sepsis led to the theorization of an early goal-directed therapy following ROSC, as a strategy of early haemodynamic optimization was shown to reduce mortality in patients with severe sepsis. However, optimal goals and targets after ROSC remain to be identified and may vary greatly between patients depending, for example, on the primary cause of arrest. The concept of early haemodynamic optimization has yet to be proven, and universal targets might not be applicable to the non-homogeneous cohort of cardiac arrest survivors.

Post-cardiac arrest myocardial dysfunction

Post-cardiac arrest myocardial dysfunction consists of reversible myocardial stunning in patients with normal coronary perfusion. In swine models, the left ventricular ejection fraction decreases from 55 to 20% as early as 30 min after ROSC. In patients who survive out-of-hospital cardiac arrest, cardiac performance reaches its nadir at 8 h after resuscitation, improves substantially by 24 h and returns to normal by 72 h after ROSC. Post-cardiac arrest myocardial dysfunction is therefore reversible, and its responsiveness to inotropic drugs has been demonstrated widely in clinical and animal studies. Awareness of post-cardiac arrest myocardial dysfunction should not reduce clinical suspicion of acute coronary syndrome in patients presenting with haemodynamic instability. In out-of-hospital cardiac arrest studies, coronary occlusion and acute myocardial infarction are present in the majority of patients; a significant percentage of these do not have a history of angina or ST elevation. When available, timely angiographic assessment of coronary perfusion is indicated in patients with haemodynamic instability in order to identify those amenable to recanalization.

Anoxic–ischaemic brain injury

Anoxic–ischaemic brain injury is the main cause of disability and mortality after cardiac arrest. In a study that looked at the mode of death of patients admitted to the ICU after ROSC (the mode of death was classified as: neurological death, cardiovascular death or multiple organ failure), the cause of death was anoxic–ischaemic neurological injury in approximately 70% of out-of-hospital and 20% of in-hospital cardiac arrest survivors admitted to the ICU but not surviving to be discharged from hospital. The mechanisms of brain injury triggered by cardiac arrest and subsequent reperfusion are complex and include excitotoxicity, free-radical formation, disrupted calcium homeostasis and apoptosis. Other factors that can impact on brain injury after cardiac arrest are pyrexia, hyper- and hypoglycaemia, and seizures. Prolonged cardiac arrest can also be followed by microvascular thrombosis and autoregulation impairment, leading to microcirculatory failure and persistent no-reflow ischaemia despite adequate cerebral perfusion pressure. All these phenomena take place over a period of hours to days after ROSC. A detailed description of the molecular pathways and physiopathological mechanisms involved in secondary anoxic–ischaemic brain injury is beyond the scope of this chapter; the important point to be made here is that it is a process rather than a single event. The existence of a broad therapeutic window for neuroprotective strategies after cardiac arrest is a concept proven by the efficacy of therapeutic hypothermia.

Clinical manifestations

The clinical manifestations of post-cardiac arrest brain injury include disorders of arousal and awareness, seizures, neuropsychological dysfunction and brain death. Coma is a common acute presentation of post-cardiac arrest brain injury, representing extensive yet potentially reversible dysfunction of the areas of the brain responsible for arousal (ascending reticular formation, pons, midbrain, diencephalon and cortex) and awareness (cortex and subcortical structures). Due to the higher vulnerability of cortical areas in comparison with the brainstem and diencephalon, many comatose survivors will eventually regain arousal with a preserved sleep–wake cycle. However, most patients 'wake up' with different degrees of long-lasting neuropsychological impairment, ranging from mild cognitive deficits to severe changes in personality or a persistent vegetative state.

Diagnosis

The diagnosis of anoxic–ischaemic coma is based on a Glasgow Coma Score of <8 (patients not opening eyes, not uttering words and not executing finalized movements) and a clinical history compatible with cerebral ischaemia caused by either global hypoperfusion (e.g. cardiac arrest, hanging) or cerebral hypoxia in the setting of adequate cerebral perfusion (e.g. respiratory failure, carbon monoxide poisoning). Differential diagnoses include toxicity (notably: neuromuscular blocking agents and sedatives administered during resuscitation), hypothermia, hyper- and hypoglycaemia and other metabolic causes of coma, non-convulsive status epilepticus and locked-in syndrome. Although CT appearances are often normal in the first hours after cardiac arrest, an early CT head scan is indicated to exclude the presence of space-occupying lesions, hydrocephalus and cerebrovascular events. CT features of anoxic–ischaemic brain injury appear 6–12 h after injury and are non-specific. After cerebral ischaemia, CT can show various degrees of brain oedema going from loss of grey/white matter differentiation to effacement of subarachnoid spaces and brain herniation. Diffusion-weighted MRI (DWI) is a more accurate method for early diagnosis of both focal and global cerebral infarction. Typically, cortical laminar hyperintensity resulting from cytotoxic oedema and restricted diffusion of free water can be demonstrated in patients with severe anoxic-ischaemic brain injury. Although these changes can be detected within the first hour after the event, MRI is unpractical and remains insufficiently specific for early prognostication. Therefore, MRI is not a priority and the transport of unstable patients is commonly deferred for 48–72 h after cardiac arrest. Early EEG studies should be performed in all patients who remain comatose despite the cessation of sedation to exclude non-convulsive status epilepticus and to inform prognosis.

Acute management

The acute management of post-cardiac arrest syndrome starts at the location where ROSC is achieved. Once stabilized, the patient should be transferred to the most appropriate intensive care area for continued monitoring and treatment (Fig. 29.2). The priorities of the acute intensive care management of cardiac arrest survivors are: (i) provision of organ support; (ii) prevention of recurrence; (iii) minimization of ongoing cerebral and cardiac injury; and (iv) prompt diagnosis and treatment of the disease that lead to cardiac arrest and underlying comorbidities.

Airway

Patients who have had a brief period of cardiac arrest responding immediately to appropriate treatment may not require tracheal intubation and ventilation; oxygen administered via a facemask may suffice in such cases. Tracheal intubation, sedation and controlled ventilation are indicated in all patients with obtunded cerebral function and/or ongoing respiratory failure. Hypoxia and hypercarbia should be prevented as they increase the likelihood of a further cardiac arrest and may contribute to secondary brain injury. The stomach is likely to be distended by mouth-to-mouth or bag–mask–valve ventilation, splinting the diaphragm and impairing ventilation. A gastric tube should routinely be inserted to allow gastric decompression and early initiation of enteral feeding.

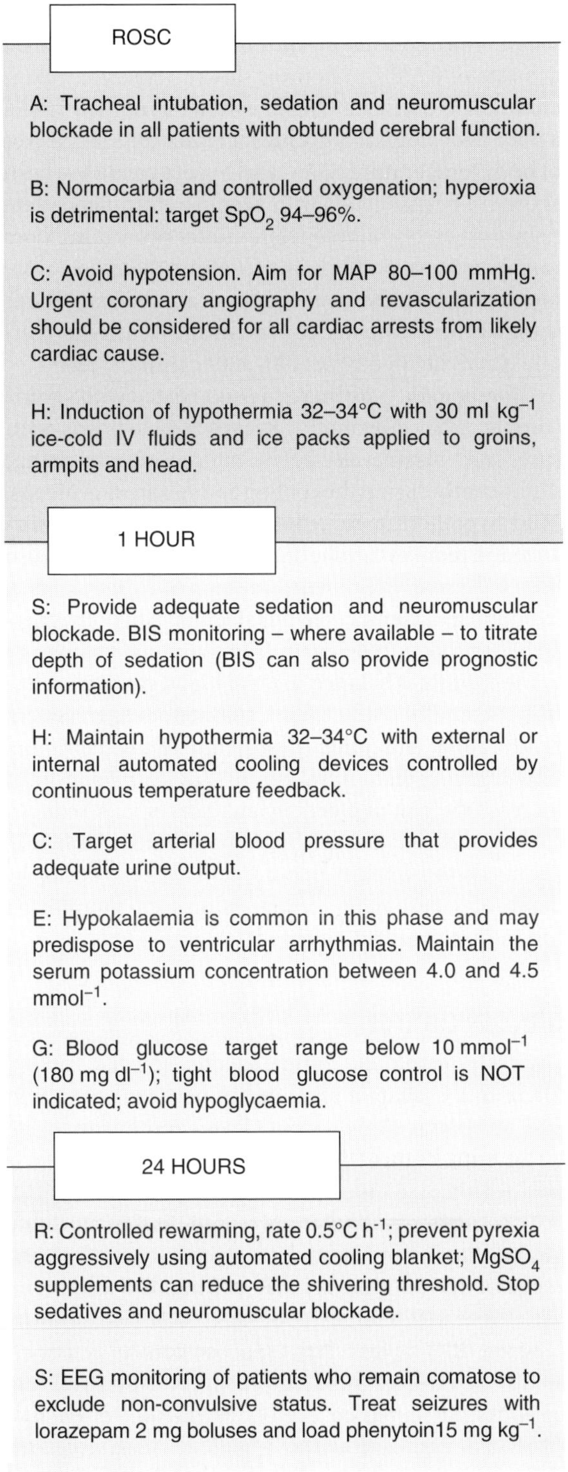

ROSC

A: Tracheal intubation, sedation and neuromuscular blockade in all patients with obtunded cerebral function.

B: Normocarbia and controlled oxygenation; hyperoxia is detrimental: target SpO_2 94–96%.

C: Avoid hypotension. Aim for MAP 80–100 mmHg. Urgent coronary angiography and revascularization should be considered for all cardiac arrests from likely cardiac cause.

H: Induction of hypothermia 32–34°C with 30 ml kg^{-1} ice-cold IV fluids and ice packs applied to groins, armpits and head.

1 HOUR

S: Provide adequate sedation and neuromuscular blockade. BIS monitoring – where available – to titrate depth of sedation (BIS can also provide prognostic information).

H: Maintain hypothermia 32–34°C with external or internal automated cooling devices controlled by continuous temperature feedback.

C: Target arterial blood pressure that provides adequate urine output.

E: Hypokalaemia is common in this phase and may predispose to ventricular arrhythmias. Maintain the serum potassium concentration between 4.0 and 4.5 $mmol^{-1}$.

G: Blood glucose target range below 10 $mmol^{-1}$ (180 mg dl^{-1}); tight blood glucose control is NOT indicated; avoid hypoglycaemia.

24 HOURS

R: Controlled rewarming, rate 0.5°C h^{-1}; prevent pyrexia aggressively using automated cooling blanket; $MgSO_4$ supplements can reduce the shivering threshold. Stop sedatives and neuromuscular blockade.

S: EEG monitoring of patients who remain comatose to exclude non-convulsive status. Treat seizures with lorazepam 2 mg boluses and load phenytoin 15 mg kg^{-1}.

Fig. 29.2. Management of post-cardiac arrest syndrome – a time-sensitive process. MAP, mean arterial pressure; BIS, bispectral index.

Breathing

Hypocarbia causes cerebral vasoconstriction and decreased cerebral blood flow and should be avoided. End-tidal carbon dioxide and arterial carbon dioxide should be monitored and ventilation should be adjusted to achieve normocarbia. A growing body of pre-clinical evidence suggests that hyperoxia during the early stages of reperfusion harms neurons by causing excessive oxidative stress. In animal models of cardiac arrest, ventilation with 100% oxygen for the first hour after ROSC resulted in a worse neurological outcome than immediate adjustment of the fraction of inspired oxygen (FiO_2) to produce an arterial oxygen saturation (SaO_2) of 94–96%. On these bases, unnecessary hyperoxia should be avoided and FiO_2 should be adjusted to the FiO_2 needed to produce an SaO_2 of 94–96%. A chest radiograph should be requested to confirm tracheal tube, gastric tube and central line positioning, and to exclude CPR complications such as rib fractures and pneumothorax.

Circulation

Adequate venous access and invasive arterial blood pressure monitoring are essential. Optimization of right-heart filling pressures should be achieved with intravenous fluids. Inotropes and vasopressors are indicated if haemodynamic instability persists despite an adequate pre-load. Choice and titration of inotropes or vasopressors should be guided by blood pressure, heart rate, echocardiographic estimates of myocardial dysfunction and by surrogate measures of tissue oxygen delivery such as mixed central venous oxygen saturations and lactate clearance. Pulmonary artery catheters and other forms of non-invasive cardiac monitoring can inform choice and titration of vasopressors and inotropic support on the basis of cardiac index and systemic vascular resistance. Haemodynamic monitoring can provide a rationale for inotropic and vasopressor titration in patients with refractory haemodynamic instability. However, a favourable impact of advanced haemodynamic monitoring on outcome in cardiac arrest survivors is not supported by evidence. The value of early goal-directed therapy in post-cardiac arrest care has also yet to be demonstrated in randomized prospective clinical trials. Reasonable targets should be determined in individual patients based on primary disease and comorbidities, presumed normal blood pressure and urinary output achieved.

Early coronary reperfusion

Coronary artery disease is present in the majority of out-of-hospital cardiac arrest patients. Early coronary angiography and percutaneous coronary intervention (PCI) after out-of-hospital cardiac arrest are feasible and have been shown to improve outcome in a number of non-randomized studies. In a recent study, the overall in-hospital mortality rate decreased from 72 to 44% after the introduction of a comprehensive post-cardiac arrest care bundle, which included intensive coronary reperfusion strategy and therapeutic hypothermia. Notably, 90% of survivors were neurologically normal. All patients resuscitated from cardiac arrest in whom acute coronary syndrome is suspected or who have ECG criteria for ST-elevation myocardial infarction should undergo immediate coronary angiography with subsequent PCI. If PCI is not available, thrombolytic therapy is an acceptable alternative for the management of ST-elevation myocardial infarction.

Therapeutic hypothermia

Unconscious adult patients with ROSC after out-of-hospital ventricular fibrillation cardiac arrest should be cooled to 32–34°C for 12–24 h. Preliminary evidence supports the idea that hypothermia may also benefit unconscious adult patients with ROSC after out-of-hospital cardiac arrest from a non-shockable rhythm or after in-hospital cardiac arrest. Although the optimal timing of initiation and duration of hypothermia has not been defined, the current consensus is to initiate cooling as soon as possible and to maintain hypothermia for at least 24 h. Rapid intravenous infusion of ice-cold 0.9% NaCl or Ringer's lactate is a simple, effective method for initiating cooling. Ice packs can be placed on the groin, armpits and head to expedite the induction of hypothermia. These low-tech methods are compatible with the transfer of patients to the angiography suite for PCI. Sedation and neuromuscular blockade should be administered to prevent shivering. Magnesium sulfate ($50 \, mg \, kg^{-1}$) reduces shivering thresholds and is a vasodilator, and can therefore expedite the cooling phase and facilitate maintenance of hypothermia. There are no data to indicate whether or not the choice of sedation influences outcome; short-acting sedatives have the theoretical advantage of allowing earlier neurological assessment. Maintenance of hypothermia is best achieved with surface or intravascular cooling devices with continuous temperature feedback. Ice packs represent a cheaper alternative but

their use is time-consuming and leads to suboptimal temperature control. Rewarming should be controlled at a rate of 0.5°C per hour or slower. Hyperthermia is common in the first 48 h after cardiac arrest. The risk of a poor neurological outcome increases for each degree of body temperature >37°C and hyperpyrexia has been shown to be associated with a temperature-dependent failure of cerebral autoregulation after rewarming from therapeutic hypothermia. Continued temperature monitoring, antipyretics and physical cooling methods should be implemented to prevent and treat hyperthermia occurring in the first 72 h after cardiac arrest.

Therapeutic hypothermia is associated with several complications. Metabolic rate, arterial blood gas pressures and plasma electrolyte concentrations change significantly during the cooling and rewarming phases. Mild hypothermia increases systemic vascular resistance and reduces cardiac output. Hypothermia can also have a diuretic effect, with subsequent hypovolaemia, hypophosphataemia, hypokalaemia, hypomagnesaemia and hypocalcaemia. It is therefore mandatory to monitor fluid balance, arterial blood gases and electrolytes, and to correct these parameters aggressively. Bradycardia and other dysrhythmias are common. Impaired coagulation and immunological response can increase the risk of bleeding and infection. A reduced clearance of sedative drugs and neuromuscular blockers needs to be taken into account. Where available, depth-of-sedation and suppression-rate monitoring can inform the titration of sedative infusions.

Glucose control

Hyperglycaemia is common after cardiac arrest. There is a U-shaped relationship between maximum and minimum blood glucose levels and hospital survival: both high and low glucose values are associated with worse outcome. A recent trial of over 6000 ICU patients reported an increased 90-day mortality among those randomized to glucose control in the range of 4.5–6.0 mmol l^{-1} (80–110 mg dl^{-1}) compared with those with a target blood glucose of 10.0 mmol l^{-1} (180 mg dl^{-1}) or less. Strict glucose control is associated with a higher incidence of severe hypoglycaemic episodes. An increased level of neuron-specific enolase (NSE) after cardiac arrest in patients managed with strict glucose controls when compared with patients with moderate (<10 mmol l^{-1}) glucose targets also suggests a detrimental effect and more severe brain injury. Patients achieving ROSC after cardiac arrest should therefore not be treated with strict glucose control targeting normoglycaemia but with a blood glucose target range of below 10 mmol l^{-1} (180 mg dl^{-1}).

Seizures

Seizures and/or myoclonus occur in 5–15% of patients who achieve ROSC and in approximately 40% of those who remain comatose. Prolonged seizure activity may cause cerebral injury and should be controlled with propofol, benzodiazepines, phenytoin, sodium valproate or a barbiturate. There is no available evidence determining the superiority of any class of anticonvulsants over another. Clonazepam, sodium valproate and levetiracetam have a role in the treatment of myoclonus refractory to phenytoin. No studies have determined the benefits of prophylactic anticonvulsant drugs or continuous EEG monitoring after cardiac arrest.

Adrenal dysfunction

Relative adrenal insufficiency occurs frequently after successful resuscitation and is associated with increased mortality. However, the use of steroids has not been studied in the post-cardiac arrest phase and remains a controversial topic. Therefore, routine use of steroids after cardiac arrest is not recommended.

Precipitating pathologies

Causes of cardiac arrest include cerebrovascular catastrophes, pulmonary embolism, sepsis, haemorrhage, hypovolaemia, respiratory failure, metabolic disorders, tension pneumothorax, cardiac tamponade and poisoning. These potential causes of cardiac arrest must be diagnosed promptly and treated according to available guidelines.

Outcome prediction in anoxic–ischaemic encephalopathy

Highly specific, poorly sensitive predictions of unfavourable outcome

Physicians caring for comatose cardiac arrest survivors often face gruelling, life-and-death decision-making moments. Continued treatment might imply survival with severe disability, including the prospect of a persistent vegetative state, while early withdrawal of organ support might deprive a patient of chances of a meaningful recovery. If physicians had prognostic tests able to predict with accuracy the whole spectrum of possible outcomes from severe disability to good recovery, they would be able to consistently manage patients' care according to patients' wishes. Unfortunately, this is not the case. In practice, the prime and only realistic objective of early prognostication after a cardiac arrest is a highly specific (and poorly sensitive) prediction of an outcome no better than death, vegetative state or severe disability with total dependency.

The brainstem is more resistant to anoxic–ischaemic damage than the cerebral cortex; thus, although compromise of brainstem reflexes suggests that the cortex must be severely damaged, the opposite is not necessarily true. Preserved brainstem reflexes do not imply intact cortical function. The absence of one or more brainstem reflexes is therefore a highly specific but poorly sensitive predictor of poor outcome. Similar considerations apply to all other available prognostic factors. Sadly, the prediction of a favourable outcome remains insufficiently accurate for use on individual patients and certainly inadequate to influence critical decision-making.

A highly specific prognostication of poor outcome can justify early withdrawal of life support in patients with a negligible chance of making a good recovery, preventing unnecessary prolonged suffering for patients and their carers while pre-empting inappropriate allocation of healthcare resources. However, the lack of sensitivity of current prognostic tests means that many patients who do not have early unfavourable features and are treated aggressively will live on in a persistent vegetative state or severely disabled. Around 10% of non-traumatic comatose patients regain consciousness at 3 months. Most, but not all, live on with severe disability. As things stand, physicians are therefore unable to provide these patients with a robust prognosis before many months of rehabilitation.

Available evidence and intrinsic pitfalls of prognostication

It is mandatory to discuss here the intrinsic limitations of the available evidence. Firstly, between-institutions differences in management protocols can affect the accuracy of generalized prognostic predictions, especially when predictive values are applied to institutions with patient populations and clinical protocols that differ greatly from those where the predictive values were derived. However, the two most dangerous pitfalls when interpreting available evidence on prognostication following anoxic–ischaemic brain injury lie in the so-called 'self-fulfilling prophecy bias' of observational studies and in the *presumed* prognostic validity of historical data in a context of ever-changing standards of care, in particular after the introduction of therapeutic hypothermia.

In observational studies, clinical care is often informed by the presence or absence of negative prognostic factors. In such cases, the presumption of an adverse outcome is likely to create self-fulfilling prophecies. If treatment is withdrawn in patients with a *presumed significant* negative prognostic factor, observational studies biased by the self-fulfilling studies will *confirm* the validity of that prognostic factor to *predict* death. Bearing this important limitation in mind, there was considered to be a sufficiently robust body of evidence coming from well-designed, blinded, prospective studies for the prognostication of cardiac arrest survivors. In 2006, the American Academy of Neurology (AAN) summarized the available evidence and published a set of guidelines for the prognostication of poor outcome in cardiac arrest survivors with anoxic–ischaemic encephalopathy, proposing a simple algorithm for clinical use. A second pitfall lies in the supposed validity – today – of historical studies that do not take into account changes in clinical practice and their impact on outcome. Current guidelines were developed before the widespread introduction of therapeutic hypothermia – nowadays considered a therapeutic standard – putting into question the validity of these historical studies in the context of profoundly changed therapeutic protocols. Firstly, the early neurological examination proposed by the AAN guidelines is unreliable in the first 24 h in patients who are cooled during CPR or early after ROSC. Furthermore, more and more evidence is building up suggesting that early prognostication (especially the motor score) is less reliable than previously thought in comatose survivors of cardiac arrest treated with hypothermia. In such cases, the AAN guidelines for neurological prognostication should be applied with great caution in order to prevent overpessimistic estimations of poor recovery and premature cessation of intensive care.

Common confounders

Clinical examination must always take into account the presence of sedatives, opioids, neuromuscular blocking agents, antimuscarinic drugs, catecholamines and all other medications that can be used during resuscitation. Testing should be postponed until there is ample evidence that these medications have been cleared from the circulation. Hypothermia, hypo- or hyperglycaemia, and electrolyte and metabolic disturbances are also common in cardiac arrest survivors and invalidate neurological examinations. As a telling example, even a strong predictor of poor outcome such as the absence of a pupillary reaction to light has an unacceptably low specificity when the examination is performed early after a cardiac arrest. Due to the aforementioned confounding factors, absence of pupillary light reflex at the time of hospital admission after a cardiac arrest has a reported estimated false-positive rate of up to 31%. This means that approximately one patient out of three admitted to hospital with fixed pupils after cardiac arrest could have an outcome better than poor. This kind of specificity is obviously inadequate to inform early withdrawal of treatment based on the absence of pupillary reflex on admission alone.

Brainstem reflexes

In patients not treated with hypothermia, the absence of one or more brainstem reflexes 72 h after cardiac arrest provides a conclusive poor prognosis. Patients with absent pupillary reflex have an outcome not better than death or severe disability, with a reported false-positive rate of 0% (95% confidence interval (CI) 0–3%). Absence of the corneal reflex (contraction of the orbicularis oculi in response to gentle corneal stimulation) and absence of the caloric vestibular–ocular reflex (eye movements in response to irrigation of the ear canal with ice water) also have a false-positive rate of 0% (with a reported 95% CI of 0–41% for both signs). A recent prospective study on 111 comatose survivors of cardiac arrest treated with therapeutic hypothermia confirmed that incomplete recovery of brainstem reflexes (defined as the inability to elicit one or more of pupillary, corneal and oculocephalic reflexes) at 72 h is an independent predictor of poor outcome. However, the reported false-positive rate was not 0%, as in patients not treated with hypothermia, but 4% (two patients out of the 45 showing incomplete recovery of brainstem reflexes at 72 h had a positive outcome at discharge).

Motor response

In patients not treated with hypothermia, a motor response to noxious stimuli that is no better than extensor posturing (decerebrate response or no response) at

72 h has a reported false-positive rate for poor outcome of 0% (95% CI 0–9%) and was therefore included in the AAN guidelines as an independent, conclusive predictor of poor outcome. In patients who were treated with hypothermia, decerebrate posturing or no motor response on day 3 was also confirmed to be an independent predictor of poor outcome; however, the reported false-positive rate for outcome better than poor in patients treated with hypothermia was a massive 16% (four patients out of the 25 patients decerebrating or not moving in response to a noxious stimulus on day 3 ultimately made a good recovery). This kind of false-positive rate is obviously inadequate to inform withdrawal of treatment based on the motor score alone. Furthermore, a small study of 37 initially comatose patients who underwent hypothermia showed recovery of awareness on day 6 in two out of 14 patients who had a motor response that was no better than extensor posturing at 72 h post-arrest. At the very least, the available evidence warrants caution when relying on the motor response alone before day 6 after rewarming for patients treated with hypothermia.

Myoclonic status epilepticus

Myoclonic status epilepticus is defined as a bilateral, synchronous twitching of limb, trunk or facial muscles. Myoclonic status epilepticus must be differentiated from generalized tonic–clonic seizures and from multifocal, asynchronous myoclonus. Tonic–clonic seizures are extremely common in cardiac arrest survivors and represent a non-specific indicator of metabolic encephalopathy without a strong prognostic value. On the other hand, when myoclonic status epilepticus is observed 24 h after arrest in patients not treated with hypothermia, it predicts a poor outcome with a false-positive rate of 0% (95% CI 0–14%). Myoclonic status epilepticus retains its significance as an independent predictor of poor outcome following therapeutic hypothermia. However, the false-positive rate is not 0% (one out of 25 patients with myoclonus in the first 24 h made a good recovery at 6 months).

Electrophysiological tests

The measurement of somatosensory evoked potentials (SSEPs), especially the absence of the N20 response (electroencephalographic upward deflection at the primary somatosensory cortex 20 ms after electrical stimulation of the median nerve at the wrist), has emerged as the most accurate predictor of a poor outcome in patients with anoxic–ischaemic encephalopathy. If the N20 responses are absent at day 1, they can be repeated at day 3 or beyond; however, if N20 responses are lost at any point, the prognosis is unequivocally poor. In a meta-analysis of studies involving 801 patients, bilateral absence of the N20 response at 72 h was associated with no false positives for poor outcome (95% CI 0–2%). The significance of SSEPs as an independent factor that could reliably, by itself, predict poor outcome was recently confirmed in patients exposed to therapeutic hypothermia; bilaterally absent N20 is currently the only variable that predicts death with a estimated false-positive rate of 0% in patients treated with hypothermia. However, SSEP results were taken into account when considering withdrawal of treatment, and the self-fulfilling prophecy bias cannot be excluded; caution is warranted for the use of SSEPs alone to inform withdrawal of treatment in patients treated with hypothermia. Preliminary evidence suggests that an unreactive EEG background in the first 72 h is a strong independent risk factor for mortality in patients treated with hypothermia following cardiac arrest. Malignant EEG patterns (such as burst suppression, or low-voltage delta, theta or alpha coma) are also ominous predictors of poor outcome. In a recent study, all post-cardiac arrest patients who had bispectral index (BIS) values of zero had a bad neurological outcome after cardiac arrest and induced hypothermia. However, insufficient data is available to put exact numbers on the accuracy of these predictors at the present stage.

Neuroimaging

CT imaging performed immediately after cardiac arrest is often normal and, with the exclusion of catastrophic cerebral swelling and herniation, cannot determine the severity of anoxic–ischaemic brain injuries. Early CT imaging is nevertheless indicated, as there may be clinically relevant information that could affect immediate management of these patients, even when non-neurological causes of cardiac arrest are suspected. Intracranial haemorrhage is detected in approximately 10% of comatose survivors of non-traumatic out-of-hospital cardiac arrest. By day 3, CT can often detect brain swelling and inversion of the grey/white densities (with the use of quantitative measures) in patients with a poor outcome. However, CT head appearances were not included in the AAN guidelines, and no evidence is available regarding the accuracy of CT prognostication in cardiac arrest survivors treated with hypothermia. Limited evidence supports the use of MRI for prognostication. It is agreed that DWI and apparent diffusion coefficient (ADC) mapping performed at some point between days 3 and 5 after arrest have optimal specificity. However, seizures can reversibly affect MRI findings and further research is required before including brain MRI in prognostication protocols.

Biomarkers

The ease of data acquisition implied in the use of biochemical markers implies intuitive practical advantages over electrophysiological tests and brain imaging. Biomarker measurement does not require time-consuming tests and does not necessitate complex electrophysiological monitoring machinery or transport of unstable patients outside the ICU. The most promising biomarker is NSE, which is released by destruction of cells with neuronal (or neuroendocrine) differentiation, and its concentration in the blood is assumed to be proportional to the extent of hypoxic brain injury after cardiac arrest. In one prospective, multicentre study involving 231 patients, an NSE level of $>33 \mu g \, l^{-1}$ (sampling occurred between 1 and 3 days after cardiac arrest) was strongly predictive of a poor outcome with no false positives. An NSE threshold of $33 \mu g \, l^{-1}$ was therefore included in the AAN guidelines with a proposed false-positive rate of 0%. However, these results may have been hampered by selection bias and the self-fulfilling prophecy bias. Although confirmed in more recent non-blinded studies, other authors have suggested that the $33 \mu g \, l^{-1}$ threshold would yield a false-positive rate of 9.6% (17/177 patients with NSE $>33 \mu g \, l^{-1}$ would have been falsely classified as having a poor neurological outcome in a recent blinded study). The diagnostic accuracy of serum NSE could be even lower in patients treated with hypothermia. Although extremely rare, the coincidental occurrence of NSE-producing tumours such as small-cell lung carcinoma, neuroblastoma and carcinoid tumours should be kept in mind when using this method for prognostic assessment after cardiac arrest. Moreover, an internationally accepted standard for serum NSE determination is still lacking. Due to all of the aforementioned limitations, we do not include serum NSE in our prognostication algorithm.

Other clinical variables

Age, gender, cause of arrest, type of arrhythmia and duration of CPR have significant but insufficient

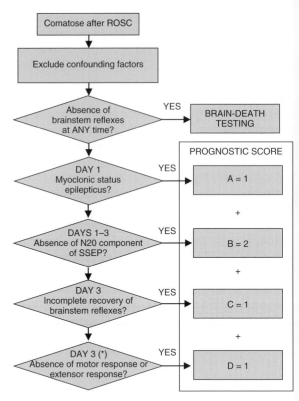

Fig. 29.3. Prognostication algorithm for anoxic–ischaemic encephalopathy derived from the AAN guidelines. A prognostic score (A + B + C + D) ≥2 can inform withdrawal of treatment in cardiac arrest survivors treated with hypothermia.

predictive value. Measures of cerebral metabolism such as positron emission tomography (PET) and determination of intracranial pressure, monitoring of brain oxygen or jugular venous oxygenation are not sufficiently discriminatory for a poor outcome to be clinically useful.

Prognostication algorithm

The emerging consensus is that after therapeutic hypothermia, prognostication should be delayed until at least 3 days after normothermia has been restored. The motor response may be delayed in hypothermia-treated patients and should not be taken into account before day 6 after rewarming. With these caveats, clinical predictors of poor outcome are reliable, regardless of whether or not hypothermia was used. However, when used by themselves in patients treated with hypothermia, clinical predictors (with the notable exception of absence of the N20 response) have a false-positive rate greater than 0. The prognostication algorithm presented here is derived from the AAN guidelines and takes into account recent evidence derived from patients treated with hypothermia (Fig. 29.3). In patients not treated with hypothermia, a single negative prognostic factor predicts poor outcome with a false-positive rate of 0%. In patients treated with hypothermia, either the absence of the N20 response or at least two other negative features should be present to exclude with certainty the possibility of a meaningful recovery. Based on the proposed algorithm, it is ethically justifiable to withdraw support from patients with a prognostic score >1 if they were not treated with hypothermia, or with a prognostic score >2 if they were treated with hypothermia. It goes without saying that every case should be considered individually in the context of all available information, the algorithm being a summary of the available evidence that should be used as the basic structure of the decision-making process. Withdrawal of treatment can also be considered for patients not fulfilling the prognostic criteria proposed here based on the severity of the primary disease and the patient's living will.

Further reading

Adrie, C., Adib-Conquy, M., Laurent, I. et al. (2002). Successful cardiopulmonary resuscitation after cardiac arrest as a "sepsis-like" syndrome. Circulation 106, 562–8.

Adrie, C., Haouache, H., Saleh, M. et al. (2008). An underrecognized source of organ donors: patients with brain death after successfully resuscitated cardiac arrest. Intensive Care Med 34, 132–7.

Al Thenayan, E., Savard, M., Sharpe, M., Norton, L. and Young, B. (2008). Predictors of poor neurologic outcome after induced mild hypothermia following cardiac arrest. Neurology 71, 1535–7.

Anon. (1994). Medical aspects of the persistent vegetative state (1). The Multi-Society Task Force on PVS. N Engl J Med 330, 1499–508.

Anon. (1999). Guidelines for intensive care unit admission, discharge, and triage. Task Force of the American College of Critical Care Medicine, Society of Critical Care Medicine. Crit Care Med 27, 633–8.

Bernard, S. A., Gray, T. W., Buist, M. D. et al. (2002). Treatment of comatose survivors of out-of-hospital cardiac arrest with induced hypothermia. N Engl J Med 346, 557–63.

Binks, A. C., Murphy, R. E., Prout, R. E. et al. (2010). Therapeutic hypothermia after cardiac arrest – implementation in UK intensive care units. Anaesthesia 65, 260–5.

Cocchi, M. N., Lucas, J. M., Salciccioli, J. et al. (2010). The role of cranial computed tomography in the immediate post-cardiac arrest period. Intern Emerg Med 5, 533–8.

Els, T., Kassubek, J., Kubalek, R. and Klisch, J. (2004). Diffusion-weighted MRI during early global cerebral hypoxia: a predictor for clinical outcome? Acta Neurol Scand 110, 361–7.

Finfer, S., Chittock, D. R., Su, S. Y. et al. (2009). Intensive versus conventional glucose control in critically ill patients. N Engl J Med 360, 1283–97.

Guérit, J. M. (2010). Neurophysiological testing in neurocritical care. Curr Opin Crit Care 16, 98–104.

Hanada, H. and Okumura, K. (2009). From 4-links to 5-links of "chain of survival". Post-resuscitation care is critical for good neurological recovery. Circ J 73, 1797–8.

Hypothermia after Cardiac Arrest Study Group (2002). Mild therapeutic hypothermia to improve the neurologic outcome after cardiac arrest. N Engl J Med 346, 549–56.

Josephson, S. A. (2010). Predicting neurologic outcomes after cardiac arrest: the crystal ball becomes cloudy. Ann Neurol 67, A5–6.

Laver, S., Farrow, C., Turner, D. and Nolan, J. (2004). Mode of death after admission to an intensive care unit following cardiac arrest. Intensive Care Med 30, 2126–8.

Lavinio, A., Timofeev, I., Nortje, J. et al. (2007). Cerebrovascular reactivity during hypothermia and rewarming. Br J Anaesth 99, 237–44.

McKinney, A. M., Teksam, M., Felice, R. et al. (2004). Diffusion-weighted imaging in the setting of diffuse cortical laminar necrosis and hypoxic-ischemic encephalopathy. Am J Neuroradiol 25, 1659–65.

Negovsky, V. A. (1972). The second step in resuscitation – the treatment of the 'post-resuscitation disease'. Resuscitation 1, 1–7.

Nolan, J. P. and Soar, J. (2010). Postresuscitation care: entering a new era. Curr Opin Crit Care 16, 216–22.

Nolan, J. P., Deakin, C. D., Soar, J., Bottiger, B. W. and Smith, G. (2005). European Resuscitation Council guidelines for resuscitation 2005. Section 4. Adult advanced life support. Resuscitation 67 (Suppl. 1), S39–86.

Nolan, J. P., Laver, S. R., Welch, C. A. et al. (2007). Outcome following admission to UK intensive care units after cardiac arrest: a secondary analysis of the ICNARC Case Mix Programme Database. Anaesthesia 62, 1207–16.

Nolan, J. P., Neumar, R. W., Adrie, C. et al. (2008). Post-cardiac arrest syndrome: epidemiology, pathophysiology, treatment, and prognostication. A Scientific Statement from the International Liaison Committee on Resuscitation; the American Heart Association Emergency Cardiovascular Care Committee; the Council on Cardiovascular Surgery and Anesthesia;

the Council on Cardiopulmonary, Perioperative, and Critical Care; the Council on Clinical Cardiology; the Council on Stroke. *Resuscitation* **79**, 350–79.

Reisinger, J., Hollinger, K., Lang, W. *et al.* (2007). Prediction of neurological outcome after cardiopulmonary resuscitation by serial determination of serum neuron-specific enolase. *Eur Heart J* **28**, 52–8.

Rossetti, A. O., Oddo, M., Logroscino, G. and Kaplan, P. W. (2010). Prognostication after cardiac arrest and hypothermia: a prospective study. *Ann Neurol* **67**, 301–7.

Rundgren, M., Karlsson, T., Nielsen, N. *et al.* (2009). Neuron specific enolase and S-100B as predictors of outcome after cardiac arrest and induced hypothermia. *Resuscitation* **80**, 784–9.

Stammet, P., Werer, C., Mertens, L., Lorang, C. and Hemmer, M. (2009). Bispectral index (BIS) helps predicting bad neurological outcome in comatose survivors after cardiac arrest and induced therapeutic hypothermia. *Resuscitation* **80**, 437–42.

Sunde, K., Pytte, M., Jacobsen, D. *et al.* (2007). Implementation of a standardised treatment protocol for post resuscitation care after out-of-hospital cardiac arrest. *Resuscitation* **73**, 29–39.

Tiainen, M., Roine, R. O., Pettila, V. and Takkunen, O. (2003). Serum neuron-specific enolase and S-100B protein in cardiac arrest patients treated with hypothermia. *Stroke* **34**, 2881–6.

Wijdicks, E. F., Hijdra, A., Young, G. B., Bassetti, C. L. and Wiebe, S. (2006). Practice parameter: prediction of outcome in comatose survivors after cardiopulmonary resuscitation (an evidence-based review): report of the Quality Standards Subcommittee of the American Academy of Neurology. *Neurology* **67**, 203–10.

Young, G. B. (2009). Clinical practice. Neurologic prognosis after cardiac arrest. *N Engl J Med* **361**, 605–11.

Zandbergen, E. G., Hijdra, A., Koelman, J. H. *et al.* (2006). Prediction of poor outcome within the first 3 days of postanoxic coma. *Neurology* **66**, 62–8.

Chapter

30

Death and organ donation in neurocritical care

Neurological determination of death, and care of the heartbeating multiorgan donor and donation after circulatory death

Paul G. Murphy

Diagnosis of death

The earth is suffocating; swear that they will cut me open so that I will not be buried alive.

Final words of Frederick Chopin, Paris, 1849

The identification of the point of death is an issue that has troubled theologians, philosophers, ethicists, physicians, lawyers and the public for thousands of years. Leaving spiritual considerations aside, the need to diagnose the moment of death was historically based on the practical need to identify the point at which an individual could be considered to be a corpse and whose body could therefore be disposed of. Current medical opinion places death within the context of the interdependencies between neurophysiology and cardiorespiratory function but is also required to be critically aware of the potential for conflict generated by the ever-increasing demands for a deceased person's organs to be made available for the purposes of transplantation. It is therefore crucial that professional guidance on the diagnosis of death is based solely on the known clinical and pathophysiological facts around loss of cardiovascular, respiratory and neurological function and not on the process of warm ischaemia (which renders organs useless for transplantation).

Some philosophers and ethicists speculate that the loss of capacity for thought, reason and feeling may indicate a state of death of the person that can be distinguished from the biological death of the organism as a whole. However, there remains a professional and indeed societal conviction that death occurs as a single phenomenon that marks the end of the biological existence of the organism and that its timing can be identified with a reasonable degree of accuracy. Despite such consensus, it should not be assumed that this implies that there is universal professional agreement over the *criteria* by which biological death can be diagnosed. For instance, a small proportion of clinicians continue to challenge the proposition that irreversible brain failure meets the standards necessary for the recognition of biological death. The various objections to such a neurological standard for the diagnosis of biological death are as follows:

1. The current methods used to diagnose total brain failure cannot possibly interrogate the functional integrity of every neuronal pathway and, if such doubt exists, then the cautious clinician should favour the recognition of life (however restricted) rather than the declaration of biological death.

2. The original proposition that brain death is associated with a failure of somatic integration that will inevitably result in cardiovascular collapse within a few days or weeks of continued critical care is false, and longer-term somatic survival is possible, at least in a proportion of cases.

3. In patients whose suspected total brain failure is the consequence of a supratentorial pressure cone and global failure of cerebral perfusion, the apnoea test used to identify the absence of respiratory drive does so at the risk of increasing intracranial pressure and reducing cerebral perfusion. In other words, the apnoea test risks

Core Topics in Neuroanaesthesia and Neurointensive Care, eds. Basil F. Matta, David K. Menon and Martin Smith. Published by Cambridge University Press. © Cambridge University Press 2011.

creating the condition that it is designed to identify.

4. The concept of brain death is an arbitrary construct designed to maintain the availability of organs for the purposes of transplantation while maintaining the dead donor rule. (The latter states that, because organ retrieval should not cause the death of the donor, the donor must be dead before organ retrieval takes place.)

Despite these objections, and recognizing that the inevitability of somatic collapse has in the past been exaggerated, the overwhelming majority of clinicians recognize the validity of a neurological standard for biological death and maintain a moral reluctance to continue to ventilate a patient in established and irreversible apnoeic coma. The original UK Code of Practice for the diagnosis of brain death placed considerable emphasis on the principle that the simultaneous and irreversible loss of both the capacity for consciousness and the capacity to breathe was a state of biological death, with the loss of the biochemical processes that maintain the apparent integrity of residual somatic physiology merely being delayed by the continuance of mechanical ventilation and nutritional support. The President's Council on Bioethics in the USA has recently expanded on these ideas, proposing that, in order to be considered to be living, an organism must be a whole, with wholeness described as follows:

> Determining whether an organism remains a whole depends upon recognizing the persistence or cessation of the fundamental vital work of a living organism – the work of self-preservation, achieved through the organism's need-driven commerce with the surrounding world. When there is good reason to believe that an injury has irreversibly destroyed an organism's ability to perform its fundamental vital work, then the conclusion that the organism as a whole has died is warranted.

The statement of the Presidential Council goes on to define the essential elements of an organism's vital work of commerce with its surroundings as follows:

1. Openness or receptivity to the signals and stimuli that emanate from the environment – consciousness.

2. The ability of an organism to interact with the environment to selectively obtain what it needs for survival, and an innate drive that compels an organism to do what it must to complete this interaction, e.g. through spontaneous respiration engage in the exchange of carbon dioxide for oxygen.

It is thereby concluded that a neurological standard that is based upon a robust identification of the simultaneous and irreversible loss of the capacity for consciousness along with the capacity to breathe meets the standard for determining the biological death of an organism.

Evolution of the concept of brain death

The natural history of a fatal intracranial catastrophe, such as a massive spontaneous intracerebral haematoma, is one of deep unresponsive coma caused by compression of the midbrain together with a critical reduction in cerebral perfusion pressure, apnoea that results from compression of respiratory centres in the pons and medulla oblongata and, in the absence of effective ventilatory support, agonal hypoxic asystole (Fig. 30.1). Although the precise sequence of events differs from death that follows a primary cardiac event, the constellation of clinical signs traditionally used to diagnose death by cardiorespiratory criteria, i.e. irreversible and simultaneous coma, apnoea and the absence of a circulation, remains the same. However, cardiopulmonary resuscitation and critical care now provide clinicians with the means to interrupt the hitherto inexorable progression from intracranial catastrophe and irreversible apnoea to cardiac death, and inadvertently generates a clinical state in which apnoeic coma is associated with at least some preservation of somatic function for as long as artificial mechanical ventilatory and nutritional support is continued.

The landmark description of this hitherto unrecognized complication of intensive care appeared in 1959, and was initially described as 'le coma dépassé' – literally, the state beyond coma. The following decade saw clinicians across the world debate the implications of this state of irreversible neurological oblivion, its relationship with the traditional form of cardiorespiratory death and the criteria by which it might be diagnosed with sufficient confidence to reassure both the medical profession and society at large. The latter was particularly important, as its close association with organ donation soon developed. Criteria in North America focused on death of the brain as a whole, i.e. (whole) brain death or total brain failure. In 1968, a report from an ad hoc committee at Harvard Medical School provided a definition of brain death that relied on the demonstration of complete loss of responsiveness and receptivity, loss of all motor activity (including spinal

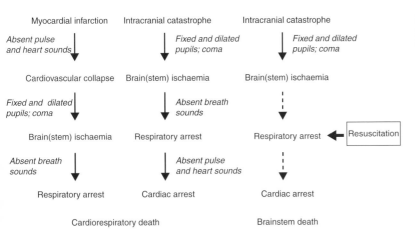

Fig. 30.1. Determination of death by cardiorespiratory and neurological criteria.

reflexes) and respiratory drive, within the overall context of a patient who was deeply unconscious and suffering from a cerebral insult of known cause. In 1971, criteria from Minnesota described the crucial importance of the loss of brainstem function as 'the point of no return' and also proposed that the diagnosis of brain death could in many circumstances be made clinically and without the need for confirmatory tests such as an EEG. Nevertheless, a report in 1981 from the Presidential Commission for the Study of Ethical Problems in Medicine and Biomedical and Behavioral Research advocated the continued use of confirmatory tests in circumstances where this would reduce the period of observation that would otherwise be necessary to make the diagnosis on clinical grounds alone. A more recent publication from the President's Council on Bioethics has continued to support the optional use of confirmatory tests such as EEG or cerebral angiography in circumstances where clinicians require independent verification that the vicious downward spiral of cerebral ischaemia and brain swelling has left a patient established on an irreversible path to total brain infarction. The Uniform Determination of Death Act established the legal basis for the diagnosis of death by neurological criteria in the USA in 1997 (Table 30.1).

The diagnosis of death has legal as well as clinical implications and, as a result, codes of practice for the diagnosis of brain death have become country or jurisdiction specific. Thus, there are variations in the criteria and codes of practice for the diagnosis of brain death around the world. While many of the differences between codes refer to operational specifics such as timing and repetition of testing, other variations are more fundamental and relate largely to the distinction between (whole) brain death and death of the

brainstem. This contrast came to the fore with the publication of the original UK criteria for the diagnosis of brain(stem) death in 1976. The original UK criteria were based on the principle that the irreversible loss of vital brainstem functions such as maintenance of consciousness and the capacity to breathe is as much a state of death as that of irreversible cardiac asystole. A further key proposition of the original UK Code was that, in the majority of circumstances at least, death of the brainstem could be determined clinically and without recourse to specialist investigations.

The original UK code clearly defines three discrete stages to the diagnosis of brain death:

1. The fulfilment of essential pre-conditions.
2. The satisfactory exclusion of potentially reversible causes of coma.
3. Clinical examination of the integrity of the brainstem and confirmation of the absence of various brainstem-hosted cranial nerve reflexes together with an apnoea test.

A completely revised Code of Practice for the Diagnosis of Death in the UK has recently been published by the Academy of the Medical Royal Colleges. This guidance builds on, rather than replaces, the original code and now recognizes a role for confirmatory testing in certain circumstances. Other important additions include guidance on biochemical tolerances for clinical testing, specific advice regarding circumstances where the validity of clinical examination may be uncertain (e.g. residual sedation), a more systematic and cautious approach to the apnoea test and a recognition that cardiorespiratory stability is an essential prerequisite for considering the diagnosis. Although the new UK code continues to refer to death of the *brainstem*,

Table 30.1 Landmarks in the evolution of criteria for the diagnosis of brain(stem) death

1894	Victor Horsley's classic description of respiratory arrest in cases of 'pathological intracranial tension'
1959	Mollaret and Goulon's landmark description of irreversible apnoeic coma ('le coma dépassé')
1968	An ad hoc committee of Harvard Medical School publishes a definition of brain death based on unresponsiveness, lack of receptivity, absence of movement and breathing, and brainstem areflexia within the context of coma of known cause
1971	Minnesota criteria emphasize the importance of loss of brainstem function in development of brain death
1971	Legislation in Finland recognizes brain death as a legal definition in death
1976	The Conference of the Medical Royal Colleges and their Faculties in the UK publish criteria for the diagnosis of brain death defined as the complete and irreversible loss of function of the brainstem
1981	The US Presidential Commission for the Study of Ethical Problems in Medicine and Biomedical and Behavioral Research publish *Defining Death: Medical, Legal and Ethical Issues in the Determination of Death*
1997	The Uniform Determination of Death Act establishes the legal basis for the diagnosis of death by neurological criteria in the USA
2008	The Academy of the Medical Royal Colleges publishes a new Code of Practice for the diagnosis of death in the UK
2008	The President's Council on Bioethics publishes *Controversies in the Determination of Death*

there seems little doubt that by endorsing the role of confirmatory tests that assess global brain function or blood flow, it has moved closer to the codes of practice used elsewhere in the world that are based on (whole) brain death.

Neurological determination of death

The diagnosis of brain death, now increasingly referred to as the neurological determination of death, requires consideration of the three discrete stages referred to above.

Pre-conditions and the causes of brain death

The neurological determination of death in an individual who is deeply unconscious and dependent on mechanical ventilation cannot be considered until a firm diagnosis of irremediable structural brain injury that is sufficient in nature and severity to explain the patient's condition has been made. Such assessments should be made only by clinicians with suitable experience in the management of patients with severe brain injury. Although not specifically required in the UK Code, it is increasingly unlikely that any clinician would consider the diagnosis of brainstem death without direct or radiological evidence of brain injury. The commonest cause of brain death is malignant intracranial hypertension, which may be consequent on a variety of diffuse or focal pathologies. It results in

axial descent of the brain through the tentorial hiatus and foramen magnum, disruption of the pontomedullary blood supply and direct compression of the brainstem by the cerebellar tonsils – so-called 'coning'. Less commonly, brain death results from direct damage to the medulla oblongata, pons and mesencephalon, usually a result of trauma or spontaneous haemorrhage. Some common causes of brain death are listed in Table 30.2.

Exclusions and irreversibility

A diagnosis of brain death cannot be made while there remains a possibility that coma is a consequence, in whole or in part, of potentially reversible influences such as hypothermia, intoxicating drugs and physiological, metabolic or endocrine disturbance.

Hypothermia

Profound hypothermia induces a reversible comatose state that mimics brain death. Although clinical confusion between this state and true brainstem death is unlikely, the contributory effects of lesser degrees of hypothermia to the profoundly injured brain are less clear. Furthermore, brain death is associated with hypothalamic failure and the inability to maintain a normal body temperature (poikilothermia). It is common for brain-dead patients to be hypothermic as a consequence. The current UK Code recommends that tests should not be performed if the body temperature is lower than 34°C.

Table 30.2 Causes of brain death

Supratentorial hypertension and medullary pressure cone	Focal pathologies: • Traumatic haematoma • Hydrocephalus • Spontaneous intracerebral haemorrhage • Ischaemic stroke • Malignancy • Cerebral abscess Diffuse brain injury (cerebral oedema): • Spontaneous subarachnoid haemorrhage • Diffuse axonal injury following trauma • Hypoxic/ischaemic brain injury • Meningitis/encephalitis
Direct brainstem injury	Trauma Malignancy Stroke

Circulatory, metabolic and endocrine disturbance

The diagnosis of brain death should not be considered in patients with cardiorespiratory instability or biochemical disturbances such as profound hyponatraemia, hypoglycaemia and acidosis. Haemodynamic instability at this stage is usually a reflection of the autonomic storm that is associated with profound brainstem ischaemia, and may be exacerbated by the hypovolaemia associated with uncorrected diabetes insipidus and diuretic therapy. Its correction with a combination of fluid resuscitation and vasopressor therapy is usually relatively straightforward. However, cardiovascular resuscitation can occasionally be challenging, particularly if there is significant neurogenic pulmonary oedema and cardiac injury.

A variety of metabolic and endocrine conditions can cause coma and/or profound flaccid paralysis. Clinicians should therefore carefully consider a patient's medical history and laboratory investigations to evaluate whether such factors are the cause of, or contributors to, apnoeic coma. Central diabetes insipidus is a common feature of brain death and, if uncorrected, results in excessive diuresis, hypovolaemia and hypernatraemia. Although many clinicians correct hypernatraemia with hypotonic solutions such as 5% dextrose or 0.45% NaCl, others only do so if they suspect that the disturbance in serum sodium preceded the patient's deterioration into a state of apnoeic coma. Disorders of plasma phosphate, calcium, potassium and magnesium may result in severe muscle weakness that can mimic some of the features of apnoeic coma and it is advised that these too should be close to their normal ranges. The revised UK Code also recommends that profound hypo- and hyperglycaemia should be excluded at the time of testing.

Drug intoxication

Drug intoxication represents a clinically significant reversible cause of coma and may complicate assessment, particularly when patients have received sedative drugs as part of their critical care treatment or when their brain injury occurred as a result of drug-induced self-harm. The most problematic circumstances are those where the identity of the intoxicating substances is unknown, where drug elimination is impaired by reduced hepatorenal function, or where agents with long context-sensitive half-lives have been used. The recommended approaches to the problem of residual sedation include the following:

- A period of observation that approximates to four times the elimination half-life of the agent, to allow effective drug elimination. This approach is best suited to circumstances where short-acting agents such as propofol and alfentanil have been administered to patients with normal hepatic and renal function.

- The administration of specific antagonists such as flumazenil or naloxone in circumstances where the residual effects of opioids or benzodiazepines is suspected.

- Analysis of plasma levels to confirm that a suspected sedative is either not detected or at a subtherapeutic level. This option is particularly suited for agents with long or unpredictable half-lives such as thiopental or phenobarbitone.

- On occasions where plasma analysis is not available, or the identity of the sedative drug is not known, a confirmatory test may be used to demonstrate the absence of cerebral blood flow. Options include cerebral angiography, transcranial Doppler ultrasonography or radioisotope perfusion scanning. It should be noted that, while confirmatory tests that examine neurological electrical activity or responsiveness may be of use in some circumstances (e.g. when access to various brainstem reflexes is restricted

Table 30.3 Cranial nerve reflexes used in the neurological determination of death

Reflex	Cranial nerves	Notes
Pupillary light reflex	II, III	Use bright light source (not that of a laryngoscope or ophthalmoscope) in a dimmed environment. Look for both direct and consensual reaction Important reflex that interrogates brainstem at level of midbrain
Corneal reflex	V, VII	Stroke edge of cornea with gauze, while gently holding eyelids open Care should be taken to avoid trauma to the cornea The various nuclei of V are found throughout the whole length of the brainstem, while that of VII (facial nerve) is in the upper medulla
Central response to deep somatic stimulation	V, VII	Apply deep pressure stimulation centrally (e.g. supraorbital ridge) and peripherally (e.g. nail bed). Look for a *central* motor response in the distribution of the facial nerve. Peripheral stimulation may illicit peripheral spinal reflexes
Cold caloric oculovestibular reflex	III, IV, VI, VIII	Establish clear access to the tympanic membrane by direct inspection with an auroscope Place the patient's head up at 30° to the horizontal unless this is contraindicated by an unstable cervical spine injury Slowly irrigate canal with 50 ml ice-cold water over 60 s. Observe for nystagmus for a further 30 s Contraindicated in trauma-related otorrhoea The nuclei of III and IV lie within the midbrain, while those of VI and VIII are in the medulla
Gag reflex	IX, X	Stimulate uvula under direct vision with throat spatula, observing for contraction of soft palate The nuclei of IX and X lie in the medulla
Tracheal cough reflex	X	Expose patient to umbilicus. Stimulate trachea to level of carina by introduction of sterile suction catheter down endotracheal tube. Observe for cough response

In circumstances where local injury or disease prevents examination of the pupillary, corneal and cold caloric reflexes on one or other side, clinical testing may nevertheless proceed. If access is prevented bilaterally, then the use of a confirmatory test should be considered.

or when a high cervical cord injury may confound interpretation of the apnoea test), they are of no value for the exclusion of drug intoxication.

Despite this general guidance, the revised UK Code of Practice remains permissive and allows clinicians latitude to dismiss the influence of sedative agents in circumstances where there is independent evidence to suggest that the patient is brain dead (e.g. on the basis of a CT head scan or a prolonged period of malignant intracranial hypertension).

Clinical testing for brain death

The confirmation of brain death requires the simultaneous demonstration of the irreversible loss of the capacity for consciousness as well as the capacity to breathe. Clinical assessment of the integrity of the brainstem has three components:

- Demonstration that a patient is in an unresponsive coma.

- Interrogation of a number of brainstem-mediated cranial nerve reflexes.
- The apnoea test.

While the conduct of testing overall is inevitably focused on this final stage of the process, it is vital to understand that the combination of deep coma, brainstem areflexia and apnoea can only be interpreted as being irreversible and therefore indicative of brain death if the essential pre-conditions have been met and the various potentially reversible influences robustly excluded. While errors in the diagnosis of brain death are extremely rare, they are invariably the result of failure to exclude inappropriate patients from testing or to identify potentially reversible influences, rather than due to errors in the performance of the clinical tests themselves.

Brainstem reflexes

Details of the brainstem reflexes incorporated into the UK Code are shown in Table 30.3. They are mediated

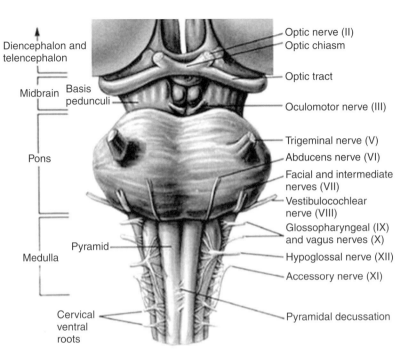

Diencephalon and telencephalon

Midbrain — Basis pedunculi

Pons

Pyramid

Medulla

Cervical ventral roots

Optic nerve (II)
Optic chiasm

Optic tract

Oculomotor nerve (III)

Trigeminal nerve (V)
Abducens nerve (VI)
Facial and intermediate nerves (VII)
Vestibulocochlear nerve (VIII)
Glossopharyngeal (IX) and vagus nerves (X)
Hypoglossal nerve (XII)
Accessory nerve (XI)

Pyramidal decussation

Fig. 30.2. Clinical anatomy of the brainstem.

by cranial nerves whose nuclei are located variously in the three components of the brainstem – the midbrain, the pons and the medulla oblongata (Fig. 30.2). Interrogation of these reflexes affords the clinician the opportunity to assess the integrity of the brainstem along much of its entire length. For example, the anatomical proximity within the midbrain of the nuclei of cranial nerves II and III to the reticular formation (the area of the brainstem that maintains consciousness) indicates the importance of being able to interrogate the pupillary light reflex, particularly as no other reflex interrogates midbrain function at such a high level. Similar importance can be attributed to the cough and gag reflexes because of the colocation of the nuclei of the glossopharyngeal and vagal nerves to the respiratory control centres within the medulla oblongata. The intervening reflex tests are the corneal reflex, the reflex that manifests central response to deep central or peripheral pain and the cold caloric oculovestibular reflex, all mediated by cranial nerve nuclei in the pons. Such overlap allows clinicians to proceed with testing even on occasions where trauma might render it impossible to test all cranial nerves reflexes, for example if one of the external auditory canals is inaccessible or facial swelling makes access to the corneas difficult.

Apnoea testing

Death of the brainstem results in irreversible and complete loss of the capacity to breathe. The apnoea test confirms the absence of respiration in a patient who has been disconnected from mechanical ventilation and who has an arterial carbon dioxide concentration ($PaCO_2$) that is above the level necessary to stimulate respiration. This level is normally set at 6.72 kPa (50 mmHg) but should be higher in patients with chronic carbon dioxide retention. Again, it is emphasized that the *irreversibility* of the condition is determined by the prior evaluation of the patient rather than by the test itself. In order to avoid exposing a patient who has residual brain activity to theoretically harmful rises in $PaCO_2$ and intracranial pressure, the apnoea test should not be performed until the complete absence of brainstem reflexes has been established and should be conducted in a fashion that allows a controlled rise in arterial carbon dioxide. The patient should be pre-oxygenated to prevent hypoxia during the period of apnoea and this can conveniently be done by administering 100% oxygen via the ventilator while examining the cranial nerve reflexes. During disconnection from the ventilator, oxygen should be delivered by bulk flow, preferably using a Mapleson C type rebreathing circuit rather than an intratracheal

Table 30.4 Revised schedule for the apnoea test (adapted from the Code of Practice for the Diagnosis and Confirmation of Death from the UK Academy of the Medical Royal Colleges)

1. Only perform after demonstration of brainstem areflexia
2. Increase FiO_2 to 1.0 and apply $EtCO_2$
3. Define relationship between arterial blood gases, SaO_2 and $EtCO_2$
4. When SaO_2 >95%, reduce ventilation until $EtCO_2$ > 6.0 kPa
5. Repeat arterial blood gas analysis and establish that $PaCO_2$ > 6.0 kPa and pH < 7.40
6. Confirm haemodynamic stability and disconnect from ventilation, maintaining oxygen delivery by bulk flow
7. Observe for 5 min, considering CPAP or recruitment manoeuvres if significant hypoxia develops during apnoeic interval
8. If apnoeic, confirm $PaCO_2$ > 6.5 kPa
9. In cases of chronic carbon dioxide retention or HCO_3^- therapy, adjust $EtCO_2/PaCO_2$ to achieve pH < 7.40

CPAP, continuous positive airway pressure; $EtCO_2$, end-tidal carbon dioxide; FiO_2, fraction of inspired oxygen; $PaCO_2$, arterial carbon dioxide tension; SaO_2, arterial oxygen saturation.

catheter. It is important to physically disconnect the patient from the ventilator during the apnoea test because the strength of cardiac pulsation is frequently sufficient to trigger ventilator-supported breaths in spontaneous breathing modes. While disconnected from the ventilator, the patient should be exposed down to the umbilicus, and their abdomen, chest and neck continuously observed for evidence of respiratory effort. Clinical observation should be supplemented by continuous palpation of the rebreathing bag and also with capnography if available. Patients with significant intrathoracic comorbidities such as pulmonary contusions or neurogenic pulmonary oedema may become hypoxaemic during the apnoeic period and it is occasionally necessary to apply continuous positive airway pressure or an occasional manual breath in such circumstances. A schedule for the conduct of the apnoea test as described in the revised UK Code is shown in Table 30.4.

Timing of testing and other organizational issues

Many clinicians offer family members the opportunity to witness the conduct of brainstem death testing. In such circumstances, it is good practice to identify whether the patient is likely to exhibit any spinal reflexes during testing and to prepare the witnesses for the tests accordingly. The UK Code does not prescribe when the tests should be performed, as this will vary considerably depending on the particular clinical circumstances. However, as a principle, the delay in performing the tests should be limited to the time required to fulfil the essential pre-conditions and exclude any reversible causes of coma and apnoea. In the UK, the tests must be performed by two experienced doctors working in a specialty with recognized experience and training in the diagnosis of brain death, at least one of whom must be a consultant. It is now mandatory that the two doctors perform the tests together and also that the tests be repeated in full, regardless of whether organ donation is being considered. In the UK, the time of death is the time at which the first set of tests is completed.

Implications of brainstem death

The brain-dead patient is dead, not dying. It is important that the patient's family understand that the neurological determination of death is not a prognosis of future (albeit inevitable) death but a diagnosis of death that is as valid as that which might be apportioned to cardiac death. Inevitably, the persistence of the circulation may prove a challenge for some families and result in conflict when the abject futility of further ventilatory support is discussed. On such occasions, it may be useful for families to understand that in circumstances where somatic function is maintained for some time after the diagnosis of neurological death (for example, to allow maturation of pregnancy), no element of neurological recovery has ever been observed. In the author's experience, allowing relatives the time to understand and accept the implications of the clinical diagnosis and prognosis of brain death is usually all that is required.

Management of the heartbeating brain-dead multiorgan donor

The ever-increasing demand for donor organs is a reflection of the effectiveness of transplantation as a treatment of end-stage organ failure, the incidence of which is rising largely because of the increasing prevalence of diabetes mellitus and hypertension in an ageing population. In contrast, the rates of brain death are falling, at least in part because of advances in the treatment of severe traumatic brain injury, ischaemic stroke and aneurysmal subarachnoid haemorrhage. Although there is no single solution to the challenge that the increasing shortage of deceased organ donors brings, it would seem appropriate to ensure that the gift of donation that is made by a deceased donor and his or her family is maximized, both in terms of the number of organs that are retrieved and in their quality and therefore longevity. There is now considerable evidence that the application of standardized donor management protocols provides an effective means of increasing the number of retrieved organs as well as increasing the proportion of brain-dead donors who are able to donate thoracic as well as abdominal organs. The role played by intensivists in organ donation should therefore not be limited to the identification and referral of potential donors but should extend to maximizing the number of organs offered for retrieval and optimizing their condition to ensure the best possible opportunity for a successful and long-lasting graft in the recipients.

Donor management requires a proactive approach that is based on a sound understanding of the physiological derangements exhibited by the brain-dead heartbeating donor. While some of these relate to the primary injury and the generic complications of critical care, there are two other processes that are specific to the severely brain-injured patient – the adverse systemic effects of brain-directed therapies and the pathophysiological consequences of brain death.

Systemic complications of brain-directed therapies

Protocols for the management of severe brain injury frequently focus on maintenance of cerebral perfusion, often to the detriment of other organ function (see Chapter 19). For example, respiratory failure is a common complication of brain injury. While this may be the result of aspiration of gastric or oropharyngeal contents at the time of the initial insult, more frequently it is a consequence of microaspiration, progressive sputum retention and dependent atelectasis in patients who are deeply sedated, pharmacologically paralysed and denied all but the most essential respiratory therapies and tracheal toilet. Furthermore, cerebral

perfusion-directed therapy incorporating fluid resuscitation and vasopressor support is also associated with a higher incidence of acute lung injury. Although cardiovascular impairment is less common, it can be equally catastrophic and has a multifactorial aetiology. Vasopressor infusions that are used to counter the hypotensive side effects of sedation may induce global subendocardial myocardial ischaemia, particularly when given in combination with infusions of propofol. Any resulting organ ischaemia will be further exacerbated by the hypovolaemia that results from aggressive osmotherapy regimens.

Pathophysiology of brain death

Haemodynamic instability is a characteristic feature of brain death. Progressive ischaemia of the brainstem leads to a massive release of catecholamines from sympathetic nerve endings and the neuroendocrine cells of the adrenal medulla. The resulting autonomic storm is characterized by a brief period of hypertension and myocardial irritability, followed by more prolonged vasoparalysis, hypotension and neurogenic pulmonary oedema (Fig. 30.3). The key contributions to the hypotension of brain death are as follows:

- Left ventricular failure consequent on the global myocardial ischaemia that follows the temporary period of extreme hypertension and systemic vasoconstriction that is the herald of the onset of brain death.
- A period of more prolonged, profound and refractory vasodilation ('vasoparalysis') that is a result of downregulation of peripheral catacholamine receptors.
- Hypovolaemia caused by the loss of blood plasma into pulmonary interstitium and alveolar air spaces across a disrupted alveolar capillary barrier.

Myocardial recovery is variable, although evidence of ongoing ischaemia and even left ventricular impairment is not uncommon.

Brain-dead patients frequently exhibit signs of hypothalamic failure. Hypothermia is almost invariable and principally a result of vasodilation (and the consequent loss of heat to cooler ambient surroundings), reduced metabolic rate and reduced heat production due to loss of muscle tone. It is frequently unrecognized because the patient's peripheries feel warm. Hypothermia may exacerbate haemodynamic and haemostatic instability and result in delays in the diagnosis of brain death. Failure of the hypothalamic–pituitary

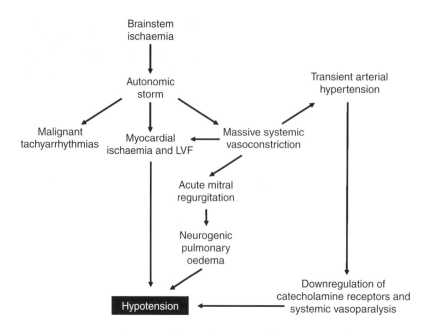

Fig. 30.3. Pathophysiology of the autonomic storm. LVF, left ventricular failure.

axis results most notably in central diabetes insipidus through failure of the release of antidiuretic hormone (ADH) from the neurohypophysis. Lack of ADH results in the excretion of large volumes of dilute urine, sometimes in excess of 1000 ml h^{-1}, and if untreated to hypovolaemia, haemodynamic instability, hypokalaemia and hypernatraemia. These changes all interfere with the diagnosis of brain death. The diuresis of central diabetes insipidus is easily terminated with 1–2 µg of parenteral desmopressin (1-deamino-8-D-arginine vasopressin or DDAVP), a synthetic analogue of ADH that has a longer half-life and which lacks the vasoconstricting properties of the endogenous hormone. It is also important to correct the existing fluid deficit with rapid intravenous infusion of an equivalent volume of 5% dextrose. The clinical significance of failure of secretion of other hormonal products of the pituitary gland is less clear, although many donor management protocols anticipate both adrenocortical insufficiency and a relative deficiency of thyroid hormones, and recommend replacement of both.

Management of the heartbeating donor

Although kidney and liver retrieval is possible from most brain-dead donors, the rate of retrieval of thoracic organs is significantly lower. While this may be an unavoidable consequence of chronic comorbidity, there is clear evidence that physiological donor optimization directed by invasive haemodynamic monitoring and lung-protective ventilatory strategies can significantly improve the likelihood of successful retrieval of the heart and lungs. It follows that the tendency to minimize critical care support for a brain-dead patient who has been identified as a potential multiorgan donor should be avoided. Rather, the management of a heartbeating brain-dead donor is an active process that is based on the recognition that continued brain-directed therapies are futile (because the brain is dead), and that they should be substituted by high-quality generic critical care that focuses on resuscitation of systemic organ systems. When planning donor management for an individual patient, it is useful to assess the potential for thoracic retrieval early because organ-specific management protocols for thoracic organs require a greater degree of intervention than those that guide splanchnic resuscitation.

The principles of donor management are based on a small number of basic observations:

- Hypotension and hypovolaemia impair renal and hepatic function and jeopardize the successful retrieval and transplantation of the splanchnic organs. Hypernatraemia is independently associated with hepatic dysfunction and graft loss.
- Infusion of high doses of catecholamine-based inotropes and vasopressors is harmful to the myocardium, may exacerbate the catecholamine-induced myocardial injury and is associated with poor post-transplant outcomes. Vasopressin

should be the first-line vasoconstrictor after brain death has been diagnosed.

- Hormone resuscitation protocols based on administration of vasopressin, methylprednisolone and possibly thyroid hormone, in association with goal-directed fluid therapy, frequently enable reduction or withdrawal of catecholamine infusions and improve the likelihood of successful heart donation.
- Invasive haemodynamic monitoring facilitates a more rational approach to the management of fluid, inotrope and vasopressor therapies, and improves the likelihood of successful heart and lung retrieval. Although this has traditionally involved the use of a pulmonary artery catheter, less invasive means of haemodynamic assessment, e.g. LiDCO, may also be of benefit.
- Brain death triggers a systemic inflammatory response that particularly targets the pulmonary microcirculation and this can impair transplant outcomes.

A detailed schedule for the various aspects of donor management is shown in Table 30.5.

Donation after circulatory death

Non-heartbeating organ donation is now referred to as donation after death circulatory death (DCD), and relates to the retrieval of organs after death that is diagnosed and confirmed using traditional cardiorespiratory criteria. The Maastricht classification of DCD describes five different circumstances in which successful organ retrieval might be possible (Table 30.6), but, in terms of process, these can be distilled into two models of donation, with the fundamental distinction being whether an individual's death is in anyway anticipated or 'controlled'. Thus, uncontrolled DCD (Maastricht criteria 1, 2 and 5) refers to donation that takes place after unexpected cardiac death, for instance following failed attempts at resuscitation in a patient with a massive acute coronary event in the emergency department. In contrast, controlled DCD (Maastricht categories 3 and 4) refers to organ retrieval that follows a cardiac death occurring as a result of planned withdrawal of futile cardiorespiratory support within an emergency department or intensive care unit (ICU).

Although these two variations of DCD are based on the same starting point, i.e. death determined using cardiorespiratory criteria, they come with a quite distinct set of operational, ethical and legal challenges, and

have rather different donation potentials. As a consequence, although donation after brain death (DBD) is supported, at least in theory, almost everywhere in the world, there is considerable variation in the practice of DCD. For example, DCD is unlawful in Germany but accounts for almost half of all deceased donation in the Netherlands. In the UK, the number of controlled non-heartbeating donations has increased tenfold over the last decade and, in 2010, accounted for almost one-third of all deceased donors. Uncontrolled DCD is declining in the UK and is now restricted to just two or three centres. In contrast to UK practice, controlled DCD is practically non-existent in Spain, even though there are established uncontrolled DCD programmes. The global variations in practice around DCD are likely to be due to a complex interaction of factors that include variations in the legal frameworks for organ retrieval, professional and societal approaches towards the concept of futility and consequent withholding or withdrawal of cardiorespiratory support (as this is an essential pre-requisite for controlled DCD), and cultural attitudes towards medical interventions after death that might be necessary to allow organ retrieval to take place.

The falling incidence of brain death, together with the ever-increasing demand for donor organs, has prompted many healthcare systems to review their potential for controlled DCD. Although it may be expected that offering patients who will not meet the criteria for brain death the option of DCD will represent a real opportunity to expand the potential deceased donor pool, more detailed analysis reveals an underlying anxiety that it might simply become an alternative for clinical staff who are supportive of donation but who face ever-increasing demands on critical care bed capacity and the professional pressure to act promptly once the futility of continued application of critical care has been recognized and accepted.

The principal steps in the controlled DCD pathway are shown in Fig. 30.4 and compared with the 'standard' pathway of death that follows withdrawal of futile life-sustaining therapies on the ICU.

Potential controlled DCD donors will typically have sustained an acute brain injury of such severity that death is considered inevitable or, more commonly, that recovery would be associated with intolerable functional disability. If warm ischaemic damage to potentially transplantable organs is to be avoided, organ retrieval must begin within minutes of the confirmation of cardiac death. It therefore follows that:

Table 30.5 Management of the multiorgan donor (adapted from the Canadian Forum recommendations on donor management)

Monitoring and laboratory investigations

- Continuous pulse oximetry, three-lead ECG and invasive intra-arterial pressure
- Hourly CVP, urine output and nasogastric drainage, fluid balance
- Point-of-care arterial blood gases, electrolytes and glucose every 4 h
- Full blood count, urea and creatinine, liver function tests and clotting screen

Maintenance of high-quality generic critical care support

- Correct acidosis, hypoxaemia, anaemia, electrolyte disturbances and hypothermia
- Initiate or continue enteral nutrition as tolerated, but discontinue once the donor is ready to be transferred to theatre. Do not initiate parenteral nutrition, but continue if it is already established
- Introduce intravenous insulin sliding scale to maintain tight control of plasma glucose at 4–8 mmol l^{-1}
- Diabetes insipidus can be defined as urine output >4 ml kg^{-1} h^{-1} that is associated with a rising serum sodium (>145 mmol l^{-1}) and rising serum osmolality and falling urine osmolality (>300 and <200 mOsm, respectively). It can be treated with an infusion of vasopressin ≤2.4 U h^{-1} and/or DDAVP, 1–4 μg IV, replacing previous urine output in full with 5% dextrose until hypernatraemia is reversed
- Continue with antibiotics and thromboembolic prophylaxis

Haemodynamic support

- Correct hypovolaemia (target CVP 6–10 mmHg) and if necessary start dopamine ≤10 μg kg^{-1} h^{-1} to achieve a MAP of 60–70 mmHg and systolic blood pressure >100 mmHg. Monitor adequacy of fluid resuscitation every 2 h with mixed venous saturation and serum lactate rather than fluid output. Add in vasopressin ≤2.4 U h^{-1} if blood pressure target is not achieved. If targets not achieved, or 2D echocardiography reveals an ejection fraction of < 40%, then (i) commence combination hormone therapy, and (ii) consider pulmonary artery catheterization, using the latter to guide additional agents such as norepinephrine, epinephrine or phenylephrine as indicated. Detailed haemodynamic targets include pulmonary capillary wedge pressure 6–10 mmHg; cardiac index >2.4 l min^{-1} m^{-2}; systemic vascular resistance 800–1200 dynes s^{-1} cm^{-5}; left ventricular stroke work index >15 g kg^{-1} min^{-1}.

Combination hormone therapy

Retrospective data from a large North American study of transplant outcomes suggests significant benefit from administration of vasopressin, thyroid hormone and methylprednisolone, although recent prospective work in the UK has questioned the value of thyroid replacement. Treatment frequently allows catecholamine infusions to be weaned off.

- Vasopressin: 1 U IV, followed by 2.4 U h^{-1}, fixed rate
- Thyroid hormone: either
  - Tetra-iodothyronine (T4), 20 μg IV bolus, followed by 10 μg h^{-1}, or
  - Tri-iodothyronine (T3), 4 μg IV bolus, followed by 3 μg h^{-1}
- Methylprednisolone: 15 mg kg^{-1}, once daily

Heart-specific management

- 12-lead ECG, troponin I/T and echocardiogram (after fluid and initial haemodynamic resuscitation)
- Insertion of pulmonary artery catheter and initiation of combination hormone therapy as indicated by
  - Haemodynamic instability despite low dose dopamine and vasopressin
  - Ejection fraction < 40%
- Cautious administration of fluids and adjustment of inotropes and vasopressors as directed by above
- Repeat echocardiography to assess response after 6 h
- Coronary angiography in selected cases (note: to lower risk of contrast nephropathy, ensure normovolaemia and administer N-acetylcysteine 150 mg kg^{-1} IV in 150 ml normal saline over 30 min immediately prior to injection of contrast, followed by 50 mg kg^{-1} in 500 ml over following 4 h

Table 30.5 (*cont.*)

Lung-specific management

- Chest X-ray, bronchoscopy, Gram stain and culture of bronchial lavage
- 30° head-up tilt and firm inflation of endotracheal tube cuff to prevent microaspiration and bronchial soiling
- Rotation to lateral position every 2 h and regular endotracheal toilet
- Intensive alveolar recruitment, e.g. periodic application of PEEP up to 15 cmH$_2$O, sustained inspiration to 30 cmH$_2$O for 30–60 s and diuresis where indicated
- Background ventilatory targets:
  - Tidal volume 8–10 ml kg^{-1}; PEEP 5 cmH$_2$O; PIP <30 cmH$_2$O
  - pH 7.35–7.45; PaCO$_2$ 4.5–6 kPa; PaO$_2$ >11 kPa SaO$_2$ >95%

CVP, central venous pressure; DDAVP, 1-deamino-8-D-arginine vasopressin; MAP, mean arterial pressure; PaCO$_2$, arterial carbon dioxide tension; PaO$_2$, arterial oxygen tension; PEEP, positive end-expiratory pressure; PIP, peak inspiratory pressure.

Table 30.6 The Maastricht classification of non-heartbeating organ donation

1	Dead on arrival at hospital
2	Unsuccessful resuscitation from cardiac arrest in hospital
3	Cardiac arrest following withdrawal of cardiorespiratory support
4	Cardiac arrest in brain-dead patient
5	Unexpected cardiac arrest in intensive care unit

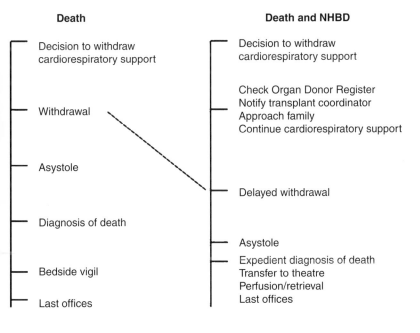

Fig. 30.4. Timeline for controlled donation after circulatory death and comparison with the 'standard' pathway of death following treatment withdrawal.

- The option of organ donation must be considered and offered to the family of the potential donor before death has occurred.
- A retrieval team must be ready in theatre before treatments are withdrawn, meaning that withdrawal must be delayed until such time as the retrieval team has travelled to the donating hospital and made their necessary preparations.
- Organ retrieval must begin as quickly as possible after death has been diagnosed and, although it must be performed in full compliance with professional and/or legal guidance, it must occur as quickly as possible after the irreversible loss of cardiac function.

In order to establish public and professional confidence in a process that poses a variety of potential ethical and legal challenges (see below), it is essential that units have written guidelines for controlled DCD that are based on national consensus and take account of the following:

- A clear separation between the declaration of the futility of continued life-prolonging support and a subsequent approach regarding organ donation.
- The requirement for continued cardiorespiratory support while the retrieval teams make their necessary preparations.
- The acceptability of any organ-directed interventions after the declaration of futility.
- The diagnosis and confirmation of death, including its documentation.

In contrast to donation after brain death, the family of the potential DCD often wish to be with their loved one following withdrawal of treatment and until death has been confirmed. Clinicians should be sensitive to the time that it takes to organize organ retrieval as this represents a delay in withdrawing treatment and the beginning of closure on what is a family tragedy. Critical care teams need to be honest in explaining the implications of DCD and give a realistic assessment of the likely time delays involved. Donor coordination and retrieval services must also be mindful of these issues and organise their support for DCD as rapidly as possible. For some units, geographical constraints may mean that the patient has to be transferred to an operating theatre area prior to treatment withdrawal, in which case attention must be given to the needs of the donor family for privacy with their loved one at the time of death.

In current UK practice, approximately 40% of potential DCD donations are stood down because the time period from treatment withdrawal to asystole extends beyond the limits set by the retrieval surgeons. These are based not only on the operational constraints of occupying a retrieval team for many hours but also on the warm ischaemic damage that occurs to organs as the dying patient becomes increasingly hypoxic and hypotensive. Families must be prepared for the possibility of stand down and, in circumstances where withdrawal of treatment takes place in the operating theatre, the critical care team should have a plan for the subsequent comfort care of the patient should donation not take place.

Original DCD programmes were restricted to kidney retrieval and, although there is a higher incidence of delayed graft function that requires a short period of post-transplant dialysis, the results from DCD kidneys are otherwise as good as those from DBD donors. While some centres now successfully retrieve liver, lung and pancreas from DCD donors, there remains significant concern about the ischaemic damage to which some of these organs might be exposed. This is particularly the case for the liver because of the associated high incidence of ischaemic cholangiography and subsequent biliary stricture. As a consequence, retrieval surgeons may be more selective when assessing a potential non-heartbeating donor than a brain-dead donor. This is particularly the case for elderly donors, those with comorbidities such as widespread arterial disease or where the time interval between withdrawal and asystole might be expected to be prolonged.

Withdrawal of therapy, consent for donation and conflict of interest

There must be a clear distinction between the recognition that further active treatments are no longer in a patient's best interests and should therefore be limited or withdrawn, and any subsequent enquiry regarding organ donation. It is advised that donation should not be considered until the family of the patient has accepted the inevitability of their loved one's death, with the key message being that donation is a potential component of end-of-life care and that the primary role of the family is to help clinical staff plan for these final acts. It is crucial that clinicians take a coherent and robust approach to withdrawal of cardiorespiratory support based on local policies that are constructed around national professional and statutory guidance. Some units consider that the request for donation should not be made by a clinician who has hitherto been involved in the care of the patient, although others do not support this view. However, under no circumstances should the discussion involve a clinician who might be involved in any subsequent transplantation. Specific mention should be made of the need to delay withdrawal of treatment to match the availability of the retrieval team, that the retrieval will be stood down if asystole does not occur within a given time interval, that the time available to be spent with their loved one immediately after death is very limited and that blood will be taken prior to death for tissue typing and virology screening to allow early identification of potential recipients. It is also important that the family understands that their permission for donation, even once offered, can be withdrawn at any time prior to the beginning of organ retrieval. While it is understandable that clinicians may fear private or public retribution from a family convinced that treatment withdrawal has been driven more by the needs of those awaiting a life-saving organ transplant than those of their dying relative, there is little if any evidence that this is a genuine concern. In the UK at least, consent rates for DCD are very similar to those for heartbeating deceased donation. Indeed, recent legal guidance from the UK Department of Health established a clear legal framework for organ donation after cardiac death. This framework does not absolve clinicians from their responsibilities but defines those responsibilities within the context of assessment of the best interests of a dying patient and gives clear guidance that donation can very often be a part of end-of-life care. Thus, if enquiry reveals that a dying patient would wish to donate after their death, and if the steps that are necessary to achieve this do not conflict with a clinician's primary duty of care to the comfort and dignity of their patient, clinicians are clearly working within the law if they take steps to facilitate donation.

Organ optimization and management of treatment withdrawal

It frequently takes several hours for an organ retrieval team to arrive at a donor hospital and cardiorespiratory support must be continued until they are ready in the operating theatre. Although the patient may be physiologically stable during this period, on occasions this will not be the case. Clinicians are then presented with a challenging dilemma – to what extent, if at all, should the potential donor's condition be stabilized through escalation of existing therapies (e.g. increasing inspired oxygen fraction or inotropic support) or by the introduction of new ones (e.g. thoracocentesis for a tension pneumothorax). Within UK practice, the answer once again lies in an assessment of the patient's best interests as described above. However, each case must be considered on an individual basis and assessed within the overall context of the support for donation from the donor's family and the experience of the primary team with DCD.

Even if a patient's condition is apparently stable up until treatment is withdrawn, anxieties over the ischaemic damage that organs may suffer as the dying patient becomes hypoxic and hypotensive limit the enthusiasm of some transplant teams for this model of donation. A variety of possible interventions to overcome or limit ischaemic damage have been proposed, although to date there is little objective evidence of their effectiveness in improving organ viability. Most commonly, blood sampling for tissue typing and virological screening prior to death is advocated, as this allows early identification of suitable recipients and thereby reduces cold ischaemia of the donor organs. It can also be argued that it is in the best interests of a donor, as it avoids an unnecessary laparotomy in a potential donor who might turn out to have a virological contraindication to donation.

To attenuate warm ischaemic damage, some protocols describe the administration of agents such as anticoagulants, vasodilators or steroids to preserve organ microcirculation. There is little clinical evidence to support such interventions and in any case they carry at least a theoretical risk of harm to the donor, e.g. by promoting rebleeding into an existing intracerebral haematoma. More contentiously, some centres advocate cannulation of the femoral vessels before death to facilitate the immediate cold perfusion of the splanchnic organs once death has been confirmed. Again, the evidence for the benefits of such interventions is lacking and there is limited support for their use. Other approaches include reviewing the need for the brief periods of respectful 'stand-off' after death that most guidelines advocate and reconsidering policies that advocate withdrawal in the ICU rather than in theatre. While such approaches and policy revisions may be justified, they should never be undertaken at the expense of the time that is needed to diagnose death or to support the donor family.

Clinical staff should also be aware that retrieval specialists will increasingly seek to explore means by which the ischaemic injury to organs might be terminated and reversed by applying some form of extracorporeal recirculation after the initial laparotomy and perfusion is complete. While any measures that increase the gift of donation that patients make in their death should be given sympathetic consideration, there must be an absolute prohibition on any intervention that risks restoring cerebral blood flow once death has been diagnosed.

Cardiorespiratory support is withdrawn once the surgical team has made the necessary arrangement for organ retrieval and is ready in the operating theatre. As noted elsewhere, although withdrawal usually takes place in the ICU, geographical factors may require that the patient be transferred to theatre prior to treatment withdrawal. However, although the location of death may necessarily be different, the mode of withdrawal of treatment should never be modified. For example, analgesia and anxiolysis should be administered according to local practice and in compliance with written local guidelines but must never be given simply to accelerate asystole and thereby facilitate donation. Similar arguments also apply to extubation or decannulation of the trachea.

Diagnosis of death and the dead donor rule

Although the proposition that organ retrieval cannot begin until death has been confirmed would appear to require no justification, the biological reality that death is usually a process rather than a discrete event in time perhaps complicates the professional framework for the diagnosis and confirmation of death. Indeed, the need to begin surgical retrieval as soon as possible after the onset of irreversible loss of cardiac function in order to minimize warm ischaemic damage has prompted a re-evaluation of the contemporary understanding of the cardiorespiratory criteria for the determination of death. The key, and interrelated, questions are:

- How should the onset of loss of mechanical cardiac function best be determined?
- At what point can clinicians be assured that the potential for spontaneous return of the circulation (autoresuscitation) has passed in circumstances when there is no intention to attempt cardiac resuscitation?
- How soon after the cessation of cardiorespiratory function can a state of simultaneous and

irreversible loss of the capacity for consciousness, and the capacity to breathe, that is sufficient to allow organ retrieval to begin be recognized?

Available evidence suggests that brain function and reactivity are completely lost within seconds of circulatory arrest and that, although full recovery can be anticipated if the circulation is restored within up to 11 min of asystole, progressive irreversible brain damage can be anticipated thereafter, at least under normothermic conditions. (Spontaneous) return of cardiac function is very unlikely after 2 min of sustained asystole and has never been reported after 11 min of continuous ECG monitoring of asystole. However, it is clear that cardiac death cannot be diagnosed within the first 120 s of asystole because of the possibility of autoresuscitation and the potential for the restoration of cerebral function if this were to occur. After 120 s, the time at which death can be declared is dependent on whether or not there is any intention to attempt cardiopulmonary resuscitation. Following the withdrawal of cardiorespiratory support within the context of futility, it is argued that death can be declared after 2 min of asystole because the chances of autoresuscitation are negligible, global brain function has been lost and there is no intention to initiate cardiopulmonary resuscitation. Despite this, most protocols prohibit any surgical intervention within the first 5–10 min after loss of mechanical cardiac function. A schedule for the diagnosis of cardiorespiratory death was recently published by the Academy of the Medical Royal Colleges of the UK and is summarized in Table 30.7.

Although the dead donor rule emerged to endorse the removal of organs from DBD donors during the development of the concept of brain death in the 1960s, it should similarly be applied to DCD donation. However, some modification that recognizes the particular concerns surrounding donation after cardiac death is required. The fundamentals of the dead donor rules that are applied within the author's institution are:

- Do nothing to accelerate death.
- Do not start retrieval until death has occurred.
- Do nothing that might restore cerebral perfusion.

Practical considerations

Non-heartbeating organ donation is not a new model of organ donation, but it is one with which the majority of the current generation of clinicians working in critical care or emergency medicine are unfamiliar. The

Table 30.7 A schedule for the diagnosis and confirmation of death after cardiorespiratory arrest prior to non-heartbeating organ donation (adapted from the Code of Practice from the Academy of the Medical Royal Colleges in the UK)

1. The patient should meet the criteria for not attempting cardiopulmonary resuscitation

2. The patient should be observed by the person responsible for confirming death for a minimum of 5 min to establish that irreversible cardiorespiratory arrest has occurred

3. Any spontaneous return of cardiac or respiratory activity during this period of observation should prompt a further 5 min observation from the next point of cardiorespiratory arrest

4. The absence of mechanical cardiac function is normally confirmed using a combination of the following:
   - Absence of a central pulse
   - Absence of heart sounds on auscultation
   - Aystole on continuous ECG display
   - Absence of pulsatile flow using direct intra-arterial pressure monitoring
   - Absence of contractile activity using echocardiography

5. After 5 min of continued cardiorespiratory arrest, the absence of the pupillary responses to light, of the corneal reflexes and of any motor response to supraorbital pressure should be confirmed

6. The time of death is recorded as the time at which these criteria are fulfilled

introduction of DCD programmes is dependent on an open, honest and respectful discussion of the potential problems among all members of the clinical teams involved and should be supported by the Executive Board of the hospital. The involvement of a hospital ethics committee is invaluable, and there should be a clear and unambiguous written operational policy that describes the process in detail. Implementation requires strong clinical leadership, with hands-on operational involvement of senior medical and nursing staff when DCD is taking place.

Some of the clinical circumstances in which DCD is possible necessitate referral of a patient's death to the Coroner or Procurator Fiscal. On such occasions, the potential for donation should not be raised with the family until a lack of coronial objection has been confirmed. Similarly, many units would consider it good practice to exclude any medical contraindication to organ donation before approaching the family of the potential donor.

In establishing DCD programmes, the practical implications of transferring the deceased from the place of death to the operating theatre in a way that maintains their dignity need to be considered. These should accommodate the needs of the family while minimizing the warm ischaemic time. Finally, staff must ensure that the usual posthumous services for the deceased and their family, such as last offices and viewing of the body, are not overlooked once organ retrieval has been completed.

Further reading

Academy of the Medical Royal Colleges (2008). *A Code of Practice for the Diagnosis and Confirmation of Death*. London. Available at http://www.aomrc.org.uk/publications/reports-guidance.html.

Ad Hoc Committee of the Harvard Medical School to Examine the Definition of Brain Death (1968). A definition of irreversible coma. *JAMA* **205**, 337–40.

Bernat, J., Capron, A., Bleck, T. *et al.* (2010). The circulatory-respiratory determination of death in organ donation. *Crit Care Med* **38**, 972–79.

British Transplant Society and Intensive Care Society (2010). Donation After Circulatory Death. Available at http://www.ics.ac.uk/intensive_care_professional/standards_and_guidelines/dcd.

Coggon, J., Brazier, M., Murphy, P., Price, D. and Quigley, M. (2008). Best interests and potential organ donors. *BMJ* **336**, 1346–7.

Conference of the Medical Royal Colleges and their Faculties in the United Kingdom (1976). Diagnosis of brain death. *BMJ* **59**, 1187–8

Department of Health (2009). *Legal Issues Relevant to Non-heartbeating Organ Donation*. London: Department of Health. Available at http://www.dh.gov.uk/en/Publicationsandstatistics/Publications/index.htm.

DeVita, M. A. (2001). The death watch: certifying death using cardiac criteria. *Prog Transplant* **11**, 58–66.

Institute of Medicine (2000). *Non-heart-beating Organ Transplantation: Practice and Protocols*. Washington DC: National Academy Press.

McLean, A. D. and Rosengard, B. R. (1999). Aggressive donor management. *Curr Opin Organ Transplant* **4**, 130–6.

Mollaret, P. and Goulon, M. (1959). Le coma dépassé. *Rev Neurol (Paris)* **101**, 3–15.

Murphy, P., Manara, A., Bell, D. and Smith, M. (2008). Controlled non-heart beating organ donation: neither the whole solution nor a step too far. *Anaesthesia* **63**, 526–30.

Pallis, C. and Harley, D. H. (1996). *ABC of Brainstem Death*, 2nd edn. London: BMJ Publishing Group.

President's Commission for the Study of Ethical Problems in Medicine and Biomedical and Behavioural Research, Report of the Medical Consultants on the Diagnosis of Death (1981). Guidelines for the determination of death. *JAMA* **246**, 2184–6.

President's Council on Bioethics (2008). *Controversies in the Determination of Death*. Washington DC. Available at http://www.bioethics.gov.

Ramos, H. C. and Lopez, R. (2002). Critical care management of the brain-dead organ donor. *Curr Opin Organ Transplant* **7**, 70–5.

Rosendale, J. D., Kauffman, H. M., McBride, M. A. *et al.* (2000). Hormonal resuscitation yields more transplanted hearts, with improved early function. *Transplantation* **75**, 1536–41.

Rosendale, J. D., Kauffman, H. M., McBride, M. A. *et al.* (2003). Aggressive donor management results in more transplanted organs. *Transplantation* **75**, 482–7.

Shemie, S. D., Doig, C., Dickens, B. *et al.* (2006). Severe brain injury to neurological determination of death: Canadian forum recommendations. *CMAJ* **174**, 1077–8.

Shemie, S. D., Ross, H., Pagliarello, J. *et al.* (2006). Organ donor management in Canada: recommendations of the forum on Medical Management to Optimize Donor Organ Potential. *CMAJ* **174**, S13–30.

Shewmon, D. A. (1998). Chronic brain death: meta-analysis and conceptual consequences. *Neurology* **51**, 1538–45.

Weber, M., Dindo, D., Demartines N, Ambühl, P. M. and Clavien, P. A. (2002). Kidney transplantation from donors without a heartbeat. *New Engl J Med* **347**, 248–55.

Wijdicks, E. F. M. (2001). The diagnosis of brain death. *New Engl J Med* **344**, 1215–21.

Chapter 3

Ethical and legal issues

Derek Duane

Prognosis after cerebral injury

When the brain is injured, the need to accurately assess the immediate and long-term outcome for the patient assumes critical importance. The reason this issue takes priority alongside medical management is the acknowledgement that survivors can be left with profound neurological and psychological deficits, which can ultimately dictate a person's quality of life. Any presumed benefit from a medical, surgical or rehabilitative intervention has to be weighed against the ultimate outcome, which is itself a probability calculation. Difficult decisions have to be made that need to take account of the pathophysiological derangement of the injured brain, treatment options that may have a weak evidence base, the known wishes of the patient and next of kin, and the consequences to society in terms of cost and the loss of the individual's contribution. These decisions encompass an appreciation of the uniqueness of every patient's clinical condition and endorse the principle that prognosis should never be the sole factor in influencing the clinical management of a severely brain-injured patient.

The range of outcomes after cerebral injury includes death, a vegetative state, a minimally conscious state, akinetic mutism, locked-in syndrome, various degrees of functional and cognitive impairment, and, possibly, complete neurological recovery. At present, determining the prognosis of a brain-injured patient is an inexact science. However, advances in this area have come from multicentre and multinational studies that have used established outcome categories and correlated these with certain features of the brain-injured patient and the early clinical course. In this process, reliance is placed on a consideration of the aetiology of injury, clinical signs, physiological parameters, biochemical and genetic data, electrophysiology and brain imaging.

All this information helps guide the type, intensity and extent of medical interventions used to treat a patient. Prognostic models may also be used to help evaluate circumstances where a decision to withhold or withdraw treatment is being considered.

Although a wide range of factors can be taken into account when assessing prognosis, in practice, only a few parameters contain the majority of the prognostic information. Poor outcome from cerebral injury is related to: (i) the depth and duration of coma; (ii) an impaired or absent pupillary light response or eye movement; (iii) patient age; (iv) the severity of secondary physiological injuries to the brain; (v) the results of investigation and imaging studies; and (vi) the impact of genetic factors. While clinical experience confirms the value and importance of these features, there remains some disagreement about their predictive utility.

In closed-head injury, the assessment of conscious level is an important index of impaired cerebral function and after the exclusion of certain confounding variables (e.g. recreational drugs, medications and cardiorespiratory instability), even brain injury severity. The Glasgow Coma Scale (GCS) score, first proposed by Teasdale and Jennett in 1974, is a useful means to monitor changes in the conscious level. It assesses awareness of the environment and cognition in patients with impaired consciousness and its purpose is to standardize documentation of changes in neurological status and aid in the assessment of prognosis. Most trained healthcare personnel can reliably measure the GCS score in a standardized way. It should be used for the purposes of prognosis once hypoxia, hypercarbia and hypotension are ruled out and sedatives and neuromuscular blocking agents have been metabolized. The probability of a poor neurological outcome is seen with a progressively decreasing or

Core Topics in Neuroanaesthesia and Neurointensive Care, eds. Basil F. Matta, David K. Menon and Martin Smith. Published by Cambridge University Press. © Cambridge University Press 2011.

Table 31.1 The Glasgow Outcome Scale

Score	Meaning
5	Good recovery: able to return to work or school
4	Moderate disability: able to live independently; unable to return to work or school
3	Severe disability: able to follow commands; unable to live independently
2	Vegetative state: unable to interact with environment; unresponsive
1	Dead

persistently low GCS score in traumatic brain injury (TBI). The recorded value is valid both as a sum score or just the motor component. It is estimated that only 20% of patients with a low initial GCS score will survive and up to 10% of these will have a limited functional state, assessed as 4–5 on the Glasgow Outcome Scale (GOS) (Table 31.1).

There is a 70% chance of a poor outcome if a patient presents with absent pupillary light reflexes bilaterally. This outcome is influenced by the level of consciousness, underlying pathology and timing of surgical evacuation of significant haematomas. Before using this parameter as a prognostic indicator, pupillary diameter should be recorded after excluding direct orbital trauma and cardiorespiratory instability. Both size and duration of dilation and fixation should be noted for each pupil. A pupillary size of >4 mm is accepted as the measure for a dilated pupil. Due to the proximity of the neural circuits controlling pupillary reflexes to the medial temporal lobe and brainstem, this clinical measurement is only an indirect indication of herniation and injury to areas of the brain controlling consciousness.

The prognosis for children after a severe cerebral injury is considerably better than for adults. It has been shown that increasing age is a strong independent factor in prognosis. There is a significant increase in poor outcome above 60 years of age, regardless of the cause of the injury. The reason for this is not clear but may relate to comorbidities seen in the older age group along with a diminished capacity for brain repair.

Post-traumatic hypotension defined as a systolic blood pressure of <90 mmHg was found to have a 67% positive predictive value for poor outcome, and when combined with hypoxia, this value increased to 79%. Both the incidence and duration of hypotension in association with hypoxia, hypercarbia, intracranial hypertension and intracranial mass lesions greatly influence outcome from brain injury. The underlying mechanism for the susceptibility of the injured brain to hypotension is not fully understood. However, from post-mortem examinations, evidence of ischaemic damage has been reported in >85% of head-injured patients. A single recording of a hypotensive episode is generally associated with a doubling of mortality and a marked increase in morbidity from a given head injury. Therefore, the immediate treatment of these secondary brain insults can decrease the frequency of poor outcomes in severely brain-injured patients.

CT scanning is now an essential investigation performed in all patients with severe TBI. It can provide valuable information that may lead to urgent neurosurgery, the placement of intraventricular drains or intracranial pressure monitors. It can also assist in the assessment of the patient's prognosis. The features of the brain CT imaging that are most useful include the presence of a mass lesion, compressed or absent basal cisterns, midline shift and traumatic subarachnoid haemorrhage. To standardize reporting of CT scans in TBI, various grading systems are used. The Marshall system (Table 31.2) is considered the standard for this purpose. It has been shown to predict mortality when used alone or in combination with other factors as part of a brain outcome injury model. Outcome is worse in TBI patients with large-volume space-occupying lesions, especially acute subdural haematomas. Mortality can be increased two- to threefold in the presence of compressed or absent basal cisterns. A midline shift of >5 mm in patients over 45 years of age is associated with a worsening prognosis, as is the extent of a traumatic subarachnoid haemorrhage, which can increase mortality twofold. Overall, an abnormal initial brain CT scan, seen in >90% of severe TBIs, has greater than a 70% positive predictive value for an adverse outcome. However, in patients with a normal brain CT scan on admission, prognosis may be related primarily to associated extracranial injuries or the later occurrence of raised intracranial pressure or the development of new lesions, which may occur in up to 40% of these patients.

Hyperglycaemia is common after TBI and, if left untreated, can result in a rise in early mortality and worsening functional recovery in adults. Studies have shown a reduction in mortality with intensive insulin therapy in critically ill patients. The improved outcome could not be extended to TBI patients with certainty, and concern remains over the high rates of hypoglycaemic episodes reported in the studies.

Table 31.2 The Marshall CT classification of traumatic brain injury

Category	Definition
Diffuse injury I	No visible intracranial pathology seen on CT scan
Diffuse injury II	Cisterns are present with midline shift <5 mm and/or lesion densities present
	No high- or mixed-density lesion >25 ml, may include bone fragments and foreign bodies
Diffuse injury III	Cisterns compressed or absent with midline shift 0–5 mm. No high- or mixed-density lesion >25 ml
Diffuse injury IV	Midline shift >5 mm. No high- or mixed-density lesion >25 ml
Evacuated mass lession	Any lesion surgically evacuated
Non-evacuated mass lession	High- or mixed-density lesion >25 ml, not surgically evacuated

Outcome after cerebral injury is increasingly being understood in terms of the interaction of an individual's genetic make-up and environmental factors. The possession of certain genes portends a worse prognosis following TBI. The gene for the apolipoprotein Eε4 variant is associated with a poorer outcome after cerebral injury. Genes that regulate interleukin-1, angiotensin-converting enzyme (ACE), transcription factor p53, dopamine receptors and catechol-O-methyltransferase are undergoing further investigations to determine their role in brain injury outcome.

The prognosis of the brain-injured patient is very much dependent on the extent of the primary injury, the cumulative effects of the secondary brain insults, the type of care offered and whether this takes place in a dedicated neuroscience centre. Prognostic indicators such as age, genetics, initial GCS score, pupillary reaction, ongoing physiological derangements and certain features of the initial brain imaging all play their part in the assessment and provision of treatment. However, this treatment may not be appropriate or desired by the patient, and it may eventually fail to offer any further benefit, thus necessitating its cessation. The ethical and legal underpinnings of our management of incapacitated brain-injured patients and their inclusion in research protocols can often present dilemmas that demand a considered approach relying as much on experience as expert knowledge.

The incompetent patient

An ethical basis for medical decisions

From Hippocratic time, medical ethics has imposed certain duties on a doctor towards his patient. These include a duty not to harm (non-maleficence) and a duty always to do good (beneficence). Embodied in these duties is a need to respect patient autonomy and welfare, both of which help form the fundamental basis of human interaction. In healthcare, promoting autonomy by practising informed consent is so important it is now central to the doctor–patient relationship. Thus, the ethical basis for treating all patients relies on the principles of beneficence, non-maleficence and respect for autonomy. Suspending any of these ethical codes weakens the moral imperative of respectful treatment of persons as ends in themselves.

Medical investigations and treatments are subject to the process of informed consent, which involves a discussion between clinician and patient about the nature, indications, benefits and risks of any proposed intervention. Intensive care unit (ICU) patients are often unable to give consent, especially if confusional states or sedative and analgesic agents impair capacity. Therefore, in these patients, the need for medical interventions or end-of-life decisions raises the issue of ethical justification. How is the promotion of their autonomy through consent managed under elective and emergency situations? Any emergency procedure performed on the unconscious ICU patient achieves justification under the ethical principle of necessity. When clinical decisions are less urgent, a doctor may seek opinions from the next of kin to help decide what is in the best interests of, or provides an overall benefit to, the patient. Although relatives cannot give a legally valid consent for any proposed intervention, their assent to medical treatment for the incompetent patient, while legally futile, adheres to the ethical principle of respect for patient autonomy as exercised through surrogates.

While every effort is made to preserve the unconscious patient's autonomy, it is clearly vulnerable in the ICU environment as the need for swift decisions, dictated by the pace of the critical illness, often arises. As a consequence, ethical standards in relation to a patient's autonomous choices may suffer, leaving the justification for non-consensual treatment reliant on the legal test of best interests and its inherent subjectivity. However, an unconscious patient who has previously issued a lasting power of attorney or has an advance directive can detail the extent of life-prolonging measures they would like taken in a severe critical illness. The right of self-determination over medical paternalism attracts such high regard that society has protected this principle by elevating the legal force of advance directives from common law to statute with the recent enactment of the Mental Capacity Act. In the absence of any known prior wishes regarding the extent of critical care intervention, most would agree that if it would harm the patient to deny them treatment without consent, then justification based on the principles of beneficence and non-maleficence serves the best interests of the patient.

Finally, one further important underlying ethical principle governing medical treatment in the incompetent unconscious patient is the need to preserve the sanctity of human life. However, this is not absolute, and a patient may choose not to be treated and convey this wish by an appropriate legal instrument. This right of choice exists regardless of whether the reasons for such a decision are rational, irrational, unknown or even non-existent. Equally important is the requirement for any clinician to discontinue treatment that is without benefit and contrary to the best interests of the patient and acknowledge that the preservation of human life at any cost is not always justified or possible.

A legal basis for medical decisions

The law upholds the position that 'every human being of adult years and sound mind has a right to determine what shall be done with his own body' (*Schloendorff v Society of New York Hospital*). The legal basis allowing touching of another person in a therapeutic context is an implied or expressed valid consent. For a valid refusal of treatment, the law demands proof of capacity. The treatment of a patient without consent is unlawful and patients may seek redress in the form of a tortious or negligence claim. However, the law has devised legal mechanisms to allow a doctor to treat, or a patient to refuse that treatment, even though contemporaneous consent is unavailable. These legal rules and procedures include the principle of necessity, declaratory jurisdiction, advance directives and the best interests test.

A doctor providing essential non-consensual treatment to an unconscious patient relies on the common law principle of necessity. The treatment undertaken must be equal to the seriousness of the patient's condition, allow immediate survival and be necessary and not just convenient. Postponement of any intervention not considered essential is preferable to continuing without consent. The doctrine of necessity is legally justified if: (i) a reasonable doctor would similarly act in the circumstances and care for the patient in their best interests; (ii) that treatment is not contrary to the known wishes of the patient; and (iii) when no suitable person is available or willing to act, officious intervention is sought.

The lawfulness of medical treatment proposed for an unconscious patient can also be decided by the Courts in England, acting through the Official Solicitor. Where doubt exists about a proposed medical intervention, good practice recommends seeking a declaration to give clarity to the rights of the patient and the duties of the doctor. By granting declaratory relief, the courts aim to protect doctors, patients' relatives and the public and reassure them that a medical intervention or omission to act is lawful.

A person can make an advance directive to refuse or limit treatment of any condition they wish to specify in the event of future incapacity. Recently, statutory recognition of advance directives followed the implementation of the Mental Capacity Act 2005. Although the patient may be unconscious and unable to give or refuse consent for medical interventions, their advance refusal of treatment is legally binding. However, any advance statement of treatment preferences is not. The Act requires a person to draft an advance statement in writing, have it witnessed and signed and contain a statement that it is to apply even where life is at risk. The usual safeguards on validity are encompassed within the Act. The validity of an advance directive depends on ensuring that: (i) patient had sufficient capacity when the directive was signed; (ii) there was absence of undue influence; and (iii) enough information was made available to the patient. A person must be assumed to have capacity unless it is established that she or he lacks capacity. The advance directive must be applicable to the circumstances that subsequently arise. A patient who has done anything clearly inconsistent with the directive, thereby questioning its applicability, will render it invalid. A Court of Protection, set up by the Act, will rule on matters of applicability and validity when doubt exists about an advanced directive. Healthcare professionals may choose to ignore the terms of a valid advance directive and treat a patient in their best interest according to the *Bolam* standard. However, liability may flow from their decisions, as patients can have recourse to the law, enabling them to bring an action in battery or negligence for non-consensual treatment.

The Mental Capacity Act 2005 established a statutory framework called a lasting power of attorney (LPA), which gives patients another way of planning ahead for a time when they might lack capacity. An individual can nominate another person (an Attorney) to make healthcare decisions on their behalf if they lose capacity. The chosen attorney must make decisions in the person's best interests but the authority does not apply to life-sustaining treatment unless stated. An LPA must be registered with the Office of the Public Guardian before it can be used, and any disputes concerning its applicability must be referred for adjudication to the Court of Protection.

To safeguard incapacitated patients who have no friends or family with whom it is practicable to consult, the services of an Independent Mental Capacity Advocate (IMCA) are required by statute. There is a legal duty on local authorities or National Health Service bodies in the UK to commission this service. The IMCA will represent and support the person who lacks capacity when serious medical decisions that may involve withdrawal of life-sustaining treatment are being made. The healthcare team involved in a patient's care must take into account the report of the IMCA in a best interests determination. The IMCA can challenge a decision made by the medical team and can ask the Official Solicitor, acting as litigation friend, to apply to the Court of Protection for dispute resolution.

The Mental Capacity Act 2005 demands that any act done to a patient who lacks capacity must be in their best interests. This determination, according to the Act, must involve a consideration of all the relevant circumstances. Those relevant to end-of-life decisions must not include a wish to bring about the patient's death but can take account of ending futile therapy. The Act also states that best interests of the unconscious patient can include recent past wishes, feelings, beliefs, values and other factors that the patient would be likely to consider if she or he were able to do so. The views of relatives, carers, a person holding an LPA, a court appointee or any other party interested in the welfare of the patient must be instrumental in defining best interests when practicable and appropriate. The point of this is not to let others decide what ought to happen but to contribute to the overall assessment of the patient's life views and values. There remains, however, some margin for interpretation of the meaning of 'values' and 'presumed wishes'. These may need judicial review if a doctor upholds a reasonable belief that his or her course of action is in the patient's best interests but others take a different view. In the future, the stage seems set for a more rational and less subjective assessment of a patient's best interests as outlined by a relatively new yet untested statute.

It is now legally important to have the rights protected under the Articles of the European Convention on Human Rights (ECHR) applied to a best interests determination of an unconscious patient unable to refuse or give consent to medical treatment. Article 2 of the Convention protects one's right to life (positive obligation) by law and prevents any intentional deprivation (negative obligation) of life. A decision to withdraw treatment in a patient's best interests is by law an omission to act and therefore consistent with Article 2, considering both the positive and negative obligations of the state to safeguard life. The positive obligation to protect the right to life is not absolute and is mitigated by the medical decision not to treat, based on the *Bolam* principle, and the patient's best interests (*NHS Trust A v M; NHS Trust B v H*). Article 3 of the ECHR forbids inhuman and degrading treatment, thus protecting a patient's dignity. When considering treatment withdrawal, any burdensome intervention not promoting a patient's best interests would be regarded as inhumane, and thus run counter to Article 3 (*A National Health Service Trust v D*). Article 8 of the ECHR encompasses a protection of one's right to personal autonomy and physical integrity. All non-consensual medical interventions are therefore contrary to the requirements of Article 8 except for patients who are unable to give consent and are treated in their best interests, when no violation of this Article occurs (*X v Austria*).

Treatment decisions in the unconscious ICU patient do not infringe Articles 2, 3 and 8 of the ECHR provided the patient is treated in their best interests and their rights enshrined within these Articles are upheld. It is a doctor's duty to treat the patient according to best practice informed by suitable professional standards while avoiding unnecessary subjective futility assessments and a rigid adherence to a principle espousing the sanctity of human life at all costs. There is optimism that the increasing use of an LPA and the higher profile given to advance directives through legislation will highlight how one's own preferences can influence care when incompetent. The net benefit resulting from all of this will be an easing of the burden of speculation about a patient's wishes for end-of-life care.

End-of-life care – withholding and withdrawing treatment

The mortality of adult patients treated on the ICU is >20%. Consequently, a significant proportion of the work of any unit is in caring for terminally ill patients, for whom >10% will have a treatment withdrawal decision preceding their death. Limiting life-prolonging treatment has a solid foundation in the ethical principles of autonomy, beneficence, non-maleficence, sanctity of life and distributive justice. A patient's wishes, values and beliefs, communicated through an advance directive or a surrogate decision-maker holding an LPA, can help guide the cessation of treatment that has no net benefit, is physiologically futile or is excessively burdensome. End-of-life decision-making benefits from an approach that shares the burden of responsibility, gives primacy to patient autonomy over medical paternalism and aims for a consensus about a patient's best interests through negotiation with the family, surrogates and all members of the healthcare team.

The principle of autonomy has a restricted role in the intensive care setting as fewer than 5% of patients are able to communicate their preferred treatment choice. End-of-life decisions are taken in a patient's best interests. Doctors aim to find out any preferences a patient may have had regarding life-sustaining treatment and their view of an acceptable quality of life after a severe critical illness. Evidence in the form of an advance directive or LPA, or from informal discussions with family members, is commonly sought. A doctor usually aims for a consensus opinion among all interested parties about the appropriateness of the decision to withdraw medical therapy. What this amounts to in essence is a unified assent. Thus, treatment withdrawal that inevitably leads to death demands the highest ethical and legal standards when no instrument exists to prove a patient's autonomous choices.

End-of-life decisions are complex and entail a balancing of medical, ethical, legal, religious, cultural, psychosocial and societal issues. In essence, these decisions focus on whether to withdraw or withhold medical treatments and, although challenging, must lead to a death with dignity and without pain. Most ethicists agree that there is no moral distinction between withholding and withdrawing therapy

when the consequence of either action is equivalent. Treatment withdrawal is a positive act often wrongly associated with a feeling of complicity in the dying process. Withholding therapy, while it may feel emotionally less burdensome, is still an act of omission that can also result in the death of a patient from the underlying illness.

Mechanical ventilation, clinically assisted nutrition and hydration, cardiovascular support drugs, antibiotics and renal replacement therapies are all interventions that when stopped will allow the patient to die of their underlying illness. A patient's underlying irreversible clinical condition, age, severity of illness, length of ICU stay and underlying chronic disorders traditionally form part of the process for end-of-life decisions. However, they are also dictated by the moral duty of the attending physician to spare the patient any undue suffering and distress. End-of-life decisions in the ICU often present unique problems. Firstly, knowledge about a patient's preferences for life-prolonging treatment is often lacking. Secondly, poor communication between caregivers and surrogates impedes understanding. Thirdly, doctors use unreliable predictive models of death and outcome data for critical illness and lastly, healthcare professionals usually have inadequate training in end-of-life care. These facts fuel the disparity in the objectivity and consistency needed in end-of-life decisions, despite ethical, legal and professional guidelines underpinning a robust framework to achieve such goals.

In keeping with the ethical principle of distributive justice, it is the duty of a physician to consider the cost of care and avoid wasting resources by ceasing ineffective therapy. End-of-life decisions are best delivered by doctors dedicated to the speciality of intensive care. Studies show that they have a timelier and rational approach to withholding or withdrawing treatment, encourage the use of advance directives and start palliative care earlier. Costs created by patients dying in ICUs are small in comparison with the overall spending of a healthcare system. Therefore, all critically ill patients should have access to intensive care facilities where resources allow. When restoration of health is not possible and is beyond technology, palliative care should be afforded the patient, regardless of cost.

Decisions on the withdrawal or withholding of treatment need careful collaboration, consideration and respect. A doctor should review all these decisions with reference to certain important tenets: (i) there is a reasonable expectation of treatment provision by the patient or society under certain circumstances; (ii) the withdrawal of treatment followed by palliative care will often hasten death; and (iii) sometimes next-of-kin dissent to treatment being withheld. Withdrawal of treatment will sometimes bring ethical principles such as respect for patient autonomy or sanctity of life into conflict. However, to effect a resolution that will synchronize with community values often demands that the important elements from each principle are blended with the concept of best interests and the views of the patient, family and physician.

Despite the recently adopted preference for a shared approach in making these difficult end-of-life decisions, there is often a willingness of families to delegate this task to doctors. It is not proper for any one group, either medical or family, to take on the sole responsibility for such decisions. Families may undergo much stress, guilt and remorse if asked, during an emotionally upsetting time, to weigh independently the complexities of medical conditions and their inherent prognostic uncertainty. In contrast, a proposal to withhold or withdraw medical treatment can also meet with disbelief and hostility from families or even other doctors. This can lead to conflict and delay a decision to end futile and burdensome treatment for the patient. Involvement of the courts in treatment abatement decisions in the ICU may be necessary to achieve a consensus opinion with all members of the healthcare team and family.

Often, the wider problem causing conflict in treatment withdrawal decisions on ICUs is denial of the inevitability of death and an unyielding view on the sanctity of life. Viewing death as a medical failure and placing an unjustified reliance on the ability of medicine and science to overcome a natural and inevitable process is a fallacy. Inappropriate treatment of critically ill patients is a deceit and should give way to a view that regards death as a natural process. Withholding or withdrawing treatment embodies the doctrine of respect for the sanctity of life. However, many hold the view that clinical practice should aim at preserving life at all costs. This would demand that patients endure all forms of interventions thought likely to succeed despite the suffering imposed and overuse of resources involved. Therefore, it becomes unworkable to adopt the sanctity-of-life principle without accepting that, under certain circumstances, stopping futile treatment and allowing a patient to die is the right thing to do. What is reasonable and practicable is to interpret the sanctity-of-life doctrine to mean an absolute prohibition on intentional killing. In doing so, there is the recognition that a doctor's conduct, which may foreseeably but not deliberately shorten life, is more acceptable. Of course, any intent or action to withdraw treatment for the sole purpose of hastening death runs counter to the fundamentals of this doctrine.

It is against accepted ethical principles not to withdraw treatments that: (i) lack benefit; (ii) preserve permanent unconsciousness; or (iii) fail to end total dependence on intensive medical care. These conditions would be unduly burdensome on the patient and hence futile. When treatment is physiologically futile, it should be stopped. End-of-life decisions based on the concept of medical futility, with its inherent paternalism, quality-of-life assessments and a consideration for resource allocation, are more difficult to see as morally or legally neutral. Many people hold differing views on the meaning of a valuable life, and this can make agreement on what is considered futile near impossible. Judgements of medical futility can always be criticized if they are based on uncertain ICU outcome data and the variety of value-laden opinions held by doctors and surrogates that infringe a patient's autonomy. The moral and legal authority for these futility judgements flows from a doctor's specific medical knowledge, professional integrity and society's expectations. As a consequence, a doctor must always act in a patient's best interest and within professional standards.

Withdrawing treatment on the ICU can begin with a decision not to perform cardiopulmonary resuscitation (CPR) on a patient while continuing all other interventions for a suitable duration. There should always be a presumption in favour of resuscitation where a reasonable chance exists for a successful outcome. When this is not the case, there is a duty on the doctor to act in the patient's best interests. A final decision to deny CPR should incorporate the results of consultations with the healthcare team, family or proxy decision-maker.

Withdrawal of treatment on the ICU may necessitate removal of the patient from the ventilator or a terminal extubation, which may lead to the immediate death of the patient. A doctor may decide to withhold further treatment or stop its escalation, thus viewing the patient's death as resulting from these omissions and not from one deliberate act. However, if the intention remains the same, the death of a patient, whether by act or omission, is morally equivalent. If the doctor's intent is to cause the death of the patient and he or she acts deliberately to make this happen, then that doctor is practising euthanasia. It is usual, once treatment is withdrawn, for the death of the patient to result from the underlying disease, and if a doctor intended this, there can be no charge of immoral conduct to answer.

Care at the end of life sometimes involves interventions that hasten the death of the patient. These actions are foreseen but unintended, yet are allowed under the ethical principle of double effect. Giving high-dose opioids, for example to treat the distress of a patient undergoing terminal ventilator weaning, is acceptable even though death is hastened. This doctrine relies heavily on a doctor's intent to distinguish between a permissible and prohibited act. Any action taken to bring about the patient's death, as in physician-assisted suicide or voluntary euthanasia, is illegal. The principle of double effect demands that: (i) the act is morally good; (ii) the good effect is intended; (iii) the bad effect is not a means to the good one; and (iv) the good effect outweighs the bad. The legitimacy of a doctor's decision to withdraw treatment and institute interventions that may unintentionally hasten an unconscious patient's death are assured by: (i) the legal principle of necessity; (ii) the best interests test; (iii) the principle of proportionality, which considers risks versus benefits; and (iv) consent, as exercised through an advanced directive or LPA.

When a patient is unconscious, a doctor may start clinically assisted nutrition and hydration to preserve the physiological function of the body's organs. If treatment fails and death is imminent, artificial nutrition and hydration (ANH) may be discontinued. Many ethicists argue that feeding methods that require some medical training and knowledge of attendant risks should be considered a form of medical treatment and thereby subject to selective provision. The House of Lords in *Airedale NHS Trust v Bland* confirmed that ANH was part of medical treatment and care. There was concurrence of opinion in this case that it was not in the best interests of the patient to die but rather that best interests were served by not giving treatment from which no benefit could be derived. Therefore, the law in the UK regards enteral tube feeding for persistent vegetative state (PVS) patients as medical treatment and its withdrawal subject to legal review. The guidance of the British Medical Association (BMA) confines a doctor's decision to withdraw ANH to extreme cases, in particular where a net benefit is absent and the patient's death is imminent. When doubt exists about the withdrawal of ANH in any clinical situation, it is prudent to enlist the advice of a senior clinician and that of the court.

The rulings in the *Bland* case form the bases for treatment withdrawal in adult patients. A convenient summary of the law as it now stands is as follows:

1. ANH is medical treatment.
2. Stopping treatment is an omission, not an act.
3. Insensate patients have no interests.
4. No duty of care exists if there are no longer any best interests.
5. It is unlawful to continue care not in a patient's best interests; therefore life-sustaining treatment can be stopped.
6. Seeking court approval to withdraw treatment in PVS cases is mandatory in England and Wales but not in Scotland.
7. The *Bolam* test should form only part of a best interests assessment.

Outside the realm of PVS patients, withdrawal of treatment needs careful application of these legal principles. Further case law (*R (on the application of Burke) v General Medical Council & Ors*) has also clarified that a doctor has no ethical or legal duty to provide treatment that a patient may want if there is no clinical indication for its provision and it is not in the patient's best interests. However, the Mental Capacity Act 2005 now governs the conduct of end-of-life decisions of patients who are incompetent. The relevant sections pertain to: (i) the best interest checklist, allowing a person's wishes, feelings, beliefs and values to be taken into consideration, along with the views of friends and family; (ii) creation of an advance directive or LPA; and (iii) representation by IMCAs of the unbefriended when decisions about serious medical treatment arise. The Court of Protection has its own special procedures, judges and jurisdiction to deal with disputes, declarations and end-of-life decisions in all incapacitated patients. Regulating end-of-life decisions in this way protects a patient's autonomous choice and clarifies the legality of these decisions taken by medical professionals.

A doctor consults different sources when deciding to withdraw treatment from a critically ill patient. These include guidelines from professional bodies such as the General Medical Council and BMA and the views of anyone with a vested interest in the patient's welfare. However, if a dispute arises and a doctor acts without seeking a satisfactory resolution, the law cannot ensure immunity from criminal prosecution, negligence claims and disciplinary proceedings. When a patient dies subsequent to treatment withdrawal, there is always a chance of a criminal investigation resulting from accusations of euthanasia or criminal negligence, but, fortunately, these are rare. However, it is well established in English law, following *R v Malcherek*, that a doctor cannot be held criminally liable for withdrawing ventilation from a patient if they have exercised good medical judgement by adhering to well-established guidelines. What establishes wrongdoing is whether a doctor continues treatment divorced from a patient's best interests. Minimizing exposure to liability for wrongful administration of treatment demands that a doctor: (i) ensures a discussion takes place with a patient or their surrogate about treatment goals while giving greater weight to patients' wishes expressed through these surrogates; (ii) establishes the existence of an advance directive or LPA when patients are unconscious; and (iii) seeks judicial review when there is a irreconcilable divergence of opinion.

End-of-life care on ICUs will continue to evolve by promoting the highest ethical and legal standards when withdrawing treatment. There should always be a presumption in favour of resuscitation and treatment unless best medical practice, informed by the professional standards and the best interests test, suggests otherwise. Clinicians, ethicists and law makers will continue to be challenged by the complexities of legitimizing appropriate end-of-life decisions. With newer proposals, there will be a need to reassure society about concerns over the right of autonomy when incapacitated, the impact of resource allocation on withdrawal decisions and the resilience of the sanctity-of-life doctrine.

Medical research on incompetent patients

Medical treatments have grown out of intuition, serendipity and, latterly, scientific methodology, which demands a systematic enquiry in the form of research to address clinical equipoise. After the Second World War, the Nuremberg Code was established in an attempt to formalize acceptable practice in research on humans. This was followed later by the publication of the Declaration of Helsinki by the World Medical Association. Over time, many nations developed their own guidelines and legislation to govern an activity that has the capability of generating great benefit but also great suffering, especially if subjects are exploited by a violation of their rights and interests. In general, therapeutic research, which offers some prospect of direct medical benefit to the patient, and non-therapeutic research, which offers no medical benefit, is carried out on competent adult patients or healthy volunteers. Minority groups such as children and incapacitated adults suffer unique medical problems that also warrant investigation. However, they are often denied the benefit of research because of their inability to give consent. Ethically, there exists a dichotomy of opinion on this subject, while legally, legislation only recently enacted permits a more reasoned basis for such research, supplementing the principle of the patient's best interests once held as the sole justification.

The ethics and legality of medical research

Using a competent patient or a volunteer to discover new information about a potential treatment may require the use of that person as a means to an end. From a utilitarian perspective, if the maximum good can be achieved, then this is justification enough for allowing experimentation on human subjects. However, other ethical views would argue that the autonomy of the individual is paramount and can never be sacrificed for the greater good of society, a philosophy that is enshrined in the Declaration of Helsinki. Overcoming some of the ethical objections to allow human subjects to participate in medical research requires that a research subject is not treated as a means to an end and is given a choice about whether to enrol in a project. Furthermore, a consideration of a subject's humanity and personhood ensures respect for their autonomy and, subject to the fulfilment of certain criteria for entry into a study, most ethicists would concede their objections to allowing competent human subjects to participate in medical research.

The principles of good ethical research are outlined in the current version of the Helsinki Declaration 2008 and the broad themes that dominate include the following:

1. A requirement for the research to be scientifically sound with independent ethical review.
2. That the risks taken by the subject are commensurate with the expected benefits.
3. That informed consent from subjects or their legal representatives is necessary.
4. That the duty of the physician is to protect the life, health and dignity of the human subject over that of science and society.

On the basis of these international ethical standards, a regulatory system in the UK has evolved to govern research on humans. Under the administrative powers of the National Health Service (NHS), the Department of Health issued its research governance framework for health and social care in 2005. This framework sets out principles, requirements and standards for research, defines mechanisms to deliver them, and describes monitoring and assessment arrangements. Supporting this policy on research are numerous guidelines and codes of practice from bodies such as the Royal College of Physicians, General Medical Council (GMC), BMA, Medical Research Council, Nuffield Council on Bioethics and many others. All of these guidelines are built on similar principles of respect for the participant's dignity, requirements for ethics committee review, informed consent, confidentiality, minimal risk, scientific soundness, monitoring arrangements and compensation.

Until recently, there was no single legal framework to ensure that all of these guidelines were followed. The general provisions of the common law as they applied to research activity were relied on for guidance. In 2001, the European Community directive 2001/20/EC was issued with its focus on clinical trials, and in 2004 the Medicine for Human Use (Clinical Trials) Regulations was implemented in the UK. It was the first comprehensive law on medical research and covered legal issues in relation to areas such as ethics committees, phase 1 trials, good practice for all clinical trials, protection for incompetent individuals, pharmacovigilance, investigational medicinal products and regulations enforcement. These regulations and other important legislation such as the Data Protection Act 1998, Human Tissue Act 2004 and the Mental Capacity Act 2005 now form an ongoing and evolving legal framework in the area of clinical research on human subjects.

The rights of the incompetent patient in medical research

There are many who believe that the medical profession behaves unethically by failing to give patients with mental incapacity the opportunity to participate in research, thereby denying others the possibility of better treatment or even disease prevention. To exclude them from any research would be discriminatory and devalue their contribution to the welfare of society. Others, fearful of the lack of appropriate safeguards in this vulnerable group, remain convinced that in relation to research on incapacitated patients, medical progress is only an optional goal and that commitment to

human dignity and autonomy is paramount and without compromise.

Guidelines, issued by authoritative medical agencies concerned with research on the incompetent individual, are unanimous in their ethical justification of the need to perform such investigations. However, this ethical stance demands robust legal instruments that will cater for the consent issue that marks the essential difference between the competent and incompetent patient. The legal protection of a competent patient who becomes involved in research is exercised through the requirement for informed consent. Without consent, an action in battery or negligence against the researcher can serve to offer legal relief to discontented competent research subjects – but what of the incompetent individual?

The Declaration of Helsinki requires that, for research on incompetent individuals to be permissible, it should be concerned with the condition the patient suffers from, that it is not possible for the research to be performed on legally competent persons and that informed consent is obtained from a legally authorized representative. The Convention on Human Rights and Biomedicine requires, in addition, that the risks are not disproportionate to the potential benefits and that consent may freely be withdrawn. This statement is also supported by the GMC who emphasize the participant's right to withdraw if there is any sign of distress, pain or any other non-verbal indication of refusal.

In the UK, different legislation applies to research on patients with incapacity undergoing either clinical trials or other research. In relation to clinical trials of medicinal products, the Medicines for Human Use (Clinical Trials) Regulations 2004 govern these studies. The Medicines and Healthcare products Regulatory Agency (MHRA) can provide advice about whether a proposed trial is covered by these regulations. In summary, this legislation states that: (i) a clinical trial must relate directly to a life-threatening or debilitating clinical condition from which the potential participant suffers; (ii) a trial must be approved by a recognized research ethics committee and licensed by the MHRA; (iii) no incentives or financial inducements may be given to a participant or their legal representative, except provision for compensation in the event of injury or loss; (iv) a legal representative or a person independent of the trial (a doctor or nominated healthcare provider) must give informed consent if consent to participate was *not* given prior to the loss of capacity; (v) that the trial has been designed to minimize pain and discomfort; and

(vi) that the product tested in the trial will produce a benefit to the subject outweighing the risks or, where no benefits for participants are anticipated, the risks should be at a minimal or negligible level.

All other research involving adults who lack mental capacity is governed by the Adults With Incapacity (Scotland) Act 2000 or the Mental Capacity Act 2005 in England and Wales. The Mental Capacity Act 2005 Code of Practice provides all of the detail for the practical application of this Act. However, the two Acts are broadly similar and detail the specific requirements to permit intrusive medical research on patients with incapacity. For the purposes of these Acts, a person must be *assumed to have capacity*. All practicable steps must be taken to help a person make a decision, and incapacity is not defined by an unwise decision. When determining capacity, an assessment should be specific to the decision needing to be made at the particular time. A person is unable to make a decision if she or he cannot (i) understand the information relevant to the decision; (ii) retain that information; (iii) use or weigh that information as part of the process of making the decision; and (iv) communicate the decision. The more serious the decision, the more formal the assessment, and this may need to be carried out by a mental health expert. The responsibility for capacity assessment belongs to those who wish to make the decision on behalf of the incapacitated person.

Once a person is deemed to lack capacity, researchers need to comply with the following:

1. All research requires approval by a research ethics committee recognized by the National Research Ethics Service.
2. The proposed research is not permitted if the study is completely unrelated to the reason for the mental incapacity.
3. It must not be possible to conduct the research with patients who can give consent.
4. The risk/benefit ratio must be in the patient's favour during research that has the potential to be of direct benefit to those taking part.
5. The risks must be negligible and restriction of basic rights kept to a minimum in non-therapeutic research.
6. To seek agreement for participation in a study, the researcher must consult with either the patient's relatives, carers, the appointed independent advocate, a court-appointed deputy or a person nominated in the patient's LPA.
7. All persons consulted must not be paid for the care they provide to the potential participant.
8. In the absence of a personal consultee, the researcher must consult a nominated consultee who has no connection with the project.
9. Any patient distress or resistance warrants immediate withdrawal from the study.

Once a participant is enrolled in a study, nothing should be done to that patient that would be contrary to their wishes as outlined in an advance directive. The interests of those taking part in research must always outweigh those of science and society, and the researcher must withdraw the incapacitated patient from the study if the inclusion criteria no longer apply. To further safeguard patients with incapacity involved in research, the level of risk that is acceptable is defined by statute. Both the Adults With Incapacity (Scotland) Act 2000 and the Mental Capacity Act 2005 in England and Wales stipulate that any intervention must impose a minimal or negligible foreseeable risk and discomfort, and any burden for the patient should not be disproportionate to the benefit. Determining the potential for direct benefit and possible risks of a research project is often difficult, especially if there is clinical equipoise in relation to a particular treatment. Judgement on this matter relies on researchers performing a careful risk/benefit analysis that satisfies the concerns of the research ethics committee.

On occasions, incapacitated patients need to be enrolled into a research project while undergoing emergency treatment, which sometimes makes a contemporaneous consultation process impossible. In relation to clinical trials, where it is not practical to meet the conditions required for consultation, the legislation stipulates that the research ethics committee needs to approve the procedure for this form of recruitment. Furthermore, it must be made clear when appropriate consent or agreement will be sought from a relative or carer and what steps will be taken if this is refused. In addition to these legal demands, the Mental Capacity Act 2005 requires that, in the emergency situation, the researcher should also have agreement from a registered doctor who is independent of the project. The law in Scotland does not at present permit recruitment without consultation in the emergency situation. Adults who lack capacity can be included in research involving human tissue samples provided there is adherence to the law as outlined in the Human Tissue Act 2004 as well as the legal requirements of the Mental

Capacity Act 2005 and Medicines for Human Use (Clinical Trials) Regulations 2004.

Medical research benefits both the individual and society, and the motivation for performing it resides in our innate altruistic nature. While the law provides the permission that society condones to conduct research on incompetent individuals, we must be forever vigilant to ensure that an overzealous pursuit does not make us treat the patient subject as a means to an end, thereby overlooking and neglecting their philanthropy, humanity and personhood.

Further reading

A National Health Service Trust v D [2000] 2 FLR 677 *per* Cazalet J.

Adults With Incapacity (Scotland) Act 2000. Office of public sector information. Available at: http://www.opsi.gov.uk/legislation/scotland/acts2000/asp_20000004_en_1.

Airedale NHS Trust v Bland [1993] 1 All ER 821, HL.

Ashby, M. A., Kellehear, A. and Stoffell, B.F. (2005). Resolving conflict in end-of-life care. *Aust J Med* **183**, 230–1.

Azoulay, E., Pochard, F., Kentish-Barnes, N. *et al.* (2005). Risk of post-traumatic stress symptoms in family members of intensive care unit patients. *Am J Respir Crit Care Med* **171**, 987–94.

Beauchamp, T. and Childress, J. (2001). *Principles of Biomedical Ethics*, 5th edn. Oxford: Oxford University Press.

Bilotta, F., Caramia, R., Paoloni, F. P. *et al.* (2009). Safety and efficacy of intensive insulin therapy in critical neurosurgical patients. *Anesthesiology*, **110**, 611–19.

Bolam v Friern Hospital Management Committee [1957] 2 All ER 118.

Brain Trauma Foundation (2000). The American Association of Neurological Surgeons. The Joint Section on Neurotrauma and Critical Care. Pupillary diameter and light reflex. *J Neurotrauma* **17**, 563–627.

British Medical Association (2007). *Withholding and Withdrawing Life-prolonging Medical Treatment: Guidance for Decision-making*. London: BMJ Books.

European Convention on Human Rights (1950). Article 8. Available at: http://www.hri.org/docs/ECHR50.html#C.Art8.

General Medical Council (2006). Withholding and withdrawing – guidance for doctors. Available: http://www.gmc-uk.org/Withholding_and_withdrawing_guidance_for_doctors.pdf_33377901.pdf.

Greenberg, M. S. (2006). Head trauma: outcome prognosticators. In *Handbook of Neurosurgery*, 6th edn. New York: Thieme Medical Publishers.

Jennett, B. (2005). Outcome after severe head injury. In P. L. Reilly and R. Bullock, eds. *Head Injury: Pathophysiology and Management*, 2nd edn. London: Hodder Arnold, pp. 441–61.

Luce, J. M. and Ruberfeld, G. D. (2002). Can health care costs be reduced by limiting intensive care at the end of life? *Am J Respir Crit Care Med* **165**, 750–4.

McLean, S. A. M. (2001). Permanent vegetative state and the law. *J Neurol Neurosurg Psychiatry* **71** (Suppl. 1), 126–7.

Medicines for Human Use (Clinical Trials) Regulations 2004. Available at: http://www.legislation.gov.uk/uksi/2004/1031/contents/made.

Mental Capacity Act 2005. Sections 24–26. Available at: http://www.legislation.gov.uk/ukpga/2005/9/contents.

Mental Capacity Act 2005 Code of Practice. Office of the Public Guardian. Available: http://www.publicguardian.gov.uk/docs/mca-code-practice-0509.pdf.

Moppett, I. K. (2007). Traumatic brain injury: assessment, resuscitation and early management. *Br J Anaesth* **99**, 18–31.

MRC CRASH Trial Collaborators (2008). Predicting outcome after traumatic brain injury: practical prognostic models based on large cohort of international patients. *BMJ* **336**, 425–9.

NHS Trust A v M; NHS Trust B v H [2001] 1 All ER 801 at [30] *per* Butler-Sloss LJ.

Patel, H. C., Menon, D. K., Tebbs, S. *et al.* (2002). Specialist neurocritical care and outcome from head injury. *Intensive Care Med* **28**, 547–53.

R (on the application of Burke) v General Medical Council & Ors [2005] QB 424.

R v Malcherek [1981] 2 All ER 422.

Research Governance Framework for Health and Social Care (2005). London: Department of Health. Available at: http://www.dh.gov.uk/en/Publicationsandstatistics/Publications/PublicationsPolicyAndGuidance/DH_4108962.

Schloendorff v Society of New York Hospital 105 NE 92 (NY, 1914).

Teasdale, G. M., Murray, G. D. and Nicoll, J. A. (2005). The association between *APOE* ε4, age and outcome after head injury: a prospective cohort study. *Brain* **128**, 2556–61.

Thompson, B., Cox, P. N., Antonelli M *et al.* (2004). Challenges in end of life care in the ICU: statement of the 5th international consensus conference in critical care: Brussels, Belgium, April 2003. *Crit Care Med* **32**, 1781–4.

Van den Berghe, G., Wouters, P., Weekers, F. *et al.* (2001). Intensive insulin therapy in the critically ill patients. *N Engl J Med* **345**, 1359–67.

Vincent, J. L. (2005). Withdrawing may be preferable to withholding. *Critical Care* **9**, 226–9.

Wardlaw, J. M., Easton, V. J. and Statham, P. (2002). Which CT features help predict outcome after head injury? *J Neurol Neurosur Psychiatry* **72**, 188–92.

Williams, G. (2001). The principle of double effect and terminal sedation. *Med Law Rev* **9**, 41–53.

Wilson, M. and Montgomery H. (2007). Impact of genetic factors on outcome from brain injury. *Br J Anaesth* **99**, 43–8.

X v Austria [1980] 18 D.R. 154.

Chapter

32

Assessment and management of coma

Nicholas Hirsch and Robin Howard

Introduction

Consciousness can be defined as a state of awareness that allows the individual to gain significance from internal and external stimuli. From a clinical perspective, it consists of two closely related components: *wakefulness* (i.e. arousal and alertness) and *content*, the result of mental processes that allow awareness of self and the environment and the expression of psychological functions of sensation, emotion and thought.

From a neuroanatomical stance, wakefulness requires a functioning ascending reticular activating system (ARAS) that comprises a network of neurons originating in the pons and midbrain that project to the thalamus and cerebral cortex. Content, and therefore awareness, requires normal functioning of both cerebral hemispheres. Thus, impairment of consciousness can occur either due to damage or suppression of the ARAS (i.e. the brainstem) or both cerebral hemispheres. Generally, unilateral hemispheric damage (e.g. following a cerebrovascular accident) does not impair consciousness.

Disorders of consciousness

Although extensively used in the past, terms such as *obtundation*, *clouding of consciousness* and *stupor* are best avoided because they lack rigorous definition. In addition, the widespread use of coma scoring scales has rendered such terms largely redundant. More definable states of impaired consciousness are now recognized (Table 32.1).

Coma

Coma is a state of unarousable unresponsiveness in which the patient lies with his or her eyes closed, i.e. both arousal and awareness are absent. They do not speak, do not follow commands, have no spontaneous movements and do not accurately localize noxious stimuli. Sleep–wake cycles are absent and respiratory patterns are variable and often abnormal. Polymorphic delta- or theta-wave activity is seen on the EEG. Coma is rarely a permanent state, and those surviving the causative insult either recover or enter a minimally aware or vegetative state.

Vegetative state

The vegetative state is caused by widespread damage to both hemispheres with preservation of brainstem function and most commonly follows traumatic or hypoxic–ischaemic cerebral injury. It is characterized by preservation of arousal mechanisms but absence of awareness of self or the environment. Patients exhibit spontaneous eye opening but have no evidence of sustained, reproducible, purposeful or voluntary responses to visual, tactile, auditory or noxious stimuli. Cardiorespiratory function and gag, cough and swallowing reflexes are usually preserved. Non-purposeful movements such as facial grimacing, smiling, frowning, vocalization and grasping can occur, often in response to auditory stimuli. Sleep–wake cycles are present and EEG shows occasional slow alpha activity on a background of polymorphic delta or theta activity.

The vegetative state may be partially or totally reversible or may progress to a persistent or permanent vegetative state or death. Although the term persistent vegetative state has been used to imply that the state has continued for at least 1 month, this definition has been questioned because this duration does not imply permanency or irreversibility. For this reason, the term 'continuous vegetative state' is being used increasingly under such circumstances. The diagnosis of a 'permanent vegetative state' is made after a patient has been in a vegetative state for 1 year and, following exhaustive testing and observation, it is thought impossible by

Core Topics in Neuroanaesthesia and Neurointensive Care, eds. Basil F. Matta, David K. Menon and Martin Smith. Published by Cambridge University Press. © Cambridge University Press 2011.

Table 32.1 States of impaired consciousness

Disorders of consciousness	Coma
	Vegetative state
	Minimally aware state
	Akinetic mutism
	Delirium
Disorders mimicking coma	Locked-in syndrome
	Guillain–Barré syndrome
	Botulism

informed medical opinion that their mental state will improve.

Minimally aware state

Patients in the minimally aware state show severe alteration in consciousness but are able to intermittently demonstrate some level of awareness of environmental stimuli or behavioural response to command that suggests some cognitive ability. EEG shows theta and alpha activity. Recovery of normal consciousness is more likely in patients who have developed a minimally aware state rather than a vegetative state.

Akinetic mutism

Akinetic mutism is a rare syndrome in which patients show wakefulness but have limited awareness and cognitive function. It probably reflects a form of the minimally aware state. Patients lie immobile and are flaccid, mute and unresponsive to pain and verbal commands. They may track movement, and blinking occurs spontaneously, as well as to visual threat. Sleep–wake cycles are preserved and the EEG shows diffuse non-specific slowing with intermittent reactive alpha and theta rhythms. The condition is usually associated with bilateral inferior frontal lobe damage but may also occur in other conditions including acute hydrocephalus.

Delerium

Delirium is characterized by the acute onset of fluctuating consciousness, impairment of attention and memory, motor restlessness, fear and irritability. It may include visual hallucinations, and the sleep–wake cycle is often disrupted. It often accompanies toxic and metabolic disorders but may also be a feature of intensive care unit (ICU) and post-operative confusional states. The EEG pattern is one of diffuse slow-wave activity.

Conditions mimicking coma

A number of conditions may mimic coma and need to be excluded when evaluating the apparently unresponsive patient. Locked-in syndrome describes a de-efferented state in which consciousness and cognition are retained but motor function is lost, thereby making movement and speech impossible. The syndrome is caused by lesions of the ventral pons that disrupt the corticospinal, corticobulbar and corticopontine tracts. The patient displays a regular unvarying rate of respiration with often total paralysis of voluntary muscle activity below the level of the third cranial nerve nuclei. Thus, the only movements possible are blinking and vertical eye movements. Other conditions causing severe motor weakness that may occasionally mimic coma include acute Guillain–Barré syndrome and botulism. EEG reveals normal activity in all these conditions.

Causes of coma

All schemes of classification of coma, and especially those based on anatomical considerations, have deficiencies because coma often has multifactorial aetiologies. Thus, a bilateral hemispheric lesion may cause unconsciousness per se or because of secondary cerebral herniation. In practical terms, the most useful working scheme is based on three observations on initial assessment – the presence of lateralizing signs, the presence of meningism and the pattern of brainstem reflexes. Using these variables, the causes of coma can be divided into four categories (Table 32.2).

In most cases, the cause of coma is associated with an obvious medical cause. In patients admitted to a general emergency department in coma of >6h duration, approximately 40% will be due to drug ingestion with or without alcohol, 25% to hypoxic–ischaemic injury secondary to cardiac arrest, 20% to stroke and the remainder to general medical disorders. Common primary neurological events causing coma include intracerebral or subarachnoid haemorrhage (SAH), pontine or cerebellar haemorrhage and basilar artery thrombosis.

Management of the comatose patient

Although the causes of coma are myriad, it is vital to implement a rapid and structured approach to diagnosis

Table 32.2 Classification and causes of coma

Classification	Cause
Coma with intact brainstem function, no meningism and no lateralizing signs	Alcohol
	Drugs: sedatives, anaesthetics, others (e.g. opioids, amphetamines, barbiturates, salicylates)
	Toxins: carbon monoxide, methanol, lead, cyanide, thallium
	Epilepsy: convulsive and non-convulsive status epilepticus, post-ictal states
	Hypoxic–ischaemic encephalopathy
	Metabolic derangements: hypoglycaemia, hyperglycaemic crises, systemic sepsis syndromes, hypoxaemia, hypercarbia, hyponatraemia, hypernatraemia, hypercalcaemia, hepatic failure, renal failure, hypothermia, hyperpyrexia, Wernicke's encephalopathy, autoimmune encephalitis
	Endocrine disorders: hypopituitarism, hypo- and hyperthyroidism, Hashimoto's encephalopathy, hypoadrenalism
	Psychiatric states: catatonia, conversion reactions, non-epileptic seizures
	Miscellaneous: porphyria, Reye's syndrome, mitochondrial disease, malaria, inborn errors of metabolism
Coma with meningism, with or without intact brainstem function and lateralizing signs	Infection: meningitis, encephalitis, malaria, human immunodeficiency virus-related
	Vascular: subarachnoid haemorrhage
Coma with intact brainstem function and lateralizing signs	Vascular: cerebral infarction (ischaemic, embolic or hypoperfusion) and haemorrhage (extradural, subdural, subarachnoid, intracerebral), vasculitis, cerebral venous thrombosis, hypertensive encephalopathy, eclampsia, endocarditis
	Traumatic brain injury
	Infection: brain abscess, subdural empyema, Creutzfeldt–Jakob disease, malaria, human immunodeficiency virus-associated
	Cerebral neoplasms
Coma with signs of focal brainstem dysfunction	Herniation syndromes
	Intrinsic brainstem disease: posterior fossa tumours, abscesses
	Advanced metabolic/toxic encephalopathy
	Vascular: vertebrobasilar occlusion or dissection, haemorrhage, arteriovenous malformations
	Traumatic brain injury
	White-matter disease: multiple sclerosis, leukoencephalopathy (chemo- or radiotherapy related), acute disseminated encephalomyelitis, toxic leukoencephalopathy, progressive multifocal leukoencephalopathy

and management in order to maximize the prospects of neurological recovery. A scheme of emergency and subsequent management is outlined in Table 32.3.

Resuscitation and emergency treatment

Although the underlying cause of coma must be treated as soon as possible, rapid and effective cardiopulmonary resuscitation is a priority to avoid further cerebral damage. The airway should be secured, oxygenation maintained and arterial blood pressure stabilized at a level that will ensure adequate cerebral perfusion. Immobilization of the cervical spine should be ensured if trauma is suspected. During resuscitation, blood samples should be taken for estimation of full blood

Table 32.3 Management of the comatose patient

Resuscitation and emergency treatment

- Secure airway: tracheal intubation if Glasgow Coma Scale score <8 or if patient not protecting airway
- Breathing: administer oxygen to maintain oxygen saturation >94%
- Circulation : administer intravenous fluids and inotropes to maintain mean arterial pressure >60 mmHg
- 25 ml 50% glucose (+ thiamine 100 mg) if hypoglycaemia present
- Naloxone if opioid overdose suspected
- Flumazenil if benzodiazepine overdose suspected
- Mannitol 0.5 g kg^{-1} if signs of cerebral herniation present

Diagnosis

- Blood for full blood count, urea and electrolytes, glucose, liver and thyroid function tests, arterial blood gas, anticonvulsant drug levels, etc.
- Blood and urine for toxicology screen
- General medical assessment: history and examination
- Detailed neurological assessment
- Subsequent management and investigations as indicated by findings of detailed history and examination, e.g. CT/MRI, examination of cerebrospinal fluid, EEG

count, electrolytes, liver and thyroid function, toxicology screen and any other relevant tests.

After baseline blood samples have been drawn, 25 ml of 50% glucose should be administered if hypoglycaemia is present. This should be accompanied by thiamine 100 mg intravenously in alcoholic or malnourished patients to prevent precipitation of Wernicke's encephalopathy. If signs of cerebral herniation are present (Table 32.4), intravenous mannitol should be administered.

Further acute management includes appropriate treatment of seizures, correction of electrolyte and acid–base disturbances, and initiation of supportive treatment including adequate nutrition and physiotherapy.

Assessment

A detailed clinical assessment should be undertaken in all comatose patients.

History

As full a history as possible should be sought from paramedical staff, family members and friends. This may reveal a predictable cause of coma (e.g. a previously diagnosed cerebral neoplasm), the presence of known risk factors (e.g. epilepsy, endocrine or metabolic disease) or may suggest an unsuspected cause (e.g. meningitis, SAH). In cases of post-cardiac arrest coma, a full resuscitation history may reveal the duration of

Table 32.4 Clinical signs of cerebral herniation

Coma

Pupillary dilation

Miosis

Lateral gaze palsy

Hemiparesis

Decerebrate posture

Hypertension, bradycardia (Cushing's reflex)

'down time', which often influences future management decisions.

Examination

A detailed general medical examination often provides important clues to the aetiology of the coma and should be conducted urgently (Table 32.5). The aim of the neurological examination is to establish the patient's level of consciousness and to identify lateralizing signs that will help determine the underlying aetiology of the coma. The scheme of neurological examination is detailed in Table 32.6 and discussed in detail below.

Assessment of level of consciousness

The level of consciousness should be assessed by the ability of the patient to respond to external stimuli in three regards – by speech, eye opening and motor movements. In order to correctly identify patients with

Table 32.5 General medical examination of the patient in coma

Examination	Possible aetiology
Breath	Alcohol, ketones, hepatic or renal fetor
Mucous membranes	Cyanosis, anaemia, jaundice, carbon monoxide poisoning
Skin	Needle tracks of iv drug abuser, rash of meningococcal septicaemia, splinter haemorrhages of bacterial endocarditis, vesicular rash of viral meningitis, barbiturate blisters, petechial rash of coagulopathy, hyperpigmentation of Addison's disease, Kaposi's sarcoma
Temperature	Hypothermia (environmental, metabolic, endocrine or drug induced), hyperthermia (systemic sepsis, thyrotoxic crisis, drug toxicity, malignant hyperthermia, neurogenic due to subarachnoid haemorrhage or hypothalamic lesions)
Cardiovascular system	Dysrhythmias, hypertension (subarachnoid haemorrhage, raised intracranial pressure, hypertensive encephalopathy), hypotension (haemorrhage, cardiac failure, sepsis, endocrine disorders), valvular disease (suggesting endocarditis)
Fundoscopy	Retinopathy (diabetes, hypertension), papilloedema (raised intracranial pressure, carbon dioxide retention), subhyaloid haemorrhage (subarachnoid haemorrhage)
Meningism	Meningitis, encephalitis, subarachnoid haemorrhage

Table 32.6 Neurological assessment of coma

Assessment	Method
Assess level of consciousness	Glasgow Coma Score
	FOUR score (Full Outline of UnResponsiveness)
Assess brainstem reflexes and activity	Pupillary responses
	Eye position and oculomotor disorders
	Eye movements:
	• Spontaneous eye movements
	• Oculocephalic reflex
	• Oculovestibular reflex
	Other cranial nerve reflexes:
	• Corneal reflex
	• Gag and cough reflexes
	Respiratory pattern
Assess motor function	Posture
	Involuntary movements
	Seizures
	Muscle tone
	Motor responses
	Tendon and plantar reflexes

locked-in syndrome, the eyelids should be held open and the patient asked to move their eyes in a horizontal and vertical plane.

Glasgow Coma Scale

The Glasgow Coma Scale (GCS) is the standard scoring system for assessment of the level of consciousness based on the best motor, verbal and eye-opening responses to external stimuli (Table 32.7).

Originally introduced in 1974 for the assessment of patients with traumatic brain injury (TBI), the GCS has gained worldwide acceptance as an easily performed and reproducible tool for the assessment of all acutely ill patients. As well as providing a quantitative documentation of the level of consciousness, it has powerful predictive value for survival and outcome in both traumatic and non-traumatic coma. However, the GCS does have limitations. The scale excludes assessment of many important neurological functions, requires serial observations to be effective and is limited to the best response in one limb. It cannot therefore identify asymmetry and has poor diagnostic value. In addition, combining the three values into a single total score can lead to disparities in assessment of true conscious level. Finally but importantly, a complete GCS cannot be obtained in patients who have eyelid swelling, are sedated and intubated with a tracheal tube or who are aphasic due to a dominant hemisphere lesion.

Table 32.7 The Glasgow Coma Score scale

Best eye-opening response	4	Spontaneous
	3	To speech
	2	To pain
	1	None
Best motor response	6	Obeys command
	5	Localizes to pain
	4	Withdrawal
	3	Flexion posturing
	2	Extensor posturing
	1	None
Best verbal response	5	Orientated
	4	Confused speech
	3	Inappropriate words
	2	Incomprehensible sounds
	1	None

Table 32.8 The Full Outline of UnResponsiveness (FOUR) score

Eye response	4	Eyelids open, tracking or blinking to command
	3	Eyelids open but not tracking
	2	Eyelids closed but open to a loud voice
	1	Eyelids closed but open to pain
	0	Eyelids remain closed with pain
Motor response	4	Thumbs-up, fist or peace sign
	3	Localizing to pain
	2	Flexion response to pain
	1	Extension response to pain
	0	No response to pain or generalized myoclonic status
Brainstem reflexes	4	Pupil and corneal reflexes present
	3	One pupil wide and fixed
	2	Pupil or corneal reflexes absent
	1	Pupil and corneal reflexes absent
	0	Absent pupil, corneal and cough reflex (using tracheal suction)
Respiration	4	Not intubated, regular breathing pattern
	3	Not intubated, Cheyne–Stokes breathing pattern
	2	Not intubated, irregular breathing pattern
	1	Breaths above ventilator rate
	0	Breaths at ventilator rate or apnoea

The FOUR score

The recently introduced Full Outline of UnResponsiveness (FOUR) score circumvents many of the limitations of the GCS (Table 32.8). The verbal score of the GCS is replaced by assessment of pupil reactions and respiratory pattern, making it more appropriate in the intubated patient.

Brainstem reflexes and activity

Pupillary responses

The normal pupillary response to light is a direct and consensual constriction and depends on functioning afferent (cranial nerve II) and efferent (cranial nerve III) pathways and the midbrain Edinger–Westphal nucleus. The presence of equal, light-reactive pupils indicates that the reflex pathway is intact. A normal pupillary reaction in a comatose patient suggests a toxic or metabolic aetiology rather than a structural one. Unilateral or bilateral miosis with normal reaction to light may be due to Horner's syndrome associated with lesions involving descending sympathetic pathways in the hypothalamus, midbrain, medulla or cervical spine (e.g. cervical carotid artery damage). Bilateral pinpoint pupils are seen with pontine lesions in the tegmentum, opioid overdose and anticholinesterase poisoning (e.g. in myasthenic cholinergic crisis). Unilateral pupillary dilation with either a sluggish or no response to light is caused by compression of the oculomotor nerve and is seen in uncal herniation, posterior communicating artery aneurysm rupture and with lesions affecting the cavernous sinus (e.g. pituitary apoplexy). Bilateral pupillary dilation with no response to light is seen in central herniation, extensive midbrain damage, hypothermia, drug intoxication (e.g. with anticholinergic agents) and brainstem death.

Eye position and oculomotor disorders

Examination of the position of the eyes can yield important lateralizing information. In the primary ocular position, the eyes may be conjugate in the

Table 32.9 Involuntary vertical eye movements in coma

Eye movement	Clinical finding	Lesion identified
Ocular bobbing	Rapid downward jerks of both eyes followed by a slow return to the mid-position Paralysis of both reflex and spontaneous horizontal eye movements	Acute pontine lesion Metabolic and toxic Extra-axial posterior fossa masses
Ocular dipping	Slow initial downward phase is followed by a relatively rapid return to the mid-position	Diffuse cerebral anoxia Following status epilepticus

midline, dysconjugate or deviated in a conjugated manner. Dysconjugate deviation is commonly seen in patients with impaired consciousness (and those on sedation) and has little localizing value.

A complete IIIrd nerve palsy is characterized by ptosis, pupillary dilation and deviation of the eye downward and laterally. It is most commonly seen as a manifestation of transtentorial herniation but may also be a feature of midbrain damage. A dysconjugate vertical gaze may be caused by IVth nerve palsy, which commonly occurs following trauma, drug intoxication or metabolic encephalopathy. VIth nerve palsy (inward deviation and failure of abduction of the eye) is often caused by trauma or raised intracranial pressure but has poor localizing value.

Tonic conjugate eye deviation is often seen in coma. In destructive hemispheric lesions, the eyes deviate towards the lesion and away from the hemiparesis and can usually be driven across the midline by vestibular stimulus. In contrast, in lesions below the pontomesencephalic junction, the eyes deviate away from the side of the lesion and do not cross the midline.

Eye movements

Spontaneous eye movements in coma tend to be either roving or involuntary, conjugate vertical movements. Roving eye movements are slow, purposeless lateral movements, either conjugate or dysconjugate. They imply intact oculomotor pathways and are usually associated with toxic or metabolic coma. A number of conjugate vertical eye movements are recognized and are classified according to the velocities of the upward and downward saccades. The most common are ocular bobbing and dipping, and they can identify anatomical and aetiological causes of coma (Table 32.9).

Oculovestibular reflexes

Oculovestibular reflexes are involuntary eye movements that occur after stimulation of the vestibular apparatus. The oculocephalic reflex is tested by sudden lateral rotation of the head while observing the motion of the eyes. Ocular responses to vertical stimulation are tested by flexing and then extending the neck. This reflex should not be tested if cervical spine instability is suspected. The oculovestibular reflex is elicited by irrigation of the tympanic membrane with cold (30°C) or warm (44°C) water. Normal and abnormal responses to oculocephalic and oculovestibular stimulation are detailed in Tables 32.10 and 32.11 respectively.

Other cranial nerve reflexes

The corneal reflex (blinking on lightly brushing the cornea with cotton wool) tests the integrity of the afferent (trigeminal nerve), efferent (facial nerve) and brainstem (trigeminal and facial nerve pontine nuclei) pathways. However, the reflex may be lost with deep sedation. The gag and cough reflexes test the integrity of the glossopharyngeal and vagus nerves and associated medullary centres.

Respiratory patterns

Although distinct abnormal respiratory patterns based on animal experiments suggest that individual patterns have localizing value, in practice early intervention with mechanical ventilation in comatose patients means that these patterns are not commonly seen in clinical practice. Primary central neurogenic hyperventilation is a rare condition characterized by rapid regular breathing that persists in the face of alkalosis, elevated arterial oxygen tension, low arterial carbon dioxide tension and in the absence of pulmonary or airway pathology. It is seen in damage to the midbrain tegmentum. Apneustic breathing consists of prolonged pauses at end inspiration and follows bilateral tegmental infarction and pontine demyelination. Cheyne–Stokes respiration consists of cyclical waxing and waning of tidal volume and respiratory rate separated by apnoeic episodes. It is seen in coma of varying aetiology and has little localizing value. Hiccups may occur as a result of structural

Table 32.10 Oculocephalic responses

Oculocephalic reflex	Response	Cause
Horizontal rotation	Eyes remain conjugate and maintain fixation (move in opposite direction to head)	Normal with reduced level of consciousness
	No movement in either eye	Low brainstem lesion Peripheral vestibular lesion Drugs Anaesthesia
	Eyes move appropriately in one direction but do not cross the midline in the other	Gaze palsy (unilateral lesion in pontine gaze centre) Pontine lesion
	One eye abducts but the other fails to adduct	IIIrd nerve palsy Internuclear ophthalmoplegia (lesion of the median longitudinal fasciculus)
	One eye adducts but the other fails to abduct	VIth nerve palsy
Vertical	Eyes remain conjugate and maintain fixation (move in direction opposite to head movement)	Normal with reduced level of consciousness
	No movement in either eye	Low brainstem lesion Peripheral vestibular lesion Drugs Anaesthesia
	Only one eye moves	IIIrd nerve palsy
	Loss of upward gaze	Pretectal or midbrain tegmental compression

Table 32.11 Oculovestibular responses

Oculovestibular reflex	Response	Cause
Cold water instilled into the right ear	Nystagmus with slow phase to right and fast phase to left	Normal
	No response	Obstructed ear canal Labyrinthine damage Low brainstem lesion
	Tonic deviation towards stimulated side (slow phase to right, no fast phase)	Supratentorial lesion with intact pons Toxic/metabolic Drugs Structural lesion above brainstem
	Dysconjugate response	Brainstem lesion (usually in region of medial longitudinal fasciculus)
	Downbeat nystagmus	Horizontal gaze palsy
	Vertical eye deviation	Drug overdose
Warm water instilled into left ear after no response to cold	Slow phase to right, fast phase to left	Peripheral VIIIth nerve lesion Labyrinthine disorder on right

or functional disorders of the medulla or its afferent or efferent connections with the respiratory muscles, and in this context may herald respiratory arrest. Ataxic breathing, characterized by irregular respiratory rate and tidal volume, is associated with severe medullary damage.

Motor responses

Assessment of motor responses involves examination of resting posture and tone, and observation of involuntary and spontaneous movements. Two characteristic resting postures are recognized. Decorticate posturing consists of flexion at the elbows and wrists with shoulder adduction and internal rotation and extension of the legs. Although it has poor localizing value, it occurs in lesions above the diencephalon (i.e. lesions of the cerebral hemispheres or thalamus). Decerebrate posturing is characterized by bilateral extension of the lower extremities, adduction and internal rotation of the shoulders and extension at the elbows. It is usually a sign of bilateral midbrain or pontine damage, although it may also be seen in metabolic coma or following bilateral supratentorial lesions involving the motor pathways. In clinical practice, the anatomical value of these classically described postures is often less clear, and more importance is attached to the response to painful stimuli, where extensor posturing is generally associated with more severe injury than flexor posturing.

The nature and asymmetry of muscle tone may also be helpful in localizing structural lesions and distinguishing between metabolic and structural coma. The presence of spasticity suggests lesions above the brainstem, whereas hypotonia is more often seen in metabolic coma.

Involuntary movements in comatose patients may be obvious or subtle and are usually due to epileptic seizures (convulsive or non-convulsive) or myoclonus, especially following hypoxic–ischaemic cerebral damage or metabolic derangement. Lance–Adams syndrome consists of multifocal and stimulus sensitive myoclonus that is most commonly identified in patients recovering from cerebral anoxia. Purposeful or semi-purposeful spontaneous movements imply intact corticospinal pathways and suggest 'light' coma.

Subsequent investigations

Following a detailed history and examination, the cause of coma can usually be attributed to one of the four categories (Table 32.2) and this will dictate appropriate further investigations. In the vast majority of patients with acute-onset coma, CT imaging is indicated urgently and will identify intracranial haemorrhage, cerebral oedema, hydrocephalus and structural shift of cerebral structures. Using modern scanners, CT allows very rapid imaging times. MRI is superior for the early detection of ischaemic stroke, hypoxic–ischaemic brain injury and venous sinus thrombosis but can be difficult to perform in critically ill and unstable patients. Lumbar puncture should be performed in patients with suspected central nervous system infection or neuroinflammation. CT imaging should be performed prior to lumbar puncture to exclude abnormalities that may predispose to cerebral herniation.

Prognosis of coma

Most patients who survive the initial insult generally emerge from coma within 4 weeks, although the outcome can range from full recovery through mild cognitive and physical disability to vegetative states. Although accurate prognostication is difficult in individual cases, a number of clinical features and investigations can help in predicting outcome:

- Aetiology of the coma.
- Depth and duration of the coma.
- Comorbidities.
- Neurophysiological testing – EEG and somatosensory evoked potentials (SSEPs).

Aetiology of the coma

Although conclusive data are lacking, it is widely believed that coma associated with drug and alcohol ingestion or metabolic disturbance carries a better prognosis than that associated with structural lesions. The prognosis for patients in traumatic coma is better than those with a similar level of coma due to non-traumatic structural lesions, but this may partly be due to the generally younger age of the former group. The poorest prognosis occurs in patients in coma due to a structural cerebral disease, such as SAH or cerebrovascular disease, with only 7% achieving moderate or good recovery. The outcome from coma due to hypoxic–ischaemic injury following cardiac arrest is even worse, with only 1% achieving good levels of recovery.

Depth and duration of the coma

The depth of the coma, as determined by the GCS score and the presence or absence of cranial nerve and other brainstem function, gives some assessment of prognosis. Better outcome is associated with a higher GCS score at presentation, preserved brainstem reflexes throughout resuscitation and in those with early recovery of speech, orientating spontaneous eye movements, ability to follow commands and normal muscle tone.

Survival following cardiac arrest is closely correlated with the duration of the coma. Only 12% of patients in coma for >6 h after cardiac arrest survive with a good or moderate outcome, and this decreases to 6% when there is no eye opening, vocal response or motor function beyond this time. Non-traumatic coma lasting for >1 week is associated with only a 3% prospect of good recovery overall.

Comorbidities

The presence of significant comorbidities is associated with poor outcome in comatose patients. These include ischaemic and structural heart disease, diabetes mellitus, hypertension, renal impairment and sepsis.

Neurophysiological testing

EEG examination can be helpful in predicting outcome in patients who have suffered cerebral traumatic or hypoxic–ischaemic injury. The presence of isoelectric, burst suppression or alpha coma activity is associated with poor outcome. These findings are often seen in patients with myoclonic status following such injuries.

Somatosensory evoked potential findings can have a high prognostic sensitivity in coma due to hypoxic injury, intracerebral haemorrhage and TBI. The bilateral absence of cortical SSEPs within the first week following anoxic injury is always associated with poor outcome. Brainstem auditory evoked potentials also have predictive value after TBI.

Prognostic value of clinical findings and investigations

The most important predictive factors for survival in patients in coma for >6 h resulting from TBI are deeper coma, defined by lower GCS score, and patient age. The extent of injury, presence of skull fractures, hemispheric damage or extracranial injury is less important in determining survival and residual disability. Secondary insults such as raised intracranial pressure and low cerebral perfusion pressure are associated with an increase in severe disability and higher mortality. In non-traumatic coma, absent brainstem reflexes and motor responses at 24 h carry a poor prognosis, but the combination of absence of SSEPs and an unreactive EEG permits a more reliable prediction of poor outcome. Poor prognosis following cardiorespiratory arrest is seen in patients with absent pupillary and corneal reflexes and motor responses at day 3. CT findings of anteroseptal shift, temporal lobe infarction and hydrocephalus also imply a poor outlook.

Conclusions

The immediate management of the comatose patient requires rapid and effective resuscitation to ensure that secondary cerebral damage is minimized. Meticulous clinical examination and subsequent directed investigations allow the aetiology of the coma to be determined and appropriate therapy to be instituted. Knowledge of the prognostic value of clinical signs and investigations allows the clinician to predict the likely outcome from coma.

In the future, it is likely that investigative tools such as functional MRI will result in a greater understanding of the mechanisms underlying coma and other disorders of consciousness, and may well result in a more accurate method of predicting outcome.

Further reading

Bates, D. (1993). The management of medical coma. *J Neurol Neurosurg Psychiatry* **56**, 589–98.

Bernat, J. L. (2006). Chronic disorders of consciousness. *Lancet* **367**, 1181–92.

Geocardin, R. G. and Eleff, S. (2008). Cardiac arrest resuscitation: neurologic prognostication and brain death. *Curr Opin Crit Care* **14**, 261–8.

Giacino, J. and Whyte, J. (2005). The vegetative and minimally conscious states: current knowledge and remaining questions. *J Head Trauma Rehabil* **20**, 30–50.

Howard, R. S. and Hirsch, N. P. (1999). Coma, vegetative state and locked-in syndrome. In Miller, D. H. and Raps, E., eds., *Critical Care Neurology*. Boston: Butterworth Heinemann.

Laureys, S., Owen, A. M. and Schiff, N. D. (2004). Brain function in coma, vegetative state, and related disorders. *Lancet Neurol* **3**, 537–46.

Posner, J. B., Saper, C. B., Schiff, N. and Plum, F. (2007). *Plum and Posner's Diagnosis of Stupor and Coma*. New York: Oxford University Press.

Stevens, R. D. and Bhardwaj, A. (2006). Approach to the comatose patient. *Crit Care Med* **34**, 31–41.

Wijdicks, E. F., Bamlet, W. R., Maramattom, B. V., Manno, E. M. and McClelland. R. L. (2005). Validation of a new coma scale: the FOUR score. *Ann Neurol* **58**, 585–93.

Young, G. B. (2009). Coma. *Ann N Y Acad Sci* **1157**, 32–47.

Young, G. B. (2009). Neurologic prognosis after cardiac arrest. *N Engl J Med* **361**, 605–11.

Index

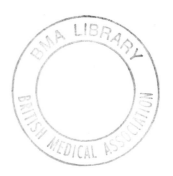